2008 Report on the global AIDS epidemic

This Book Belongs to Nana F

UNAIDS
UNHCR UNICEF WFP UNDP UNFPA UNODC ILO UNESCO WHO WORLD BANK
JOINT UNITED NATIONS PROGRAMME ON HIV/AIDS

Table of contents

Figures

Acknowledgements

The *2008 Report on the global AIDS epidemic* is a report from the Joint United Nations Programme on HIV/AIDS (UNAIDS). It includes contributions from the Office of the United Nations High Commissioner for Refugees (UNHCR), the United Nations Children's Fund (UNICEF), the World Food Programme (WFP), the United Nations Development Programme (UNDP), the United Nations Population Fund (UNFPA), the United Nations Office on Drugs and Crime (UNODC), the International Labour Organization (ILO), the United Nations Educational, Scientific and Cultural Organization (UNESCO), the World Health Organization (WHO), the World Bank, the Global Fund to Fight AIDS, Tuberculosis and Malaria, and the UNGASS Civil Society Steering Committee.

UNAIDS brings together in the AIDS response the efforts and resources of ten UN system organizations.

UNHCR
The UN Refugee Agency

The OFFICE OF THE UNITED NATIONS HIGH COMMISSIONER FOR REFUGEES (UNHCR) is mandated to lead and coordinate international action to protect refugees and other persons of concern. UNHCR strives to ensure that everyone can exercise the right to seek asylum and find safe refuge in another State. UNHCR is at the forefront of responding to HIV among conflict-affected and displaced populations. Refugees, asylum seekers and internally displaced persons are are vulnerable to HIV infection as conflict and displacement expose them to poverty, family disintegration, social disruption and increased sexual violence. HIV prevention, care and treatment, including access to antiretroviral treatment, are central to the overall protection of refugees and other persons of concern to UNHCR.

unicef

For more than 60 years the UNITED NATIONS CHILDREN'S FUND (UNICEF) has been working with partners around the world to promote the recognition and fulfilment of children's human rights. This mandate was established in the Convention of the Rights of the Child, and is achieved through partnerships with governments, nongovernmental organizations and individuals in 162 countries, areas and territories. UNICEF brings to UNAIDS this extensive network and its ability for effective communication and advocacy. HIV is one of UNICEF's core priorities within its Medium-Term Strategic Plan 2006–2009. In line with the Plan, through the *Unite for Children, Unite against AIDS* campaign, and the UNAIDS Technical Division of Labour, UNICEF focuses its support to countries on "Four P" priority areas: prevention of mother-to-child transmission of HIV (PMTCT Plus); paediatric treatment; protection, care and support for children affected by HIV; and prevention among adolescents.

WFP

The WORLD FOOD PROGRAMME (WFP) is the world's largest humanitarian agency. It helps poor households affected by hunger and AIDS by using food aid and other resources to address prevention, care and support. WFP's food assistance helps keep parents alive longer, enables orphans and vulnerable children to stay in school, permits out-of-school youth to secure viable livelihoods and enables tuberculosis patients to complete their treatment. WFP works in partnership with governments, other United Nations agencies, nongovernmental organizations and communities and helps people—regardless of their HIV status—who lack adequate food to secure nutrition and food security.

UNDP

The UNITED NATIONS DEVELOPMENT PROGRAMME (UNDP) the UN's global development network, advocates for change and connecting countries to knowledge, experience and resources to help people build a better life. Working on the ground in 166 countries, the organization supports national partners to address development challenges and achieve the Millennium Development Goals. Responding to AIDS is one of UNDP's priorities. As a cosponsor of UNAIDS, UNDP focuses on responding to the development and governance dimensions of the AIDS epidemic, protecting the rights of people living with HIV and vulnerable groups, and promoting gender equality.

UNFPA

Through strengthening the linkages between HIV and sexual and reproductive health the UNITED NATIONS POPULATION FUND (UNFPA), focuses its response to AIDS in over 140 countries on HIV prevention among young people and women (including the most marginalized) and comprehensive male and female condom programming including in humanitarian concern and post-conflict settings. UNFPA further contributes through helping nations and communities meet the reproductive health rights and needs of women and adolescents living with HIV, promoting confidential voluntary HIV testing and counselling, supporting training and services which prevent HIV transmission from mother-to-child, and improving access to HIV information and education. UNFPA also provides demographic and sociocultural support and studies to guide programme and policy development.

UNITED NATIONS
Office on Drugs and Crime

The **UNITED NATIONS OFFICE ON DRUGS AND CRIME (UNODC)** is mandated to assist countries in their struggle against illicit drugs, crime and terrorism. With this area of expertise within the UN system, UNODC has been given the responsibility to lead the UNAIDS response to HIV among injecting drug users and in prison settings. UNODC is also responsible for facilitating the development of a UN response to HIV for people vulnerable to human trafficking. These marginalized populations are often subjected to discrimination and violation of their human rights. Only few have access to HIV prevention, treatment, care and support services. UNODC assists countries to provide injecting drug users, prisoners and people vulnerable to human trafficking with evidence-informed comprehensive HIV prevention, treatment and care services through support in developing effective legislation and policies and building capacity of national stakeholders including civil societies and community organizations to ensure optimum coverage of these population groups with HIV services.

The **INTERNATIONAL LABOUR ORGANIZATION (ILO)** works to meet the aspirations of people in their working lives for opportunity and income; rights, voice and recognition; family stability and personal development; fairness and gender equality. The concept of decent work reflects the priorities of governments, workers and employers, who together provide the ILO with its unique tripartite identity. The ILO brings to the AIDS response direct access to the workplace, where AIDS policies and programmes help the achievement of universal access to prevention, treatment, care and support. By integrating AIDS in world of work structures, the ILO helps ensure protection against discrimination in labour laws, promotes comprehensive approaches to prevention through occupational safety and health mechanisms, and supports the livelihoods of those affected by AIDS through training provision, employment opportunities and social protection.

The distinctive mix of competencies in education, natural science, social and human sciences, culture and communication and information give the **UNITED NATIONS EDUCATIONAL, SCIENTIFIC AND CULTURAL ORGANIZATION (UNESCO)** an interdisciplinary, organizational and technical capacity suited to contributing to the achievement of universal access to comprehensive HIV prevention programmes, treatment, care and support. As the lead agency in the UNAIDS division for HIV transmission prevention with young people in educational institutions, UNESCO continues to promote comprehensive, scaled-up education sector responses to AIDS and deepened education sector engagement in national responses to AIDS. Its leadership of EDUCAIDS (the UNAIDS Global Initiative on Education and HIV and AIDS) and its coordination of the UNAIDS Inter-Agency Task Team (IATT) on Education are two mechanisms supporting strengthened strategic partnerships and cooperation among ministries of education, UNAIDS' cosponsors, bilateral agencies and civil society groups at global, regional and country levels to ensure maximum synergy and impact.

World Health Organization

The objective of the **WORLD HEALTH ORGANIZATION (WHO)** is the attainment by all peoples of the highest possible level of health. Its work in HIV is focused on the rapid scale up of treatment and care while accelerating prevention and strengthening health systems so that the health sector response to the epidemic is more effective and comprehensive. WHO defines and develops effective technical norms and guidelines, promotes partnership and provides strategic and technical support to Member States. The Organization also contributes to the global AIDS knowledge base by supporting surveillance, monitoring and evaluation, reviewing the evidence for interventions and promoting the integration of research into health service delivery.

THE WORLD BANK

The **WORLD BANK'S** mission is to fight poverty. It is one of the world's largest sources of funding and knowledge for developing countries. The World Bank's work on AIDS contributes to scaling up towards universal access to prevention, care and treatment through supporting efforts to strengthen national AIDS strategies and monitoring and evaluation, funding comprehensive AIDS programmes, and helping ensure that AIDS is part of the broader development agenda. By December 2007, the World Bank had committed more than US$ 3.6 billion for AIDS programmes globally. Most of the resources have been provided on highly concessional terms including grants for the poorest countries. The World Bank works in partnership with governments, donor agencies, UNAIDS' cosponsors and the Secretariat, civil society and the private sector on comprehensive AIDS responses encompassing prevention, care, treatment and impact mitigation.

Foreword

The *2008 Report on the global AIDS epidemic* confirms that the world is, at last, making some real progress in its response to AIDS.

Governments are acting on their promises at the 2006 United Nations High Level Meeting on HIV/AIDS, to scale up towards universal access to HIV prevention, treatment, care, and support by 2010. As of 2008, a small number of countries are already providing universal access to antiretroviral treatment and to services to prevent mother-to-child transmission of HIV. Others are well on the way to doing so. In more and more countries, HIV infection levels are falling.

But this is only the beginning. Twenty-seven years into the epidemic, AIDS continues to challenge all of our efforts. Today, for every two people who start taking antiretroviral drugs, another five become newly infected. Unless we take urgent steps to intensify HIV prevention we will fail to sustain the gains of the past few years, and universal access will simply be a noble aspiration.

This 2008 global report is the most comprehensive ever, based on country inputs with unprecedented scope and detail. It contains valuable information about what works and why, as well as highlighting the key challenges we face in our quest to respond effectively to AIDS—now and in the decades to come.

AIDS is a supremely complex issue that demands an unparalleled response from all sectors of society, worldwide. But as this report shows, it is increasingly evident that—given the will and given the resources—we can do it.

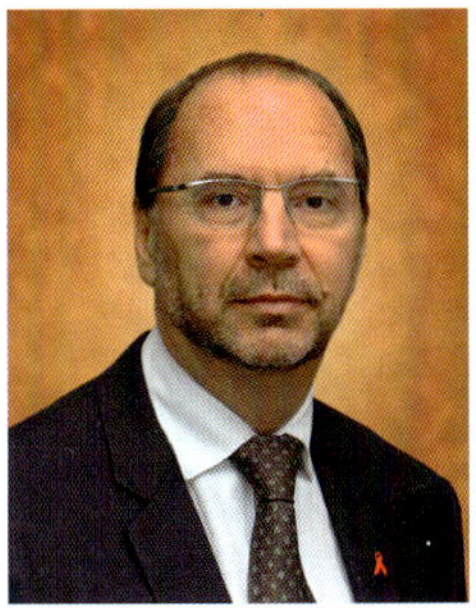

Dr Peter Piot

UNAIDS Executive Director and

Under-Secretary-General of the United Nations

The global HIV challenge: assessing progress, identifying obstacles, renewing commitment

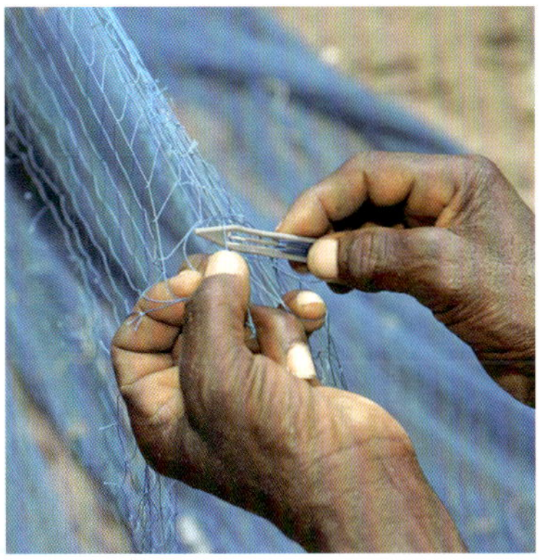

1

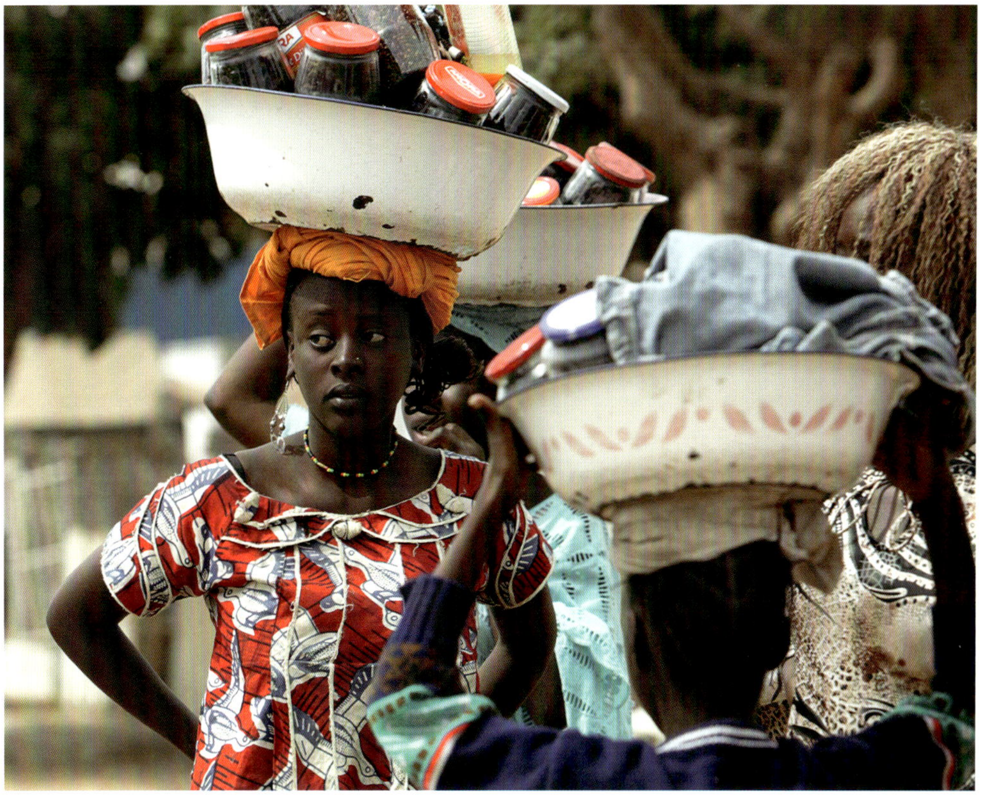

Chapter 1

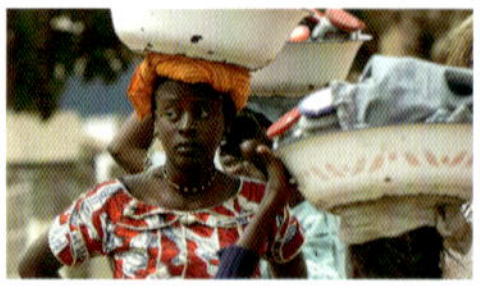

FIGURE 1.1 Selected events in the global response to the epidemic

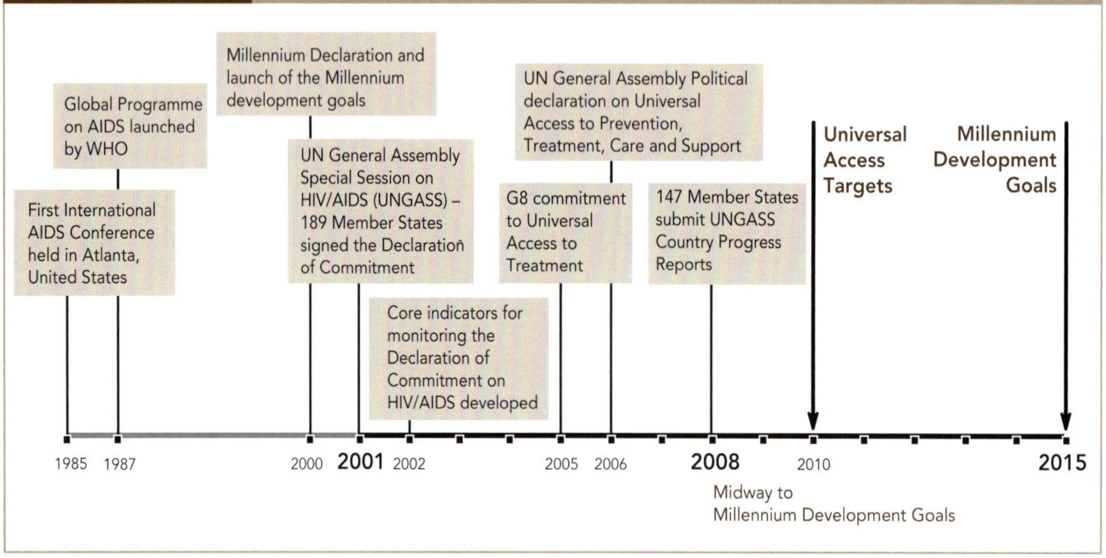

Key Findings

- This report provides the most comprehensive global assessment ever undertaken of the response to HIV, being based on reports from 147 countries on national progress in implementing the 2001 *Declaration of Commitment on HIV/AIDS.*
- Unprecedented numbers of civil society groups have joined their government counterparts and participated in this reporting process, using their participation as a means to communicate to the world on the situation within their country.
- The HIV response is critical to progress across the breadth of the global development agenda.
- A 6-fold increase in financing for HIV programmes in low- and middle-income countries is beginning to bear fruit, with many countries making major progress in lowering AIDS deaths and preventing new infections.
- Progress remains uneven, however, and the epidemic's future is still uncertain, underscoring the need for intensified action to move towards universal access to HIV prevention, treatment, care, and support.
- Achieving the many political commitments made on HIV will require stronger leadership, building on recent successes, taking account of lessons learnt, increased financial resources, improved coordination of effort, and effective action to address societal determinants of HIV risk and vulnerability.
- Monitoring and evaluation systems are being strengthened, largely with external funds, because countries are only beginning to avail themselves of the standard provision that up to 10% of programme funds can be directed to strengthening such systems.

The HIV epidemic has changed our world

In the countries most heavily affected, HIV has reduced life expectancy by more than 20 years, slowed economic growth, and deepened household poverty. In sub-Saharan Africa alone, the epidemic has orphaned[1] nearly 12 million children aged under 18 years. The natural age distribution in many national populations in sub-Saharan Africa has been dramatically skewed by HIV, with potentially perilous consequences for the transfer of knowledge and values from one generation to the next. In Asia, where infection rates are much lower than in Africa, HIV causes a greater loss of productivity than any other disease, and is likely to push an additional 6 million households into poverty by 2015 unless national responses are strengthened (Commission on AIDS in Asia, 2008). According to the United Nations Development Programme (UNDP), HIV has inflicted the "single greatest reversal in human development" in modern history (UNDP, 2005).

At the same time, the epidemic has heightened global consciousness of health disparities, and catalysed unprecedented action to confront some of the world's most serious development challenges. No disease in history has prompted a comparable mobilization of political, financial, and human resources, and no development challenge has led to such a strong level of leadership and ownership by the communities and countries most heavily affected. In large part due to the impact of HIV, people throughout the world have become less willing to tolerate inequities in global health and economic status that have long gone unaddressed.

In 2000, global leaders embraced a series of Millennium Development Goals that reflected newfound resolve to make the world safer, healthier, and more equitable. Millennium Development Goal 6 provides that, by 2015, the world will have halted and begun to reverse the global HIV epidemic. By making the HIV response one of the overriding international priorities for the 21st century, world leaders acknowledged the centrality of the HIV response to the future health and well-being of our increasingly interconnected planet.

At the first-ever Special Session on HIV/AIDS of the United Nations General Assembly (UNGASS) in 2001, UN Member States strengthened the response to Millennium Development Goal 6 by unanimously endorsing the *Declaration of Commitment on HIV/AIDS*. This *Declaration* included time-bound pledges to generate measurable action and concrete progress in the AIDS response. At the five-year review of implementation of the *Declaration of Commitment* in 2006, UN Member States reaffirmed the pledges made at the 2001 Special Session. Also, in the *Political Declaration on HIV/AIDS*, they committed to taking extraordinary action to move towards universal access to HIV prevention, treatment, care, and support by 2010.

This *Report on the global AIDS epidemic* emerges at the halfway mark between the 2001 UNGASS *Declaration of Commitment* and the 2015 target for Millennium Development Goal 6, and only two years before the agreed target date for universal access. This juncture provides an opportunity to assess the HIV response and to understand what must be done to ensure that nations are on course to achieve the HIV commitments they have made.

[1] Contrary to traditional usage, UNAIDS uses "orphan" to describe a child who has lost either one or both parents; the organization uses the terms "maternal orphan", "paternal orphan", and "double orphan" to describe a child who has lost its mother, father, or both parents, respectively.

An effective HIV response: vital to achievement of the Millennium Development Goals

Although one of the Millennium Development Goals (Goal 6) specifically addresses the HIV epidemic, an effective HIV response will also support achievement of other Millennium Development Goals embraced by the world community, as shown below.

Millennium Development Goal 1: *Eradicate extreme poverty and hunger.* Especially in high-prevalence settings, HIV deepens household poverty, slows economic growth, and undermines vital sectors on which economic development depends. In rural areas with high HIV prevalence, the epidemic degrades agricultural sectors and exacerbates food insecurity (see Chapter 6). Alleviating the epidemic's burden helps countries to grow their economies, reduce income inequalities, and prevent acute hunger.

Millennium Development Goal 2: *Achieve universal primary education.* The HIV response promotes universal education initiatives; these provide an essential venue for HIV prevention education for young people, and reduce girls' vulnerability to HIV (see Chapter 4). School attendance is a central focus of initiatives to address the needs of children orphaned or made vulnerable by HIV (see Chapter 6). Better access to treatment helps to minimize the epidemic's impact on fragile educational systems; it also reduces the likelihood that young people will be withdrawn from school in response to HIV in the household.

Millennium Development Goal 3: *Promote gender equality and empower women.* The HIV response is helping to drive efforts to reduce inequalities between the sexes (see Chapter 3). Countries are now monitored on the degree to which gender equity is a component of national HIV responses. Thus, the epidemic has increased the urgency of initiatives to forge new gender norms, and extensive worldwide efforts are under way to develop new HIV prevention methods that women may initiate (see Chapter 4). HIV has prompted parents, communities, and governments alike to approach the sexual and reproductive health needs of women, girls, and sexual minorities with renewed commitment.

Millennium Development Goal 4: *Reduce child mortality.* At the beginning of this decade, AIDS accounted for 3% of all deaths in children aged under 5 years—a toll that is likely to be much larger today in light of the high level of mother-to-child HIV transmission in the intervening years (WHO, 2005). A key component of a comprehensive HIV response is the scaling up of prevention strategies that can nearly eliminate the risk of mother-to-child HIV transmission (see Chapter 4).

Millennium Development Goal 5: *Improve maternal health.* Women now account for about half of all people living with HIV, and for more than 60% of infections in Africa (see Chapter 2). Greater access to antiretroviral medicines is improving the health and well-being of women, through programmes that couple prevention of mother-to-child transmission with continuing treatment to help mothers remain alive and in good health to care for their children. Integration of HIV initiatives with programmes addressing sexual and reproductive health is helping to ensure that women have access to the information and services they need to make informed reproductive decisions.

Millennium Development Goal 6: *Combat HIV/AIDS, malaria, and other diseases.* A strong HIV response yields health benefits that extend well beyond HIV itself. For example, HIV is an important contributing factor in the continued spread of tuberculosis. The push to expand access to HIV treatment in resource-limited settings is helping to strengthen fragile health infrastructures and is driving improvements in human capacity in low- and middle-income countries (see Chapter 5).

Millennium Development Goal 8: *Develop a global partnership for development.* Perhaps more than any other issue in our time, HIV has highlighted global and economic inequities, and has galvanized action on international development. HIV has helped place people at the centre of development; it has also helped to ensure that development strategies are inclusive, respectful of human rights, and country owned.

Promising progress, but enduring challenges

The 6-fold increase in financing for HIV activities in low- and middle-income countries during this decade is beginning to yield results. For the first time since what we now know as AIDS was recognized 27 years ago, signs of major progress in the HIV response have become apparent. The annual number of AIDS deaths has declined in the past two years from 2.2 million [1.9 million–2.6 million] in 2005 to 2.0 million [1.8 million–2.3 million] in 2007, in part as a result of the substantial increase in access to HIV treatment in recent years. In a number of heavily affected countries—such as Kenya, Rwanda, Uganda, and Zimbabwe—dramatic changes in sexual behaviour have been accompanied by declines in the number of new HIV infections, contributing to a global stabilization, beginning in the late 1990s, in the percentage of people aged 15–49 who are infected with HIV.

But these gains have not been consistent within and between regions, and favourable epidemiological and behavioural trends have not been sustained in some countries (see Chapter 4). Infections are on the rise in a number of countries including China, Germany, Indonesia, Mozambique, Papua New Guinea, the Russian Federation, Ukraine, the United Kingdom, and Viet Nam. In other countries—such as Lesotho, Namibia, South Africa and Swaziland—HIV prevalence appears to have stabilized at extraordinarily high levels. Although the number of people on antiretroviral drugs in low- and middle-income countries has risen, most of those who need such therapies are not currently receiving them (see Chapter 5). Moreover, the epidemic is outpacing the rate at which these drugs are being delivered. In 2007, the estimated number of new HIV infections was 2.5 times higher than the increase in the number of people on antiretroviral drugs in that year, underscoring the need for substantially greater success in preventing new HIV infections.

The recent stabilization of the global epidemic cannot obscure its most important aspect—its profound human toll. Since the beginning of the epidemic, 25 million people have died of HIV-related causes. Collectively, these deaths represent an incalculable loss of human potential. Individually, each is associated with enduring trauma in households and communities.

There is also a risk that the important progress achieved in recent years might lull some into complacency. Indications that the annual global number of new HIV infections may have peaked

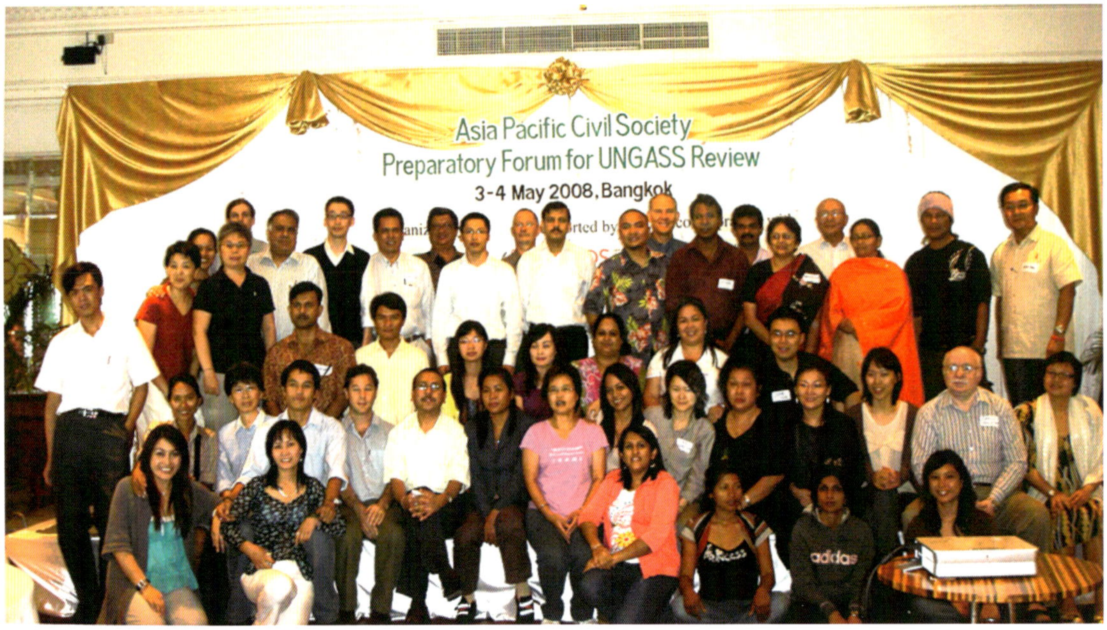
Asia Pacific Civil Society
Preparatory Forum for UNGASS Review
3-4 May 2008, Bangkok

around the beginning of the century have generated speculation in the popular media that the epidemic may have entered a long-term decline (McNeil, 2007). Yet the history of infectious disease suggests that epidemics are often cyclical, characterized by waves of infection that make it difficult to predict the epidemic's future course (Commission on AIDS in Asia, 2008; May & Anderson, 1979). Indeed, the HIV epidemic has repeatedly defied predictions derived from epidemiological modelling. A decade ago, few would have predicted that one million or more people would be living with HIV in the Russian Federation alone. If the epidemic's history is any indication, HIV is likely to have additional surprises in store that the world must be prepared to address.

Above all, the dimensions of the epidemic remain staggering. In 2007 alone, 33 million [30 million–36 million] people were living with HIV, 2.7 million [2.2 million–3.2 million] people became infected with the virus, and 2 million [1.8 million–2.3 million] people died of HIV-related causes.

Purpose and contents of the report

This report examines the current status of the global HIV response in a series of chapters devoted to key thematic areas. For each of these themes, the report assesses the response by seeking to answer a series of related questions:

- Are the right actions being taken?
- Are the right actions being undertaken in the right manner?
- Have these actions been sufficiently scaled up to make a difference?

To answer these questions, the report relies heavily on data reported to UNAIDS by 147 UN Member States in early 2008; the data relate to 25 core UNGASS indicators (Table 1) developed to measure progress in implementing the *Declaration of Commitment*.[2] The number of countries reporting on these indicators, and the completeness of national reports, have steadily improved since reporting began in 2003 (Figure 1.2). This improvement underscores increased national commitment to HIV monitoring and evaluation; it also shows

[2] Copies of the reports submitted by countries are available on the UNAIDS web site (http://www.unaids.org/en/KnowledgeCentre/HIV-Data/CountryProgress/2007CountryProgressAllCountries.asp).

TABLE 1 National indicators for the implementation of the *Declaration of Commitment on HIV/AIDS*

National Commitment and Action
1. Domestic and international AIDS spending by categories and financing sources
2. National Composite Policy Index (Areas covered: gender, workplace programmes, stigma and discrimination, prevention, care and support, human rights, civil society involvement, and monitoring and evaluation)
National Programmes (blood safety, antiretroviral therapy coverage, prevention of mother-to-child transmission, co-management of Tuberculosis and HIV treatment, HIV testing, prevention programmes, services for orphans and vulnerable children, and education)
3. Percentage of donated blood units screened for HIV in a quality assured manner
4. Percentage of adults and children with advanced HIV infection receiving antiretroviral therapy
5. Percentage of HIV-positive pregnant women who received antiretrovirals to reduce the risk of mother-to-child transmission
6. Percentage of estimated HIV-positive incident Tuberculosis cases that received treatment for Tuberculosis and HIV
7. Percentage of women and men aged 15-49 who received an HIV test in the last 12 months and who know their results
8. Percentage of most-at-risk populations that have received an HIV test in the last 12 months and who know their results
9. Percentage of most-at-risk populations reached with HIV prevention programmes
10. Percentage of orphaned and vulnerable children aged 0–17 whose households received free basic external support in caring for the child
11. Percentage of schools that provided life skills-based HIV education in the last academic year
Knowledge and Behaviour
12. Current school attendance among orphans and among non-orphans aged 10–14*
13. Percentage of young women and men aged 15–24 who both correctly identify ways of preventing the sexual transmission of HIV and who reject major misconceptions about HIV transmission*
14. Percentage of most-at-risk populations who both correctly identify ways of preventing the sexual transmission of HIV and who reject major misconceptions about HIV transmission
15. Percentage of young women and men aged 15–24 who have had sexual intercourse before the age of 15
16. Percentage of women and men aged 15–49 who have had sexual intercourse with more than one partner in the last 12 months
17. Percentage of women and men aged 15–49 who had more than one sexual partner in the past 12 months reporting the use of a condom during their last sexual intercourse*
18. Percentage of female and male sex workers reporting the use of a condom with their most recent client
19. Percentage of men reporting the use of a condom the last time they had anal sex with a male partner
20. Percentage of injecting drug users reporting the use of a condom the last time they had sexual intercourse
21. Percentage of injecting drug users reporting the use of sterile injecting equipment the last time they injected
Impact
22. Percentage of young women and men aged 15–24 who are HIV infected*
23. Percentage of most-at-risk populations who are HIV infected
24. Percentage of adults and children with HIV known to be on treatment 12 months after initiation of antiretroviral therapy
25. Percentage of infants born to HIV-infected mothers who are infected

* Millennium Development Goals indicator

FIGURE 1.2 Percentage of UN Member States reporting by region, 2004–2008

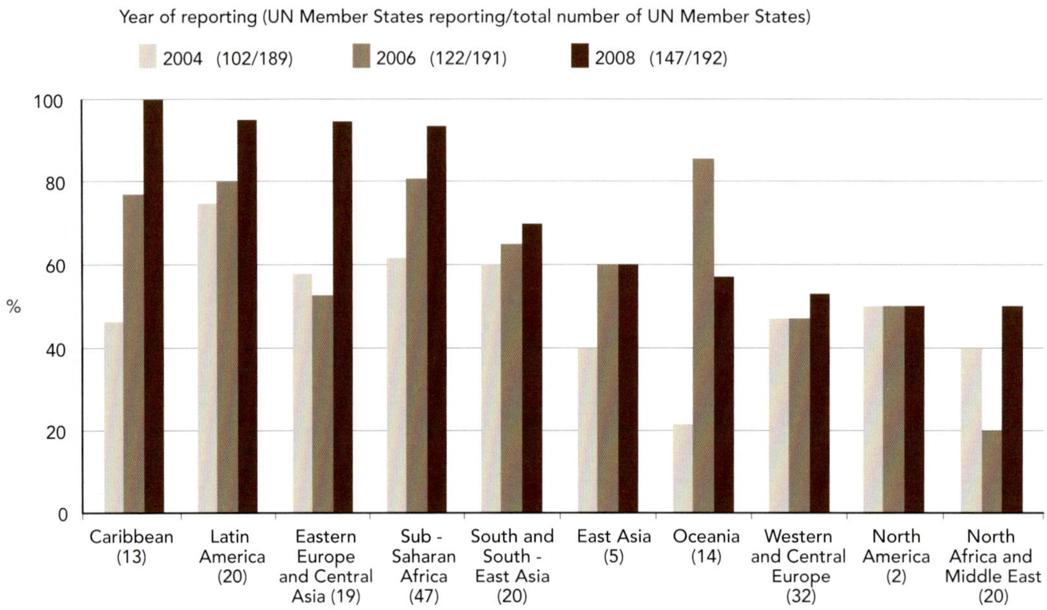

Source: UNGASS Country Progress Reports 2008.

increased global ownership of the tracking of HIV commitments made by countries earlier this decade. In 2008, all Caribbean countries reported on core indicators; reports were also received from nearly all countries in Latin America, Eastern Europe and Central Asia, and sub-Saharan Africa. Reporting rates were notably lower in other regions.

Based on the specific time-bound pledges made by countries at the 2001 Special Session of the UN General Assembly on HIV/AIDS, the core UNGASS indicators cover a broad array of variables, such as HIV prevalence among young people aged 15–24, coverage of antiretroviral therapy and key HIV prevention initiatives, services to support children orphaned or made vulnerable by HIV, and national adoption of recommended HIV policies. Information from national progress reports is supplemented by other data sources such as household surveys, civil society reports, and the budgets and programme-monitoring data of donor governments, UNAIDS Cosponsors, philanthropic foundations, and biomedical research agencies.

Civil society engagement in monitoring progress in the HIV response

The participation of civil society is an essential part of the reporting process. UNAIDS engaged a consortium of civil society organizations, led by the International Council of AIDS Service Organizations and the International Women's Health Coalition, to support civil society organizations in national reporting.[3]

[3] For a full description of the methods used for national reporting of progress in implementing the *Declaration of Commitment*, including the extent of civil society involvement in national reporting, see Annex 2.

Important progress has been made since the last reporting round regarding inclusion of civil society in national reporting. National HIV authorities, which were responsible for submitting data on core indicators for the *Declaration of Commitment*, indicated that civil society provided input in 82% of countries, and people living with HIV provided input in 75%. In Indonesia, for example, civil society agreed to include a "community report" representing civil society's perspectives in the official submission to UNAIDS.

Civil society has an important, formal role in the completion of the National Composite Policy Index (NCPI). This index assesses progress in development and implementation of sound national HIV policies and strategies. It is an extensive questionnaire completed through a review of relevant documents and through interviews with people most knowledgeable about the topics covered. Part A of the NCPI is completed by government officials, whereas Part B is completed by representatives from civil society and by bilateral and multilateral organizations.

In all countries, civil society participated in the completion of the nongovernmental component of the NCPI.[4] Altogether, more than 700 local nongovernmental organizations (represented by many more individuals) served as key informants on the NCPI, far outnumbering the international nongovernmental and bilateral and multilateral organizations involved. UN agencies participated in completion of the nongovernmental part of the NCPI in 65% of countries, and bilateral donor agencies assisted in 29% of countries.

Civil society groups in 19 countries submitted additional parallel information on the national HIV response. This information included complementary or qualitative data to supplement national reports, such as survey data on sexual and reproductive health and rights (Gestos, 2008). In some of these countries, where civil society was not included in national reporting or where countries failed to submit a national report, "shadow" reports were submitted.

Using evidence to assess progress

Altogether, the body of data assembled in 2008 on national efforts permits the most comprehensive evaluation ever undertaken of global, regional, and national progress in addressing the epidemic. The information presented in this report enables the reader to assess progress made since 2001, identify the strengths and weaknesses of the response to date, and better understand the magnitude of the challenges facing the world in its quest to begin to reverse the epidemic by 2015. A closing chapter on scaling-up (see Chapter 7) specifically examines the main obstacles to accelerated success on HIV and describes the most promising strategies for overcoming these obstacles.

The report also includes profiles of individuals from different regions who are living with, affected by, or responding to, HIV. These profiles are a reminder of the human dimensions of the global HIV response—that attached to each number cited in this report is a person who possesses an inalienable human right to dignity, respect, and effective health care. They also underscore one of the enduring lessons of HIV—that international health and development efforts must ultimately be owned and led by the people who are most affected.

[4] Not all Member States submitted NCPI data (130/192), and four countries did not indicate who provided the NCPI responses.

Improved country-level monitoring and evaluation: facilitating an evidence-informed response to the epidemic

Since HIV was first recognized, approaches and methodologies to monitor the epidemic and the response have continuously improved. As a result, the world is better equipped than ever to estimate HIV prevalence or the rate of new HIV infections, to determine the extent of programme coverage, to characterize and evaluate national responses, and to gauge the level of funding available for HIV programmes in low- and middle-income countries.

Country reports on progress

By the time this report went to press, 147 UN Member States had reported national information against the 25 core UNGASS indicators developed by UNAIDS and its partners to track implementation of the *Declaration of Commitment on HIV/AIDS*. As country progress reports were submitted early in 2008, UNAIDS made them available in unedited form on the Internet.

For the first time, this report permits an understanding of the main trends in the HIV response for key indicators that have not changed significantly. For example, the report examines trends in HIV prevalence and knowledge among young people, access to antiretroviral therapy, and national adoption of relevant human rights protections. It also highlights regional and subregional variations in epidemiological trends, behaviours, and national responses, in recognition of the limited usefulness to national decision-makers of global numerical values on HIV indicators.

This report provides an initial assessment of the latest information on the epidemic and on national responses. UNAIDS and its research partners plan to follow up the indicator data summarized in this global report with more in-depth analytical papers in particular thematic areas and with studies that more exhaustively examine data pertinent to various regions.

Increasing national capacity on monitoring and evaluation

This report reflects some of the improvements that have occurred in national and global information systems in recent years. Beginning in 2004, UNAIDS embarked on a long-term effort to strengthen national systems for HIV monitoring and evaluation. By 2008, almost 60 monitoring and evaluation advisers had been placed in national and regional UNAIDS offices. These advisers:

- provide continuing technical support for the building of national monitoring and evaluation capacity;
- work with national AIDS programmes to develop and monitor measurable indicators to assess implementation of national strategies; and
- help countries to extend monitoring and evaluation activities from the national to the district level.

Countries receive continuing support in the development and maintenance of a comprehensive national HIV monitoring and evaluation system. They also benefit from a growing array of other sources of technical assistance, including the Global AIDS Monitoring and Evaluation Team housed at the World Bank, and the United States President's Emergency Plan for AIDS Relief (PEPFAR). Individual UNAIDS cosponsors, such as the United Nations Children's Fund (UNICEF) (UNICEF, UNAIDS & WHO, 2008) and the World Health Organization (WHO), have also intensified their technical assistance on monitoring and evaluation.

The increased assistance to countries is intended to facilitate improved coordination of national stakeholders under a single monitoring and evaluation framework. This is in line with the "Three Ones" principles for effective country-level action—one national strategic framework, one national coordinating body, and one monitoring and evaluation system (see Chapter 7).

As indicated in Figure 1.3, the percentage of countries with a central HIV database increased from 41% in 2005 to 68% in 2007, and endorsement of the monitoring and evaluation plan by key partners also increased from 54% in 2005 to 78% in 2007 (UNGASS Country Progress Reports, 2008).

FIGURE 1.3 Percentage of countries with monitoring and evaluation components in place, 2005 and 2007

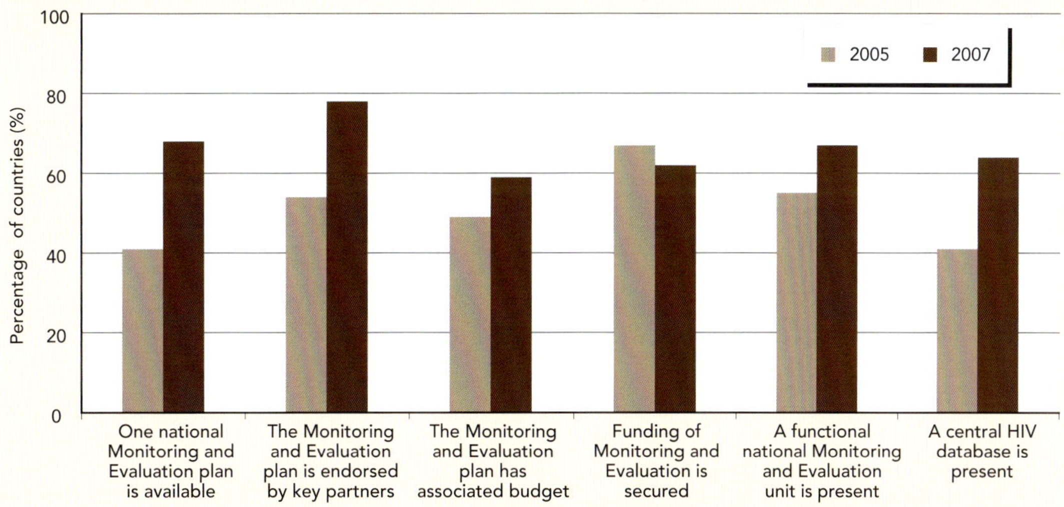

Source: UNGASS Country Progress Reports 2008.

Between 2005 and 2007, the number of countries having one costed national monitoring and evaluation plan with secured funding, as well as a functional national monitoring and evaluation unit or national technical working group, and a centralized HIV database, increased from 14 to 44 (UNGASS Country Progress Reports, 2008).

The Global Fund to Fight AIDS, Tuberculosis and Malaria has played a key role in driving improvements in national monitoring and evaluation systems. Proposals for assistance from the Global Fund must be based on sound country-level information. In addition, timely and accurate national progress reporting is essential for securing continued funding under the performance-based approach of the Global Fund.

Not only are systems for monitoring and evaluation stronger, but available methods to track key aspects of the epidemic have improved. In countries with generalized epidemics, increased use of national household surveys has increased the accuracy and reliability of national estimates of HIV prevalence, incidence, and mortality (see Chapter 2). Figure 1.4 shows global trends in strengthening of monitoring and evaluation systems.

FIGURE 1.4 Global trends in monitoring and evaluation system strengthening, 2005 and 2007

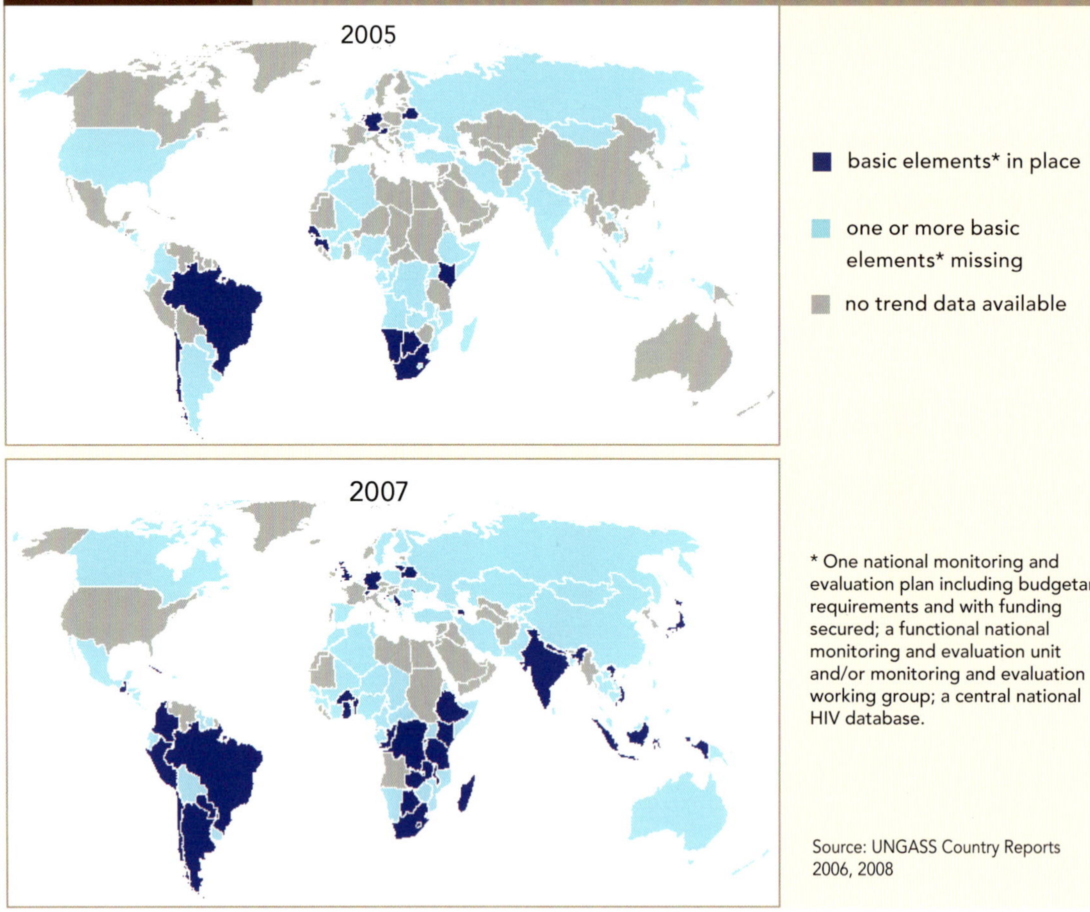

* One national monitoring and evaluation plan including budgetary requirements and with funding secured; a functional national monitoring and evaluation unit and/or monitoring and evaluation working group; a central national HIV database.

Source: UNGASS Country Reports 2006, 2008

Moving towards universal access to HIV prevention, treatment, care, and support

To quicken progress towards the 2015 deadline for the Millennium Development Goals, the global community has embraced the goal of moving towards universal access to HIV prevention, treatment, care, and support by 2010. This step is of historic significance in global health and development. Converting aspirations into achievements will require unprecedented commitment and resources, as well as innovative ways of approaching challenges and bottlenecks

Key weaknesses and gaps in monitoring and evaluation

Although improvements in national monitoring and evaluation capacity are evident, critical gaps and weaknesses remain. One in four countries with a national monitoring and evaluation plan have not calculated the budgetary requirements, and one in three have not secured funding to implement the plan. More than one third of countries with a monitoring and evaluation plan have no centralized HIV database. To build the national capacity needed to provide a robust information base for decision-making on policies and programmes, countries require ready access to financial and technical resources for monitoring and evaluation, including HIV surveillance. Although the Global Fund, the World Bank, and PEPFAR permit as much as 10% of any grant to be earmarked for monitoring and evaluation, countries are just beginning to avail themselves of this provision.

Reported expenditures[5] on monitoring and evaluation range from 0.1% of national HIV expenditures to 15.6% (median 0.9%, UNGASS indicator 1, 2006-2007 data). In more than half of countries (54%), monitoring and evaluation activities are exclusively financed through external sources. Only one in 10 countries report financing of HIV monitoring and evaluation exclusively through domestic funding. The imbalance in financing for monitoring and evaluation raises concerns about the sustainability of this essential function in future years. In addition, external funding for monitoring and evaluation is not necessarily supporting the national monitoring and evaluation system. For example, Guyana indicates considerable progress in monitoring and evaluation, but several donor-funded projects with monitoring and evaluation components are not linked to the national monitoring and evaluation plan (Guyana UNGASS Country Progress Report 2008).

As national monitoring and evaluation capacity continues to grow, countries and national partners must ensure that they actually use the information generated to improve decision-making. Evaluation of resource flows has found that national allocation of prevention resources is sometimes sharply at odds with the picture of the epidemic generated by national surveillance systems (UNAIDS, 2004). Similarly, inertia and bureaucratic pressures sometimes work against the discontinuation or revision of particular programmes or strategies, even when evaluation data indicate that these approaches are ineffective.

[5] A total of 48 countries reported expenditures for 2006 or 2007 on monitoring and evaluation.

What is universal access?

Universal access signifies both a concrete commitment and a renewed resolve among people the world over to reverse the course of the epidemic. It is a process that builds on past initiatives and infuses existing efforts with greater momentum.

Universal access does not imply that there will be, or should be, 100% coverage of HIV prevention, treatment, care, and support services—even in high-income countries where health care is universally available, some patients who are medically eligible for antiretroviral drugs are not receiving them for various reasons (e.g. a deliberate decision not to undergo testing or a decision to initiate therapy at a later time). Rather, by moving towards nationally set targets for universal access, the world has committed to make concrete, sustained advances towards a high level of coverage for the most effective programmes needed to manage diverse epidemics in all regions. The basic principles for scaling up towards universal access emphasize that services must be equitable, accessible, affordable, comprehensive, and sustainable over the long-term.

Because different settings often have distinctly different needs, universal access cannot fit a standardized time frame or approach, and countries will adopt varying time lines and strategies to achieve scale-up. For example, countries with generalized epidemics (see Chapter 4) require very high coverage for initiatives aimed at the general popuation (e.g. mass media awareness campaigns, school-based education, and workplace prevention programmes). In contrast, countries with low-level and concentrated epidemics may require less intense coverage for initiatives aimed at the general population, but high coverage for programmes addressing populations most at risk of HIV exposure. By setting national targets, countries are holding themselves accountable to reach universal access within a time frame that is both urgent—galvanizing support and momentum around this goal—and feasible, and that will set them on the way to reach the 2015 Millennium Development Goals.

that have long impeded swifter progress on human development in resource-limited settings.

In 2005-2006, 123 countries and 7 regions, with assistance from UNAIDS, implemented consultative processes to determine the challenges associated with moving towards universal access to HIV prevention, treatment, care, and support. Results of these consultations informed deliberations at the High Level Meeting on HIV/AIDS at the UN General Assembly in June 2006.

This meeting resulted in a formal, unanimous endorsement by UN Member States of the goal of moving towards universal access by 2010 (UN General Assembly, 2006).

With normative guidance from UNAIDS (UNAIDS, 2006), countries in all regions initiated evidence-informed processes for achieving a national, multisectoral consensus on targets for universal access. As of March 2008, 105 countries had established targets for universal access to

HIV prevention, treatment, care, and support—including 76 countries that had incorporated these targets into their national strategic AIDS plans or broader development instruments (e.g. Poverty Reduction Strategy Papers, Medium Term Expenditure Frameworks). A total of 41 countries have defined the actions and costs required to achieve universal access—a key step in mobilizing the necessary resources to meet defined goals. Some countries have established especially ambitious targets, sometimes exceeding feasibility estimates for HIV treatment or other initiatives.

Following up on the target-setting processes, countries are now supporting universal access initiatives at subnational levels. In Nigeria, for example, strategic plans for universal access are being elaborated in six states.

Civil society advocacy for universal access

The movement towards universal access to HIV prevention, treatment, care, and support is serving as an effective vehicle for mobilizing civil society.

At country level, civil society has participated in the establishment of national targets for universal access, and is monitoring implementation of national plans to ensure greater accountability in the national response. In Malawi and Cambodia, for example, concerted advocacy by civil society organizations helped spur national decision-makers to establish ambitious targets for universal access. Similarly, in Nigeria, eight civil society networks have joined together to forge a civil society action plan on universal access—the "People's AIDS agenda"—released on World AIDS Day 2007.

Globally, the World AIDS Campaign is using the cause of universal access to mobilize diverse constituencies and civil campaigners. In July 2007, civil society campaigners from 35 regions convened under the World AIDS Campaign umbrella in Nairobi to share perspectives and coordinate efforts on promoting universal access. National AIDS campaigns are now active in five of the eight countries that comprise the Group of Eight (G8) leading industrialized nations, and these national campaigns are coordinating advocacy to ensure that HIV remains a priority for the G8.

The Coalition of Asia Pacific Regional Networks on HIV/AIDS developed a toolkit on 'Minimum Standards for Civil Society Participation in Universal Access Initiatives', drawing on regional and national consultations of civil society organizations. The toolkit is designed to be used by civil society representatives and other stakeholders to assess and promote greater civil society involvement in national universal access initiatives. In keeping with the principles outlined in the toolkit, UNAIDS sponsored a civil society consultation to inform the development of technical recommendations for scaling up HIV testing and counselling in the Asia and Pacific region. Regional forums for populations most at risk have also been convened to ensure strong civil society involvement in efforts to plan and implement scaled-up prevention programmes.

Activism to achieve results

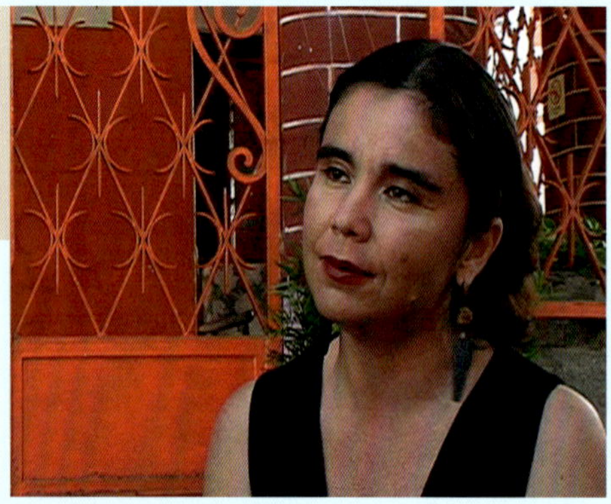

Alessandra Nilo is co-founder and co-coordinator of GESTOS, a nongovernmental organization based in Brazil

For Alessandra Nilo, a Brazilian-based activist, her work on HIV is part of a broader struggle for social justice and human rights. "Over time it has become clearer that the issues of poverty, gender inequality, but above all, the cultural differences and challenges are all points which need to be addressed and dealt with once and for all", she says.

Alessandra and others joined together in 1993 to establish GESTOS, with the aim of providing psychosocial support and leadership training for people living with HIV in the Brazilian city of Recife. In subsequent years, GESTOS has become increasingly engaged in public policy analysis and advocacy, including monitoring the Brazilian government's progress in meeting its HIV commitments. In the second half of the 1990s, GESTOS began developing links with other groups in Latin America. In collaboration with other civil society groups, GESTOS was an active participant in the 2001 UN General Assembly Special Session on HIV/AIDS. Today, GESTOS works in 16 different countries and in 2008 reported on the status of sexual and reproductive health in these countries as a complement to national reporting on core indicators for the *Declaration of Commitment*.

Notwithstanding the epidemic's complexity, Alessandra says one of the most satisfying aspects of HIV activism is that solutions actually exist for many of the most important challenges. "What drives me to pursue my work as an activist is the possibility to find solutions and to deal with inequalities that are configured in a macrostructure of society in a somewhat more tangible manner. Here, in my community, I have taken action to ensure that those who were very poor before and who had never had the possibility of gaining access to adequate treatment for HIV/AIDS now have a chance to benefit from it, as well as gaining access to food aid, decent living conditions, and, above all, that the community may learn how to live with this epidemic."

Alessandra believes now is the time for the HIV response to show results. "Since 2001, there have been considerable investments concerning HIV/AIDS", she says. "What we need to do now is to show how this money is invested, show the results of this large number of investments and show clearly that it is necessary to make even more investments... In my opinion, we won't get there unless civil society is committed and involved."

For Alessandra, HIV activism is more than a cause, it is a way of life. "This is not a kind of work where one can just drop the pen and go home... We are people who are fighting for a cause, a social-welfare cause which mobilizes us 24 hours a day, seven days a week!"

Beginning to reverse the epidemic by 2015

A principal finding of this report is that, although some countries are on course to meet the 2010 targets in the *Declaration of Commitment*, others are not. Without a substantial strengthening and acceleration of the HIV response, many countries will not achieve universal access to HIV prevention, treatment, care, and support by 2010 or begin to reverse the epidemic by 2015. The global community should renew and strengthen its commitment to work with countries to expedite progress towards universal access to HIV prevention, treatment, care, and support.

Throughout the subsequent chapters, this report emphasizes a number of key factors that will affect the world's ability to meet the challenges ahead.

- *Building on success.* There has been recent progress across many regions in bringing essential HIV services to scale—reducing HIV incidence, stabilizing mortality rates, and in caring for children made vulnerable by the epidemic; this progress demonstrates that dramatic results are achievable, even in the most resource-limited settings.
- *Making the money work.* Despite the concrete progress achieved in recent years in gaining dramatically greater resources for HIV, countries are often struggling to translate new funding into scaled-up national programmes for HIV prevention, treatment, care, and support. The actions of diverse national stakeholders are often poorly coordinated, and infrastructure weaknesses are slowing the capacity of countries to absorb new financing. Important steps have been taken in recent years to address the factors that blunt the impact of increased funding; however, substantially stronger action is urgently needed to close the access gap for essential HIV programmes.
- *Tailoring the response to national and local needs.* What is referred to as the "global epidemic" is actually an amalgam of an almost infinite number of individual epidemics—in communities, districts, countries, subregions, and regions. No single pattern is sufficient for an effective response. Different countries may learn from one another in crafting, implementing, and revising their national strategies. However, national efforts need to be informed by evidence and carefully tailored to national needs and circumstances if they are to be optimally effective. National decision-makers and partners must "know their epidemic and their response" in order to develop national plans that will achieve maximum impact.
- *Addressing societal factors that increase HIV risk and vulnerability*, and deepen the epidemic's impact. Scale-up of programmes must be coupled with an intensified effort to address cross-cutting issues that impede an effective response. This is especially important in hyperendemic settings where marginal changes in risk behaviour are likely to have only limited impact on the epidemic's trajectory. All stakeholders should work to promote gender equality and women's empowerment, reduce HIV stigma and discrimination, and alleviate the social marginalization of groups at highest risk of exposure to HIV. Throughout this report, gender, social marginalization, and income inequality will be addressed as cross-cutting issues that play critical roles across the entire breadth of the HIV response.
- *Planning for the long-term.* Even were the world to begin to halt the epidemic by 2015, as envisioned in the Millennium Development Goals, the epidemic would remain an overriding global challenge for decades to come. While responding on an emergency basis with efforts to bring essential HIV prevention, treatment, care, and support to scale, an effective response needs to be sustained for the long-term. This will require novel mechanisms and the creation of capacity that does not currently exist; it will also require thoughtful planning, because some of the challenges

the epidemic will pose 10 or 20 years from now are likely to be quite different from those faced today.

- *Placing people at the centre of health and development.* One of the great lessons of the HIV epidemic is the central role of civil society—especially of people living with HIV and those most at risk of HIV exposure—in effective national and local responses. Yet the people most heavily affected by the epidemic continue to remain on the periphery of decision-making in many countries. To overcome the daunting obstacles hindering efforts to move towards universal access, countries urgently need the knowledge, passion, and commitment of those who possess the best insight on how to reach those in greatest need of HIV services.

Status of the global HIV epidemic

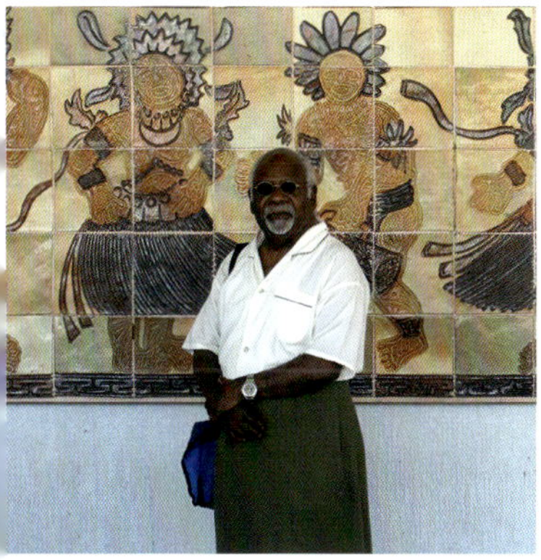

2

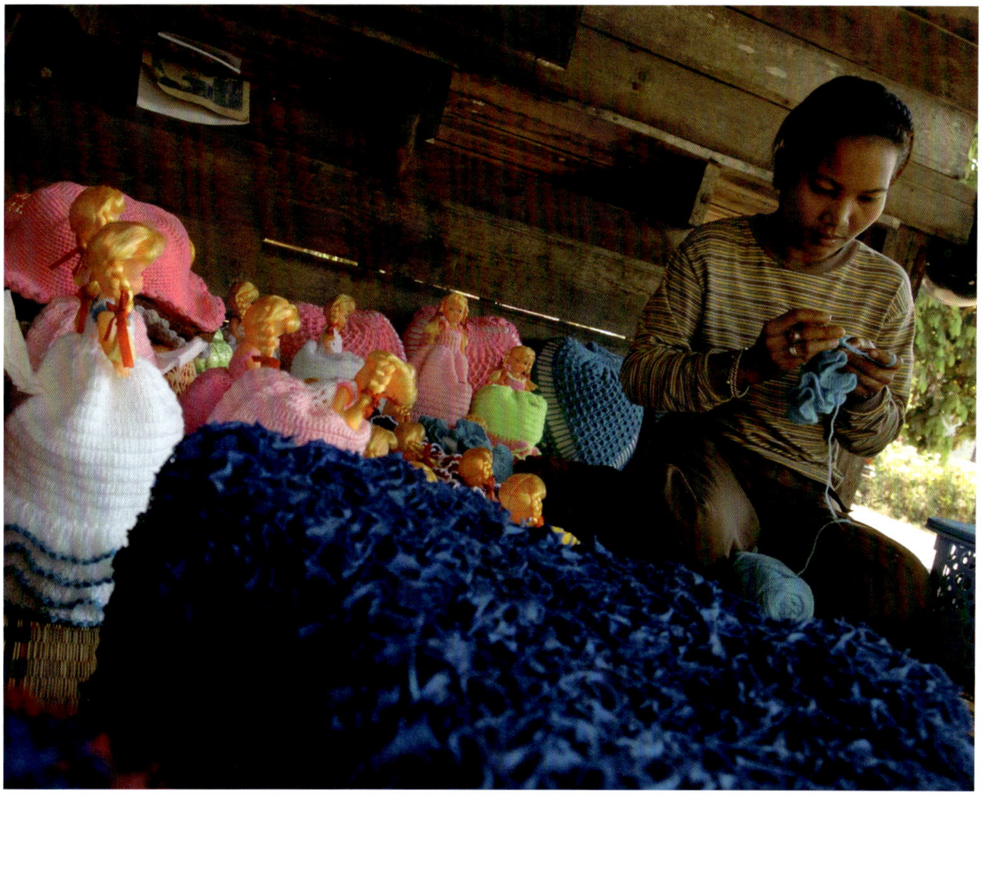

Chapter 2

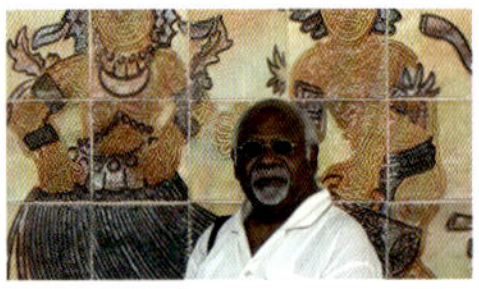

FIGURE 2.1 Selected events in tracking the epidemic

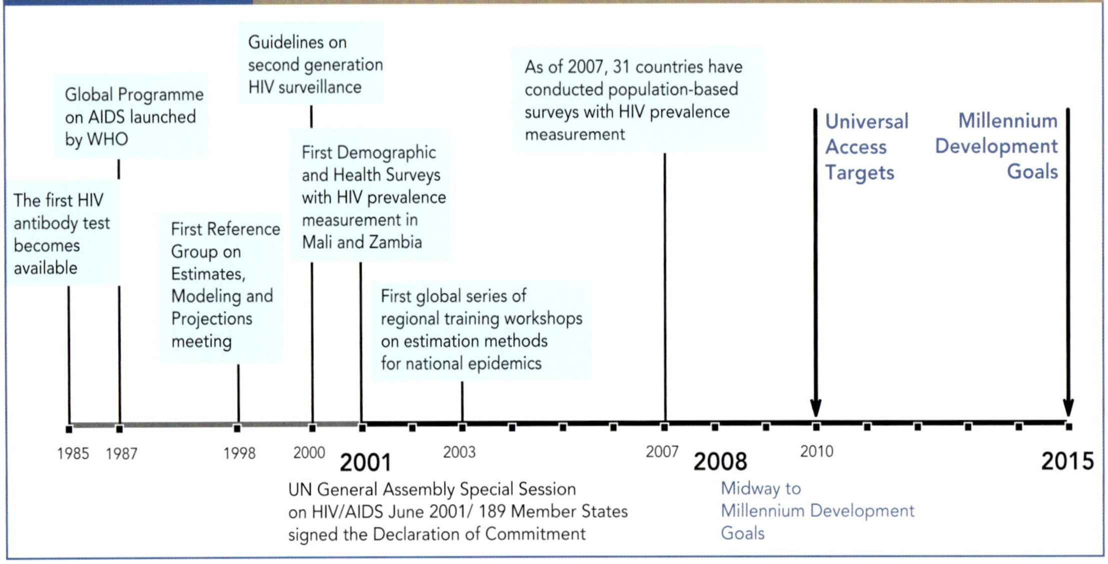

Key Findings

- The global percentage of adults living with HIV has leveled off since 2000.
- In 2007 there were 2.7 million new HIV infections and 2 million HIV-related deaths.
- The rate of new HIV infections has fallen in several countries, but globally these favourable trends are at least partially offset by increases in new infections in other countries.
- In 14 of 17 African countries with adequate survey data, the percentage of young pregnant women (ages 15–24) who are living with HIV has declined since 2000-2001. In 7 countries, the drop in infections has equalled or exceeded the 25% target decline for 2010 set out in the *Declaration of Commitment*.
- As treatment access has increased over the last ten years the annual number of AIDS deaths has fallen.
- Sub-Saharan Africa remains the region most heavily affected by HIV, accounting for 67% of all people living with HIV and for 75% of AIDS deaths in 2007. However, some of the most worrisome increases in new infections are now occurring in populous countries in other regions, such as Indonesia, the Russian Federation, and various high-income countries.
- Globally, the percentage of women among people living with HIV has remained stable (at 50%) for several years, although women's share of infections is increasing in several countries.
- In virtually all regions outside sub-Saharan Africa, HIV disproportionately affects injecting drug users, men who have sex with men, and sex workers.

HIV remains a global health problem of unprecedented dimensions. Unknown 27 years ago, HIV has already caused an estimated 25 million deaths worldwide and has generated profound demographic changes in the most heavily-affected countries.

The most recent international epidemiological data contain some good news. In some countries in Asia, Latin America and sub-Saharan Africa, the annual number of new HIV infections is falling. The estimated rate of AIDS deaths has also declined, in part as a result of success in expanding access to antiretroviral drugs in resource-limited settings. Yet these favourable trends are not uniformly evident, either within or between regions, underscoring the need for more comprehensive progress in implementing effective policies and programmes.

This chapter summarizes the current status of the epidemic—analysing broad global trends and providing regional snapshots of the epidemic's path. It draws on the latest epidemiological data from countries; in many cases, these data have significantly improved (see box "Improving HIV estimates"). Annex I provides specific epidemiological information for 168 countries.

Improving HIV estimates

HIV surveillance in designated sites ("sentinel surveillance") has expanded and improved considerably (especially in sub-Saharan Africa and Asia), leading to more reliable estimates of the HIV epidemic and its impact. In addition, a growing number of countries have conducted national population-based surveys that include HIV testing. Together, these data sources provide complementary information on both adult HIV prevalence and on epidemiological trends over time.

UNAIDS and WHO primarily use three tools to generate HIV estimates for countries and regions: the Estimation and Projection Package (EPP), WORKBOOK, and Spectrum.[1] These models generate estimates of HIV prevalence[2] over time, the number of people living with HIV, new infections, deaths due to AIDS, children orphaned by AIDS, and treatment needs. The estimates are based on data from sentinel surveillance, surveys, and special studies; the models and assumptions used in these tools are regularly updated on the basis of the latest available research.

HIV prevalence data collected in national population-based surveys, in particular in countries with generalized epidemics, have improved the reliability of national HIV estimates. These surveys are geographically more representative than sentinel surveillance, and include both men and women. Since 2001, 30 countries in the Caribbean, sub-Saharan Africa, and Asia have conducted national population-based surveys with HIV prevalence measures. In almost all of those surveys, new estimates of HIV prevalence were lower than estimates of prevalence published before the new survey data became available.

Such surveys have also made it possible to update and revise assumptions in the EPP and Spectrum software tools. For example, national population-based HIV surveys

---

[1] More information about these tools can be found at: http://www.unaids.org/en/KnowledgeCentre/HIVData/Methodology/

[2] HIV prevalence refers to the total number of infections at a given time. Incidence or new infections refers to the percentage or number of people who have become newly infected over a period of time, traditionally a given year.

have found HIV prevalence to be approximately 20% lower than the prevalence among antenatal clinic attendees, in both rural and urban areas (Gouws et al., in press). Some countries in sub-Saharan Africa have not conducted such surveys—notably Angola, Eritrea, Gambia, Guinea-Bissau, Mozambique, Namibia, Nigeria, Somalia, and Sudan. To develop the estimates included in this report, HIV prevalence data from antenatal clinic attendees in these countries have been adjusted downward to a level of approximately 0.8 times the prevalence found in antenatal clinic surveillance. The level of adjustment varies, based on the proportion of urban to rural populations within a country.

New research has also led to important revisions in the assumptions used in the models developed by UNAIDS and WHO. One such revision relates to estimates of HIV incidence and AIDS mortality. Central to these is an assumption about the average time people survive from HIV infection to death in the absence of antiretroviral treatment (Stover et al. in press). Longitudinal studies (Marston et al., 2007; Todd et al., 2007) indicate that, in the absence of such treatment, the estimated net median survival time after infection with HIV is 11 years (UNAIDS Reference Group on Estimates, Modelling and Projections, 2006), instead of the previously estimated 9 years (UNAIDS Reference Group on Estimates, Modelling and Projections, 2002).[3]

Improved surveillance systems and data sources, together with the changes in assumptions, have enabled more reliable epidemiological estimates. Since revisions also affect historical trends, latest estimates should not be compared directly with estimates published in previous reports. Where this report cites epidemiological trends, revisions to historical estimates are given.

The UNAIDS Secretariat and WHO will continue to update the HIV and AIDS estimation methods as new scientific data and research become available.

On a global scale, the HIV epidemic has stabilized, although with unacceptably high levels of new HIV infections and AIDS deaths.

- Globally, there were an estimated 33 million [30 million–36 million] people living with HIV in 2007 (Figure 2.2).
- The annual number of new HIV infections declined from 3.0 million [2.6 million–3.5 million] in 2001 to 2.7 million [2.2 million–3.2 million] in 2007.
- Overall, 2.0 million [1.8 million–2.3 million] people died due to AIDS in 2007, compared with an estimated 1.7 million [1.5 million–2.3 million] in 2001.
- While the percentage of people living with HIV has stabilized since 2000, the overall number of people living with HIV has steadily increased as new infections occur each year, HIV treatments extend life, and as new infections still outnumber AIDS deaths (Figure 2.3).
- Southern Africa continues to bear a disproportionate share of the global burden of HIV: 35% of HIV infections and 38% of AIDS deaths in 2007 occurred in that subregion. Altogether, sub-Saharan Africa is home to 67% of all people living with HIV.

[3] This applies to all countries except those where HIV subtype E accounts for most infections. In the latter countries, the median net survival time is estimated to be nine years (UNAIDS Reference Group on Estimates, Modelling and Projections, 2006).

FIGURE 2.2 A global view of HIV infection, 2007
33 million people [30 – 36 million] living with HIV, 2007

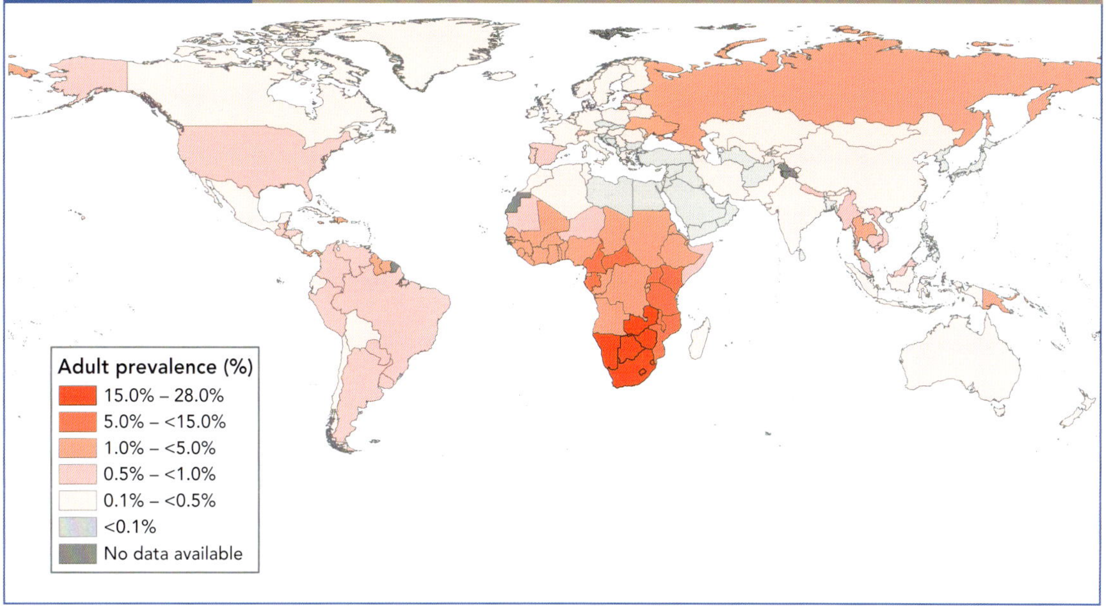

- Women account for half of all people living with HIV worldwide, and nearly 60% of HIV infections in sub-Saharan Africa. Over the last 10 years, the proportion of women among people living with HIV has remained stable globally, but has increased in many regions (Figure 2.4).
- Young people aged 15–24 account for an estimated 45% of new HIV infections worldwide.
- An estimated 370 000 [330 000–410 000] children younger than 15 years became infected with HIV in 2007. Globally, the number of children younger than 15 years living with HIV increased from 1.6 million [1.4 million–2.1 million] in 2001 to 2.0 million [1.9 million–2.3 million] in 2007. Almost 90% live in sub-Saharan Africa (see box "HIV among children").

Young people: recent HIV infection and sexual behaviour trends

The *Declaration of Commitment* established a target of reducing HIV prevalence by 25% in young people (ages 15–24) in the most-affected countries by 2005. To assess progress towards this goal, 35 high-prevalence countries (with national prevalence that exceeded 3%) and four additional countries in Africa with notable prevalence levels (Table 2) were asked to compile data on recent trends in HIV and sexual behaviour among young people.

Given the practical difficulties of conducting HIV incidence studies,[4] serial HIV prevalence over time in young women (ages 15–24) attending antenatal clinics serves as a proxy measure for incidence, providing important indications of recent epidemiological trends.

[4] As most people are unaware when they become infected and are diagnosed only months or years later, tracking HIV incidence typically requires special epidemiological studies that are complex and expensive. Certain high-income countries are using new epidemiological technologies to help public health agencies to gauge HIV incidence, but these technologies have not been validated for use in high-prevalence settings.

TABLE 2

Analysis of trends among 15–24-year-olds in high-prevalence countries (all countries with national prevalence that exceeded 3% and four additional countries in Africa with notable prevalence levels): HIV prevalence among pregnant women (2000–2007) in sentinel surveillance systems, and selected sexual behaviours among women and men (1990–2007) from national surveys

COUNTRY	Time period for which prevalence data were available	Prevalence trend[a]		Percent of young people (15–19 years) having had sex before age 15[b]		Proportion having sex with more than one partner in the last 12 months[c]		Condom use during last sex among those with more than one partner in the last 12 months[d]	
		Urban	*Rural*	*Females*	*Males*	*Females*	*Males*	*Females*	*Males*
Angola[a]		ID	ID						
Bahamas		↓							
Benin[b]	2000–2006	↓*	↔	↔	↓*	↓*	↑	↑	↑
Botswana	2001–2006	↓*	↓*						
Burkina Faso	2000–2006	↓*	↓	↓*	↓*	↓*	↓*	↔	↑*
Burundi	1999–2004	↓	↔	↑*					
Cameroon[a]		ID	ID	↓*	↓*	↓*	↓*	↑*	↑*
Central African Republic[b]				↑	↓				
Chad[a]		ID	ID	↓*	↑	↓	↓*	↓	↑
Congo[a]		ID	ID						
Côte d'Ivoire	2000–2004	↓*	ID	↓*	↑	↓*	↓*	↑*	↔
Democratic Republic of the Congo[a]		ID	ID						
Djibouti[b]									
Ethiopia[b]				↓*	↓*	↓*	↓*		↓
Gabon[b]									
Gambia[b]									
Ghana[b]				↓*	↓*	↔	↔	↑*	↑
Haiti[b]				↑*	↑*	↑	↓	↓	↑*
Kenya	2000–2005	↓*	↓*	↔	↔	↓*	↓*	↓	↑*
Lesotho[a]	2003–2007	↔	↓						
Liberia[b]									
Malawi[e]	1999–2005	↓*	↔	↓*	↓*	↑	↓*	↔	↑
Mozambique[f]	2000–2007	↔		↔	↑*				
Namibia	2002–2006	↓	↓	↔	↓*	↔	↓*	↑*	↑
Nigeria[a]									
Rwanda	1998–2003	↓	ND	↑*	↑*	↓*	↓		
Sierra Leone[a]		ID	ID						
South Africa[g]	2000–2006	↔				↓*	↔		
Sudan[a]									
Swaziland	2002–2006	↓	↓						
Togo[a]									
Uganda[b]				↓*	↓	↔	↔	↑*	↑*
United Republic of Tanzania	2000–2006	↔	↓	↔	↓*	↓*	↓*	↑*	↑*
Zambia[h]	1998–2004	↔		↓*	↓*	↓*	↓*	↑	↑
Zimbabwe	2000–2004	↓*	↓	↔	↓*	↓*	↓*	↔	↔

Notes:

[1] *Highlighted cells indicate positive trends in prevalence or behaviour.*

[2] ** Consistent sites only were used in the analysis of change in HIV prevalence over time, for a minimum of three years. Significance test based on H_0: slope =0*

Legend:

a Prevalence obtained from pregnant women attending antenatal clinics in selected countries.

b Among 15–19-year-olds, proportion reported having had sex by age 15. Analyses based on DHS, MICS or national surveys conducted between 1990 and 2007.

c Among 15–24-year-olds, proportion reported having had sex with more than one partner in the last 12 months. Analyses based on data from repeat DHS or national surveys conducted between 1990 and 2007.

d Among 15–24-year-olds, proportion of those with more than one partner reporting having used a condom the last time they had sex. Analyses based on data from repeat DHS or national surveys conducted between 1990 and 2007.

↑ Observed increase in HIV prevalence or behaviour.

↓ Observed decrease in HIV prevalence or behaviour.

↓* Statistically significant decrease in HIV prevalence of more than 25% or significant decrease in measured behavioural indicator. Analysis of prevalence based on regression analysis; analysis of behaviour based on Chi-square or Chi-square test for trend.

↑* Statistically significant increase in measured behavioural indicator. Analysis of behaviour based on Chi-square or Chi-square test for trend.

↔ No evidence of change.

*ID Insufficient data, i.e. less than three years of data received.

**ND Data not received.

e Semi-urban and urban areas were combined in analysis of urban data.

f Analysis in Mozambique combined for South, North and Central.

g No data received in response to working group process; analyses based on data in South Africa surveillance report.

h No data received in response to working group process; analyses based on data reported in Zambia 2005 surveillance report. Analysis based on urban and rural data combined.

HIV prevalence among young women attending antenatal clinics in urban or rural areas (or both) has declined since 2000-2001 in 14 of the 17 countries with sufficient data to analyse recent trends in the most-affected countries (sufficient prevalence data from three different years). These countries include the Bahamas, Benin, Burkina Faso, Burundi, Côte d'Ivoire, Kenya, Lesotho, Malawi, Namibia, Rwanda, Swaziland, the United Republic of Tanzania, and Zimbabwe. Declines in HIV prevalence exceeded 25% in seven countries. In two of these countries—Botswana and Kenya—declines occurred in both urban and

FIGURE 2.3 Estimated number of people living with HIV and adult HIV prevalence. Global HIV epidemic, 1990–2007; and, HIV epidemic in Sub-Saharan Africa, 1990–2007

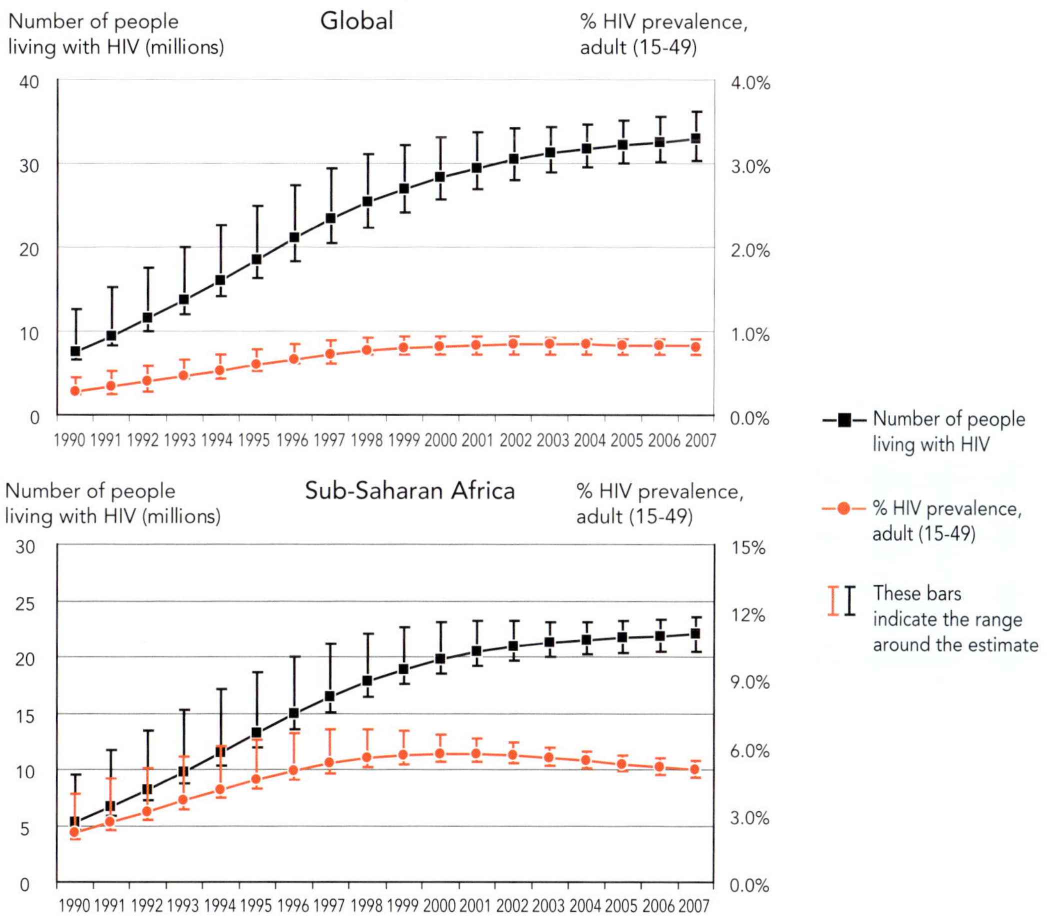

Note: Even though the HIV prevalence stabilized in sub-Saharan Africa, the actual number of people infected continues to grow because of ongoing new infections and increasing access to antiretroviral therapy.

FIGURE 2.4 Percent of adults (15+) living with HIV who are female, 1990–2007[5]

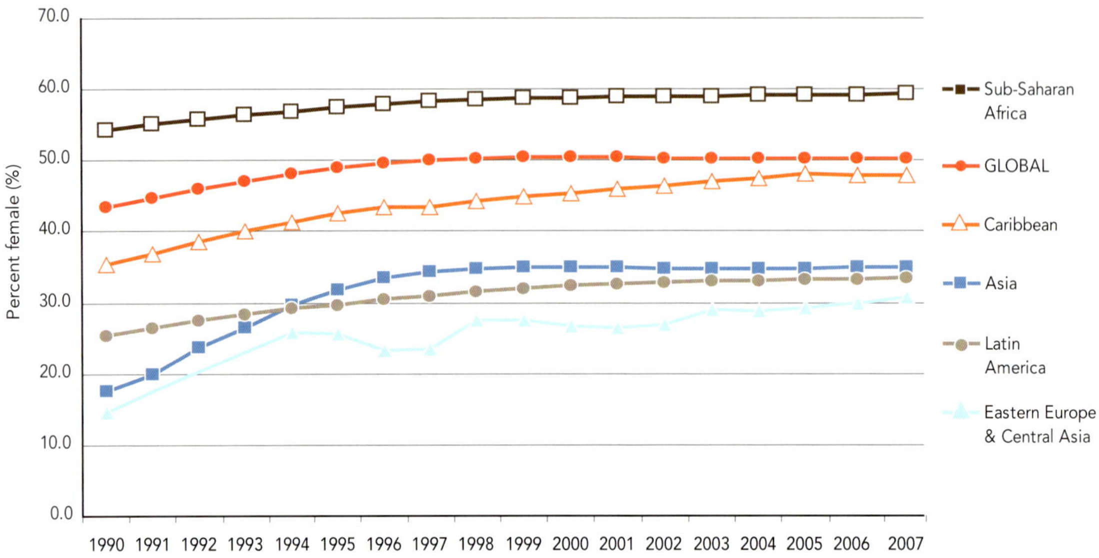

rural areas. In five countries—Benin, Burkina Faso, Côte d'Ivoire, Malawi, and Zimbabwe—declines were significant only in urban areas.

In addition to HIV prevalence data, a number of countries have also tracked sexual behaviours among young people. Among the 35 high-prevalence countries, 19 countries conducted national surveys between 1990 and 2007 that provided sufficient comparative data to assess sexual behaviour trends. The percentage of both young women and men (ages 15–19) who became sexually active before their 15th birthday declined in seven countries, but increased in Haiti and Rwanda. The proportion of both young women and men (ages 15–24) who had more than one partner in the previous 12 months decreased in 10 countries and remained unchanged in two, but increased among young women in two countries and among young men in one.

Condom use has increased among young people. Among young men (ages 15–24) who had more than one partner in the previous 12 months, rates of condom use increased in 12 countries. Among their female counterparts, rates of condom use increased in eight countries. Although observed changes in behaviour are not statistically significant in every instance, overall trends show that reductions in risky behaviour have been occurring in several countries.[6]

[5] The global proportion of women versus men who are infected has remained at approximately 50% since the late 1990s. In this figure of proportional rates, even though the proportion of women versus men has been increasing in each region, in most regions, the overall number of men infected is still far greater than the number of women.

[6] 24 out of the 35 countries had insufficient or no data on HIV prevalence and/or sexual behaviour trends, or both, among young people—including several countries with exceptionally high HIV prevalence in southern Africa.

FIGURE 2.5 Children living with HIV globally, 1990–2007

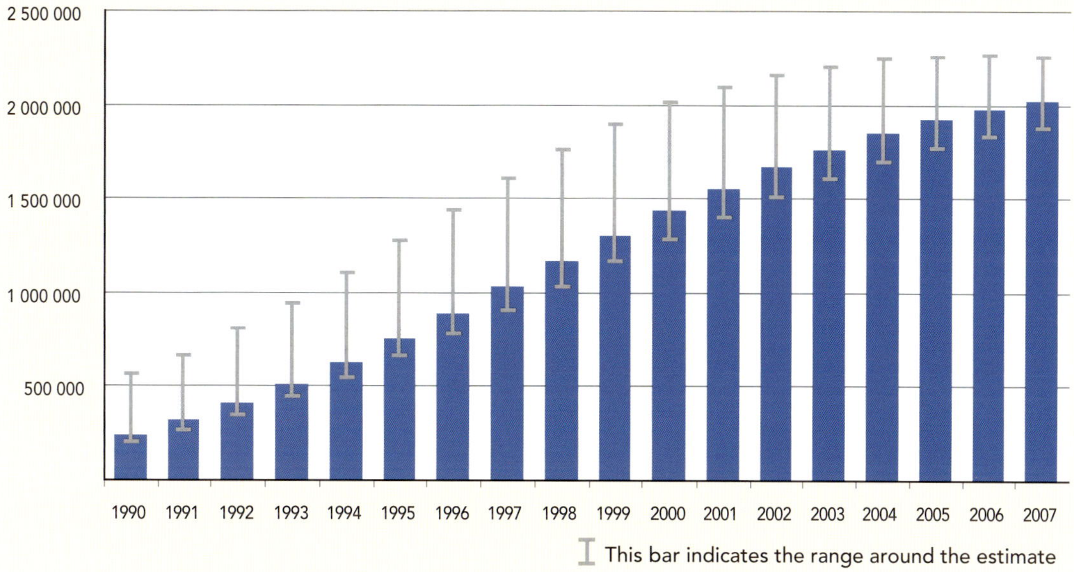

HIV among children

Few direct HIV surveillance data are available for children. Antenatal clinic surveys typically capture data for pregnant girls and women 15 years or older; most national population-based surveys with HIV testing include only adults. HIV estimates for children are obtained through modelling that is based primarily on HIV prevalence in adult women (ages 15–49), fertility rates, and assumptions about the survival of HIV-positive children (Stover et al., 2006; Stover et al., in press). Such estimates show that the number of children living with HIV globally continues to increase steadily (Figure 2.5).

It is estimated that more than 90% of children living with HIV acquired the virus during pregnancy, birth or breastfeeding—forms of HIV transmission that can be prevented. A small fraction of HIV infections in children are caused by contaminated injections, the transfusion of infected blood or blood products, sexual abuse, sexual intercourse (although this is a significant mode of transmission among adolescents), or scarification (Kengeya-Kayondo et al., 1995; Mulder et al., 1996; Hauri, Armstrong & Hutin 2004; Kiwanuka et al., 2004; Schmid et al., 2004).[7]

As shown in Figure 2.6, new HIV infections in children appear to have peaked in 2000–2002. This is believed to be due mainly to the stabilization of HIV prevalence among women overall, and to increasing coverage of programmes for preventing mother-to-child transmission of HIV (see Chapter 4).

In 2007, an estimated 270 000 [250 000–290 000] HIV-infected children younger than 15 years died because of AIDS—more than 90% of them in sub-Saharan Africa. In the

[7] The role of child sexual abuse as a source of HIV infection in children is poorly documented, but this mode of transmission is of particular concern in countries where both HIV and child sexual abuse are major public health problems.

FIGURE 2.6 New HIV infections among children, 1990–2007

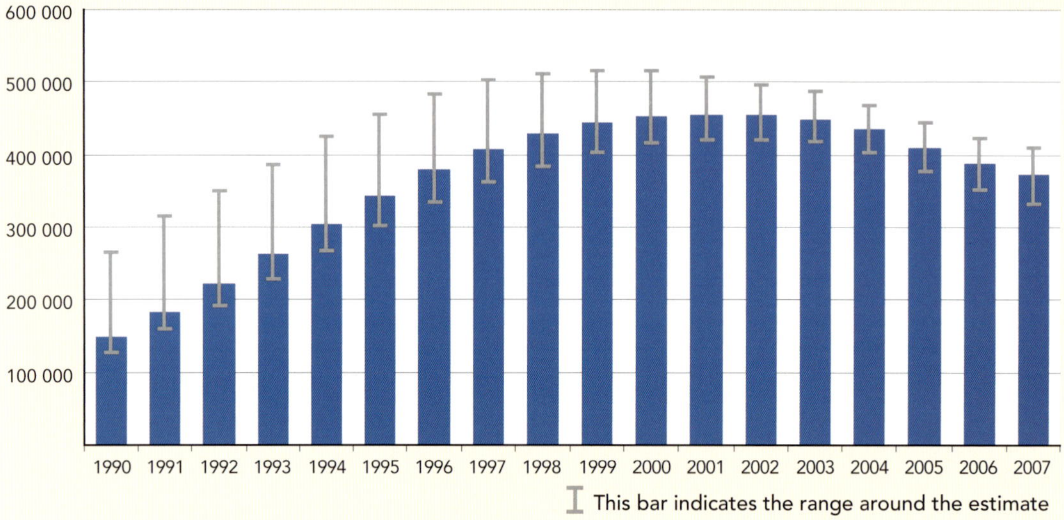

most heavily-affected countries, such as Botswana and Zimbabwe, HIV is the underlying reason for more than one third of all deaths among children under the age of five (Mason, 2006). Indeed, without antiretroviral treatment, the progression of HIV infection in children is particularly aggressive, and many children die at a young age (Taha et al., 2000; Newell et al., 2004; Brahmbhatt et al., 2006).

As Figure 2.7 illustrates, the total number of AIDS deaths in children peaked around 2003 and has decreased since. This decline mainly reflects the drop in new infections in children seen earlier (visible in Figure 2.6), as well as increased access to antiretroviral treatment.

FIGURE 2.7 Child deaths due to AIDS, 1990–2007

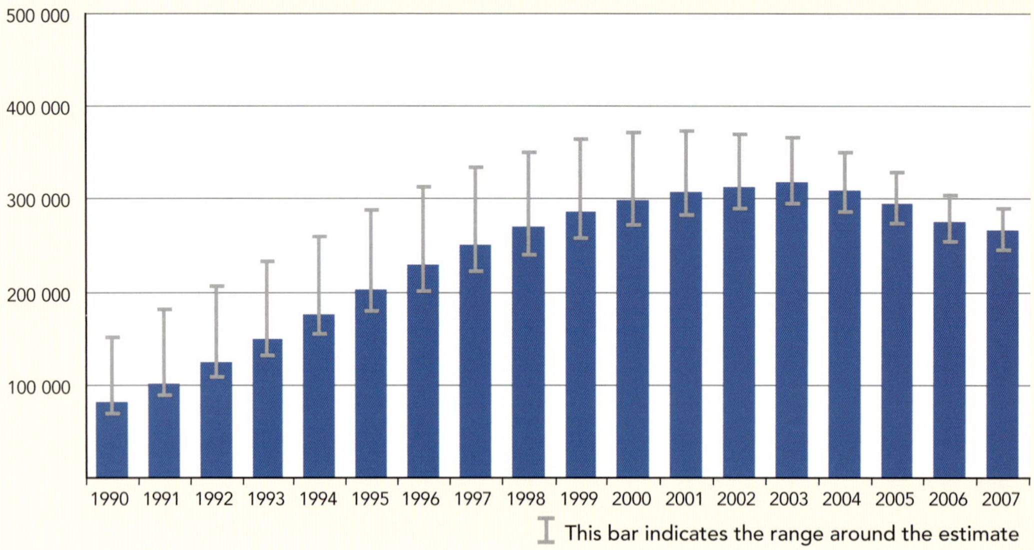

FIGURE 2.8 HIV prevalence (%) in adults (15–49) in Africa, 2007

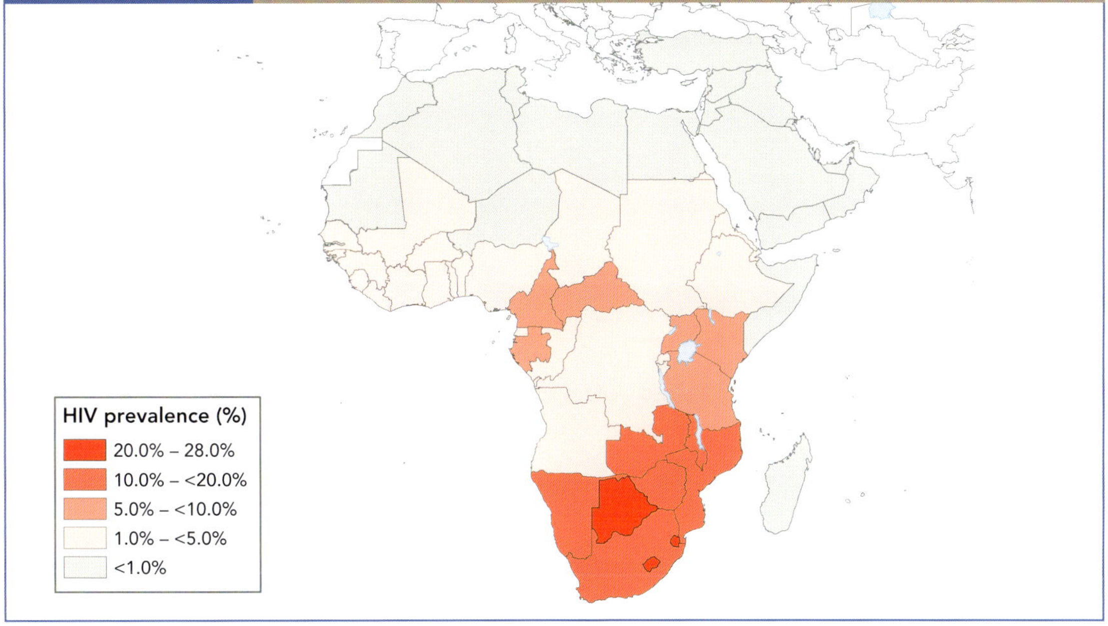

Sub-Saharan Africa

An estimated 1.9 million [1.6 million–2.1 million] people were newly infected with HIV in sub-Saharan Africa in 2007, bringing to 22 million [20.5 million–23.6 million] the number of people living with HIV. Two thirds (67%) of the global total of 33 million [30 million–36 million] people with HIV live in this region, and three quarters (75%) of all AIDS deaths in 2007 occurred there.

Sub-Saharan Africa's epidemics vary significantly from country to country in both scale and scope (Figure 2.8). Adult national HIV prevalence is below 2% in several countries of West and Central Africa, as well as in the horn of Africa, but in 2007 it exceeded 15% in seven southern African countries (Botswana, Lesotho, Namibia, South Africa, Swaziland, Zambia, and Zimbabwe), and was above 5% in seven other countries, mostly in Central and East Africa (Cameroon, the Central African Republic, Gabon, Malawi, Mozambique, Uganda, and the United Republic of Tanzania).

Recent epidemiological trends

Most epidemics in sub-Saharan Africa appear to have stabilized, although often at very high levels, particularly in southern Africa. Additionally, in a growing number of countries, adult HIV prevalence appears to be falling. For the region as a whole, women are disproportionately affected in comparison with men, with especially stark differences between the sexes in HIV prevalence among young people (Figure 2.9 and Figure 2.10).

In southern Africa, reductions in HIV prevalence are especially striking in Zimbabwe, where HIV prevalence in pregnant women attending antenatal clinics fell from 26% in 2002 to 18% in 2006 (Ministry of Health and Child Welfare [Zimbabwe], 2007).[8] In Botswana, a drop in HIV prevalence among pregnant 15–19-year-olds (from 25% in 2001 to 18% in 2006) suggests that the rate of new infections could be slowing (Ministry of Health [Botswana], 2006). The epidemics in Malawi and Zambia also appear to have

[8] This development is discussed in detail in the 2006 and 2007 editions of the AIDS epidemic update, available at http://www.unaids.org

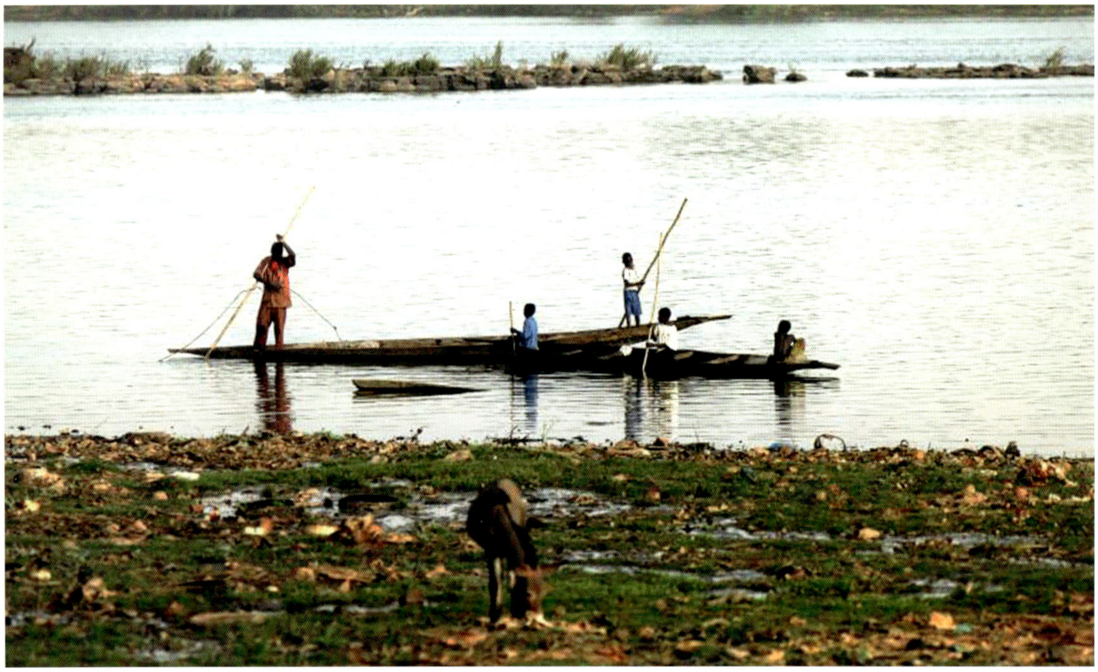

stabilized, amid some evidence of favourable behaviour changes (Heaton, Fowler & Palamuleni, 2006; Sandoy et al., 2007) and signs of declining HIV prevalence among women using antenatal services in some urban areas (Ministry of Health and Population [Malawi], 2005; Ministry of Health [Zambia], 2005; Michelo et al., 2006; National AIDS Commission [Malawi], 2007).

HIV data from antenatal clinics in South Africa suggest that the country's epidemic might be stabilizing (Department of Health [South Africa], 2007), but there is no evidence yet of major changes in HIV-related behaviour. The estimated 5.7 million [4.9 million–6.6 million][9] South Africans living with HIV in 2007 make this the largest HIV epidemic in the world. Meanwhile, the 26% HIV prevalence found in adults in Swaziland in 2006 is the highest prevalence ever documented in a national population-based survey anywhere in the world (Central Statistical Office [Swaziland] & Macro International Inc., 2007).

In Lesotho and parts of Mozambique, HIV prevalence among pregnant women is increasing. In some of the provinces in the central and southern zones of the country, adult HIV prevalence has reached or exceeded 20%, while infections continue to increase among young people (ages 15–24) (Conselho Nacional de Combate ao HIV/SIDA, 2006).

HIV prevalences in the comparatively smaller epidemics in East Africa have either reached a plateau or are receding. After dropping dramatically in the 1990s (Asamoah-Odei, Garcia-Celleja & Boerma, 2004; Kirungi et al., 2006), adult national HIV prevalence in Uganda has stabilized at 5.4% [5.0%–6.1%]. However, there are signs of a possible resurgence in sexual risk-taking that could cause the epidemic to grow again. For example, the proportion of adult men and women who say they had sex with a

[9] All estimates of the total number of people living with HIV in a given country are for 2007.

FIGURE 2.9 HIV prevalence (%) among pregnant women attending antenatal clinics in sub-Saharan Africa, 1997–2007

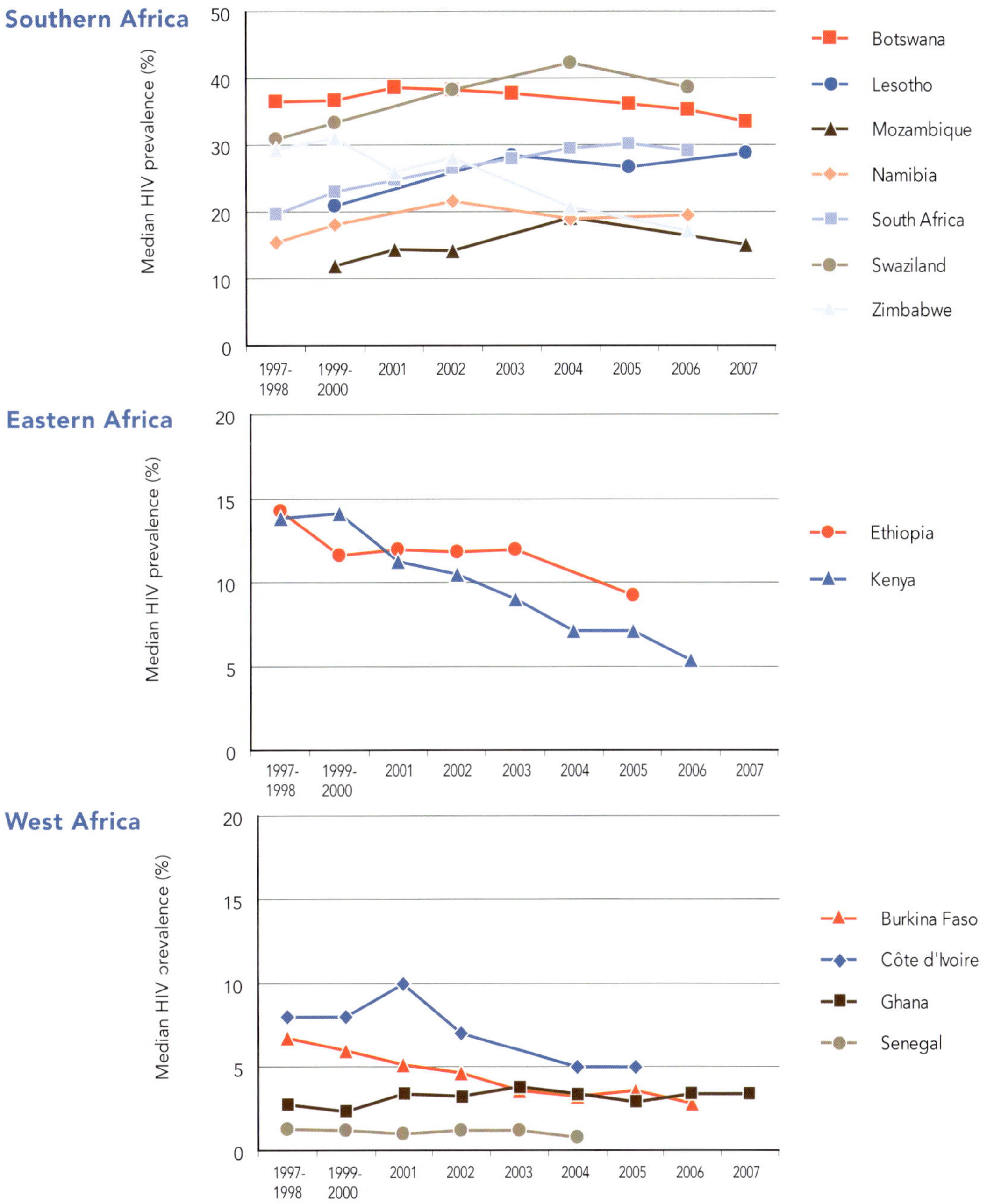

Note: Analysis restricted to consistent surveillance sites for all countries except South Africa (by province) and Swaziland (by region).
Source: National surveillance reports and UNAIDS/WHO/UNICEF, Epidemiological Fact Sheets on HIV and AIDS. July 2008.

FIGURE 2.10 HIV prevalence (%) among 15–24 years old, by sex, selected countries, 2005–2007

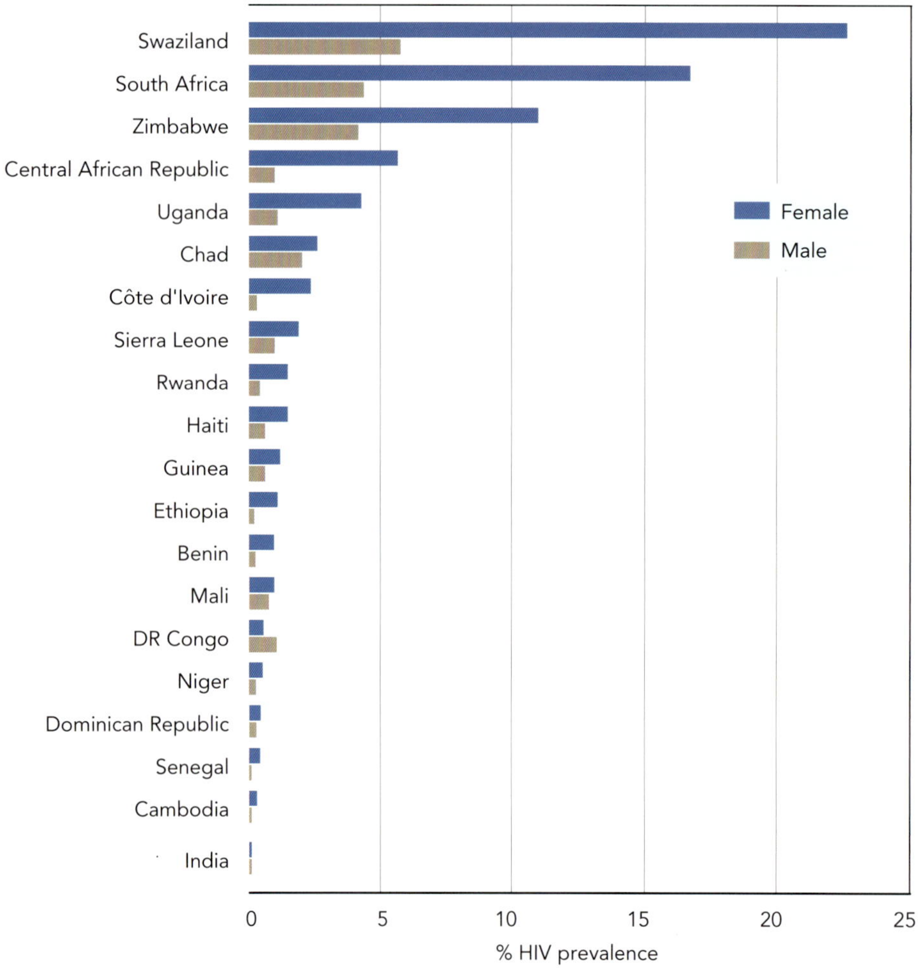

Source: Demographic and Health Surveys and other national population-based surveys with HIV testing.

person who was not a spouse and did not live with the respondent has grown since 1995 (from 12% to 16% for women and 29% to 36% for men) (Kirungi et al., 2006; Ministry of Health [Uganda] & ORC Macro, 2006; Uganda Bureau of Statistics & Macro International Inc, 2007).

Most of the comparatively smaller HIV epidemics in West Africa are stable or are declining—as is the case for Burkina Faso, Côte d'Ivoire, and Mali. In Côte d'Ivoire, HIV prevalence among pregnant women in urban areas fell from 10% in 2001 to 6.9% in 2005

(Ministère de la Santé et de l'Hygiene Publique de la Côte d'Ivoire & CDC/RETRO-CI/ MEASURE Evaluation, 2007). The largest epidemic in West Africa—in Nigeria, the continent's most populous country—appears to have stabilized at 3.1% [2.3%–3.8%], according to HIV infection trends among women attending antenatal clinics (Federal Ministry of Health [Nigeria], 2006).

Main modes of HIV transmission

Heterosexual intercourse remains the epidemic's driving force in sub-Saharan Africa. The high rate of sexual transmission has also given rise to the world's largest population of children living with HIV. However, recent epidemiological evidence has revealed the region's epidemic to be more diverse than previously thought.

Heterosexual intercourse related to serodiscordant couples

According to Demographic and Health Surveys in five African countries (Burkina Faso, Cameroon, Ghana, Kenya, and the United Republic of Tanzania), two thirds of HIV-infected couples were serodiscordant, that is only one partner was infected. Condom use was found to be rare: in Burkina Faso, for example, almost 90% of the surveyed cohabiting couples said they did not use a condom the last time they had sex (de Walque, 2007). A separate, community-based study in Uganda has shown that, among serodiscordant heterosexual couples, the uninfected partner has an estimated 8% annual chance of contracting HIV (Wawer et al., 2005). Strikingly, in about 30%–40% of the serodiscordant couples surveyed, the infected partner was female. Indeed, it appears that more than half of the surveyed HIV-infected women who were married or cohabiting had been infected by someone other than their current partner (de Walque, 2007).

Sex work

Sex work is an important factor in many of West Africa's HIV epidemics. More than one third (35%) of female sex workers surveyed in 2006 in Mali were living with HIV (Ministère de la Santé du Mali, 2006), and infection levels exceeding 20% have been documented among sex workers in Senegal (Gomes do Espirito Santo & Etheredge, 2005) and Burkina Faso (Kintin et al., 2004). Sex work plays an important, but less central, role in HIV transmission in southern Africa, where exceptionally high background prevalence results in substantial HIV transmission during sexual intercourse unrelated to sex work.

Injecting drug use

Injecting drug use is a factor to some extent in several of the HIV epidemics in East and southern Africa, including Mauritius, where the use of contaminated injecting equipment is the main cause of HIV infection (Sulliman, Ameerberg & Dhannoo, 2004). In various studies, about half of the injecting drug users tested in the Kenyan cities of Mombassa (50%) (Ndetei, 2004) and Nairobi (53%) were HIV-positive (Odek-Ogunde, 2004).

Sex between men

Several recent studies suggest that unprotected anal sex between men is probably a more important factor in the epidemics in sub-Saharan Africa than is commonly thought. In Zambia, one in three (33%) surveyed men who have sex with men tested HIV-positive (Zulu, Bulawo & Zulu, 2006). In the Kenyan port city of Mombasa, 43% of men who said they had sex only with other men were found to be living with HIV (Sanders et al., 2007). HIV prevalence of 22% was found among the 463 men who have sex with men who participated in a study in Dakar, Senegal (Wade et al., 2005).

The role of concurrent partnerships in HIV epidemics

The concept of concurrent partners has received increasing attention in the scientific literature and in the media. It has been argued that concurrent partnerships—in conjunction with high viral load during acute HIV infection and the low level of male circumcision—have contributed to the rapid spread and the high prevalence levels of HIV in southern Africa (Halperin & Epstein, 2007). Few epidemiological and mathematical modelling studies have investigated the prevalence of concurrency and its effect on the transmission of HIV and other sexually transmitted infections. Early modelling work concluded that, for the same number of partners per person, sexual partner networks that include concurrent partnerships lead to larger HIV epidemics than do networks without concurrent partnerships (Morris & Kretzschmar, 1997).

While researchers and prevention progamme experts agree that having multiple sexual partners is an important risk factor in the transmission of HIV (Malamba et al., 1994; Wawer et al., 1994; McFarland, Mvere & Katzenstein, 1997; Chen et al., 2007; Mishra et al., 2007), the comparative impact of concurrent multiple relationships as opposed to serial multiple relationships in the spread of HIV is less clear. For example, a study in five cities in sub-Saharan Africa found no association between concurrency and HIV prevalence level (Lagarde et al., 2001), and a small study in Malawi also found no association between the density of sexual networks and HIV prevalence (Helleringer & Kohler, 2007). Multiple concurrent partnerships are often linked to mobility (including labour-related mobility), in that people may have different partners at their different residences; also, those staying behind may themselves have other partners (Lurie et al., 2003; Coffee, Lurie & Garnett, 2007).

Most authors define concurrency as "sexual relationships that overlap in time" (Garnett & Johnson, 1997; Lagarde et al., 2001; Adimora et al., 2003; Adimora et al., 2004; Carael et al., 2004; Helleringer & Kohler, 2007). However, others have considered multiple partnerships in a short time period to be a proxy measure of concurrency (Halperin & Epstein, 2007). Important issues for the epidemiological assessment of concurrent partnerships include the length of overlap of sexual relationships, how the number of partners is categorized (more than one, more than five, etc.), and the length of the period during which concurrency is assessed (the last month, last six months, last year, etc.). Also important for measurement in surveys are a host of behavioural and social factors ranging from local terminology to factors influencing recall and reporting bias for different types of sexual contacts.

Understanding sexual networks is crucial to understanding the HIV epidemic. Considerable work is needed to refine methods for measuring and comparing sexual norms, behaviours and networks in diverse cultural contexts and risk settings worldwide. Standard definitions and further collection and analysis of primary behavioural, network and context data are needed to understand and quantify the relationship between concurrency and the spread of HIV.

Prevention programmes should aim to reduce the occurrence of multiple sexual partnerships, whether or not they are concurrent, and to communicate the likely additional risk of concurrent sexual relationships—including those that are long term and socially accepted (see Chapter 4 pp. 117 and 119-121). In the countries in southern Africa where HIV prevalence is extremely high, the probability that one's sexual partner is infected with HIV is around one in four to six, making it extremely risky to have unprotected sex with anyone whose HIV status is unknown. More effective interventions are needed to overcome the denial and misunderstandings of HIV risk in concurrent and age-disparate relationships that are impeding prevention in the region.

The most significant demographic impact of HIV occurs in sub-Saharan Africa

Ideally, the assessment of the epidemic's demographic impact would be based on data from death certificates. However, such vital registration is poor in many of the countries most affected by the global AIDS epidemic. Even where death notification systems function relatively well (e.g. in South Africa), deaths due to AIDS are seldom documented as such.

FIGURE 2.11 Life expectancy at birth, selected regions, 1950–1955 to 2005–2010

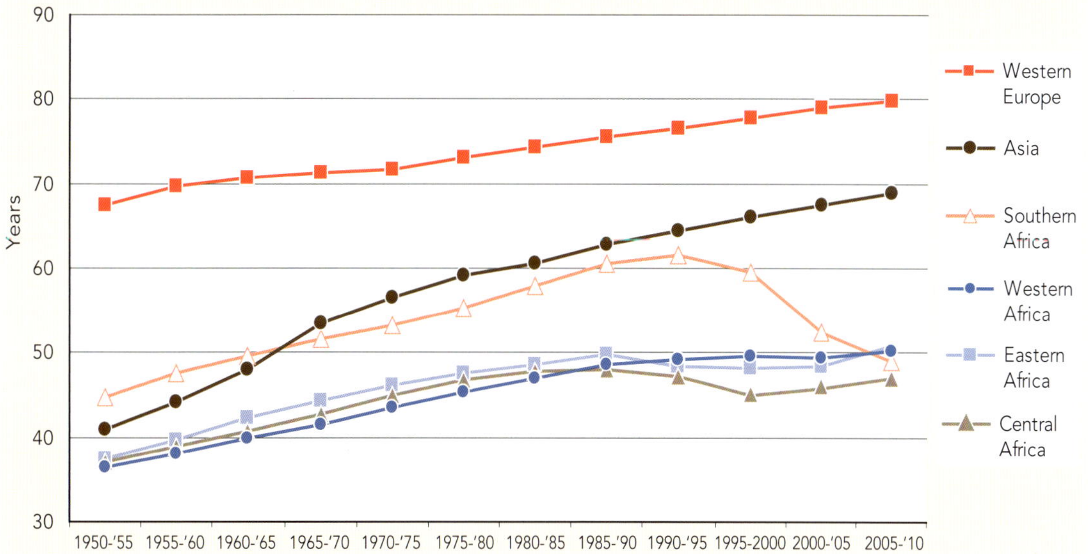

Source: Population Division of the Department of Economic and Social Affairs of the United Nations Secretariat, World Population Prospects: The 2006 Revision, http://esa.un.org/unpp

In countries with high HIV prevalence, life expectancy at birth has fallen, sometimes dramatically. In southern Africa, average life expectancy at birth is estimated to have declined to levels last seen in the 1950s; it is now below 50 years for the subregion as a whole, as Figure 2.11 shows, and below 40 years in Zimbabwe (WHO, 2006). Steady gains in life expectancy experienced in East Africa since the early 1950s stalled in the late 1980s, although falling HIV prevalences in some East African countries are expected to lead to an increase in life expectancy in that subregion. By contrast, the comparatively smaller HIV epidemics in Western Europe and Asia have scarcely affected life expectancy trends in those regions.

FIGURE 2.12 Changes in population structure: Ghana and Lesotho

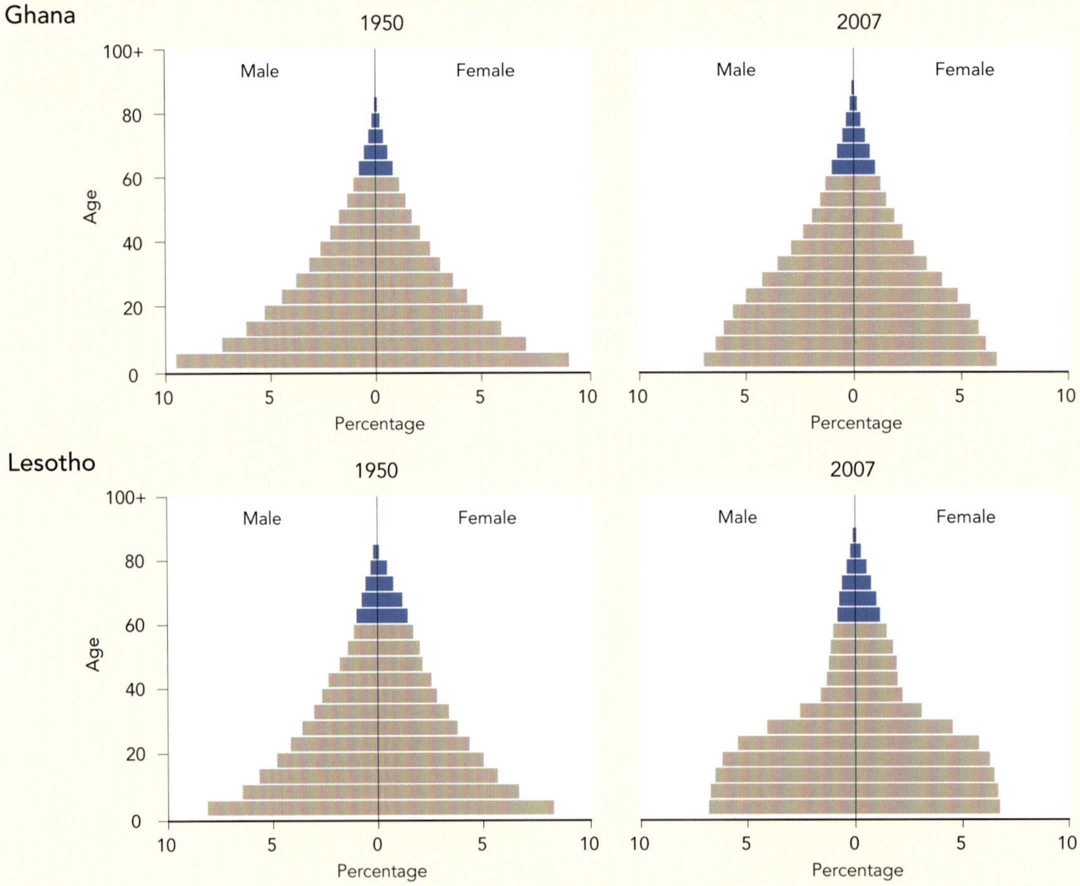

Source: Population Division of the Department of Economic and Social Affairs of the United Nations Secretariat, World Population Prospects: The 2006 Revision, http://esa.un.org/unpp

In southern Africa, the combined effects of premature death and reduced fertility among HIV-positive women have lowered population growth rates and dramatically reshaped the population structure. In a high-prevalence country such as Lesotho, the groups most heavily affected by HIV are infants and young children, and the 30–50 age group. The latter normally constitute the core of countries' economically active and child-raising populations. By contrast, the population pyramid of Ghana, where HIV infection levels are much lower, reflects a more conventional structure in a low-income country (Figure 2.12).

In South Africa, total deaths (from all causes) increased by 87% between 1997 and 2005 (Statistics South Africa, 2005; Statistics South Africa, 2006). During this period, death rates more than tripled for women aged 20–39, and more than doubled for males aged 30–44, with at least 40% of deaths believed to be attributable to HIV (Dorrington et al., 2001; Bradshaw et al., 2004; Actuarial Society of South Africa, 2005; Medical Research Council, 2005; Anderson & Phillips, 2006). The rate of population growth in the country fell from 1.25% in 2001–2002 to slightly more than 0.97% in 2006-2007) (Statistics South Africa, 2007).

In eastern Zimbabwe, the demographic impact has been more acute than was anticipated in the early 1990s. Total fertility is now 8% lower than would be expected without an HIV epidemic, due to the effects of HIV infection on fertility, early mortality, and behaviour. In the worst affected areas (towns with HIV prevalence of 33% in 1998–2005), the population growth rate is now considerably lower than it would have been without an epidemic (1% instead of 2.9%) (Gregson et al., 2007). In northern Namibia, mortality rates tripled from 1991 to 2003, according to parish registers (Notkola, Timaeus & Siiskonen, 2004).

Meanwhile, the estimated number of maternal, paternal, and double orphans due to AIDS in Malawi, South Africa and the United Republic of Tanzania rose from 1.2 million in 2001 to 2.9 million in 2007. However, a recent study found no evidence of an increase in the prevalence of child-headed households in these three countries (Hosegood et al., 2007), which suggests that all but a small minority of orphaned children are being absorbed into kinship, community, and other support networks.

Outside sub-Saharan Africa, the demographic impact tends to be less severe because HIV prevalence is comparatively low. Nevertheless, in the Caribbean, AIDS is one of the leading causes of death in adults aged 15–44 (Caribbean Epidemiology Centre, PAHO & WHO, 2004).

FIGURE 2.13 HIV prevalence (%) in adults (15–49) in Asia, 2007

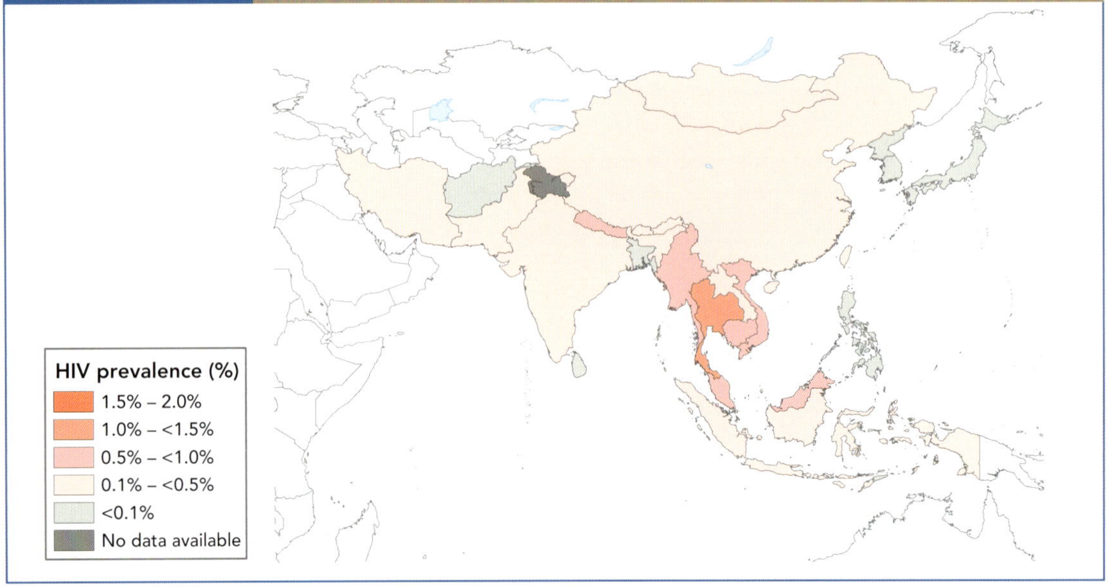

Asia

In Asia, an estimated 5.0 million [4.1 million–6.2 million] people were living with HIV in 2007, including the 380 000 [200 000–650 000] people who were newly infected that year. Approximately 380 000 [270 000–490 000] died from AIDS-related illnesses. National HIV infection levels are highest in South-East Asia (Figure 2.13), where there are disparate epidemic trends.

Recent epidemiological trends

The epidemics in Cambodia, Myanmar and Thailand all show declines in HIV prevalence, with national HIV prevalence in Cambodia falling from 2% in 1998 to an estimated 0.9% in 2006 (National Center for HIV/AIDS, Dermatology and STIs, 2007). However, epidemics in Indonesia (especially in its Papua province), Pakistan, and Viet Nam are growing rapidly. In Viet Nam, the estimated number of people living with HIV more than doubled between 2000 and 2005 (Ministry of Health [Viet Nam], 2005). New HIV infections are also increasing steadily, although at a much slower pace, in populous countries such as Bangladesh and China.

Main modes of HIV transmission

The several modes of HIV transmission make Asia's epidemic one of the world's most diverse.

Injecting drug use

Injecting drug use is a major risk factor in the epidemics of several Asian countries. Slightly fewer than half the people living with HIV in China in 2006 are believed to have been infected through use of contaminated injecting equipment (Lu et al., 2006; Ministry of Health [China], 2006). High infection levels have been detected among injecting drug users in the north-eastern part of India and in several large cities outside the north-east, including in Tamil Nadu, where 24% of drug users were believed to

FIGURE 2.14 HIV prevalence among injecting drug users, men having sex with men, and female sex workers in Pakistan, 2004–2007*

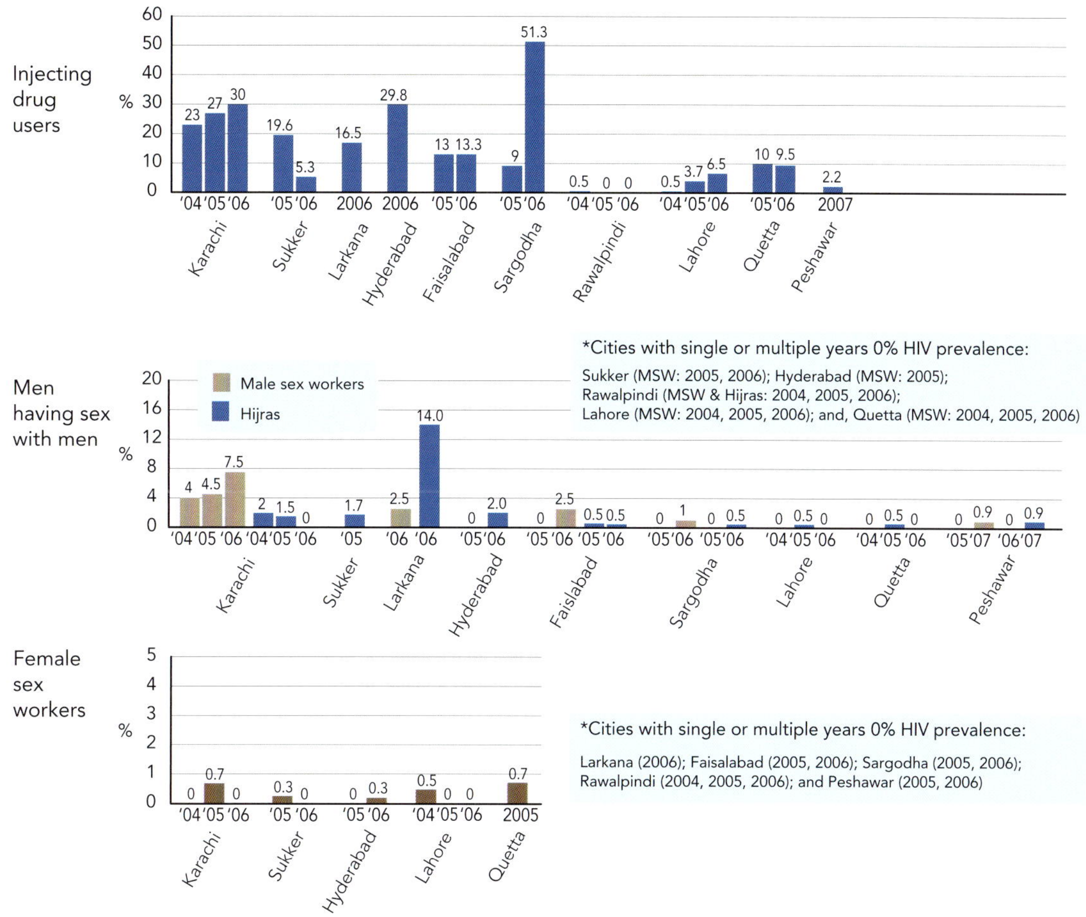

Source: Ministry of Health Pakistan. HIV Second Generation Surveillance in Pakistan, National Report Rounds I and II.

be infected in 2006 (National Institute of Health and Family Welfare & National AIDS Control Organisation, 2007). Use of contaminated injecting equipment (as well as unprotected sex between injecting drug users and their regular partners) is also the driving force of the epidemic in Viet Nam (Tuang et al., 2007), and in Malaysia, where more than two thirds of HIV infections to date have been among injecting drug users (Reid, Kamarulzaman & Sran, 2007).

Overlap of sex work and injecting drug use

An increasing number of women are injecting drugs in China, and substantial proportions of them (about 56% in some cities) also sell sex (Choi, Cheung & Chen, 2006; Liu et al., 2006). Many male injecting drug users also buy sex, and often do not use condoms (Hesketh et al., 2006). For example, in a 2005-2006 survey in Viet Nam, between 20% and 40% of injecting drug users (depending on the area surveyed) said that they had bought sex in the previous 12 months, and up to 60% said that they regularly had sex with a steady partner. Between 16% and 36% said that they consistently used condoms with regular partners (Ministry of Health [Viet Nam], 2006). The overlap of injecting drug use and sex work is also a potentially worrisome phenomenon in India and Pakistan (Chandrasekaran et al., 2006; Ministry of Health [Pakistan], 2006). An example of the complexity of transmission dynamics is presented for Pakistan in Figure 2.14.

Figure 2.15 projects the long-term effects of the intersection between injecting drug use and sex work in Jakarta, Indonesia—a metropolis in which an estimated 40 000 people inject drugs (Commission on AIDS in Asia, 2008). Although the epidemic was initially powered by HIV transmission among injecting drug users, about 15 years later, injecting drug users no longer comprise the majority of people infected with HIV. Indonesia's fast-growing epidemic is spreading quickly into sex-work networks (Statistics Indonesia & Ministry of Health [Indonesia], 2006; Ministry of Health [Indonesia] & Statistics Indonesia, 2007).

The most recent HIV outbreak has been in Afghanistan, where narcotics are now also being injected (opium traditionally was either inhaled or ingested orally) (UNODC, 2005). In Kabul, 3% of injecting drug users surveyed were HIV-positive, although this number may well rise because half of the survey participants said they had shared needles or syringes (Todd et al., 2007).

Sex work

Unprotected sex (commercial and otherwise) is the most important risk factor for the spread of HIV in several parts of Asia. Sex-trafficked women and girls face especially high risks of HIV infection. HIV prevalence of 38% has been found among sex-trafficked females who have been repatriated to Nepal, while up to a half of the women and girls trafficked to Mumbai, India, who have been tested were HIV-positive (Silverman et al., 2006; Silverman et al., 2007). In India's Karnataka State, HIV prevalence of

FIGURE 2.15 Projected total number of HIV infections in various population groups, 2000–2020, in Jakarta, Indonesia

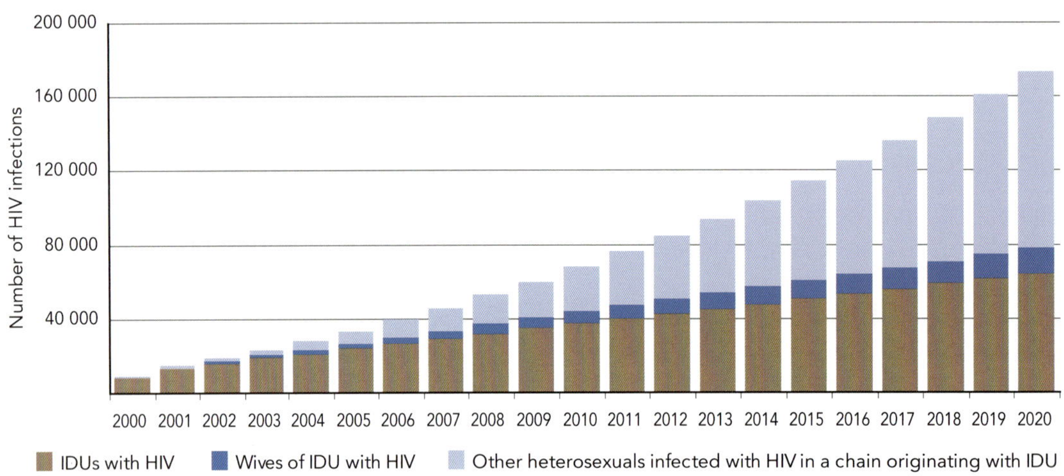

Source: Asian Epidemic Model projections using Jakarta data.

16% has been found among home-based sex workers, 26% among their street-based peers, and 47% among those working in brothels (Ramesh et al., 2006).

Some countries with epidemics driven by sex work have experienced declines in infections, due in part to an increase in the use of condoms during paid sex. For example, Cambodia's decline in HIV prevalence occurred at the same time that consistent condom use during commercial sex rose from 53% in 1997 to 96% in 2003 in Battambang, Kampong Cham, Phnom Penh, Siem Reap, and Sihanoukville (Gorbach et al., 2006). HIV prevalence among sex workers dropped significantly—from 46% in 1998 to 21% in 2003—among brothel-based sex workers, and from 44% to 8% over the same period among sex workers older than 20 (Ministry of Health [Cambodia], 2006). Similar trends have been observed in Thailand and Tamil Nadu (in southern India), over the past decade.

The serious epidemic under way in Indonesia's Papua province is somewhat anomalous in Asia, in that HIV transmission appears to be occurring mainly due to both unprotected sex with a regular partner and paid sex. In a province-wide population-based survey in 2006, adult HIV prevalence was 2.4% (2.9% among men and 1.9% among women). Given that only 14% of men who buy sex say that they use condoms with sex workers (Ministry of Health [Indonesia] & Statistics Indonesia, 2007), it is not surprising that high HIV infection levels (14%–16%) have been found among sex workers in parts of the province (National AIDS Commission [Indonesia], 2006).

Heterosexual intercourse

Although paid sex has become safer in Cambodia, the spouses and regular partners of people infected during commercial sex now account for a growing percentage of new infections (National Centre for HIV/AIDS, Dermatology and STIs, 2004). Similarly, Thailand's epidemic has diminished but has also become more heterogeneous (Over et al., 2007), and HIV is increasingly affecting people traditionally considered to be at lower risk of infection. About 43% of new infections in 2005 were among women, most of whom were infected by husbands or partners who had had unprotected sex or had used contaminated injecting equipment (WHO, 2007). In India, a significant proportion of women with HIV have probably been infected by regular partners who paid for sex (Lancet, 2006).

Sex between men

As in most other regions in the world, unprotected anal sex between men is a potentially significant but under-researched factor in the HIV epidemics in Asia. In Bangkok, HIV prevalence among men who have sex with men rose from 17% in 2003 to 28% in 2005 (van Griensven et al., 2006), and it is estimated that as many as one in five (21%) new HIV infections in Thailand in 2005 were attributable to unprotected sex between men (Gouws et al., 2006). In China's younger epidemic, it has been estimated that up to 7% of HIV infections might be attributable to unprotected sex between men (Lu et al., 2006).

Male sex workers face a particularly high risk of HIV infection. In Viet Nam, one in three (33%) male sex workers recruited from more than 70 sites in Ho Chi Minh City tested HIV-positive (Nguyen et al., in press). Studies earlier this decade documented high HIV infection levels among transgender sex workers in Jakarta, Indonesia, and Phnom Penh, Cambodia, in 2003 (Girault et al., 2004; Pisani et al., 2004).

FIGURE 2.16 HIV prevalence (%) in adults (15–49) in Eastern Europe and Central Asia, 2007

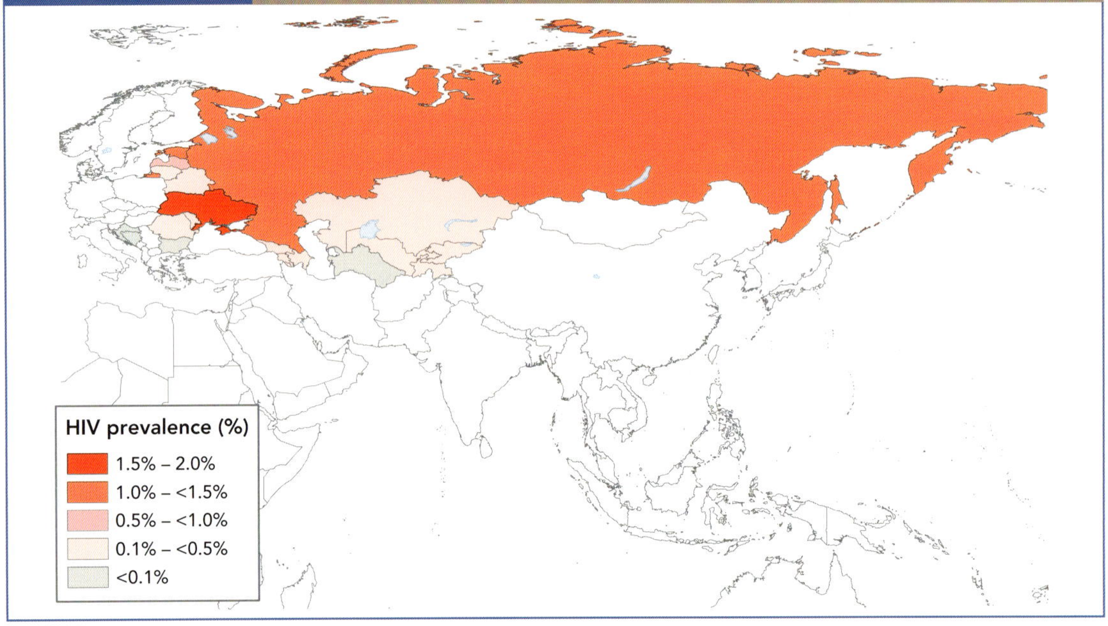

Eastern Europe and Central Asia

The estimated number of people living with HIV in Eastern Europe and Central Asia rose to 1.5 million [1.1 million–1.9 million] in 2007; almost 90% of those infected live in either the Russian Federation (69%) or Ukraine (29%). It is estimated that 110 000 [67 000–180 000] people in this region became infected with HIV in 2007, while some 58 000 [41 000–88 000] died of AIDS.

Recent epidemiological trends

The HIV epidemic in the Russian Federation (already the largest in this region) continues to grow, although apparently at a slower pace than in Ukraine, where annual new HIV diagnoses have more than doubled since 2001 (UNAIDS Reference Group on Estimates, Modelling and Projections, 2006; EuroHIV, 2007a). The annual numbers of newly reported HIV diagnoses are also rising in Azerbaijan, Georgia, Kazakhstan, Kyrgyzstan, the Republic of Moldova, Tajikistan, and Uzbekistan (which now has the largest epidemic in Central Asia).

Main modes of HIV transmission

Each of the HIV epidemics in this region is concentrated largely among injecting drug users, sex workers, and their various sexual partners.

Injecting drug use

Of the new HIV cases reported in this region in 2006 for which information is available on the mode of transmission, about 62% were attributed to injecting drug use.[10] In the Russian Federation, HIV prevalence among injecting drug users ranges from 3% in Volgograd to more than 70% in Biysk (Pasteur Scientific and Research Institute of Epidemiology, 2005). Prevalence is also high among injecting drug users in Ukraine; among surveyed injecting drug users in national diagnostic studies prevalence increased from 11% in 2001 to 17% in 2006 (EuroHIV, 2007a); also, local HIV prevalence as high as 63% has been found (Ministry of Health [Ukraine], 2007). High infection levels have been detected among injecting drug users in Tashkent, Uzbekistan (30%, 2003–2004) (Sanchez et al.,

[10] Officially documented HIV cases represent only those persons who have been in direct contact with a country's HIV reporting system. The actual number of people infected with HIV is considerable higher.

2006; EuroHIV, 2007a); in Zlobin, Belarus (52%) (EuroHIV, 2007a); and in Kazakhstan (Ministry of Health [Kazakhstan] et al., 2005).[11]

The overlap of sex work and injecting drug use

The overlap of sex work and injecting drug use features prominently in the region's epidemics. For example, 39% of female sex workers in the Samara oblast, Russian Federation (Population Services International, 2007), 37% in a St Petersburg study (Benotsch et al., 2004), and up to 30% of sex workers participating in other studies (Rhodes et al., 2004) said that they had injected drugs. Nowhere in this region have HIV epidemics reached a stage where they are likely to evolve independently of HIV transmission among injecting drug users and sex workers.

Heterosexual intercourse

As the epidemics in this region evolve, the proportion of women infected with HIV is growing. About 40% of newly registered HIV cases in Eastern Europe and Central Asia in 2006 were among women (EuroHIV, 2007a). Exceptionally high HIV prevalence was reported among pregnant women in several regions of central and eastern Ukraine. Three large, densely populated regions reported HIV prevalence among pregnant women exceeding 1% including Odess oblast, Kiev oblast and Mykolaev oblast (Ministry of Health [Ukraine], 2008). Most of these women were probably infected during sex with a partner who had been infected through use of contaminated drug injecting equipment (Scherbinska, 2006; EuroHIV, 2007a). In the region overall, it is estimated that some 35% of HIV-positive women were infected through use of contaminated injecting drug equipment, and about 50% acquired the virus during unprotected sex with drug-injecting partners (EuroHIV, 2006a).

Sex between men

In 2006, less than 1% of newly registered HIV cases (where the mode of transmission was known) were attributed to unprotected sex between men (EuroHIV, 2007a); this is probably an underestimate of the role of this mode of HIV transmission. In the Russian Federation, HIV prevalence found in this population group has varied from 0.9% in Moscow (Smolskaya et al., 2004; Smolskaya, 2006) to 9% in Nizhni Novgorod in 2006 (Ladnaya, 2007). Of men who have sex with men who participated in a study in Tashkent, Uzbekistan, 11% tested HIV-positive in 2005 (Ministry of Health [Uzbekistan], 2007), as did 5% of their peers in a study in Georgia (EuroHIV, 2006b).

Caribbean

An estimated 230 000 [210 000–270 000] people were living with HIV in the Caribbean in 2007 (about three quarters of them in the Dominican Republic and Haiti), while an estimated 20 000 [16 000–25 000] people were newly infected with HIV in this region, and some 14 000 [11 000–16 000] people died of AIDS.

Recent epidemiological trends

HIV surveillance systems are still inadequate in several Caribbean countries, but available information indicates that most of the epidemics in the region appear to have stabilized, while a few have declined in urban areas. The latter trend is especially evident in the Dominican Republic and Haiti.

Main modes of HIV transmission

The main mode of HIV transmission in the Caribbean is unprotected heterosexual intercourse, paid or otherwise. However, sex between men, although generally denied by society, is also a significant factor in several national epidemics.

Heterosexual intercourse

In Haiti, which has the biggest epidemic in the Caribbean, HIV prevalence among pregnant

[11] Not all countries in this region apply the same definition of "injecting drug users" or of "men who have sex with men". As a result, prevalence data such as these are not necessarily comparable between different countries.

FIGURE 2.17 HIV prevalence (%) in adults (15–49) in the Caribbean, 2007

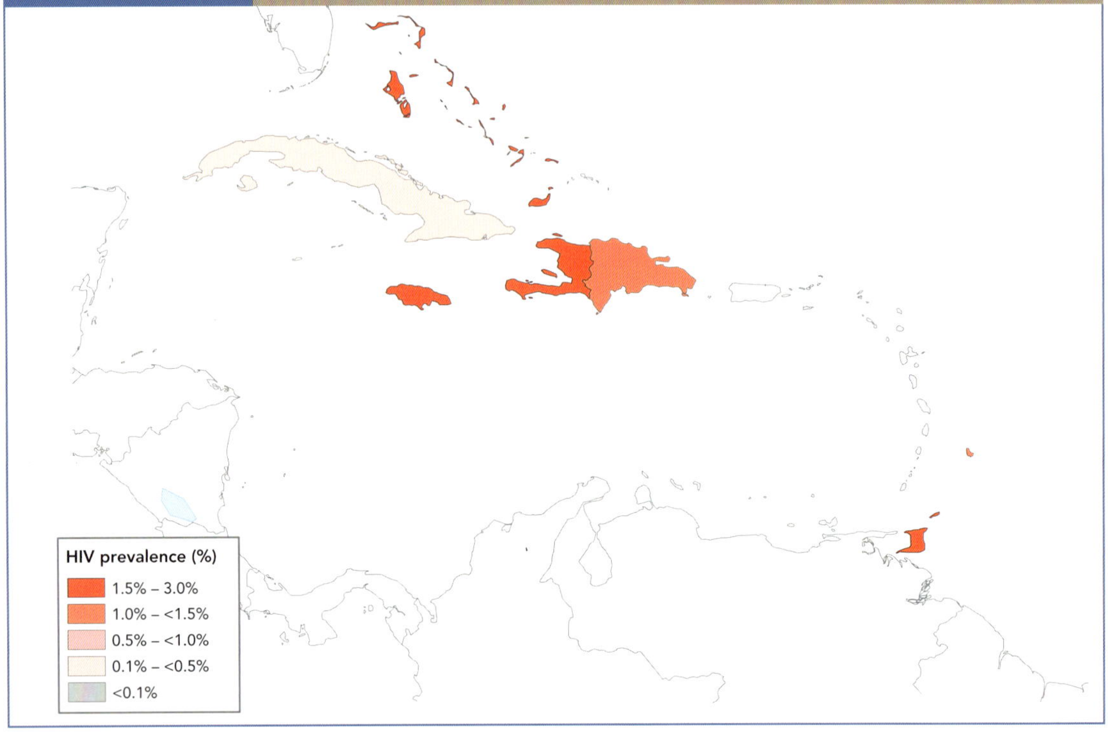

women attending antenatal clinics declined from 5.9% in 1996 to 3.1% in 2004 (Gaillard et al., 2006), and has subsequently remained stable (Ministère de la Santé Publique et de la Population, 2007). Although positive behaviour changes appear to be at least partly responsible for the decline (Cayemittes et al., 2006; Gaillard et al., 2006; Hallett et al., 2006), significant levels of high-risk behaviour have been documented in Haiti's rural areas and among young people (Cayemittes et al., 2006; Centre d'Evaluation et de Recherche Appliquée et Family Health International, 2006; Gaillard et al., 2006).

Sex work

As HIV prevalence has declined in the Dominican Republic, surveys have indicated that more sex workers are protecting themselves (and their clients) against HIV infection, especially in the main urban and tourist centres (Kerrigan et al., 2006). Among female sex workers, HIV prevalence of 9% has been documented in Jamaica and 31% in Guyana (Secretaría de Estado de Salud Pública y Asistencia Social de Republica Dominica, 2005; Allen et al., 2006; Gebre et al., 2006; Gupta et al., 2006; Pan American Health Organization, 2007).

Sex between men

As many as one in eight (12%) reported HIV infections in the region occurred through unprotected sex between men (Caribbean Commission on Health and Development, 2005; Inciardi et al., 2005). Unprotected sex between men is the main mode of HIV transmission in Cuba, where men account for more than 80% of all reported HIV cases (Programa Nacional de Prevención y control de las ITS/VIH/Sida, 2006), and in Dominica, where almost three quarters (71% of the 319 HIV infections reported to date) have been in men (Ministry of Health and Social Security [Dominica], 2007). Studies have found HIV prevalence of 20% among men who have sex with men in Trinidad and Tobago (Lee et al., 2006), 21% in Guyana's Region 4 (Ministry of Health [Guyana], 2005), and 11% in the Dominican Republic (Toro-Alfonso & Varas-Díaz, 2008).[12]

Latin America

New HIV infections in 2007 totalled an estimated 140 000 [88 000–190 000], bringing to 1.7 million [1.5 million–2.1 million] the number of people living with HIV in this region. An estimated 63 000 [49 000–98 000] people died of AIDS last year.

Recent epidemiological trends

The overall levels of HIV infections in Latin America have changed little in the past decade.

Main modes of HIV transmission

HIV transmission in this region is occurring primarily among men who have sex with men, sex workers, and (to a lesser extent) injecting drug users.

Sex between men

High HIV prevalence has been documented among men who have sex with men in several countries:

- 18%–22% in Peru, in studies conducted between 1996 and 2002 (Ministerio de Salud de Peru, 2006; Sanchez et al., 2007);
- 14% in Buenos Aires, Argentina, in 2000–2001 (Pando et al., 2006);
- 22% in Montevideo, Uruguay (Montano et al., 2005);
- 15% in four Bolivian cities and in Quito, Ecuador (Montano et al., 2005); and
- 10%–25% in some cities in Colombia (Mejía et al., 2006; Ministerio de la Protección Social de Colombia & ONUSIDA Grupo Tematico, 2006).

FIGURE 2.18 HIV prevalence (%) in adults (15–49) in Latin America, 2007

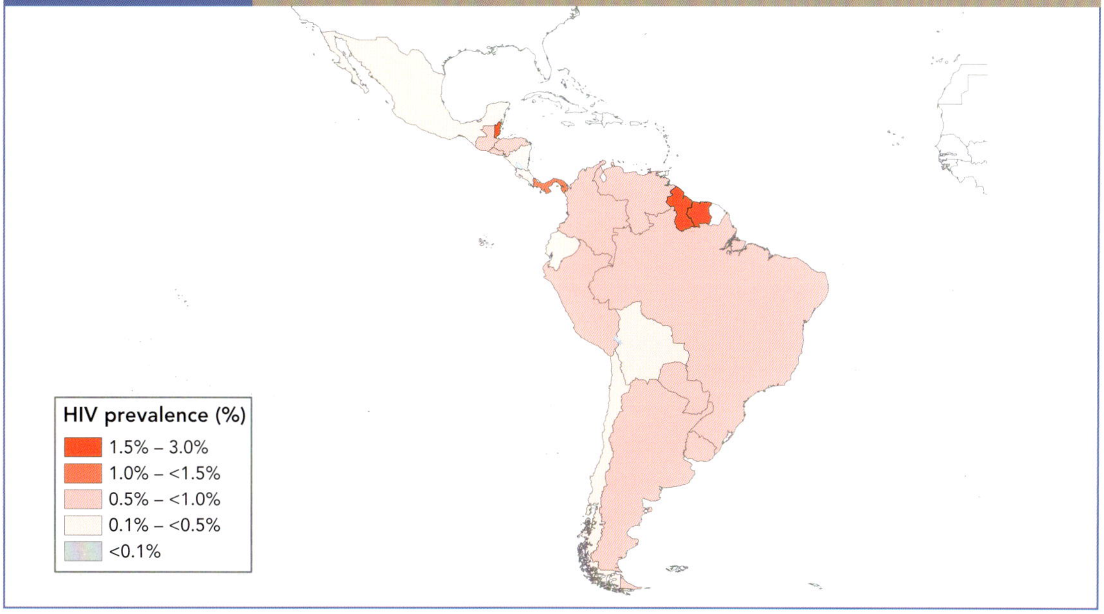

[12] Because the level and nature of HIV risk behaviours of men who have sex with men sometimes differ from study to study, direct comparisons between HIV prevalence data such these are not necessarily valid.

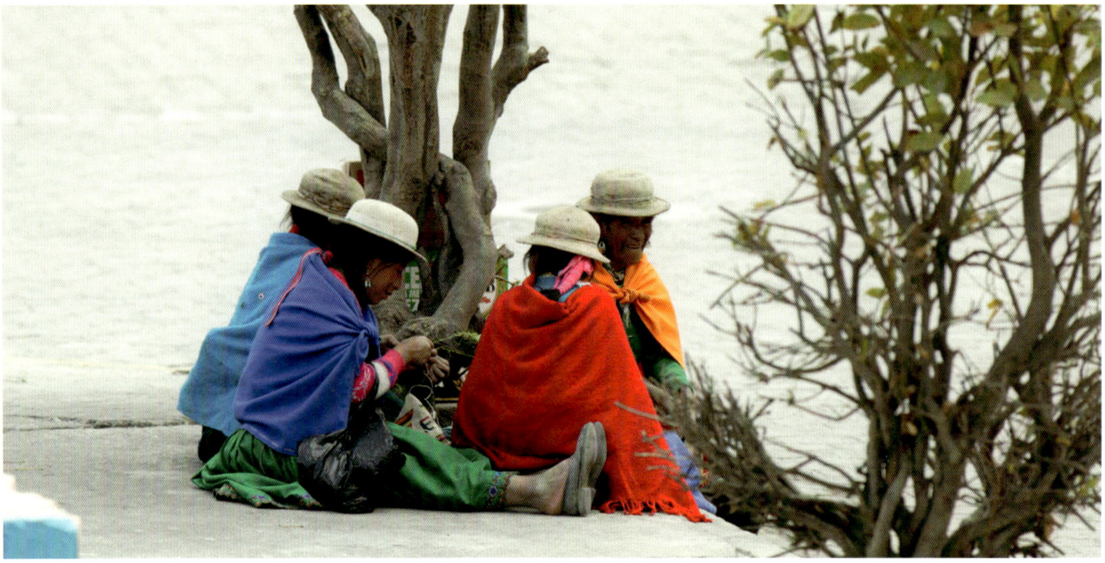

Research has uncovered hidden epidemics of HIV among men who have sex with men in several Central American countries, including Belize, Costa Rica, El Salvador, Guatemala, Mexico, Nicaragua, and Panama (Magis et al., 2006; Soto et al., 2007). More than half (57%) of the HIV diagnoses to date in Mexico have been attributed to unprotected sex between men (Bravo-Garcia, Magis-Rodriquez & Saavedra, 2006). Between one quarter and one third of men who have sex with men in those countries (except for Panama) also have sex with women—and between 30% and 40% of those men said that they had had unprotected sex with both men and women in the previous month (Soto et al., 2007).

Sex work

Across South America, levels of HIV infection among female sex workers tend to be much lower than those among men who have sex with men (Bautista et al., 2006a). HIV prevalence among female sex workers has been found to be 10% in Honduras, 4% in Guatemala, and 3% in El Salvador (Soto et al., 2007). However, there is recent evidence of a steep decline in HIV prevalence among female sex workers in Honduras, where condom promotion efforts were stepped up in recent years. (Secretaría de Salud de Honduras et al., 2007a; Secretaría de Salud de Honduras et al., 2007b).

Injecting drug use

HIV transmission as a result of injecting drug use still features in several of South America's epidemics. Regionally, this mode of transmission appears to be accounting for a smaller number of new infections than was the case previously. In Argentina, injecting drug use accounted for only about 5% of new HIV infections in Buenos Aires between 2003 and 2005 (Cohen, 2006), and HIV infection levels in injecting drug users have declined in some Brazilian cities (Fonseca et al., 2006; Okie, 2006; Rossi et al., 2006). Notable HIV transmission has been occurring among injecting drug users in the capitals of Paraguay (12% HIV-positive in various surveys) and Uruguay (19% HIV-positive) (IDES et al., 2005; National AIDS Program [Paraguay], 2006).

Heterosexual intercourse

Increasing numbers of women are becoming infected in several countries in the region, including Argentina, Brazil, Peru, and Uruguay (Ministerio de Salud de Peru, 2005; National AIDS Programme [Argentina], 2005; Cohen, 2006; Martínez et al., 2006; Dourado et

FIGURE 2.19 HIV prevalence (%) in adults (15–49) in North America, Western and Central Europe, 2007

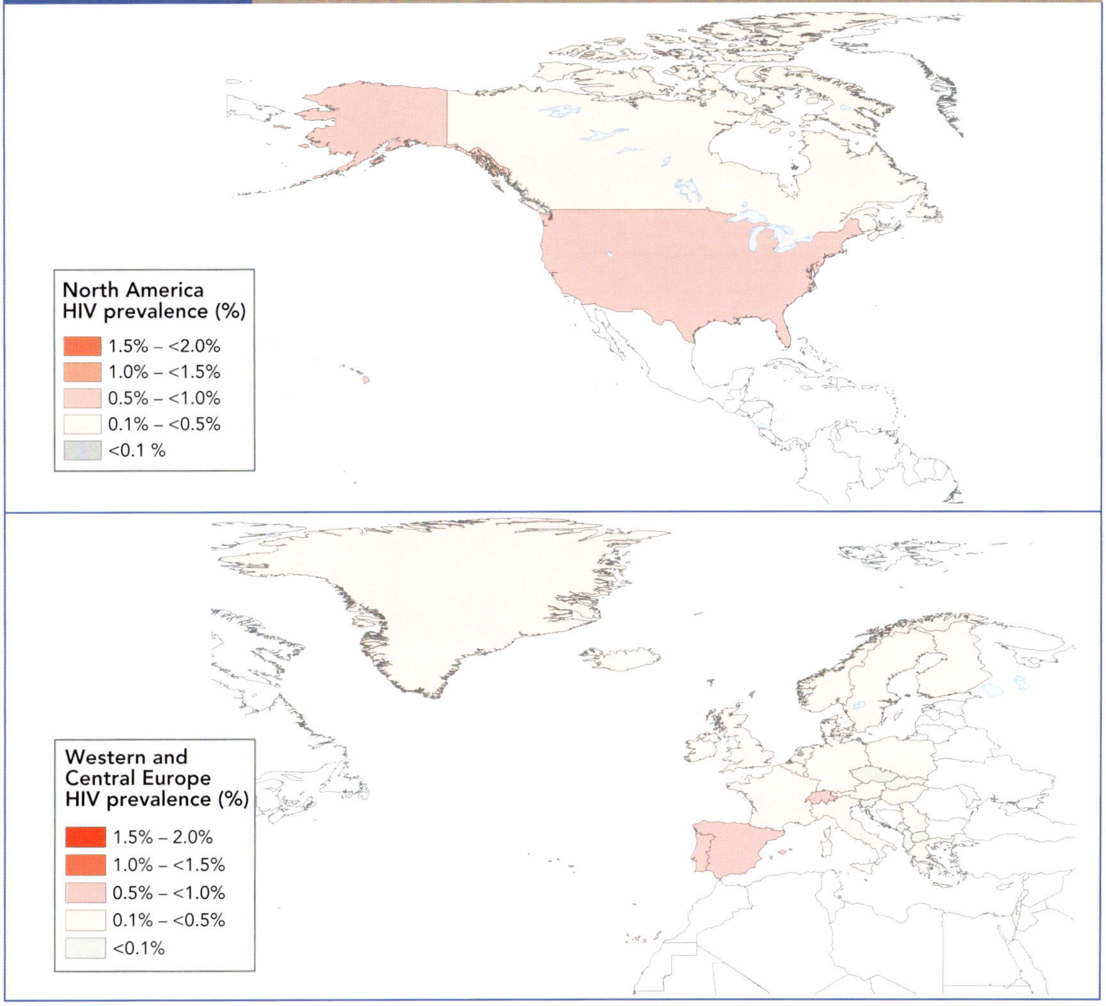

al., 2007). In Uruguay, for example, unprotected sex (mostly heterosexual) is believed to account for approximately two thirds of newly reported HIV cases (Montano et al., 2005). Most of the women are being infected by male sexual partners who acquired HIV during unprotected sex with another man or through use of contaminated drug injecting equipment (Ministerio de Salud de Peru, 2005; Cohen, 2006; Silva & Barone, 2006).

North America, Western and Central Europe

The United States of America accounted for an estimated 1.2 million [690 000–1.9 million] of the 2.0 million [1.4 million–2.8 million] people living with HIV in North America, and in Western and Central Europe in 2007. Overall in those regions, 81 000 [30 000–170 000] people were newly infected with HIV in 2007. Comparatively few people—31 000 in a range of 16 000–67 000—died of AIDS last year.

FIGURE 2.20 HIV infections newly diagnosed in injecting drug users and men who have sex with men, by country, and year of report, 2002–2006

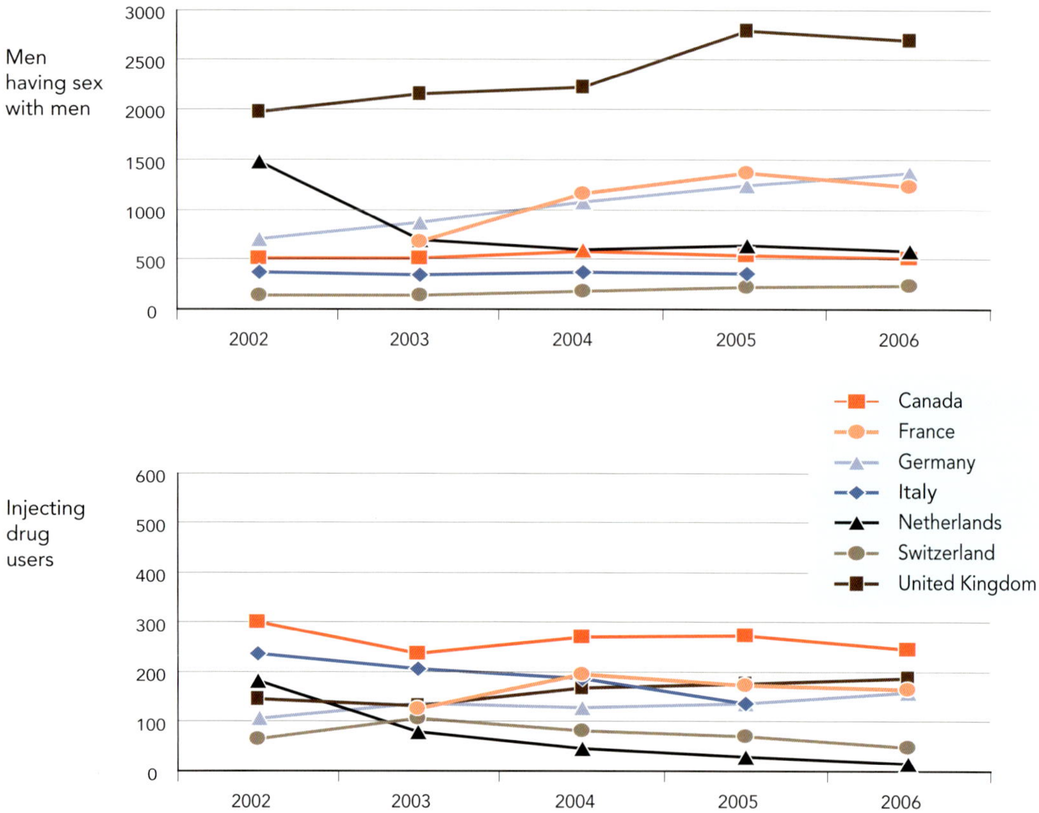

Sources:
(1) Public Health Agency of Canada. HIV and AIDS in Canada. Selected Surveillance Tables to June 30, 2007. Surveillance and Risk Assessment Division, Centre for Infectious Disease Prevention and Control, Public Health Agency of Canada, 2007. (2) Epidemiologisches Bulletin (5. Oktober 2007/ Sonderausgabe B aktuelle daten und informationen zu infektionskrankheiten und public health). (3) The UK Collaborative Group for HIV and STI Surveillance. Testing Times. HIV and other Sexually Transmitted Infections in the United Kingdom: 2007. London: Health Protection Agency, Centre for Infections. November 2007. (4) EuroHIV. HIV/AIDS Surveillance in Europe. End-year report 2006. Saint-Maurice: Institut de veille sanitaire, 2007. No. 75. (5) EuroHIV. HIV/AIDS Surveillance in Europe. Mid-year report 2007. Saint-Maurice: Institut de Veille Sanitaire, 2007. No. 76.

Recent epidemiological trends

In North America, annual numbers of new HIV diagnoses have remained relatively stable over recent years, but access to life-prolonging antiretroviral therapy has led to an increase in the estimated number of people living with HIV (Public Health Agency of Canada, 2006; US Centers for Disease Control and Prevention, 2007).[13] In Western Europe, new HIV diagnoses are increasing, as is the total number of people living with HIV (the latter also because of wide access to antiretroviral treatment).

Main modes of HIV transmission

These high-income countries have diverse epidemics, although their epidemiological profiles have diverged as the epidemic has evolved. In general, injecting drug use is accounting for a smaller share of new HIV infections than before.

Sex between men

Unprotected sex between men is still the main mode of HIV transmission in both

[13] This analysis is based mainly on reported HIV diagnoses. A significant limitation of using annual HIV diagnoses to monitor the HIV epidemic is that this yardstick does not represent the total incidence (because it may include infections that occurred several years earlier) and it only captures those people that have been tested for HIV. As a result, HIV trends based on reported HIV cases can be skewed by changes in the HIV testing intake or by changes in patterns of reporting. As far as possible, this analysis alerts readers to instances where such changes have occurred.

Canada and the United States—40% of new HIV diagnoses in Canada in 2006 and 53% in the USA in 2005 (Public Health Agency of Canada, 2007; US Centers for Disease Control and Prevention, 2007). Men who have sex with men continue to be the population group most at risk of acquiring HIV within most Western European countries. Indeed, the number of new HIV diagnoses attributed to unprotected sex between men has increased sharply in recent years in Western Europe, and appears to be associated with reported increases in higher-risk unprotected sex between men in several countries (Dodds et al., 2004; Balthasar, Jeannin & Dubois-Arber 2005; Moreau-Gruet, Dubois-Arber & Jeannin, 2006; Hamouda et al., 2007). In Germany, for example, the number of new HIV diagnoses among men who have sex with men rose by 96% (to 1370) between 2002 and 2006 (Robert Koch Institut, 2007).

Heterosexual intercourse

About one third (32%) of newly diagnosed HIV infections and AIDS cases in the United States in 2005 were attributable to high-risk heterosexual intercourse (US Centers for Disease Control and Prevention, 2007), as were 33% of new HIV infections in Canada in 2006. However, in Canada, a substantial proportion of those infections were in people born in countries with high HIV prevalence (mainly sub-Saharan Africa and the Caribbean) (Boulos et al., 2006; Public Health Agency of Canada, 2007). A similar situation was seen in Western Europe, where unprotected heterosexual intercourse accounted for the largest share (42%) of new HIV diagnoses in Western Europe in 2006 (compared with the 29% that were attributed to unprotected sex between men). Unprotected heterosexual intercourse is the main reported mode of transmission in most countries of Central Europe, except for Estonia, Latvia, Lithuania, and Poland, where the main mode is injecting drug use, and Croatia, the Czech Republic, Hungary, and Slovenia, where it is unprotected sex between men (Hamers, 2006; Rosinska, 2006; Brucková et al., 2007; EuroHIV, 2007a).

Injecting drug use

Transmission by multiple use of contaminated injecting equipment accounts for 18% of new HIV diagnoses in the United States (2005) and 19% in Canada (2006) (Public Health Agency of Canada, 2007; US Centers for Disease Control and Prevention, 2007). In Western Europe, a diminishing proportion of HIV diagnoses (6%) are related to the use of contaminated injecting equipment in 2006 (EuroHIV, 2007b). In Denmark and the Netherlands, the number of new HIV diagnoses among injecting drug users fell by 72% and by 91%, respectively in 2002–2006 (EuroHIV, 2007b). In Central Europe, too, newly reported HIV diagnoses in injecting drug users have decreased (EuroHIV, 2007b).

Middle East and North Africa

The limited HIV information available for the Middle East and North Africa indicates that approximately 380 000 [280 000–510 000] people were living with HIV in 2007, including the 40 000 [20 000–66 000] people who were newly infected with the virus last year.

Recent epidemiological trends

With the exception of the Sudan, the epidemics in this region are comparatively small.

Primary sources of HIV transmission

Varying combinations of risk factors are associated with the epidemic; chief among them are unprotected paid sex and the use of contaminated drug injecting equipment (Obermeyer, 2006).

Injecting drug use

The Islamic Republic of Iran is home to a serious drug-related epidemic, with HIV prevalence of

CHAPTER 2

FIGURE 2.21 HIV prevalence (%) in adults (15–49) in Middle East and North Africa, 2007

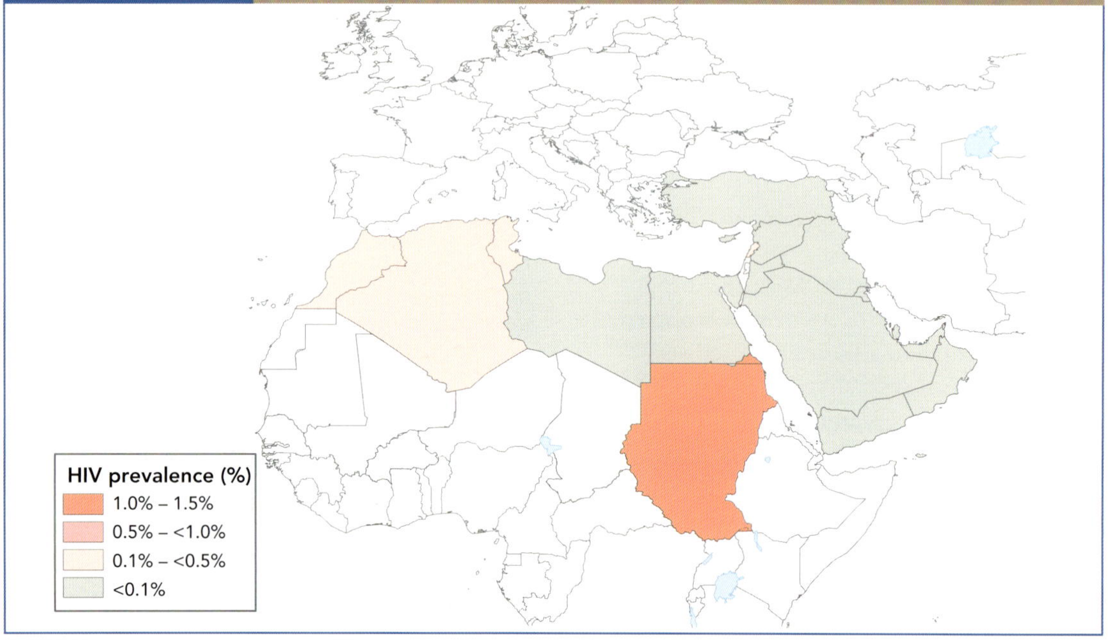

between 15% and 23% documented among male injecting drug users who make use of drop-in or drug-treatment services in Tehran (Zamani et al., 2005; Zamani et al., 2006). Exposure to contaminated drug injecting equipment is also the main route of HIV transmission in the Libyan Arab Jamahiriya and Tunisia, and it features in the epidemics of Algeria, Morocco, and the Syrian Arab Republic (Kilani et al., 2003; Ministry of Health and Medical Education [Iran], 2005; Mimouni & Remaoun, 2006; Obermeyer, 2006).

Overlap of injecting drug use and sex work

A combination of injecting drug use and sex work may be facilitating the spread of HIV in Algeria, Egypt, Lebanon, and the Syrian Arab Republic, where one third or more of surveyed injecting drug users said that they recently either bought or sold sex. In the Syrian Arab Republic, more than half (53%) of the drug users interviewed in one study said they sold sex, and 40% of those users said they never used condoms (Ministry of Health [Syria] et al., 2007).

Heterosexual intercourse

Unprotected heterosexual intercourse is the main factor in Sudan's epidemic—the most extensive in the region—with national adult HIV prevalence estimated at 1.4% [1.0%–2.0%] in 2007. In several other countries, increasing numbers of women are being diagnosed with HIV, most of them infected by husbands or boyfriends who had acquired HIV through injecting drug use or paid sex In Morocco, for example, one third (33%) of women diagnosed with AIDS were married (Ministére de la Santé [Maroc], 2007).

Sex between men

Although socially stigmatized and officially censured throughout the region, unprotected sex between men is probably a factor in several of the region's epidemics. A recent study in Egypt, for example, found that 6.2% of men who have sex with men were infected with HIV (Ministry of Health [Egypt] et al., 2006), while 9% prevalence was found among their counterparts in Khartoum State, Sudan (Elrashied, 2006).

Oceania

Overall, an estimated 74 000 [66 000–93 000] people were living with HIV in Oceania in 2007, about 13 000 [12 000–15 000] of whom were newly infected in the same year.

Recent epidemiological trends

Most of the region's epidemics are small, except in Papua New Guinea, where the annual number of new HIV diagnoses more than doubled between 2002 and 2006, when 4017 new HIV cases were reported (National AIDS Council Secretariat [Papua New Guinea], 2007).

Primary sources of HIV transmission

Heterosexual intercourse

Unprotected heterosexual intercourse is the main mode of HIV transmission in Papua New Guinea (National HIV/AIDS Support Project, 2006; National AIDS Council Secretariat [Papua New Guinea] & National HIV/AIDS Support Project, 2007), and unprotected paid sex in particular appears to be a central factor. In one recent survey, 60%–70% of truck drivers and military personnel, and 33% of port workers, said they had bought sex in the previous year (National AIDS Council Secretariat [Papua New Guinea] & National HIV/AIDS Support Project, 2007). Community-based studies in 10 provinces have shown that about 40% of participants were infected with at least one sexually transmitted infection (Institute of Medical Research, 2007).

FIGURE 2.22 HIV prevalence (%) in adults (15–49) in Oceania, 2007

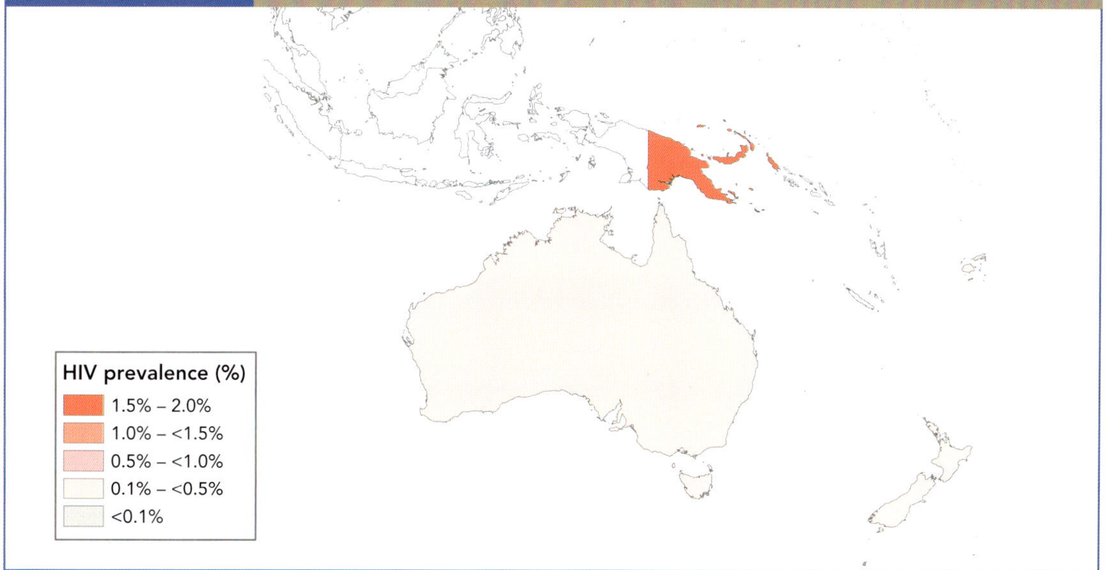

FIGURE 2.23 Annual diagnoses of HIV infections and AIDS in Australia, 1981–2006

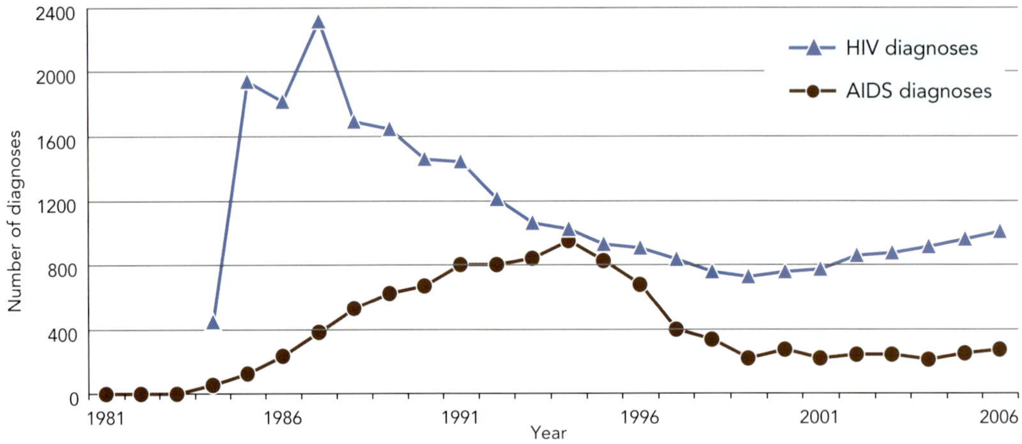

Source: National Centre in HIV Epidemiology and Clinical Research, 2007. Data available at http://www.nchecr.unsw.edu.au/NCHECRweb.nsf/resources/SurvRep07/$file/ASR2007.PDF

Sex between men

Unprotected sex between men is the primary cause of HIV infection in Australia (National Centre in HIV Epidemiology and Clinical Research, 2007a) and New Zealand (Ministry of Health [New Zealand], 2007). After declining sharply in the 1990s, new HIV diagnoses in Australia have increased, from the 763 reported in 2000 to 998 reported in 2006 (Figure 2.23). There is evidence that the prevalence of unprotected sex between men has increased or remained at high levels in recent years in several cities including Adelaide, Brisbane, Canberra, Perth (National Centre in HIV Epidemiology and Clinical Research, 2007b), and Sydney (Prestage et al., 2006). Unprotected sex between men also could be a factor in Papua New Guinea's epidemic. When surveyed, more than one in ten (12%) young men said they had had sex with men, and condom use was rare (Maibani-Michie & Yeka, 2005).

Addressing societal causes of HIV risk and vulnerability

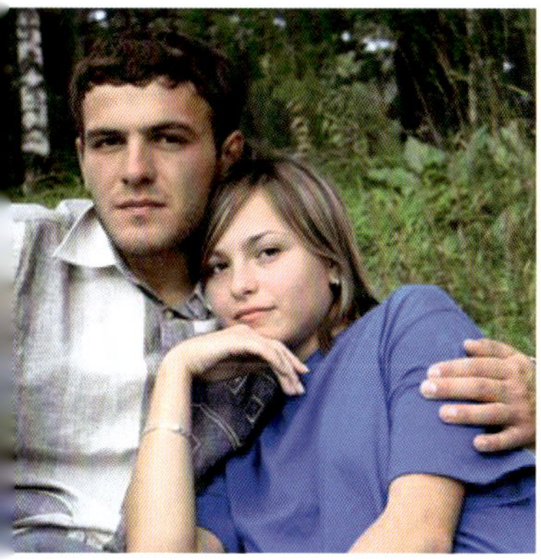

3

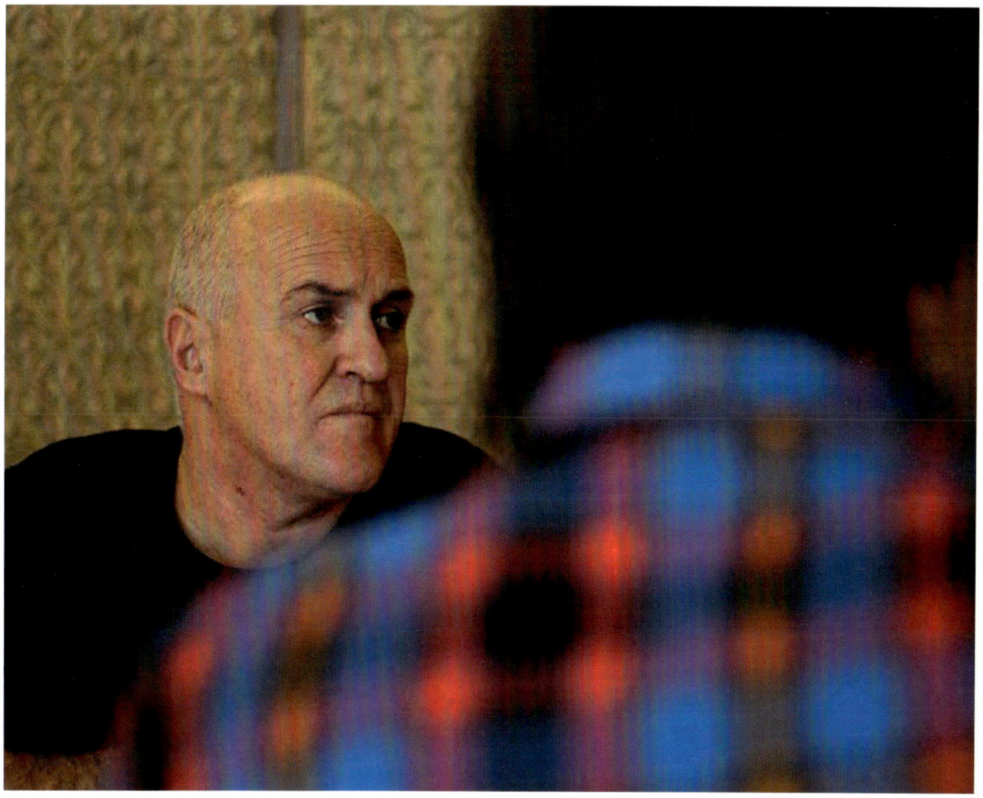

Chapter 3

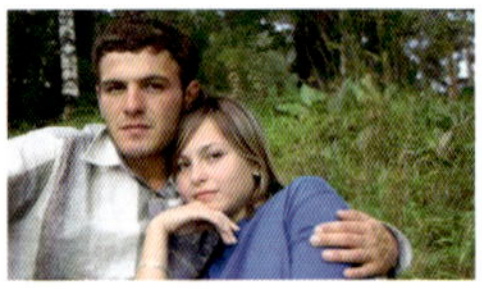

FIGURE 3.1 Selected events related to social determinants of the HIV epidemic

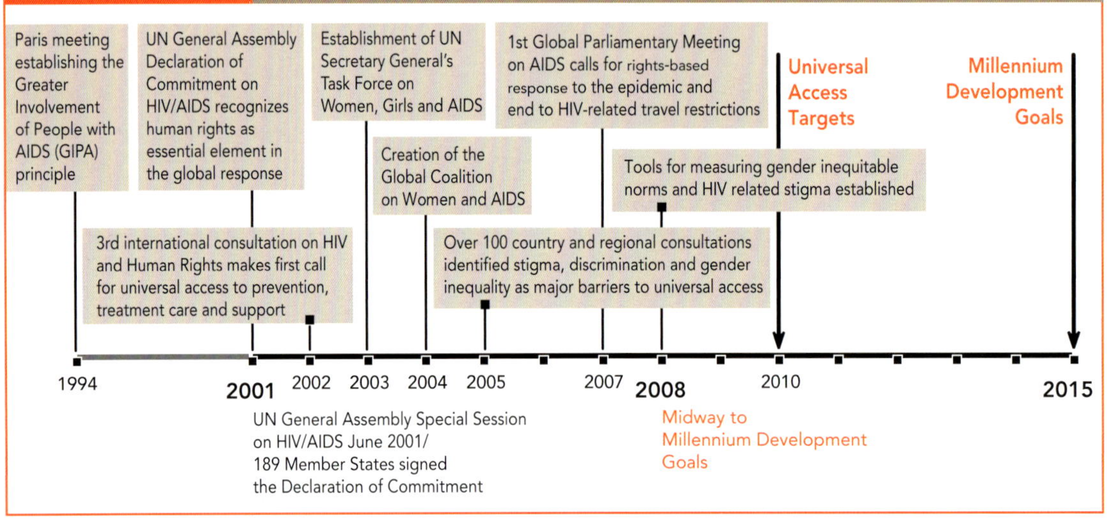

Key findings

- Long-term success in responding to the HIV epidemic will require sustained progress in addressing human rights violations, gender inequality, stigma, and discrimination.
- Significant investment in girls' education, supported by policies mandating universal primary and secondary education, would substantially reduce HIV risk and vulnerability for women and girls.
- Evidence-informed programmes to forge norms of gender equity should be brought to scale, with particular attention to initiatives focused on men and boys.
- National governments and international donors should prioritize strategies to increase women's economic independence and legal reforms to recognize women's property and inheritance rights.
- All countries should ensure rigorous enforcement of antidiscrimination measures to protect people living with HIV. The one third of countries that lack legal protections against HIV-based discrimination should immediately enact such laws. Countries should also protect populations most at risk from discrimination and ensure their equal enjoyment of human rights.
- Countries should include anti-stigma strategies as integral components of their national AIDS plans, investing in a broad range of activities, including public awareness and "know your rights" campaigns, legal services for people living with HIV, expansion of access to antiretroviral drugs, and expressions of national solidarity in the HIV response.
- Much stronger financial and technical support is needed for capacity-building for organizations and networks of people living with HIV, and groups most at risk of HIV infection.

HIV is a biological entity that is responsive to medical interventions, but the epidemic has continued to expand, largely due to the failure to tackle societal conditions that increase HIV risk and vulnerability. This chapter examines two sets of societal factors that affect HIV risk and vulnerability but have not been effectively addressed in most countries:

- gender inequality and the lack of empowerment of women and girls; and
- discrimination, stigma, and social marginalization.

This chapter also includes a brief discussion of the role of economic inequality in the HIV epidemic. The social factors differ in their manifestation, intensity, and impact between and within regions, but they are present to some degree worldwide, and in all cases impede an effective, evidence-informed and rights-based response to the epidemic (Mann & Tarantola, 1996).

Relatively few studies have rigorously examined strategies to minimize these and other societal sources of HIV risk and vulnerability. Nevertheless, sufficient evidence exists to guide national initiatives that aim to minimize the societal sources of HIV risk and vulnerability and to create more enabling environments for the human rights, health, and well-being of all people, including those most at risk of exposure to HIV. In particular, tools have been developed in recent years to measure gender inequality and HIV-related discrimination and stigma, facilitating improved social science research and programme evaluation. Efforts to change the contextual influences that increase HIV risk and vulnerability using a variety of initiatives—including a new generation of social change communication strategies—should constitute an integral part of any comprehensive national HIV strategy. This chapter is complementary to Chapter 4, which discusses the components of effective, comprehensive programmes to prevent new HIV infections.

Attempting to change the societal determinants of HIV risk and vulnerability could be

CHAPTER 3

Defining HIV risk and vulnerability

Risk is defined as the probability or likelihood that a person may become infected with HIV. Certain behaviours create, increase, and perpetuate risk. Examples include unprotected sex with a partner whose HIV status is unknown, multiple sexual partnerships involving unprotected sex, and injecting drug use with contaminated needles and syringes.

Vulnerability results from a range of factors outside the control of the individual that reduce the ability of individuals and communities to avoid HIV risk. These factors may include: (1) lack of knowledge and skills required to protect oneself and others; (2) factors pertaining to the quality and coverage of services (e.g. inaccessibility of service due to distance, cost or other factors); and (3) societal factors such as human rights violations, or social and cultural norms. These norms can include practices, beliefs and laws that stigmatize and disempower certain populations, limiting their ability to access or use HIV prevention, treatment, care, and support services and commodities. These factors, alone or in combination, may create or exacerbate individual and collective vulnerability to HIV.

Based on: UNAIDS (2007a).

considered beyond the resources, time frame or mandate of public health programmes. Yet the HIV epidemic has already led to major alterations in international development and global public health practice, dramatic changes in attitudes, and monumental shifts in social norms. The history of the epidemic demonstrates the pitfalls of a response that is too narrow and focused only on the short term. Far-reaching changes in social norms and practices are possible if there is sufficient political leadership, community engagement, programme direction, and international solidarity. In recent years, the attitudes, behavioural patterns, and laws that cause, reflect, and reinforce the societal determinants of HIV risk and vulnerability have been exhaustively mapped in diverse settings. A growing body of scientific evidence is available to guide policy responses and programmes.

Moreover, now is the time to address the root causes of HIV risk and vulnerability. Important, if uneven, progress has been made in expanding access to many HIV prevention strategies (see Chapter 4), but efforts to curb the spread of HIV are being undercut by gender inequality, stigma, and discrimination. Especially in hyper-endemic settings—where modest changes in risk behaviour that might keep low-level epidemics in check would be unlikely to have sufficient impact—broader social changes are required to bring the epidemic under control (SADC, 2006).

Rights-based approaches to HIV

A human rights-based approach to HIV ensures that matters often considered discretionary are recognized as legitimate entitlements of all individuals. This approach also ensures that governments, the UN system, donors, and the private sector are obligated and empowered to assist in the realization of the rights necessary to respond to HIV. It brings human rights standards and principles into the heart of all HIV programming processes, and empowers people to know and claim their rights. It helps stakeholders to address power imbalances that exist at household, community, and national levels. In particular, a human rights-based approach to HIV ensures:

- a focus on the vulnerable and marginalized in the HIV epidemic (e.g. women, young people, people living with HIV, orphans, men who have sex with men, drug users, sex workers, mobile populations, ethnic and indigenous groups, and refugees);
- equality and non-discrimination in expenditure on HIV programmes and applications;
- programmes to empower those vulnerable to, or living with, HIV, including law reform, legal aid, human rights education, social mobilization, social change communication, and support for civil society;
- programmes designed to achieve human rights standards relevant to HIV (e.g. protection from sexual violence, gender equality, education, information, health, employment, access to scientific progress);
- informed, active, free, and meaningful participation by those affected by HIV in HIV-related programme design, implementation, monitoring, and evaluation; and
- accountability mechanisms for governments, intergovernmental organizations, donors, and the private sector (e.g. UNGASS and the "Three Ones" principles).

Gender inequality and harmful gender norms

The many and varied links between gender inequality and increased vulnerability to HIV infection among women and adolescent girls have been well documented.[1] Cultural or social norms often restrict women's access to basic information about sexual and reproductive health. Even if women have access to information and commodities (e.g. condoms), gender norms that prescribe an unequal and more passive role for women in sexual decision-making undermine women's autonomy, expose many to sexual coercion, and prevent them from insisting on abstinence or condom use by their male partners.

Gender inequality has a clear, demonstrable impact on the epidemic. In Botswana, individuals who held three or more discriminatory gender beliefs (e.g. extramarital sex is less permissible for women than for men, a husband is justified in beating his wife if she has sex outside the marriage) were nearly three times more likely to have had unprotected sex with a non-marital partner in the previous year than those without such beliefs. A related study in Swaziland found that people who had six or more discriminatory gender attitudes were more than twice as likely to have multiple sex partners than those without such attitudes (Physicians for Human Rights, 2007).

Traditional expectations related to masculinity and male sexual behaviour also increase the risk of infection among men and boys. Typical male roles that call for men and boys to be tough, aggressive, sexually dominant, and risk-taking are often associated with behaviours that increase men's risk of HIV infection. Such behaviours include a high number of sexual partners, use of drugs or alcohol, and refusal to seek medical care for sexually transmitted infections (ICRW, 2007; WHO, 2007). The mutually harmful nature of some gender norms underscores the importance of involving men and boys in any effort towards change.

FIGURE 3.2 Percentage of countries in regions reporting that women are addressed as a specific component of their multisectoral HIV strategy with a specific HIV budget for their activities

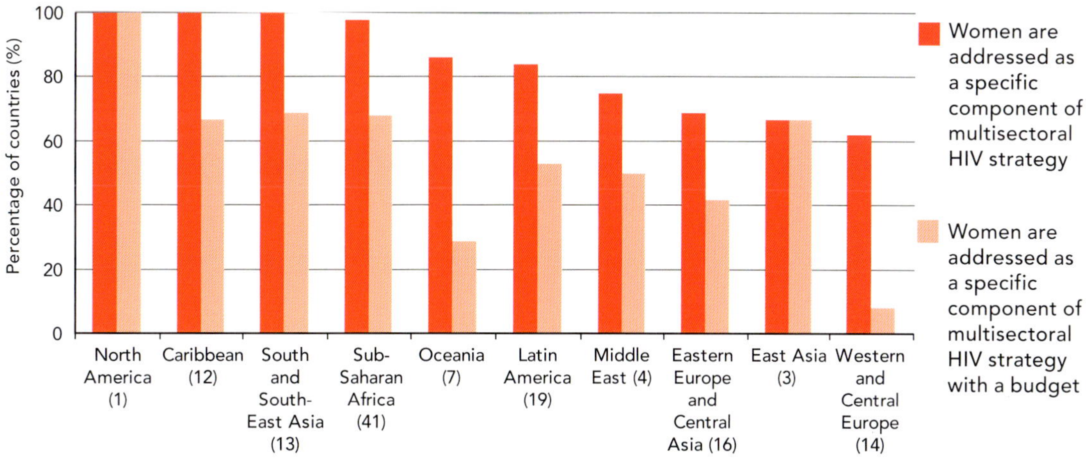

Source: UNGASS Country Progress Reports 2008.

[1] For a summary of what is known about how gender inequality increases HIV risk and vulnerability, see Global Coalition on Women and AIDS (2006a).

National policy responses to gender inequality

Although a large majority of countries have begun to recognize gender issues in their HIV planning processes, a substantial number lack budget and policy support for such issues. More than 80% of national governments report a focus on women as part of their multisectoral strategy for HIV, but only 52% report having a dedicated budget allocation for programmes addressing women's issues (UNGASS Country Progress Reports, 2008). The largest proportions of countries with reported budgets for such efforts are in Asia (69%) and sub-Saharan Africa (68%) (Figure 3.2).

In 2007, nongovernmental respondents in 82% of countries reported having policies in place to ensure equal access to HIV prevention, treatment, care, and support for women and men, with important regional variations, as shown in Figure 3.3 (UNGASS Country Progress Reports, 2008). This is an increase from 2003, when 69% of national governments reported that such policies were in place. Despite the large number of countries with such policies in place, nongovernmental informants in 12% of these countries report the existence of other laws and policies that present obstacles to the delivery of services to women (UNGASS Country Progress Reports, 2008).

Based on countries' responses to 14 questions about policies related to women, UNAIDS rated each country on a policy index ranging from 0 (for those with none of the equitable policies in place) to 14 (for those with all of them). As Figure 3.4 illustrates, the lowest scores on policies ensuring equal access to women were in Eastern Europe and Centralo Asia, and the highest were in sub-Saharan Africa.[2]

FIGURE 3.3 Percentage of countries (by region) reporting policies in place to ensure equal access to HIV prevention, treatment, care, and support for women and men

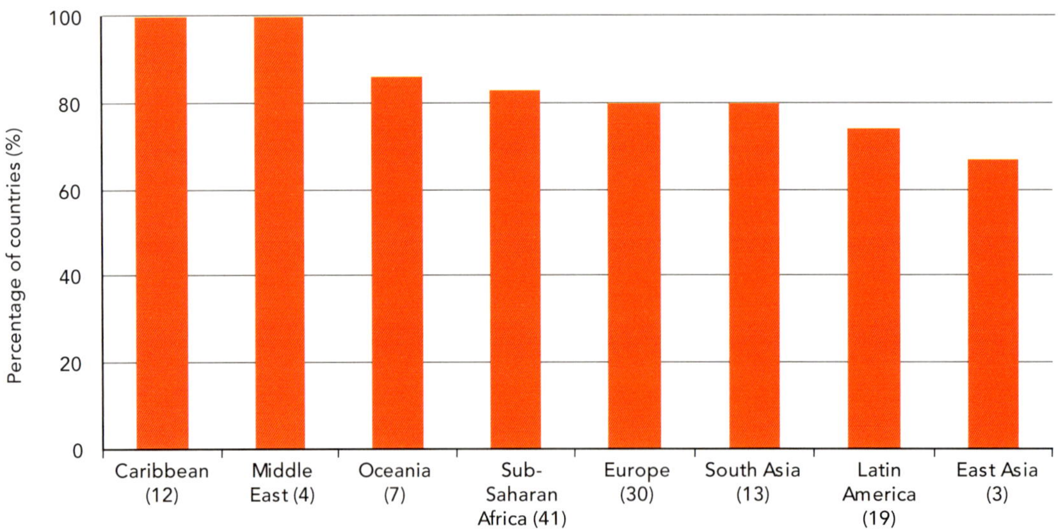

Source: UNGASS Country Progress Reports 2008.

2 The 130 responding countries were rated according to their replies to 14 policy questions in NCPI. Each country was given a score of 1 for each policy in place. Questions related to inclusion of specific women's issues in national strategic plans and in development plans, in HIV prevention (government response) and in human rights (nongovernmental response). A value of –1 was given if a country responded positively to the question on whether there are laws, regulations or policies that present obstacles to HIV programmes for women.

FIGURE 3.4 Index of policies related to women's vulnerability to HIV

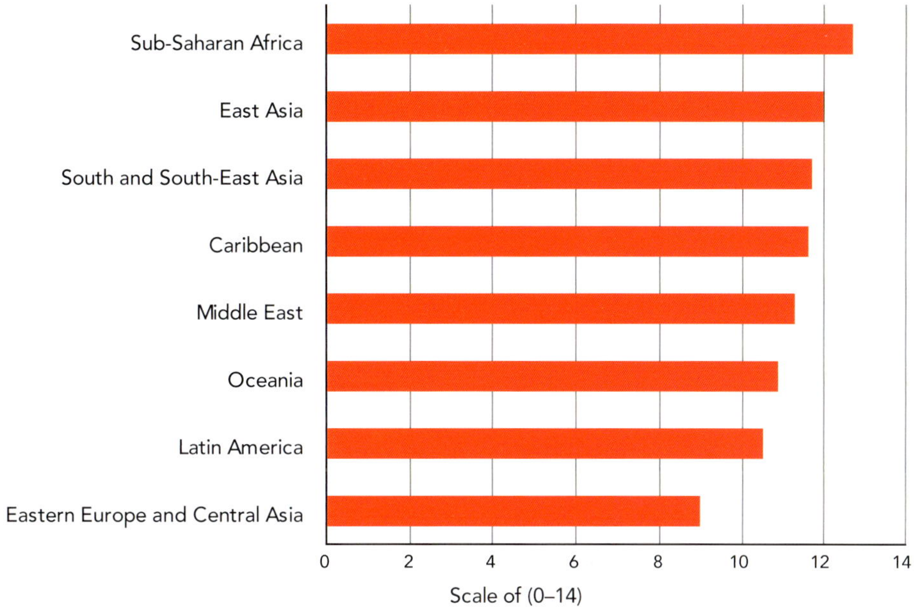

Source: UNGASS Country Progress Reports 2008.

Despite important progress in developing national policy frameworks related to women's vulnerability and HIV, key gaps remain in many countries. For example, nongovernmental informants reported that nearly one third of countries (31%) do not have non-discrimination laws or regulations in place that explicitly mention women (with a range across regions of 12%–50%) (UNGASS Country Progress Reports, 2008). According to government reports, 32% of countries lack information, education, and communication policies or strategies to encourage the involvement of men in reproductive health programmes (UNGASS Country Progress Reports, 2008).

Effective strategies to reduce gender inequality and change harmful gender norms

A growing number of strategies, discussed below, can reduce gender inequality and change harmful gender norms. These strategies are:

- education;
- multicomponent efforts to change harmful gender norms;
- reduction in gender-based violence;
- income-generating strategies; and
- advocacy and support.

Promoting universal education

Earlier in the epidemic, evidence about the relationship between educational attainment and risk of HIV infection was ambiguous, but more recent data from 11 African countries clearly link higher educational levels with lower HIV prevalence (Hargreaves, 2008). A recent study in rural South Africa found that each additional year of educational attainment reduced the risk of HIV infection by 7% (Bärnighausen et al., 2007). In particular, schooling offers an excellent means of reducing girls' HIV risk and vulnerability.

Measuring changes in normative beliefs relating to gender between men and women

The global history of women's empowerment demonstrates that it is feasible to radically alter gender norms. Until recently, however, it has been difficult to establish whether particular initiatives to promote equity between men and women have led to changes in gender norms and practices. This shortcoming has stemmed primarily from the absence of reliable, measures in this area.

Fortunately, this barrier has been overcome, creating the potential for easier and more rigorous programme evaluation studies. Developed and tested by the Horizons project in Brazil, and subsequently tested in Asia and Africa, the Gender Equitable Men scale provides HIV programmes with a practical and reliable way to measure key beliefs and norms that contribute to gender inequality.

Horizons researchers found they could characterize prevalent gender norms by asking respondents if they agreed with a small set (15–25) of questions, such as "There are times when a woman deserves to be beaten" and "A man should have the final word about decisions in his home." The resulting scale enables programmes in widely varying contexts to demonstrate their impact on equitable gender norms. In Brazil and India, for example, the scale was used to evaluate a six-month programme of peer-led, interactive sessions with young men that included role play, dialogue, and other techniques to prompt critical reflection on gender norms and their consequences. The study also evaluated an intensive arm of the programme that supplemented the standard activity with a "lifestyle social marketing campaign" to promote sexually responsible, non-violent male behaviour. In both Brazil and India, both the standard and the intensive activities significantly reduced support for inequitable gender norms at 6 and 12 months, in comparison with a control group that had not participated in these activities. In Brazil, the young men who abandoned inequitable gender norms after taking part in the programme were less likely to report a sexually transmitted infection and more likely to use condoms with their regular partners. In Mumbai, India, men who took part in the programme were twice as likely to have used a condom with their most recent sexual partner, and were significantly less likely to engage in violence with their intimate partners. Verma et.al., 2006; Pulerwitz et al., 2006).

Girls who complete primary education are more than twice as likely to use condoms, while girls who finish secondary education are between four and seven times more likely to use condoms, and are less likely to be infected with HIV (Hargreaves & Boler, 2006).

Unfortunately, in many low- and middle-income countries, girls are systematically denied equal educational opportunities. In the least developed countries, girls are 11% less likely to attend primary schools than boys (UNDP, 2007). By the time girls reach secondary school age, their educational opportunities are even further diminished. In least developed countries, girls are 19% less likely than boys to be in school. In Benin, Côte d'Ivoire, and Guinea, girls are only slightly more than half as likely as boys to attend secondary school (UNDP, 2007).

Since 1999, the global disparity in school attendance between the sexes declined, from a 9% deficit among girls to a 6% deficit in 2005 (UNESCO, 2007). However, 113 countries lacked gender parity in primary and secondary school attendance in 2005, and UNESCO projections suggest that only 18 of these countries are likely to achieve equal access to education by 2015 (UNESCO, 2007). Gender disparities in schooling are much larger in secondary and tertiary education than in primary education. Of 144 reporting countries, only Botswana, China, Mexico, and Peru had achieved parity in tertiary education (UNESCO, 2007).

Strategic national efforts can close gender gaps in education. For example, in Burkina Faso, Ethiopia, and a number of other countries, strong national commitment to push towards global Education for All[3] goals has been associated with a significant narrowing of educational gaps between girls and boys (UNESCO, 2007). In parts of Africa, the elimination of school fees has led to dramatic increases in girls' primary school enrolment (Burns, Mingat & Rakotomalala, 2003; Deininger, 2003; UNICEF, 2005). In India, young women (both in and out of school) who participated in skills building and vocational training, and received referrals to comprehensive age-appropriate reproductive health services, were more likely to delay marriage until age 18, to report more consistent condom use, and to exhibit stronger health-seeking behaviour (CEDPA, 2001).

Multicomponent efforts to change harmful gender norms

National leadership and intervention programmes can help accelerate the process of forging more equitable gender norms. All such efforts should aim to promote dialogue at national and community levels, to examine the costs of inequitable gender norms to both women and men, and to explore new ways of thinking about gender.

A wide array of promising programmes have arisen to help communities develop equitable gender norms. Stepping Stones workshops[4], used in more than 40 countries, have helped to reduce the acceptability and prevalence of violence against women and promoted HIV awareness and condom use by fostering community dialogue (Jewkes et al., 2007). Participants in the Men as Partners programme in South Africa, implemented through Engender Health, were more likely to believe men and women should have equal rights, and that wife-beating was wrong (Kruger, 2003; Peacock & Levack, 2004; Bott, Morrison & Ellsberg, 2005). In Brazil, Instituto Promundo's Program H has demonstrated improvements in young men's attitudes toward gender equality and reductions in risk of HIV and sexually transmitted infections. Program H used small group sessions, reinforced by a social marketing campaign, to replace community norms of male dominance with attitudes of respect and trust (Pulerwitz, 2006).

Confronting learned, shared attitudes is an important element of success in promoting gender equality. A meta-analysis of programmes to promote gender equality found that 29% were effective in producing changes in relevant attitudes or behaviour (Barker, Ricardo & Nascimento, 2007). Programmes that expressly aimed to transform gender roles through critical reflection, role play, and other interactions were

[3] The 'Education for All' movement began in 1990 at the World Conference on Education for All. At the World Education Forum in Dakar, Senegal, in 2000, governments pledged to achieve quality basic education by 2015, with particular attention to girls' education.

[4] Stepping Stones is a workshop that aims to alter behaviours and norms pertaining to HIV, gender and relationships. (See Welbourn, 1995)

most likely to be effective in producing changes in the targeted attitudes and behaviours.

Reducing gender-based violence

Widespread violence against women not only represents a global human rights crisis but also contributes to women's vulnerability to HIV. Between 40% and 60% of women surveyed in Bangladesh, Ethiopia, Peru, Samoa, Thailand, and the United Republic of Tanzania said they had been physically and/or sexually abused by their intimate partners (Garcia-Moreno et al., 2005). In conflict situations, rape and other forms of sexual coercion are often used as weapons of war (Raise Initiative, 2007). In parts of the Democratic Republic of the Congo affected by conflict, the prevalence of rape is believed to be the highest in the world (McCrummen, 2007).

In several African countries, the risk of HIV among women who have experienced gender-based violence may be up to three times higher than among those who have not (Global Coalition on Women and AIDS, 2004). Fear of violence can be a barrier to HIV disclosure (Medley et al., 2004); for example, in Cambodia, fear of violence contributes to the low numbers of women accessing counselling and testing services in antenatal clinics (Duvurry & Knoess, 2005).

International experience has shown that rates of violence can be lowered. However, 29% of national governments report that they lack laws or policies to prevent violence against women. To be successful, efforts to reduce gender violence must reverse social norms that hold violence to be natural and acceptable. Norm-changing programmes should be supported by legal reform, enhanced law enforcement to hold perpetrators of violence to account, and activities to address the attitudes and conditions that may contribute to gender-based violence.

In February 2007, Zimbabwe enacted legislation that expands protections for survivors of domestic violence and imposes penalties of up to 10 years in prison for offenders. Police stations are required by law to have personnel on duty

Addressing cultural practices that increase risk and vulnerability of women and girls

Globally, between 100 million and 140 million girls and women have undergone partial or total removal of the external female genitalia, or other injury to the female genital organs for non-medical reasons. An additional 3 million girls are affected each year by such practices (UNAIDS et al., 2008). In addition to reflecting and reinforcing women's subordinate status, female genital mutilation also exposes women to considerable health risks. In 2008, UNAIDS joined with nine other UN agencies to urge rapid implementation of laws and policies to eliminate the many forms of female genital mutilation (UNAIDS et al., 2008).

National laws and community awareness initiatives are increasingly addressing female genital mutilation and other cultural practices that can increase women's risk and vulnerability. Legislation passed in Zimbabwe in 2007 prohibits forced marriages or servitude, and in 2005 the Zambian Government amended the penal code to prohibit "widow cleansing", a practice whereby women whose husbands have died submit to sex with a village leader in order to be re-accepted into the community (UN Office for the Coordination of Humanitarian Affairs, 2005; Gable, 2007).

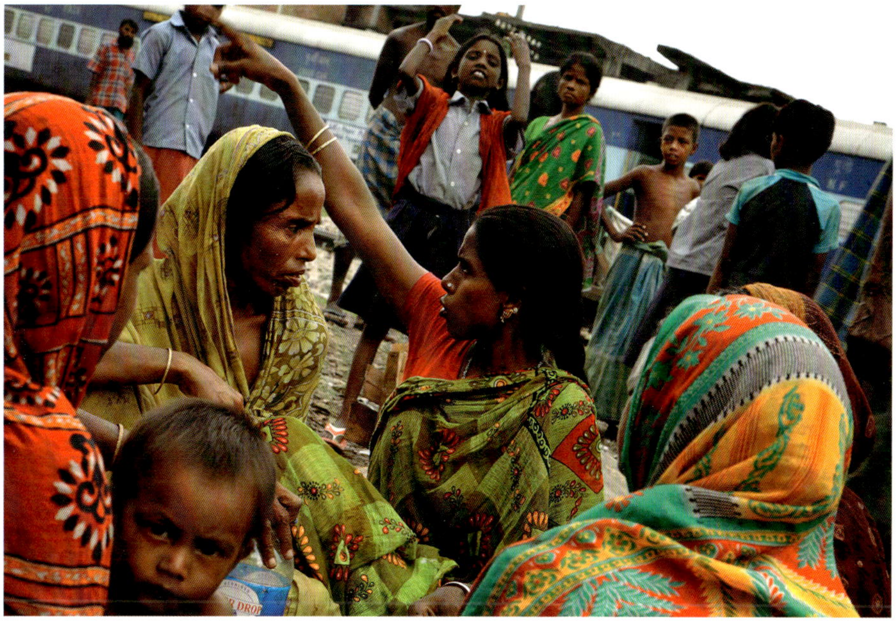

Women's ability to negotiate for safer sex is severely limited in many countries

with expertise in domestic violence. The law also grants law enforcement personnel the authority to arrest alleged perpetrators without a warrant if harm appears reasonably imminent. In support of this initiative, UNICEF has partnered with the national government and the Zimbabwe Women Lawyers Association to train more than 300 chiefs and traditional healers on how to apply the act to support survivors of violence and prevent abuse in their communities.

Countries are advised to approach violence prevention in the same way as other public health problems. Steps include developing a national action strategy, improving data collection and analysis, evaluating programmes to assess their results, reporting strategies and results through mass media, and investing in care and support services for survivors (Mercy, 2007). In general, research on the prevention of violence in low- and middle-income countries has attracted meagre financial support (Institute of Medicine, 2008).

In addition to programmes to encourage men to regard gender-based violence as unacceptable (whether directed at men or women), national and local laws can also help to reduce women's vulnerability to violence. However, laws against gender-based violence are meaningful only if they are effectively enforced. For example, Zambia established specialized police units to respond to reports of gender-based abuses (Human Rights Watch, 2007).

Income-generating strategies

In many regions, gender inequality may result in women's economic dependence on men, which may in turn heighten their vulnerability to HIV. In places where laws or social customs deprive women of an independent means to generate income, and permit husbands to abandon their wives if they are disobedient, women often have little, if any, means to insist on abstinence or condom use by their husbands.[5] According to a recent study in Botswana and Swaziland, women who lack sufficient food are 70% less likely to perceive personal control in sexual relationships, 50% more likely to engage in intergenerational sex, 80% more likely to engage in survival sex,

[5] For a discussion of the contribution of economic inequities to the disproportionate HIV infection rates among adolescent females in sub-Saharan Africa, see Chapter 4.

and 70% more likely to have unprotected sex (Weiser et al., 2007).

Women who own property or control other economic assets have higher incomes, a secure place to live, and greater bargaining power within their households. With a heightened sense of self-efficacy, women are better able to remove themselves from domestic violence, or to leave a relationship that threatens them with HIV infection. With greater ownership and control over economic assets, women are more empowered to negotiate abstinence, fidelity, and safer sex, and can avoid exchanging sex for money, food, or shelter (Strickland, 2004; Gupta, 2005; Global Coalition on Women and AIDS, 2006b). Young women with higher socioeconomic status also are more likely to delay sexual debut, have fewer sexual partners, and to use condoms (Hallman, 2004; Hallman, 2005).

In many countries heavily affected by HIV, however, laws do not recognize women's right to own or inherit property. Such institutionalized discrimination is often compounded by cultural norms, such as the practice in some communities that requires widows to marry a male relative of the deceased (Carpano, Izumi & Mathiesobn, 2007). The Canadian HIV/AIDS Legal Network is collecting "best practices" in the area of legislative reform to empower women, with the goal of drawing up model legislation and a legal toolkit to aid country-level advocacy (Carpano, Izumi & Mathieson, 2007).

In settings where women's economic rights are recognized, efforts are often required to acquaint women with their rights and to assist them in protecting those rights. In several African countries, grass-roots organizations help women to navigate the legal process, and train paralegals and others in the enforcement of women's property, inheritance, and legal rights (ICRW, 2006b). For example, Women's Land Link Africa links grass-roots organizations in 10 African countries to improve women's access to land and property ownership, and to advocate greater inclusion of women in policy-making processes (Carpano, Izumi & Mathieson, 2007). In India, the Lawyers Collective integrates training in HIV prevention and care into its legal services for women (Global Coalition on Women and AIDS, 2006b). Women who participated in a World Vision programme combining HIV education and microfinance showed greater economic resilience, higher levels of HIV awareness and prevention behaviours, and improved educational attainment and nutrition among their families (World Vision, 2008). A multiyear project in Mozambique aims to increase the gender sensitivity of judicial officers (Carpano, Izumi & Mathieson, 2007). However—according to a survey of nongovernmental organizations in Bangladesh, India, Nepal, and Sri Lanka—efforts to link women's property rights to HIV initiatives have largely been fragmented and ad hoc (ICRW, 2007).

In addition to legal reform to increase property ownership by women, substantially greater international support is needed for women-focused microfinance initiatives that provide direct financial support for women's economic independence. A study of the IMAGE project in South Africa, which combines microfinance with gender and HIV training, demonstrated a 55% reduction in intimate partner violence against women (Pronyk et al., 2006).[6]

Advocacy and support

Globally, many organizations and networks are actively working to build solidarity among women living with HIV, and to undertake joint advocacy to address the epidemic's disproportionate impact on women and girls. National governments and international donors should increase their capacity-building support for women's organizations that are working to advance women's rights and reduce women's vulnerability.

In Kenya, for example, GROOTS (Grassroots Organizations Together in Sisterhood) is a network of women's self-help groups that works to build the capacity of women to protect their

Finding support in an HIV microcredit programme

Imane, a 27-year-old woman in Algeria, believes her story "might seem to be the story of millions [of] HIV-positive women in the Arab world" *

When she was married five years ago, her husband did not disclose that he was HIV-positive. When Imane showed the medicines he took to one of her sisters, the sister urged Imane to take an HIV test. Although her 4-year-old daughter tested negative, tests showed that Imane had become infected with HIV. "When my doctor asked me if I knew about my disease I couldn't believe him," Imane says. "HIV! The disease of the prostitutes. This was my thinking then. This is the thinking in my culture!"

Today, Imane knows better. "The majority of HIV-positive women I know are women who never get out of their houses... more than 60% of the HIV-positive women I know are infected by their husbands."

Imane's physician explained that HIV had become a chronic disease and that she could live a normal life with antiretroviral drugs. Still, she had difficulty accepting the diagnosis and became depressed. Her husband displayed little empathy for her situation, and her best friend cut off contact after learning that Imane was living with HIV. Caring for her daughter became Imane's sole concern.

Eventually, a woman at her local hospital, who had been living with HIV for 10 years, invited Imane to visit El Hayet, a network of people living with HIV. El Hayet helps HIV-positive people to generate income by enabling them to obtain a diploma in one of a number of vocational fields, such as traditional pastry making, sewing, or painting. The organization links its members with microcredit opportunities generated through El Hayet's partnership with the Ministry of Solidarity and Social Affairs.

Through participation in El Hayet's income generation programme, Imane found a group of people who understood her and who gave her support. "I went several times until I felt totally relaxed when being there, and less and less lonely as days went through... There is a very positive atmosphere and so great relationship between the trainers and the trainees. What I found great here is that you may learn or teach... and speak freely about your disease with no fear."

"Today, with El Hayet, my wounds have healed."

* Iman requested that her photograph not be used.

legal and economic rights. In Nigeria, 150 women's groups joined together in August 2007 to launch the National Coalition on Women and AIDS. The aim was to address the root causes of women's vulnerability to infection, under the leadership of the country's First Lady.

Globally, the Huairou Commission links grass-roots women's organizations to share resources, information, and political and community organizing strategies (Carpano, Izumi & Mathieson, 2007).

Stigma, discrimination, and vulnerability to HIV

Stigma, discrimination, and social marginalization are causes of HIV risk and vulnerability, and consequences of being HIV-positive. Human beings are inherently social animals, and their physical and psychological health is damaged when they are isolated and cut off from their social group (Jenkins & Sarkar, 2007).

Stigmatizing attitudes to HIV and those most at risk of HIV infection derive from two principal sources. The first is fear of contagion, which has been a source of disease-related stigma through the ages. The second is negative, values-based assumptions about people living with HIV, which fuels prejudice and discrimination (ICRW, 2006a). In some cases, discrimination against people living with HIV is enshrined in national and local laws. According to the European AIDS Treatment Group, 74 countries restrict the entry or stay of people based on their HIV status, including 12 countries that ban people living with HIV from entering for any reason or for any length of time.

HIV-related stigma and discrimination undermine HIV prevention efforts by making people reluctant to be tested (Ford et al., 2004; Wolfe et al., 2006; Ma et al., 2007; Pulerwitz & Barker, 2008); to seek out information about how to protect themselves from infection; and,

Stigma and discrimination

HIV-related stigma is defined as: "...a 'process of devaluation' of people either living with or associated with HIV and AIDS" (UNAIDS, 2003).

Discrimination refers to action based on stigma. HIV-related discrimination follows stigma, and is the unfair and unjust treatment of an individual based on his or her real or perceived HIV status (UNAIDS, 2003).

Discrimination against people living with HIV and those perceived to be living with HIV occurs within families and other social networks, and is often institutionalized. Examples of institutionalized discrimination include government laws, policies, and procedures that negatively target people living with HIV or groups perceived to be living with HIV, and discrimination in workplace settings or health-care settings. Omission can also be a form of discrimination where, for example, the needs and interests of people living with HIV or stigmatized populations are ignored or minimized.

Discrimination is a human rights violation and is prohibited by international human rights law. The Commission on Human Rights, now the Human Rights Council, has stated that discrimination on the basis of "other status" includes health status, including HIV.

[6] For a discussion of the role of microfinance in mitigating the epidemic's impact on women, see Chapter 6.

in some cases, reluctant to use condoms for fear of being identified with the disease or with marginalized populations that are most heavily affected (Nyblade et al., 2003). Fear of stigma and discrimination also makes people living with HIV less likely to seek care and treatment, adhere to treatment, and disclose their HIV status to their sexual partners (White & Carr, 2005; Liu et al., 2006; Mills, 2006). In some cases, family members, caregivers, and the children of people living with HIV are also subject to discrimination and shame. Far too often, the health-care system itself—including doctors, nurses, and staff responsible for the care and treatment of people living with HIV—are prime agents of HIV-related stigma and discrimination (Reis et al., 2005; Mahendra et al., 2007; USAID, 2007a). In 2006, UNAIDS-facilitated consultations with civil society and government stakeholders in 122 countries consistently identified HIV-related stigma and discrimination as one of the top five barriers to achieving universal access to HIV prevention, treatment, care, and support.

Law can be a force to change or to legitimizing distinctions made about groups. Laws can protect people living with HIV from discrimination or can increase discrimination against them. For example, broadly applying the criminal law to HIV transmission sends the message that people living with HIV are potential criminals. The law can also protect other groups (e.g. men who have sex with men, drug users, or sex workers) from human rights violations, particularly violence, vilification, discrimination, and lack of due process. However, where the activities of some groups are criminalized (e.g. men who have sex with men, drug users, or sex workers) the law and its enforcement can become a major barrier to access and uptake of HIV prevention, treatment, care, and support. Institutionalized discrimination is also reflected in acts of omission, such as when the level of HIV resources directed towards the needs of men who have sex with men, injecting drug users, or sex workers is not commensurate with local epidemiology, or when HIV surveillance systems fail to track such groups.

Reducing stigma, discrimination and social marginalization

Over the past few years, the harmful effects of stigma and discrimination have become even more clearly understood, and a growing number of institutions and organizations have focused greater attention on these effects. A number of successful approaches and strategies have emerged and are discussed below. Successful approaches include:

- preventing HIV-based discrimination;
- promoting HIV knowledge and awareness, tolerance, and compassion;
- increasing involvement and visibility of people living with HIV;
- scaling up treatment;
- prohibiting discrimination against populations most at risk;
- empowering the community among populations most at risk.

Preventing HIV-based discrimination

Legal protections against HIV discrimination are an essential prerequisite for a sound national HIV response. A large majority of countries (67%) report that laws and regulations are in place to protect people living with HIV from discrimination. Namibia's 2008 report to UNAIDS indicates that, following advocacy by the AIDS Law Unit, the Namibian parliament included HIV as a prohibited basis for discrimination in the country's Labour Bill passed in 2007. Laws in the Bahamas, Malawi, South Africa, and Zimbabwe prohibit mandatory HIV testing as a condition of private employment (Gable et al., 2007). Cambodia, Guyana, and other countries have laws specifying the right of people living with HIV to equal access to high-quality health care (Gable et al., 2007). However, the degree to which these laws are enforced or

Measuring stigma

As with gender inequality, a challenge to effective action to reduce stigma historically has been the absence of agreed methods for measuring stigma.

In more than 10 studies conducted over eight years, the Horizons project demonstrated that stigma and discrimination can be recognized and measured in widely diverse settings in Latin America, Asia and Africa. Focusing both on people who experienced stigma and also on "the stigmatizers", Horizons developed a practical conceptual framework that applies in different cultural settings. This framework recognizes that people living with HIV struggle with internalized stigma (self-stigma), perceived stigma, and enacted stigma (discrimination).

In-depth qualitative research revealed that the problem becomes manageable, measurable, and changeable when it is broken down and addressed in four parts. The first part is to undertake formative research, which involves defining specific attitudes, beliefs and behaviours, and documenting the problem locally. This is essential for part two, which involves helping people to recognize the issue. Horizons' baseline studies showed that people who discriminate and shame people they believe are associated with HIV often do not realize they are doing anything harmful. The third part is to provide accurate information on HIV and create a supportive environment, to counter the fear-based drivers of stigma (e.g. fear of infection through casual contact). The fourth part is to facilitate reflection on the social judgements that are entailed in HV stigma ("blame and shame"), and to confront people with the fact that those judgements are often inaccurate and unfair to the realities of people affected (e.g. assumptions about reckless pleasure-seeking or sexual excess). An essential part of the strategy is to partner with people living with HIV as educators and facilitators. To guide and document these efforts, Horizons' partners developed stable measures of stigmatizing attitudes (recognition, fear, and "blame and shame" components) events (isolation, verbal stigma, loss of identity and status, and loss of access to resources), and tools for measuring improvements in the environment that can be adapted and applied worldwide.

Building on a common knowledge base, other promising tools to track HIV-related stigma have been developed. People Living with HIV Stigma Index, developed by the Global Network of People Living with HIV/AIDS and the International Community of Women Living with HIV/AIDS, is being implemented in the Dominican Republic, and in Asia and the Pacific, with studies in additional areas planned for 2008 (IPPF et al., 2008a; IPPF et al., 2008b). Other indices have been used to measure stigma and discrimination among medical providers and within HIV facilities in Kenya (USAID, 2007b), India (Mahendra et al., 2006), and Ukraine (USAID, 2007a).

In 2007, Tajikistan undertook its first national effort to identify the level and types of HIV-related stigma and discrimination. Tracking HIV-related stigma is consistent with UNAIDS' *Practical guidelines for intensifying HIV prevention*, which encourage policy-makers and programmers to "know your epidemic" and "match your response to the epidemic" (UNAIDS, 2007a).

to which people have access to them has not been documented.

Moreover, in the third decade of the epidemic, one third (33%) of countries still do not report having such laws. Though governments report a significant improvement in the availability of legal services for people living with HIV since 2003, nongovernmental informants indicate that less than half (47%) of countries reported the availability of such services in 2007 (UNGASS Country Progress Reports, 2008) for the nearly 9.6 million in need of treatment. Nongovernmental informants in three quarters of all countries (75%) report the existence of programmes designed to educate and raise awareness among people living with HIV of their human rights (UNGASS Country Progress Reports, 2008). The quality, scale, and coverage of such programmes have not been measured or evaluated.

Prioritizing the reduction of HIV-related stigma and discrimination within a national HIV plan is important, but without a specific effort to track stigma and discrimination over time, progress will be difficult, if not impossible, to measure. However, according to nongovernmental reports, only 33% of countries use performance indicators or benchmarks for the reduction of HIV-related stigma and discrimination (UNGASS Country Progress Reports, 2008;) (Figure 3.5). In early 2007, the Brazilian Government created a mechanism for confidential reporting to authorities of violations of the country's law prohibiting HIV-based discrimination.

Similarly, nongovernmental informants indicate that countries have not systematically implemented mechanisms to report, document, and address cases of discrimination against people living with HIV or populations most at risk (UNGASS Country Progress Reports, 2008) (Figure 3.6).

Civil society can play an important role in enforcing antidiscrimination laws. In Belize, for example, the Alliance Against AIDS celebrated its 10th anniversary of work to reduce HIV-related stigma and discrimination in 2007. Over the last

FIGURE 3.5 Percentage of countries (by region) reporting programmes designed to change societal attitudes of stigmatization associated with HIV and/or using indicators for reduction of HIV-related stigma and discrimination

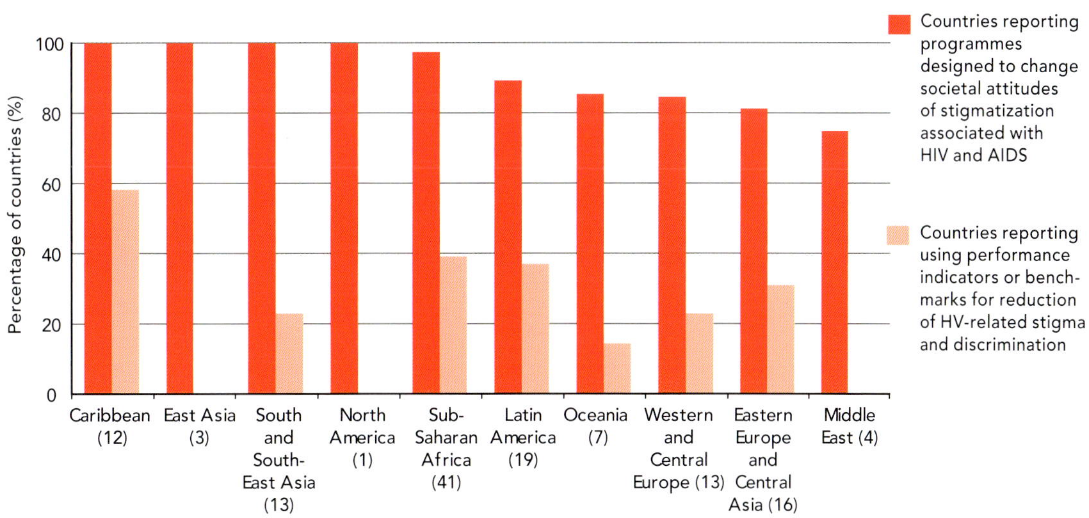

Source: UNGASS Country Progress Reports 2008.

two years, this nongovernmental organization has successfully united a broad civil society coalition to undertake intensified anti-stigma efforts, including a public awareness campaign highlighting continuing discrimination against people living with HIV in health-care settings.

Promoting HIV knowledge and awareness, tolerance, and compassion

Three root causes of stigma and discrimination that can be successfully addressed through programming include:

- lack of awareness and knowledge of stigma and discrimination and their harmful effects;
- fear of acquiring HIV through everyday contact with infected people because of lack of detailed knowledge and information;
- linking people living with HIV with behaviour that is considered improper and immoral (UNAIDS, 2008).

Programmes that address such issues should be an integral part of national strategic plans, and should be supported by other nongovernmental stakeholders. Interactive programmes that foster greater understanding of the harm caused by stigma and discrimination are particularly effective. Active involvement of people living with HIV and of representatives from other affected populations in planning and implementation will help ensure that their needs are addressed.

Because stigma and discrimination are multifaceted, programmes to address these issues need to operate at various levels (individual, family, community, organizational, institutional, government, and legal) and use a range of approaches to engage many different groups. Successful programmes often include the following components: empowerment of people living with HIV, education about HIV, and activities that foster interaction between people living with HIV and key audiences, including policy-makers and high-profile celebrities (UNAIDS, 2008).

In India, researchers worked in partnership with national HIV authorities to implement an anti-stigma programme in three major hospitals where people living with HIV reported having been badly treated. After educating hospital staff

FIGURE 3.6 Percentage of countries (by region) reporting legal protections against discrimination and relevant mechanisms

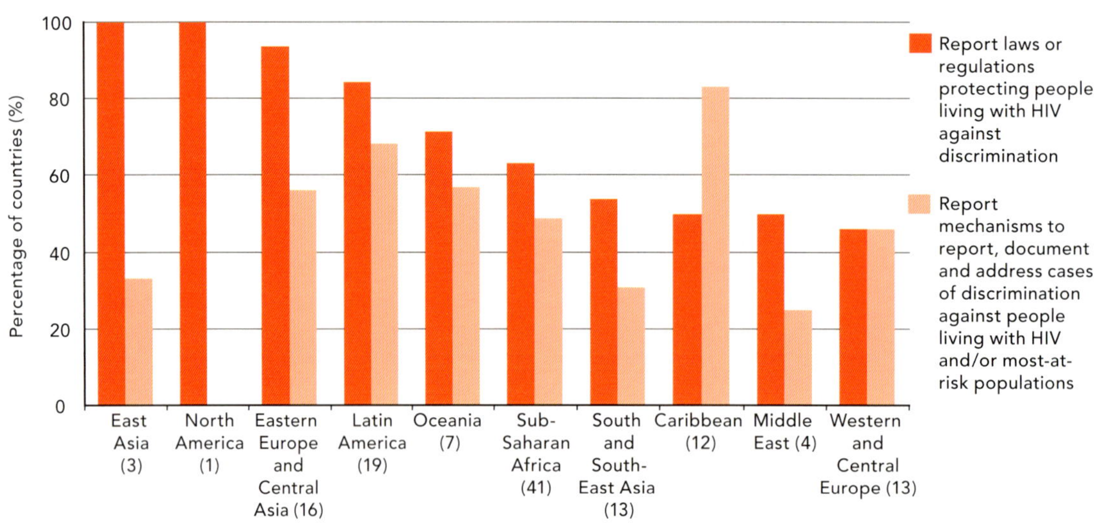

Source: UNGASS Country Progress Reports 2008.

about the presence of stigmatizing attitudes, the programme implemented a series of policies that improved safety for providers (e.g. gloves, ready availability of post-exposure prophylaxis in case of blood exposure) and prohibited discriminatory practices, such as segregation or delay of treatment for patients with HIV. Selected staff members of all levels participated in interactive training workshops for two hours, every other day, for two weeks. All levels of hospital workers (from ward staff to department heads) were provided with information and the opportunity to participate in small-group discussions within the hospital. This multifaceted programme led to significant decreases in stigmatizing attitudes and practices by all levels of health-care workers, and to significant improvements in adherence to guidelines on confidentiality and informed consent for HIV testing and counselling (Population Council, 2006). Comparable improvements in quality of care were achieved in Viet Nam following implementation of an anti-stigma programme in four hospitals (Oanh et al., 2008).

National governments in nearly all countries (98%) report addressing stigma and discrimination as part of their national HIV strategy, including all countries with a generalized HIV epidemic reporting this data (UNGASS Country Progress Reports, 2008). Nongovernmental informants in the vast majority of countries (92%) say programmes are in place to change societal norms to reduce stigma and discrimination. Most of these efforts involve the use of various strategies including the media, school-based education, and personalities speaking out about AIDS (UNGASS Country Progress Reports, 2008). However, the UNGASS indicators do not measure the scale or effectiveness of such programmes.

The media can play a critical role in reducing HIV stigma and discrimination. In 2007, the Zambia National AIDS Network trained more than 300 journalists to report on HIV issues. Ghana's National Campaign Against HIV-Related Stigma, launched in January 2007,

Criminalization of HIV transmission

The recent increase in the use of criminal law in cases of HIV transmission where other, less punitive public health programmes would be more appropriate, is a dangerous trend that fuels the perception that people living with HIV are criminals, and undermines the goal of universal access (UNAIDS, 2002). Laws criminalizing HIV transmission exist at the national or subnational level in at least 36 countries (GNP+ & TGT, 2005; Chan, 2006; Burris, 2007; Klein, 2007; Pearhouse, 2007).

Though such laws may stem from frustration at the continuing high rates of new infections, they are short-sighted strategies that fail to give people any meaningful ways, legal or otherwise, to reduce their vulnerability to HIV. Investment in evidence-informed HIV prevention programmes for both HIV-positive and HIV-negative individuals is a more rational and effective way to reduce infection than implementation of laws criminalizing HIV transmission, which fan the flames of HIV stigma. Where countries retain criminal penalties for transmission, UNAIDS recommends that the criminal law only be applied to cases involving the *intentional* transmission of HIV, that is, where someone intended to transmit HIV, acted with such intent, and did transmit HIV.

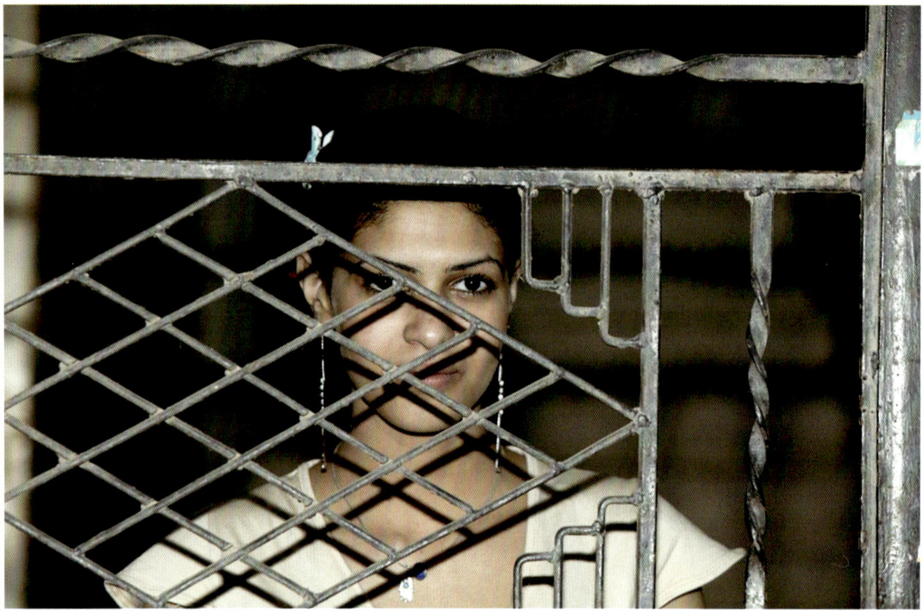

Women and girls become sex workers for many different reasons.

included advertisements on national television and radio that asked, "Who are you to judge? People living with HIV are just like you".

Greater involvement and visibility of people living with HIV

Silence, fear, and shame are some of the factors that enable HIV stigma and discrimination to flourish. To reverse these conditions, it is necessary to:

- promote the visibility of people living with HIV;
- ensure their integral involvement in the planning and implementation of strategies and programmes;
- invest in strategies that empower people living with HIV to work to change the social conditions that facilitate HIV stigma and discrimination.

Networks of people living with HIV can help to foster leadership; also, social mobilization coupled with legal advocacy, can enable social change. In South Africa, for example, the Treatment Action Campaign has used a supporting legal framework and strategic litigation to promote access to HIV treatment (Heywood, 2002; Jones, 2005). In Malawi, the Malawi Network for People Living with AIDS and its many partners in the human rights field create awareness of people's rights and of where to go for redress. In Belize, the Alliance Against AIDS has forged a broad-based alliance to advocate against stigma and discrimination in health-care settings, and to promote education on sexual and reproductive health.

Between 1996 and 2007, the Network of Zambian People Living with AIDS (NZP+) grew from 28 members to more than 50 000. NZP+ operates on an empowerment model, expressly rejecting the notion that its members are vulnerable "patients" who must depend exclusively on charity. Through more than 3000 self-help groups, NZP+ mobilizes its members to combat HIV stigma and to demand better access to high-quality services.

Unfortunately, in only 20% of countries do nongovernmental respondents indicate that civil society organizations have meaningful access to financial support (UNGASS Country Progress Reports, 2008). National governments and international donors should prioritize capacity-building to support networks of people living with

Increasing the visibility and involvement of people living with HIV in the UN system

UN Plus, the advocacy group of UN staff living with HIV, has significantly increased the visibility of people living with HIV in the UN system. Formed in 2005 to provide support and an effective voice for UN staff living with HIV, UN Plus developed an e-workspace to facilitate online discussions on relevant topics. UN Plus meets with decision-makers in the UN system to address key concerns of staff living with HIV. The group has also partnered with UN Cares, the system's HIV workplace programme, to ensure that all staff know the facts about HIV prevention, treatment, care and support, including the UN codes of conduct that require equal treatment and respect for all staff, regardless of their health status.

Hosted by UNAIDS, UN Plus helps other international organizations to establish and strengthen advocacy groups for HIV-positive staff. UN Plus is an example of "UN reform in action", in that it brings together staff from 37 countries in 27 different UN agencies and associated programmes.

HIV. In particular, donors should examine their decision-making processes to assess the degree to which they are helping to empower people living with HIV to lead the response to HIV. An instructive example is the Collaborative Fund for HIV Treatment Preparedness, a joint project of the Tides Foundation and the International Treatment Preparedness Coalition. Funding and policy decisions for the Collaborative Fund are made exclusively by people living with HIV, who work in regional groupings to identify funding priorities and project recipients for treatment preparedness work.

Scaling up treatment

In addition to saving lives and reducing suffering, public investment in antiretroviral treatment helps to mitigate HIV stigma by underscoring the value attached to the lives and well-being of people living with HIV, and reflecting the inclusion of HIV-positive people in the body politic. Scale-up of treatment increases incentives for people to be tested for HIV, which can in turn promote more open public discussion of HIV issues. A longitudinal study in Mombasa, Kenya, found that individuals on antiretroviral drugs had lower levels of internalized stigma 12 months after starting therapy and were more likely to disclose their HIV infection to family members (Kaai et al., 2007).

However, introduction of treatment on its own is unlikely to eradicate negative attitudes towards people living with HIV. In the United States, for example, where HIV treatments have been widely available for more than a decade, 68% of Americans say they would be uncomfortable having an HIV-positive dentist, and 27% would prefer not to work closely with a woman living with HIV (Blumenthal, 2008).

Prohibiting discrimination against populations most at risk

Few countries report having non-discrimination laws or regulations that specify protections for populations most at risk of HIV. Nongovernmental informants in 26% of countries report the existence of laws that protect men who have sex with men; also, anti-discrimination laws for sex workers and injecting drug users are reported in 21% and 16% of countries, respectively (UNGASS Country Progress Reports, 2008). Figure 3.7

illustrates the legal and regulatory environment regarding non-discrimination in countries that reported good-quality coverage data for HIV prevention programmes serving different populations most at risk. Among countries submitting coverage data, the reach of HIV prevention programmes for populations most at risk is generally better in countries with non-discrimination laws in place than countries without such laws.

In addition, an international nongovernmental organization reports that, in 2007, 91 countries (mostly low- and middle-income) had laws prohibiting sexual activity between consenting adults of the same sex (Ottosson, 2007). Seven countries impose the death penalty for men who have sex with another man. However, in recent years, several countries have repealed laws criminalizing same-sex sexual relations, sometimes in response to judicial rulings. In 2003, the Supreme Court of the United States struck down all state anti-sodomy laws on the grounds that they were a human rights violation under the country's constitution. South Africa's post-apartheid constitution specifically prohibits discrimination on the basis of sexual orientation (Gable et al., 2007).

Overall, nongovernmental sources report that a significant minority of countries have laws that interfere with their ability to provide services to injecting drug users (40%), men who have sex with men (32%), and sex workers (45%) (UNGASS Country Progress Reports, 2008).

Most jurisdictions worldwide prohibit the sale and purchase of sex, making protection of the human rights of sex workers (including

FIGURE 3.7 Median percentage of population reached with HIV prevention services within the specified legal environment

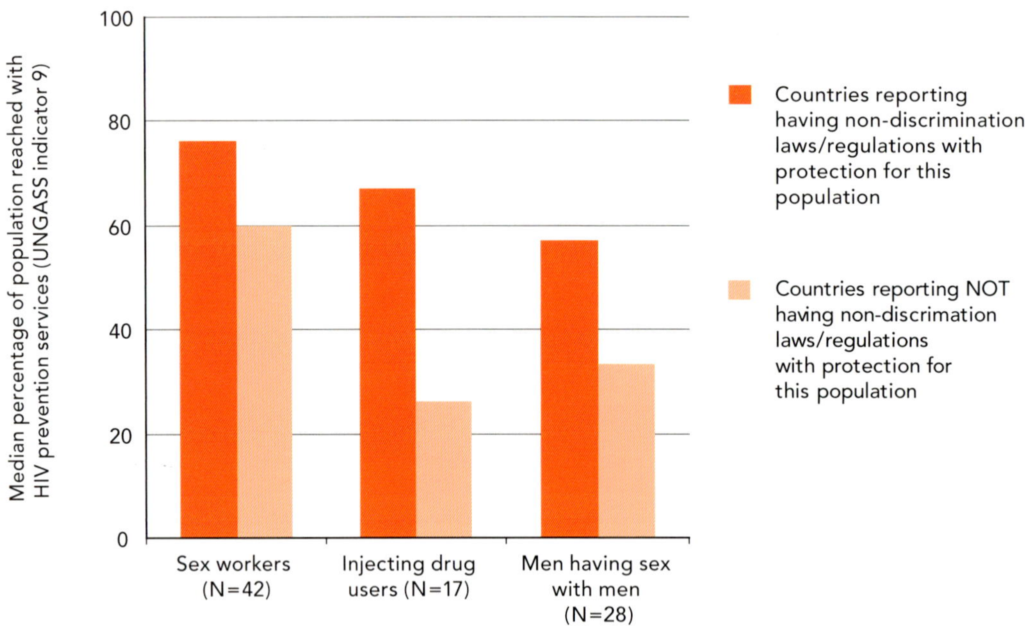

Source: UNGASS Country Progress Reports 2008.*

* Between one third and a half of the countries did not provide information on non-discrimination laws/regulations for most-at-risk populations. Information from NCPI: a different data set (from different countries) from that reflected in Figure 4.10.

Brazil without homophobia

In 2004, the Brazilian Government launched the "Brazil Without Homophobia" programme to reduce stigma and discrimination against people who engage in same-sex sexual activity. Building on the national commitment to address homophobia, the government launched a national initiative in 2008 to address HIV and sexually transmitted infections among men who have sex with men and transgender individuals. The 2008 initiative was prompted by the government's concern over continued high infection rates among men who have sex with men, who accounted for 40% of all reported AIDS diagnoses among males between 2000 and 2005.

The initiative aims to involve civil society—as well as federal, state, and local governments—to address the role of stigma and discrimination in increasing HIV risk and vulnerability of Brazilian men who have sex with men. In mid-2008, the Brazilian President is convening the first National Gay, Lesbian, Bisexual, Transvestite and Transsexual Conference, to promote a national dialogue on homophobia and HIV. The 2008 initiative, which sets forth concrete targets to be achieved by 2011, will also be discussed.

their rights to HIV prevention, treatment, care, and support) a daunting challenge (Gable et al., 2007). Even where sex work is not prohibited, sex workers are often the target of police harassment. Since decriminalizing sex work in 2003, New Zealand has taken steps to promote condom use during sex work (Gable et al., 2007). A key aim of progressive legal reform for sex work is to reduce the stigmatization and harassment of sex workers, and to prevent workers from being placed in situations that threaten their health and safety. Some advocates for legal reform have favourably cited the "Swedish model", which penalizes the purchaser of sex but not the sex worker. However, critics of this approach say that criminal surveillance and official harassment of sex workers continue under such laws (Open Society Institute, 2006a). Involvement and sensitization of police is a critical component of an effective long-term response that aims to increase sex workers' access to HIV prevention, treatment, care, and support.

Hostility towards populations most at risk, often abetted by laws that do not expressly pertain to HIV, may undermine otherwise sound and progressive policy reforms. For example, Ukraine began implementing buprenorphine-based substitution therapy programmes for injecting drug users in 2005, but the continuing high prevalence of stigmatizing and discriminatory attitudes and practices stops many people from using these programmes. Stigmatizing and discriminatory practices include criminalization of drug use and requirements that users be registered in law enforcement agencies and health-care facilities. According to surveys of drug users and sex workers in Ukraine, police officers frequently harass outreach workers from harm-reduction projects, and health-care providers often actively discriminate against drug users. Many Ukrainian drug users avoid seeking treatment for their addiction or their HIV infection due to legal requirements that their names be reported to the police (Human

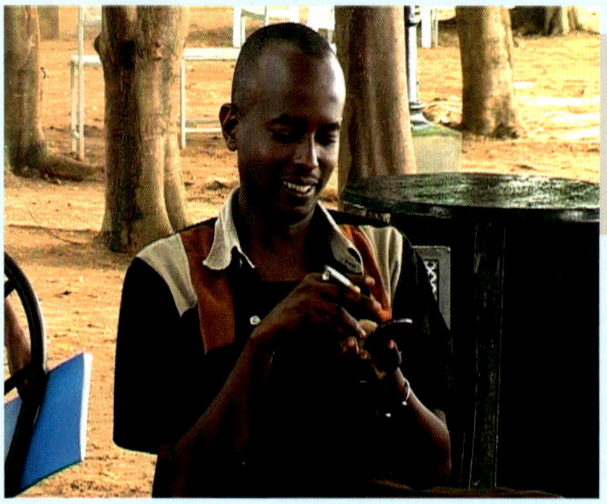

Building community among men who have sex with men in Burundi

Georges Kanuma is the president and founder of the Association for the Respect of Homosexuals' Rights in Burundi

Georges Kanuma was 18 years of age by the time he realised that he must be gay.

But most people in his home town of Bujumbura do not believe that there are African homosexuals. As a result, many gays and lesbians in Burundi suffer secret shame and isolation, and those who are open about their sexual orientation are discriminated against at every level of society.

These problems led Kanuma to start an organization called the Association for the Respect of Homosexuals' Rights (ARDHO), which now has 25 members. "We are here to demonstrate that homosexuality is an evident reality in Burundi," says Kanuma. "We founded ARDHO in order to fight for our social integration, to claim understanding from the society, and to fight against our marginalization, and [against] HIV/AIDS within our community."

In a hostile world, the association provides a supportive community. It also defies taboos by conducting HIV education and safer sex workshops, in which the risks of unprotected anal sex are openly discussed. The association has found that few men who have sex with men are aware of their physical vulnerability to the virus, wrongly believing that they can only be infected by penile–vaginal sex. "We try to organize information sessions on the ways of HIV infection and modes of prevention," says Kanuma. "We meet twice a month and we mobilize our homosexual fellows and our partners on the use of gel and of condoms."

The climate of homophobia seems to extend to other organizations involved in the response to HIV. Apart from UNAIDS, only two nongovernmental organizations support the association. This means that ARDHO remains unregistered, and experiences a continuing shortage of educational materials, condoms, and other resources. Targeted HIV services for men who have sex with men—particularly those who have suffered gender-based violence—are also much in need, but remain a distant dream.

All the members of the association have their own tales to tell about the stigma and discrimination that they have experienced. "Our parents refuse to pay for our school fees for example, and they refuse to take care of us when we are ill," says Flaviana, an association member. "Our brothers and sisters insult us and mock at us… and we suffer from this discrimination even at the work place. The religious people incite the population against us, saying we are a precursory sign of the end of the world."

One member of the group was beaten by his father and thrown out of the family home; another was forced to drop out of school because his teachers believed that he was cursed by God. Kanuma says that this kind of treatment leads to alcohol and drug abuse, which in turn increases the risk of HIV.

Despite all of these challenges, Kanuma and his friends are happy with their lives. "Finally I've got a boyfriend," he says, "I accept my life and I'm proud of it."

Rights Watch, 2006). However, experience in Asia demonstrates that anti-drug laws need not permanently prevent the introduction of harm-reduction programmes. Various countries including China, the Islamic Republic of Iran, and Viet Nam have recently introduced or expanded evidence-informed initiatives to prevent HIV transmission among injecting drug users (see Chapter 4).

As with HIV-based discrimination, enactment of laws prohibiting discrimination against the groups most at risk of HIV exposure should be supported by energetic efforts to enforce these laws. In Peru, for example, the national government has attempted to improve reporting and redress of violations under the country's human rights laws by mapping the determinants of stigma and discrimination against men who have sex with men, sex workers and prisoners, and capacity-building initiatives for subnational ombudsperson offices. However, nongovernmental informants indicate that a majority of countries in most regions lack mechanisms to record, document, and address cases of discrimination experienced by people living with HIV and populations most at risk of HIV. Countries in the Caribbean and Latin American regions are most likely to have such mechanisms in place (UNGASS Country Progress Reports, 2008).

Community empowerment among populations most at risk

Access to social support—sometimes referred to as "social capital"—is vital to reducing vulnerability of marginalized or disempowered groups. In nearly all countries where the HIV epidemic has been reversed, grass-roots community mobilization was at the heart of the national HIV response (Merson, 2008). However, not all countries have a tradition of community engagement and empowerment. In populations whose risk behaviours may be criminalized, there is little capacity to mobilize in response to the epidemic. Despite these obstacles, communities across the globe have organized to address the HIV challenge, often with few resources and at considerable risk to the individuals involved. International donors have been slow to support these efforts, highlighting a serious gap in the global HIV response that should be rectified.

The situation with sex workers exemplifies the need for social support. Hundreds, perhaps thousands, of grass-roots groups and nongovernmental organizations either represent or serve sex workers throughout the world . In general, however, financial support for these groups is scarce, although certain funders have prioritized assistance for community-building, mutual support, and advocacy activities among sex workers (Open Society Institute, 2006b). HIV prevention funding has supported programmes to reach sex workers in all regions, but often such programmes are not run by and for sex workers (Open Society Institute, 2006a). Some HIV-prevention initiatives that focus on sex workers have primarily regarded workers as "vectors of transmission", but the most successful initiatives have empowered sex workers. For example, the Sonagachi project in Calcutta, India, which used an empowerment approach to strengthen health services for sex workers, was associated with significant increases in condom use and declines in incidence of HIV and sexually transmitted infections (Pardasani, 2005; Jenkins & Sarkar, 2007). Unfortunately, the laws of national governments and rules of multilateral organizations often make it difficult to register nongovernmental organizations representing sex workers (Open Society Institute, 2006a).

In high-income countries in the epidemic's early years, gay men were able to build strong community-based responses to HIV based on community infrastructures that existed before the HIV epidemic (Shilts, 1987). Group consciousness and community organization among men who have sex with men are increasing in many countries, but community infrastructures remain weak in most low- and middle-income countries, especially in

FIGURE 3.8 HIV Prevalence by wealth status: men

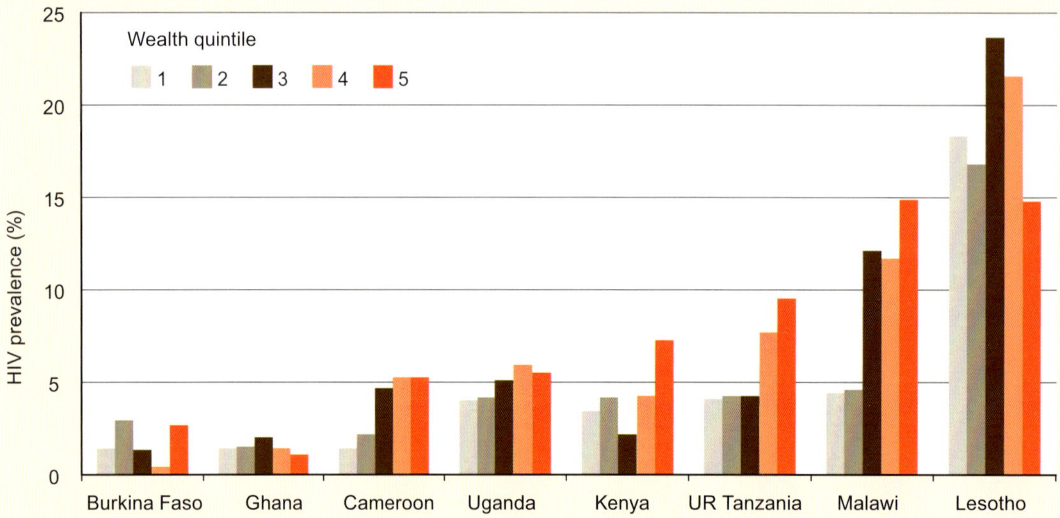

Source: Mishra V, Bignami-Van Assche S, Greener R, Vaessen M, Hong R, Ghys P, Boerma T, Van Assche A, Khan S, Rutstein S, "HIV infection does not disproportionately affect the poorer in sub-Saharan Africa", 2007, AIDS, Vol 21 Supplement 7, November 2007

Poverty, income inequality and vulnerability to HIV

The relationship between socioeconomic status and health is well documented, with higher income individuals generally enjoying better health status than those with lower socioeconomic status. This has been shown to be the case for most measures of health, including nutrition, morbidity and mortality, and for health-care use. Variations in health status often run along a gradient, with individuals in each successive income level having better health than those directly below them (Marmot, 2006; Commission on the Social Determinants of Health, 2007).

HIV has no socioeconomic boundaries; however, the vast majority of people living with HIV in the world are in low- and middle-income countries, and poorer regions of the world bear a substantially greater burden of HIV disease. For example, sub-Saharan Africa—which has one of the highest rates of extreme poverty in the world—is home to just over 10% of the world's population but accounts for more than two thirds (68%) of all people living with HIV (Population Reference Bureau, 2007; UNAIDS, 2007d). More than 40% of the region's population live on less than one US dollar per day (Chen & Revaillon, 2004).

The disproportionate burden of HIV in low-income countries, and the more severe impact of the disease on poor households, often lead to the assumption that HIV is a "disease of poverty", and that poor people are at greater risk for infection. In fact, the relationship between absolute poverty and risk of infection is more nuanced, being also highly dependent on context.

In sub-Saharan Africa, for example, HIV prevalence is highest not in the poorest countries, but in two of the wealthiest—South Africa and Botswana—where prevalence is 18.8% and 24.1%, respectively (UNAIDS, 2007b). In this same region, a recent analysis of eight national surveys found greater HIV prevalence among adults with higher levels of wealth than among those with the lowest levels of wealth (Mishra et al., 2007) (Figure 3.8). This finding is tied to the fact that wealthier and better educated individuals tend to have greater sexual autonomy and higher rates of partner change (due to their greater mobility) and greater likelihood of living in cities (where HIV prevalence is generally higher) (Gillespie, Kadiyala & Greener, 2007). These findings highlight the importance of prevention strategies that target all socioeconomic strata.

Some researchers speculate that this dynamic may be shifting in later stages of the epidemic, because wealthier individuals are more likely to have access to HIV prevention information and condoms, and to adopt behaviour changes (Lopman et al., 2007). A recent review of the relationship between educational attainment and risk of HIV documents a shift over time towards higher HIV prevalence among the least educated in sub-Saharan Africa (Hargreaves et al., 2008).

Although poorer individuals, as a group, are not necessarily at greater risk of infection, there are situations where the combination of gender and poverty confers risk. For example, food insecurity is associated with increased chances of risky sexual practices among women, including increased likelihood of selling sex for money or resources, and of engaging in unprotected or intergenerational sex (Weiser et al., 2007). Women who are poor or economically dependent on their male partners may also be less likely to avoid or leave a relationship that threatens them with infection.

Other studies point to a potential relationship between income inequality and HIV risk, with greater risk (as measured at the population level by HIV prevalence) in countries with more income inequality (Gillespie, Kadiyala & Greener, 2007; Piot, Greener & Russell, 2007). The exact pathways through which income inequality contributes to HIV risk and vulnerability—and, indeed, whether such a causal relationship exists—are still not fully understood. However, some researchers suggest that income inequality may reflect the level of social cohesion in a society, with greater income disparities reflecting greater social stratification between socioeconomic groups. Additional subnational and community-level research is required before sound policy formulation in this regard would be possible.

settings where homosexuality remains highly stigmatized. In 2005, funding for lesbian, gay, bisexual, transgender, and intersex organizations in low- and middle-income countries totalled less than US$ 10.5 million (Funders for Lesbian and Gay Issues, 2007). In 2005, the average annual budget for such organizations in low- and middle-income countries was US$ 7600. In a global mapping exercise, Latin America accounted for more than half (54%) of lesbian, gay, bisexual, transgender, and intersex organizations identified in low- and middle-income countries (Funders for Lesbian and Gay Issues, 2007).

Among drug users facing the world of HIV initiatives, the slogan has become "Nothing About Us without Us" (Canadian HIV/AIDS Legal Network 2008). Community empowerment initiatives can help drug users, and their advocates and service providers, to overcome institutional barriers to service access. In the Philippines, for example, early support for a peer-based initiative of drug users from the International HIV/AIDS Alliance and the Philippine NGO Support Programme was leveraged to obtain longer-tem support from the Global Fund. The project trains injecting drug users as harm reduction advocates, and promotes alliances with local government officials. In addition to providing sterile needles, and condoms, the project has formed a peer educator group that has helped bring drug users out of the shadows, and has increased public awareness and acceptance of harm reduction services. Although quantitative data on the project are still limited, the number of local 'shooting galleries' has dramatically declined since the project began, and the visibility of current and former drug users has significantly increased.

Leadership for change

It has long been recognized that the response to HIV must be both evidence-informed and rights-based. In this regard, the HIV epidemic has shown time and again that effective responses are those that also empower individuals and groups through the realization of their human rights—the rights to education, expression, privacy, health, and gender equality, and the rights to freedom from discrimination and gender-based violence. But changing harmful gender norms to reduce vulnerability to HIV, and eliminating stigma and discrimination, will require bold leadership on the part of many stakeholders. Issues that are often considered private or secretive must be brought out into the open and discussed, and laws, government policies, and programme priorities may need to change. In particular, women, young people, people living with HIV, and key populations at risk—particularly men who have sex with men, sex workers, and injecting drug users—need to have a more meaningful role in collaborative decision-making, planning, and continued monitoring of progress towards the goal of universal access.

There is an urgent need to develop greater technical capacity on issues of gender and human rights, to move from conceptual support for a rights-based approach to practical implementation of such an approach. The adoption of policies to address these societal level causes of HIV vulnerability is an important first step. However, it is ultimately the allocation of sufficient resources and the use of proven programmes (including social change communication strategies to change social norms) that will determine success.

Implementation will require a long-term view of the epidemic, recognizing that the impact of some programmes will only be measurable over time. Existing efforts to integrate HIV programming into broader poverty alleviation and development frameworks must also be accelerated. There is also important synergy to be gained from stronger partnerships between those working in the field of HIV and others working on human rights, including the rights of women and children.

At the national level, the prioritization of vulnerable populations may lead to calls for shifts in funding between programme areas or populations, and for the implementation of strategies that not only have an impact on HIV but also on society as a whole, and may therefore be considered politically controversial. However, the use of HIV funding on strategies that do not go to the core of HIV vulnerability and risk among women, young people, people living with HIV, and key populations at risk is inefficient, and it is this approach that should be considered most controversial.

Emerging evidence from the field has helped to identify effective strategies for reducing gender inequality and HIV-related stigma and discrimination. These factors are outside the direct control of the individual, but have a profound effect on HIV risk and vulnerability. In the past few years, understanding of the complex association between HIV, income inequality, and poverty has also evolved. More research and additional models of successful programmes are needed, but the time for action is now.

Social change communication

Social change communication involves the strategic use of advocacy, communication, and social mobilization strategies to facilitate or accelerate social change. In the context of HIV, Social change communication strategies can help to change underlying social attitudes and behaviours that contribute to HIV risk and vulnerability.

Successful communication programmes blend mass media approaches, community engagement strategies, and empowerment strategies with other forms of informational and motivational communication and advocacy. The goal of Social change communication is to act as a catalyst for action at the individual, community, and policy levels.

Social change communication programmes work. They have been rigorously evaluated and have been shown to make significant and durable change in deeply rooted practices. In August 2007, UNAIDS held a Technical Consultation on Social Change Communication to develop a better understanding of the role of Social change communication in the global response to HIV (UNAIDS, 2007e). In 2008, UNAIDS will develop practical guidance and technical support on Social change communication for national AIDS programmes.

Source: Based on a UNAIDS definition of social change communication developed with a group of international stakeholder during a Technical Consultation in August 2007. The meeting report and a background discussion paper are available online at http://www.unaids.org.

Evidence for action

Are the right actions being taken?

- A total of 80% of countries specifically address women as a component of their national HIV strategy, and 83% of countries report having a policy to ensure equal access for women and men to HIV services.
- About two thirds (67%) of countries report have laws protecting people with HIV from discrimination.
- A majority (67%) of countries report having laws, regulations, or policies that provide protection against anti-discrimination to people living with HIV.

Are the right actions being undertaken in the right manner?

- Only about half (53%) of countries report budget allocations specifically devoted to HIV-related programmes for women and girls.
- Less than half (47%) of countries report supporting the provision of legal services to assist people living with HIV in enforcing their rights under anti-discrimination protections.
- Nearly two thirds (63%) of countries report having laws, regulations, or policies in place that impede access to HIV prevention, treatment, care, and support among populations most at risk.

Have these actions been sufficiently scaled up to make a difference?

- Civil society organizations have meaningful access to financial assistance in one in five countries.
- Few countries have legal protections for the populations most at risk of HIV infection. A total of 26% of countries report having laws that protect men who have sex with men, 21% have anti-discrimination laws for sex workers, and fewer than one fifth (16%) protect injecting drug users from discrimination.
- There is still insufficient data on the scale, quality, coverage, or impact of the programmes reported by countries above.

Source: UNGASS Country Progress Reports, 2008.

Camp Goodtime

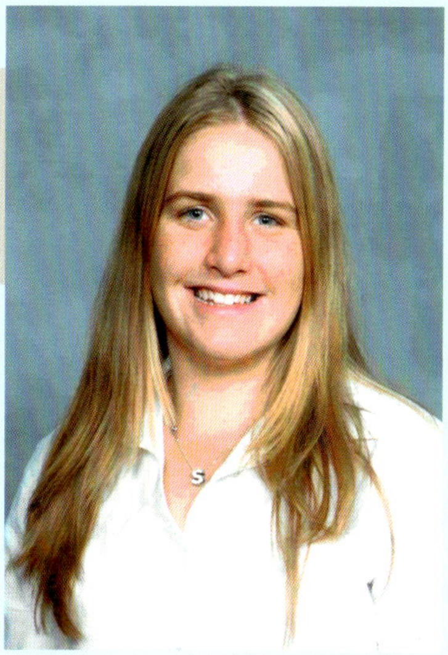

"I'm not like other schoolgirls", says Stephanie, an Australian teenager living with HIV. "Well, I am... but I also have to deal with secrecy, discrimination, uneducated attitudes at school, what to tell my negative friends, and the constant fear of being found out..."

Stephanie was born with HIV when Australia was in the grip of terror about the condition. Although a first-rate medical system has kept her healthy and strong, she has suffered at the hands of an otherwise caring community.

"For any teenager, high school is hard, but the cloud of secrecy looms over my head every day", she says. "A fairly normal activity for an Aussie teenager—sleeping over at a friends' house—demands more consideration than simply packing pyjamas and a toothbrush. It becomes a major issue, with having to hide medications from friends and their family."

At school, Stephanie has experienced the full extent of people's fear and ignorance about HIV—from cruel jokes to active discrimination. At her previous high school she disclosed her HIV status to the Vice Principal and was told that unless she informed the whole school, she would have to leave. So she left—but not before the staff was informed of her HIV status.

"There are many heart-breaking stories of little kids being humiliated because of a disease they inherited. But the HIV teenagers of Australia are not going down without a fight", she says. "The very fact that people like me are still here shows that people with HIV are some of the strongest people in the world... "

There is only one brief period in the year when Stephanie does not have to fear discrimination: that is when she goes to Camp Goodtime, the annual national camp for HIV-positive children and their families. "There is nothing like the bond between positive teenagers. When we get together there is no stopping the laughter, tears, support, and stories of past camps and members who have died", she says.

The camp means more to positive teenagers than their medicine. "Camp Goodtime means acceptance, love... and the power of being able to speak freely, without fear", she says.

Stephanie feels that she owes her survival to the camp, and to the support and strength she has received from her mother and HIV-positive friends. An inspired mentor who introduced her to a support group for HIV-positive women also helped her define her role as an advocate for teenagers living with HIV. "She opened my eyes to making the change for yourself instead of waiting for someone else to."

When she was 15 years old Stephanie addressed a group of HIV-positive women at the International Women's Summit. She challenged them with the words "My name is Stephanie. I have lived through the war of HIV and I have something to say to the world. Do you?"

Preventing new HIV infections: the key to reversing the epidemic

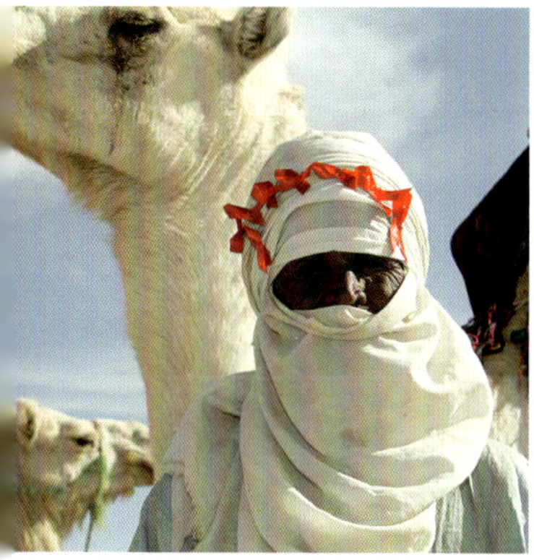

4

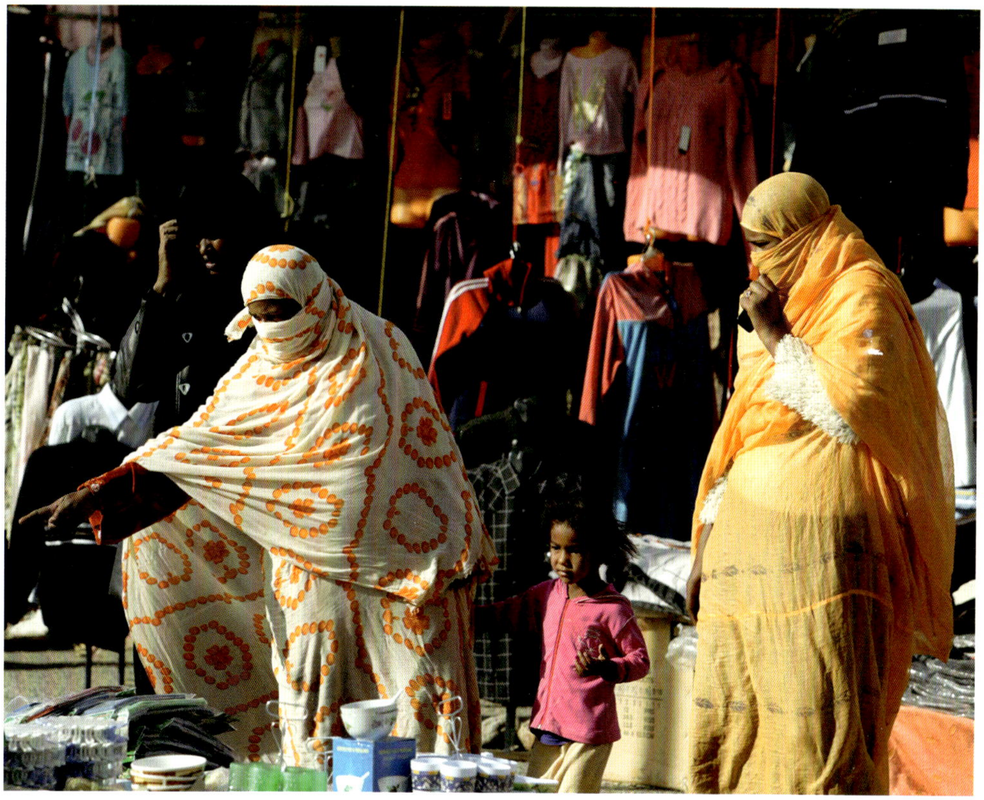

Chapter 4

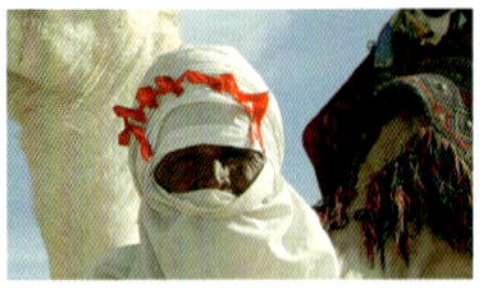

FIGURE 4.1 Selected events related to HIV prevention

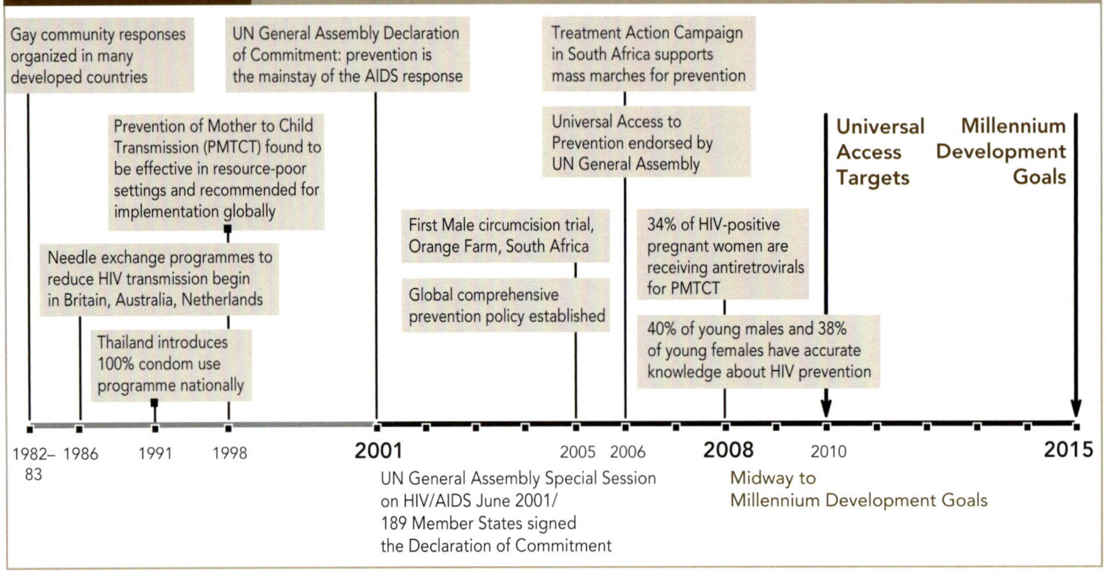

Key findings

- The global HIV epidemic cannot be reversed, and gains in expanding treatment access cannot be sustained, without greater progress in reducing the rate of new HIV infections.
- Existing prevention strategies can be effective in reducing the risk of HIV exposure, but prevention programmes, especially in countries with concentrated epidemics, fail to reach many people at high risk of exposure to HIV, including a majority of men who have sex with men and injecting drug users.
- Young people aged 15–24 account for 45% of all new HIV infections in adults, and many young people still lack accurate, complete information on how to avoid exposure to the virus.
- In the last two years, major progress has been made to expand access to services to prevent mother-to-child transmission. This progress suggests that in future sufficient financing, commitment, and strategic action could render this mode of HIV transmission rare.
- Prevention efforts should become more strategically focused on sexual partnerships, especially those that increase the risk of HIV exposure; these include serodiscordant relationships and multiple concurrent partners.
- Prevention programmes will not be optimally effective unless they are supported by effective initiatives to address the social factors that increase risk and vulnerability, including gender inequality, HIV stigma and discrimination, and the social marginalization of the populations most at risk of HIV exposure.
- Sustaining prevention gains represents one of the great challenges in HIV prevention. To maintain a robust prevention response, countries need to nurture a "prevention movement", build the human and technical capacity needed to sustain prevention efforts, and work to stimulate greater demand for prevention services.

The HIV epidemic cannot be reversed without strong, sustained success in preventing new HIV infections. HIV prevention remains—in the words of the *Declaration of Commitment on HIV/AIDS*—"the mainstay of the response". Treatment access has steadily expanded in recent years, but efforts to prevent new HIV infections have lagged. While 87% of countries with targets for universal access have established goals for HIV treatment, only about 50% of these countries have targets for key HIV-prevention strategies.

Between 2005 and 2007, substantial new funding became available for HIV-related programmes in low- and middle-income countries; and, as the discussion below reveals, access to certain components of comprehensive HIV prevention improved. However, at the halfway mark towards the deadline for the Millennium Development Goals, many people at risk of HIV infection lack meaningful access to evidence-informed prevention services.[1]

This chapter focuses on HIV prevention activities. It complements Chapter 3, which describes the societal factors that must be addressed to maximize the impact of HIV-prevention programmes. After briefly summarizing the evidence base for available HIV prevention tools and strategies, this chapter provides information on programme coverage and identifies key actions required to amplify the strategic impact of HIV prevention efforts. A closing section examines the challenge of sustaining gains in HIV prevention, emphasizing the need to build national and local prevention capacities, and to create a broad-based social movement that generates ongoing demand for prevention services.

The evidence base for HIV prevention

Extensive experience in diverse regions has demonstrated the effectiveness of a broad range of HIV-prevention strategies. Effective strategies exist to prevent every mode of HIV transmission—sexual, bloodborne (including through injecting drug use or in health-care settings), and mother-to-child (see Wegbreit, 2006). Available HIV prevention approaches include strategies to:

- change sexual and drug-using behaviours;
- promote correct and consistent use of male and female condoms;
- reduce the number of sexual partners;
- improve the management of sexually transmitted infections;
- broaden access to HIV testing and counselling;
- increase access to harm-reduction programmes for drug users;
- promote medical male circumcision; and
- ensure effective infection control in health care settings (UNAIDS, 2005).[2]

In recent years, male circumcision has been confirmed as a potentially valuable technology for HIV risk reduction in men. Other recent developments include the emergence of a cluster of HIV prevention strategies centred on antiretroviral treatment; strategies include prevention of mother-to-child transmission, post-exposure prophylaxis, experimental regimens for pre-exposure prophylaxis[3], and probable secondary-prevention benefits from therapeutic administration of antiretroviral drugs. Prevention efforts are most effective when they involve strategic combinations of evidence-informed strategies that meet the specific needs of people at risk. Bringing combination HIV prevention to scale would avert more than half of all new HIV infections projected to occur between 2005 and 2015 (Stover et al., 2006).

---

1 Evidence-informed prevention strategies are those having a basis in sound scientific evidence. Factors relevant to national decision-making on HIV prevention strategies include not only evidence but also appropriateness, cost, feasibility, and equity.

2 Observational studies indicate that—in countries that implemented HIV prevention programmes in the early years of the epidemic—population-based behaviour changes lowered HIV incidence by an average of 50%–90% (Auerbach, Hayes & Kandathil, 2006).

3 Trials for eight different experimental approaches to pre-exposure prophylaxis were either under way or planned as of March 2008. Two of these trials are studying topical formulations, including CAPRISA 004, the first microbicide trial of a product incorporating antiretroviral drugs.

Likewise, clear guidelines have been established for national identification of prevention priorities. Essential programmes required for HIV prevention have been identified, ranging from tailored programmes to prevent sexual and drug-related transmission to strategies to protect the safety of national blood supplies. Normative guidance is available to countries on essential policy actions to support national HIV prevention strategies (UNAIDS, 2005).

Selection of the particular combination of prevention strategies best suited to national conditions should be guided by evidence. Countries are advised to "know your epidemic and your response". Using a strong and constantly improving evidence base, countries are able to:

- identify the behaviours and settings linked to HIV transmission, and populations most at risk of exposure to HIV;
- understand key epidemiological trends;
- assess the scope, scale, quality, and focus of prevention programmes;
- address contextual factors that increase risk and vulnerability to HIV; and
- close gaps in access to critical prevention services (see UNAIDS, 2005; UNAIDS, 2007a).

Maximizing the strategic impact of HIV prevention

In previous years, the *Report on the global AIDS epidemic* has summarized the evidence for the effectiveness of the individual components of comprehensive HIV prevention (see UNAIDS, 2006a). The remainder of this chapter focuses on a selected number of high-impact steps for maximizing the impact of existing HIV prevention approaches. By using evidence-informed HIV prevention more strategically—and by finally addressing many key issues that have been ignored or under-prioritized—accelerated progress can be achieved towards the ultimate goal of reversing the global epidemic by 2015, as stated in Millennium Development Goal 6.

Frank, accurate, and comprehensive HIV prevention programmes for young people

The global epidemic cannot be reversed without sustained success in reducing new HIV infections among young people. Nearly half the world's population is under 25 (UNFPA, 2006). Globally, it is estimated that young people under age 25 accounted for an estimated 45% of all new HIV infections in adults in 2007.

Addressing inadequate knowledge of HIV

While knowledge alone is often insufficient to produce long-lasting behaviour change, an accurate understanding of the risks of HIV and how to prevent exposure is a prerequisite to risk reduction. Tragically, many young people lack basic knowledge about HIV prevention. Survey data from 64 countries indicate that 40% of males and 38% of females aged 15–24 had accurate and comprehensive knowledge about HIV and about how to avoid transmission (UNGASS Indicator 13).[4] Although this represents an improvement, especially for females, over 2005 knowledge levels, when 37% of males and 28% of females were found to have a basic knowledge of HIV, knowledge levels in 2007 are still well below the *Declaration of Commitment's* goal of ensuring comprehensive HIV knowledge in 95% of young people by 2010.

While more than 70% of young men know that condoms can protect against HIV exposure, only 55% of young women cite condom use as an effective prevention strategy (UNGASS Indicator 13). In Somalia, only 4% of young women (ages 15–24) report accurate knowledge of HIV, and only 11% of adult females are aware that condoms can prevent HIV transmission.

[4] This indicator uses population-based survey data (preferably from the last two years) to assess young people's ability to correctly identify ways of preventing sexual HIV transmission (e.g. condom use) and to reject major misconceptions about HIV transmission (e.g. that HIV may be transmitted by mosquito bites). Young people are asked five pertinent questions and are deemed to have accurate and comprehensive knowledge of HIV if they can answer all five questions accurately.

Does national leadership on HIV prevention make a difference? The case of Namibia

In recent years, the Government of Namibia has taken steps to strengthen the country's HIV response, which is guided by a five-year strategic plan that has an overriding goal of reducing HIV incidence. Over the last two years, the country more than doubled its domestic spending on HIV programmes; it has also been successful in mobilizing substantially greater external support. In 2007, the country enacted legislation to stimulate and guide greater effort on HIV by a broad array of national ministries and sectors.

These efforts are bearing fruit in the form of improved coverage for essential prevention initiatives, and favourable behavioural and epidemiological trends. Life-skills based HIV education is now taught in 79% of secondary schools, a national campaign has targeted HIV risk and alcohol abuse, and more than 25 million male condoms are distributed for free each year by the public sector (equivalent to seven condoms per male aged 15–49). Namibia has the highest rate of HIV testing of the 38 countries recently surveyed by the Demographic and Health Survey programme, with 29% of women and 18% of men aged 15–49 having received the results of an HIV test within the last 12 months (MEASURE DHS, 2008). Levels of knowledge about HIV and condom use have increased, while rates of sex before the age of 15 and sex with more than one partner in the last 12 months have decreased (Figure 4.2). Adult HIV prevalence appears to have stabilized, while HIV prevalence in young women attending antenatal clinics declined from 18% in 2003 to 14% in 2007.

FIGURE 4.2 Namibia: HIV related knowledge and behaviour in the general population, 2000–2006

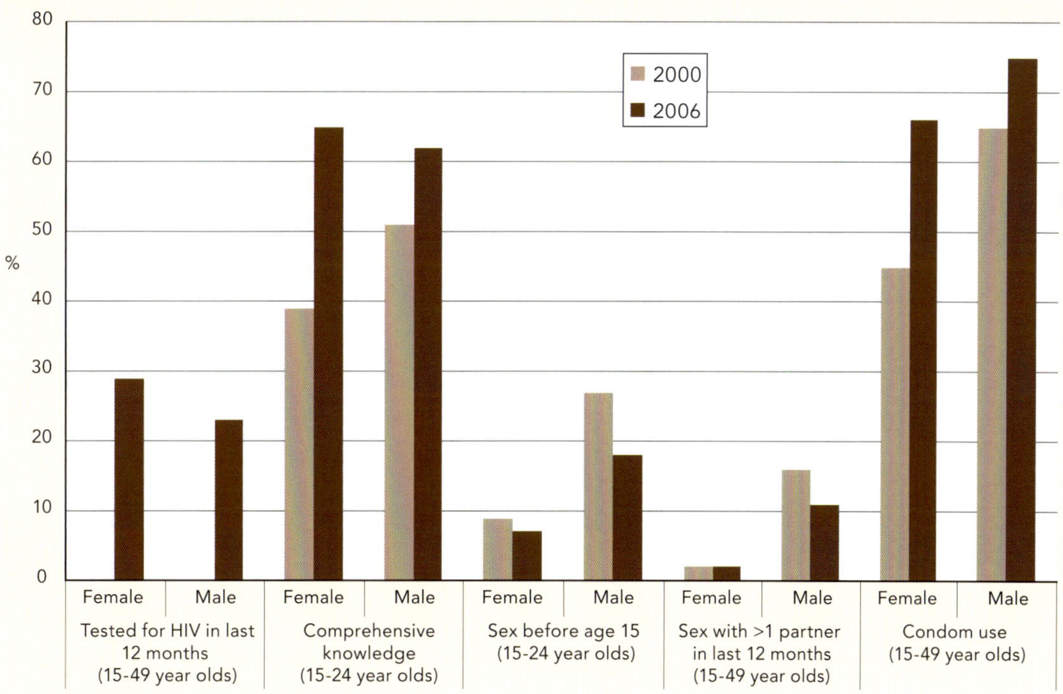

Source: Namibia Country Progress Report 2008.

Tailoring prevention efforts to diverse settings

Countries with different epidemic patterns will inevitably require different national strategies for implementing effective HIV prevention programmes. HIV epidemics have been classified as low-level, concentrated, generalized, or hyperendemic, as outlined below.

- In a low-level epidemic, HIV infection may have existed for many years but has never spread to significant levels in any subpopulation.
- In a concentrated epidemic, HIV has spread rapidly in a defined subpopulation, but is not well established in the general population. This pattern suggests active networks of risk within the subpopulation. The future course of the epidemic is determined by the frequency and nature of links between highly infected subpopulations and the general population.
- In a generalized epidemic, HIV is firmly established in the general population. Although subpopulations at high risk may continue to contribute disproportionately to the spread of HIV, sexual networking in the general population is sufficient to sustain an epidemic, independent of subpopulations at higher risk of infection.
- In a hyperendemic country, the overall prevalence of adult HIV infection exceeds 15%.
- Of 135 low- and middle-income countries, UNAIDS estimates that 97 countries have low-level or concentrated epidemics and 38 have generalized epidemics, of which 7 are categorized as hyperendemic.

In countries with low-level and concentrated epidemics, the central prevention focus will be on populations at greatest risk. Unfortunately, 69% of countries with low-level or concentrated epidemics report having laws, regulations, or policies that pose barriers to use of HIV services for populations most at risk. Countries should work to repeal these legal barriers and to actively promote prevention access. To reduce the likelihood that a low-level or concentrated epidemic will become generalized, prevention programmes should also focus on potential epidemiological bridges, such as the sex partners of injecting drug users or men who have sex with men.

In generalized epidemics, where infection extends beyond discrete populations at elevated risk, greater investment is required in broader, population-based interventions, such as mass media, school-based education, community mobilization, workplace interventions, and strategies to alter social norms. In contrast, hyperendemic countries require broad-based societal mobilization to address the sociocultural and economic practices that contribute to unsafe sexual behaviour. This expanded focus should complement intensive knowledge and behaviour change interventions, to reduce the number of people who have sex with a nonregular partner or multiple concurrent sexual partnerships. Access to medical male circumcision should also be scaled up (UNAIDS, 2007a).

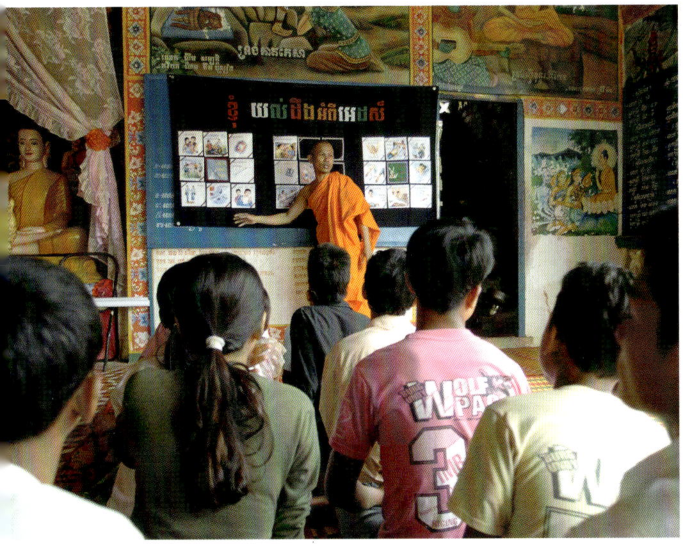

A Buddhist monk conducts an HIV education session with local youth. Potential sources of HIV prevention services for young people are numerous, including schools, peers, media, parents and religious leaders.

Effective strategies for reaching young people

Numerous channels exist to educate young people about HIV, to ensure their access to prevention commodities and health services, and to encourage them to take steps to avoid HIV transmission.[5]

- *School-based programmes.* In a meta-analysis of 22 studies of school-based prevention education programmes in low- and middle-income countries, 16 programmes that involved curriculum-based, adult-led interventions had positive effects on age of first sex, frequency of sex, number of partners, use of condoms or contraceptives, and frequency of unprotected sex (WHO et.al., 2006b; Biddlecom et al., 2007).[6]
- *Community-based programmes for young people who are not in school.* Evaluation studies have determined that strong behavioural results may be achieved among out-of-school

FIGURE 4.3 Comprehensive knowledge of HIV among young people (ages 15–24), 1999–2007

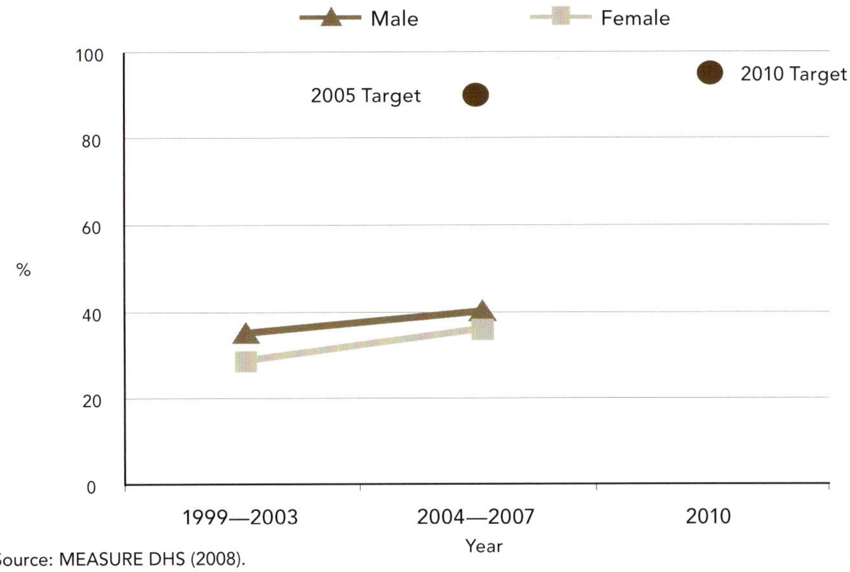

Source: MEASURE DHS (2008).

---

5 For a recent summary of the evidence of behaviour change programmes focused on young people, see World Association for Sexual Health, 2008.

6 Kenya and Zimbabwe—countries where significant positive changes in sexual behaviours among young people have been reported in recent years—made major early investments in school-based HIV prevention programmes.

FIGURE 4.4 Comprehensive knowledge of HIV among young people, by type of question

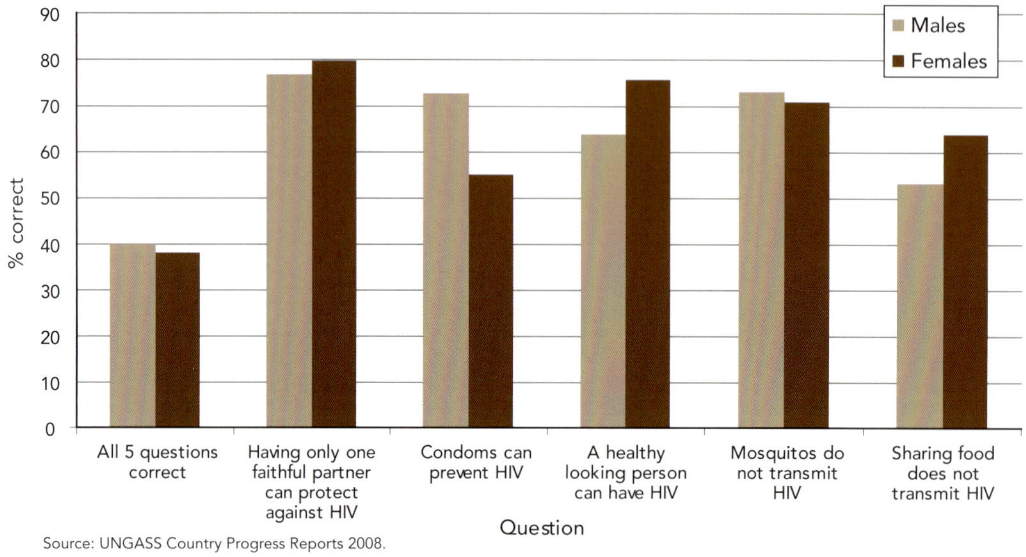

Source: UNGASS Country Progress Reports 2008.

youth, especially when they are delivered by established youth service organizations (Maticka-Tyndale & Brouillard-Coyle, 2006).

- *Mass media.* According to a meta-analysis, five of six youth-oriented media campaigns in various low- and middle-income countries had a measurable impact on HIV-related risk behaviours (National Research Council, et.al., 2005).
- *Youth services.* Youth services provide a "hook" to connect young people with HIV prevention information and services. Such services also address factors that may increase young people's risk of exposure to HIV, such as unemployment, poverty, or lack of access to health care (Akhmedov et al., 2007).[7]

Many countries are failing to make use of available channels for delivering HIV prevention information and services to young people. Most countries (89%) indicate having integrated HIV education into their secondary school curricula, but only 65% address HIV education in primary schools, with countries in sub-Saharan Africa being most likely to do so (Figure 4.5). National governments in 67% of countries with generalized epidemics report having implemented school-based HIV education in most or all districts in need, and 42% have put in place HIV prevention programmes for out-of-school youth in most or all districts in need. Nongovernmental responses indicated even lower levels of implementation, at 51% and 28%, respectively (UNGASS Country Progress Reports, 2008). This low level of implementation is reflected in the paucity of data on this intervention. Of the 147 countries that submitted national progress reports in 2008, only 34 reported on the percentage of schools that taught life-skills based HIV

[7] Young people are over-represented among the world's poor (ILO, 2006). Poverty or the lack of decent work opportunities may deprive young people of a sense of purpose or belonging, and potentially subject them to coercive sex and other conditions that increase their risk of HIV exposure.

prevention in the last academic year. Among the reporting countries, this intervention was, on average, provided in less than 40% of schools. In addition, nongovernmental informants in 36 countries (28%) state that they have laws, policies, or regulations that actually impede young people's access to HIV prevention and other services (UNGASS Country Progress Reports, 2008).

All young people have the right to be educated about how to avoid HIV transmission, but the need for HIV-prevention services is especially pressing for those who are particularly at risk of HIV exposure. This includes young people experiencing displacement, migration, poverty, or imprisonment; and sex workers, injecting drug users, and men who have sex with men.

Providing accurate, comprehensive HIV prevention for young people

A central weakness of many prevention initiatives for young people is that they do not speak frankly or provide the accurate, comprehensive information that young people need. Many countries that require HIV education in schools have curricula that prioritize abstinence-focused programming, discouraging forthright discussions about condoms and safer sex. However, no study in low- and middle-income countries has found this approach to be effective, and studies in the United States indicate that youth-oriented prevention programmes that exclusively promote abstinence do not reduce the risk of HIV infection (Underhill, Montgomery & Operario, 2007).

FIGURE 4.5 Percentage of countries with AIDS education as part of the school curriculum

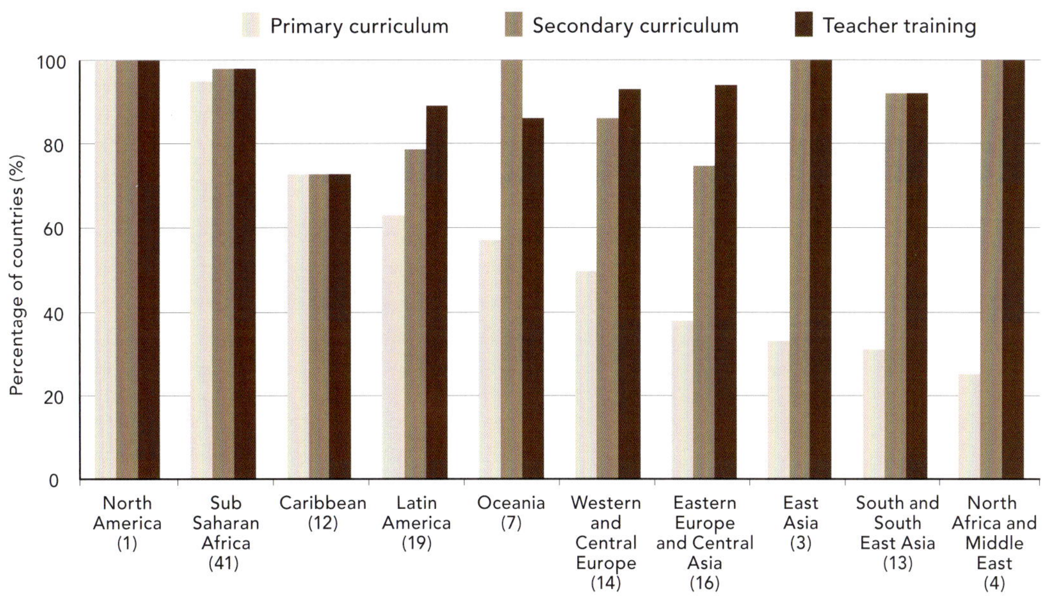

Source: UNGASS Country Progress Reports 2008.

Educating young peers about HIV

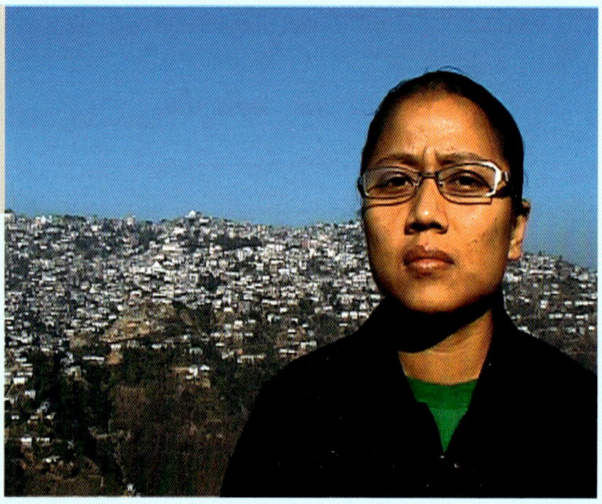

Champuii (24) is a former drug user and peer educator in Aizwal, Mizoram, India

Champuii's troubles began early. Abandoned by her parents when she was just six years old, she was brought up by foster parents, but she never felt at home. By early adolescence, she was drinking alcohol, and before long she was using hard drugs.

"Since I did drugs, my life became upside down", she says. "My schoolteachers expelled me and when my parents knew that I was into such things they kicked me out." With no place to live, the streets became her home, and her drug-using friends became her only family. She began selling drugs to support herself and her habit.

Champuii also struggled with her sexual identity. "My parents forbade me to wear boys' clothes and play with boyish toys", she says. "They forced me to live a girl's life. But that didn't convince me. When I was out of the house, it was a young man's life that I led."

She was arrested many times and sent to rehabilitation centres and camps. The last time she was put in lockup she realized that her days were numbered. Her body and mind were rapidly deteriorating, and she became afraid she was going to die. A painful sore on her leg kept her awake all night. By morning she had decided that she would change her life, and stop taking drugs. "At the last minute, I said, why should I die of drugs? This life has been given to me by God, so I should give it back to him", she says.

Champuii has not taken drugs for over two years. She works as a peer educatorunder UNODC for CHARCA, a local nongovernmental organization, offering support, information, and advice to drug users who are at risk of HIV. She also works with local youth groups and associations. Champuii always speaks about her own experiences. "This gives people faith in me", she says. "They are able to tell me their problems and I can give them counselling. That is the advantage of being open about my life."

Champuii and the other peer educators use music to reach out to young people. She gives regular performances in church and has also sung on local television. Each time she uses the opportunity to educate listeners about drug use and HIV.

She has come a long way from her days of drug use. "Earlier, people looked down on me", she says. "Today when I perform and sing in church, I feel accepted by them. I am the happiest when they praise my songs."

Champuii has become a role model and a leader in her town. When she is not educating her peers, Champuii is taking care of them at the centre where she lives. It is a commune for young people who have given up drugs and sex work, which houses up to 25 people.

"After all I've gone through, all the ups and downs, I feel empowered", she says. "I'm looking at life from a better place. I'm very optimistic."

FIGURE 4.6 Percentage of young people who have first sex before age 15, by sex

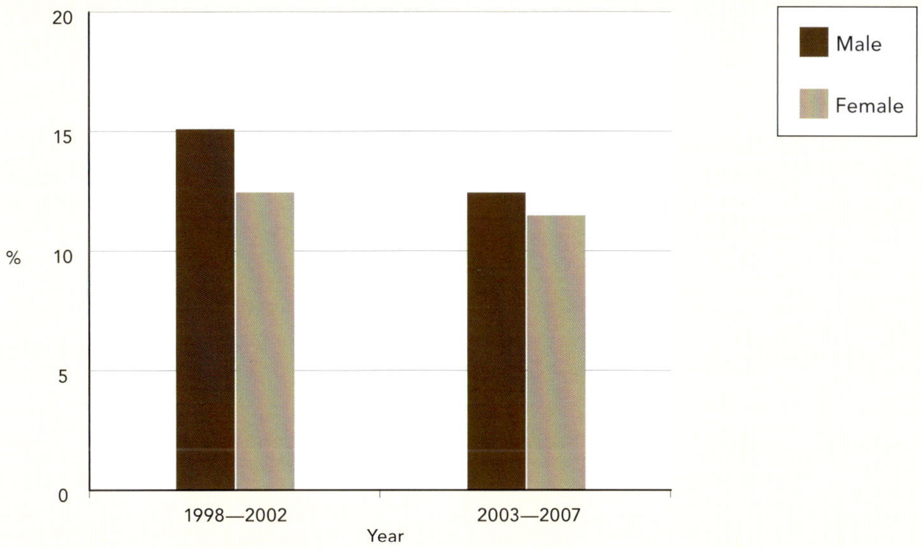

Source: MEASURE DHS.

Increasing age of sexual debut for young people

In low- and middle-income countries, the percentage of young people having sex before age 15 is declining in all regions—a continuation of trends detected earlier this decade (Figure 4.6). Males are significantly more likely to report sex before age 15, except in sub-Saharan Africa, where adolescent girls under 15 are almost 50% more likely than boys to be sexually active. While the global trend toward delayed sexual debut is clear, surveys reveal substantial variations between countries. In a comparison of young men's sexual behaviours in six African countries, average age of first sexual intercourse fell in Ethiopia, Nigeria, and the United Republic of Tanzania between 1996–2001 and 2002–2006, but increased in Mozambique, Rwanda, and Uganda (UNGASS Indicator 15).

In much of the world, many young people become sexually active as adolescents. For example, in Kenya, the United Republic of Tanzania, Uganda, and Zambia, most young people have become sexually active by age 18 (Zaba et al., 2004). Such rates are comparable to those reported in high-income countries, such as the United States, where 47% of young people have initiated sex by the time they finish high school (CDC, 2006a). Parents, health authorities, school systems, and youth service providers have an interest in encouraging young people to delay initiation of sexual activity and they also have an obligation to provide sexually active young people with potentially life-saving information and support.

Curbing the delivery of human sexuality and HIV prevention information to young people is inconsistent with a critical element of effective youth-focused HIV prevention efforts—the

The search for new prevention tools

While national programmes work to bring available HIV prevention strategies to scale and to improve their strategic application, the search continues for additional tools to strengthen prevention efforts. In particular, new prevention technologies are urgently needed for women who currently lack access to female-initiated prevention methods.

In 2007, results from the HIV biomedical prevention research field were sobering. In September 2007, efficacy trials of the most promising HIV vaccine candidate—a product by Merck & Co. that aimed to elicit strong cell-mediated immune responses to viral exposure—were discontinued after the vaccine appeared not to be efficacious. Similarly, studies of early generation vaginal microbicides found that they were also not efficacious (Nelson, 2007). Trials also determined that female diaphragms (used in concert with a lubricant gel) had no additive benefit to condoms (Padian et al., 2007), and studies of acyclovir treatment for herpes simplex virus type 2 failed to demonstrate additional protection against HIV infection (Watson-Jones et al., 2008).

Disappointment is natural when clinical trials fail to confirm effectiveness, but the magnitude and severity of the HIV epidemic compel continued emphasis on research, including research into innovative social behavioural strategies and new prevention technologies. Researchers are investigating new prevention approaches, such as vaccines that aim to generate broadly neutralizing HIV antibodies (see Montefiori et al., 2007) and microbicides that incorporate antiretroviral compounds, two of which have now entered clinical trials. Some next-generation microbicides are especially attractive, because they

FIGURE 4.7 Annual investment in preventive HIV vaccine research and development by source between 2000 and 2006

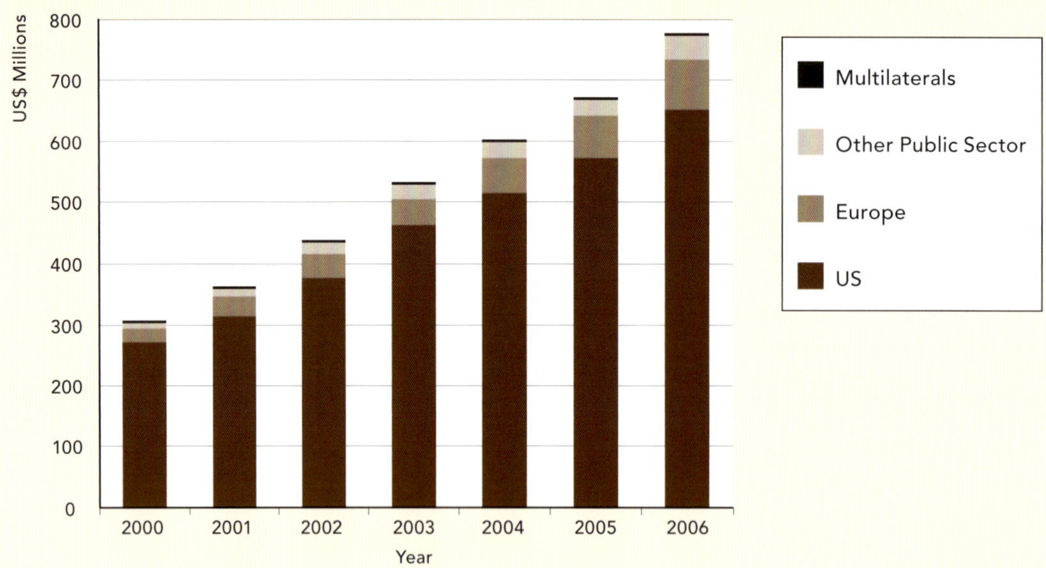

Source: HIV Vaccines and Microbicides Resource Tracking Working Group, 2007.

do not require application immediately before sexual intercourse. In addition, studies are investigating whether pre-exposure antiretroviral prophylaxis and improved treatment of herpes simplex virus type 2 can reduce the risk of sexual HIV transmission.

Noncommercial spending on research on new prevention technologies rose sharply between 2000 and 2006—by 153% for vaccines, and by 430% for microbicides (Figure 4.7). During this period, public sector funders invested approximately US$ 67 million in research and development on a range of other experimental biomedical prevention approaches, including adult male circumcision, suppression of herpes simplex virus type 2, cervical barriers to prevent HIV transmission, and pre-exposure antiretroviral prophylaxis.

Well-designed prevention trials are complex and costly (Global HIV Prevention Working Group, 2006). Trials must enroll thousands of participants to assess the efficacy of new prevention technologies, and often suffer from complications, including low adherence to trial protocols by participants and insufficiently high incidence of HIV to provide the statistical power needed to render results meaningful. HIV incidence tends to fall over time in trial cohorts—perhaps as a result of trial sponsors' regular provision of a strong HIV prevention package—further complicating the ability of trials to reliably detect the effect of interventions (Gray & Wawer, 2007). It is also clear that prevention trials are unlikely to succeed without meaningful, ongoing involvement and ownership by the communities in which such research is taking place (UNAIDS & AVAC, 2007).

encouragement of open discussion of sex and the consequences of early sexual behaviour. In South Africa, the most significant predictors of condom use among young adults were condom use at sexual debut, and talking with one's first partner about condoms (Hendriksen et al., 2007).

In addition to providing basic information and encouraging discussion about safer sex, prevention programmes for young people should promote social norms that protect young people and reduce their risk of infection. This often means that programmes must address sensitive topics that some may find uncomfortable. Such topics include gender norms that idealize "machismo" and multiple sexual partnerships for men and boys, and increase the risk of exposure to HIV for girls. For example, in Burkina Faso, Ghana, Malawi, and Uganda, nearly one in five adolescent females (ages 15–19) reported that their first sexual experience involved force or coercion (Biddlecom et al., 2007).

Another sensitive topic that youth-focused HIV prevention efforts must address is the role of intergenerational sex in HIV transmission to girls and young women. Adolescent women in southern Africa are two to four-and-a-half times more likely to be infected than their male counterparts (Bearinger et al., 2007). The extent of sexual contact between adolescent females and adult men is often an important factor in the gender disparities in HIV prevalence among teenagers in Africa (Dupas, 2006). According to recent surveys in Uganda, three out of four unmarried, sexually experienced adolescent girls reported having received gifts or money in exchange for sex, usually from an older man (Darabi et al., 2008).

The median age difference between spouses in Africa ranges from 5.5 years to 9.2 years—significantly greater than the median age difference among married couples in other regions (Wellings et al., 2006). In low- and middle-income countries, early marriage represents the most common factor that increases risk of HIV exposure for adolescent girls; young married women have more frequent unprotected intercourse than their unmarried counterparts, typically with husbands

FIGURE 4.8 Country reporting on prevention services for populations most at risk, 2005 and 2007

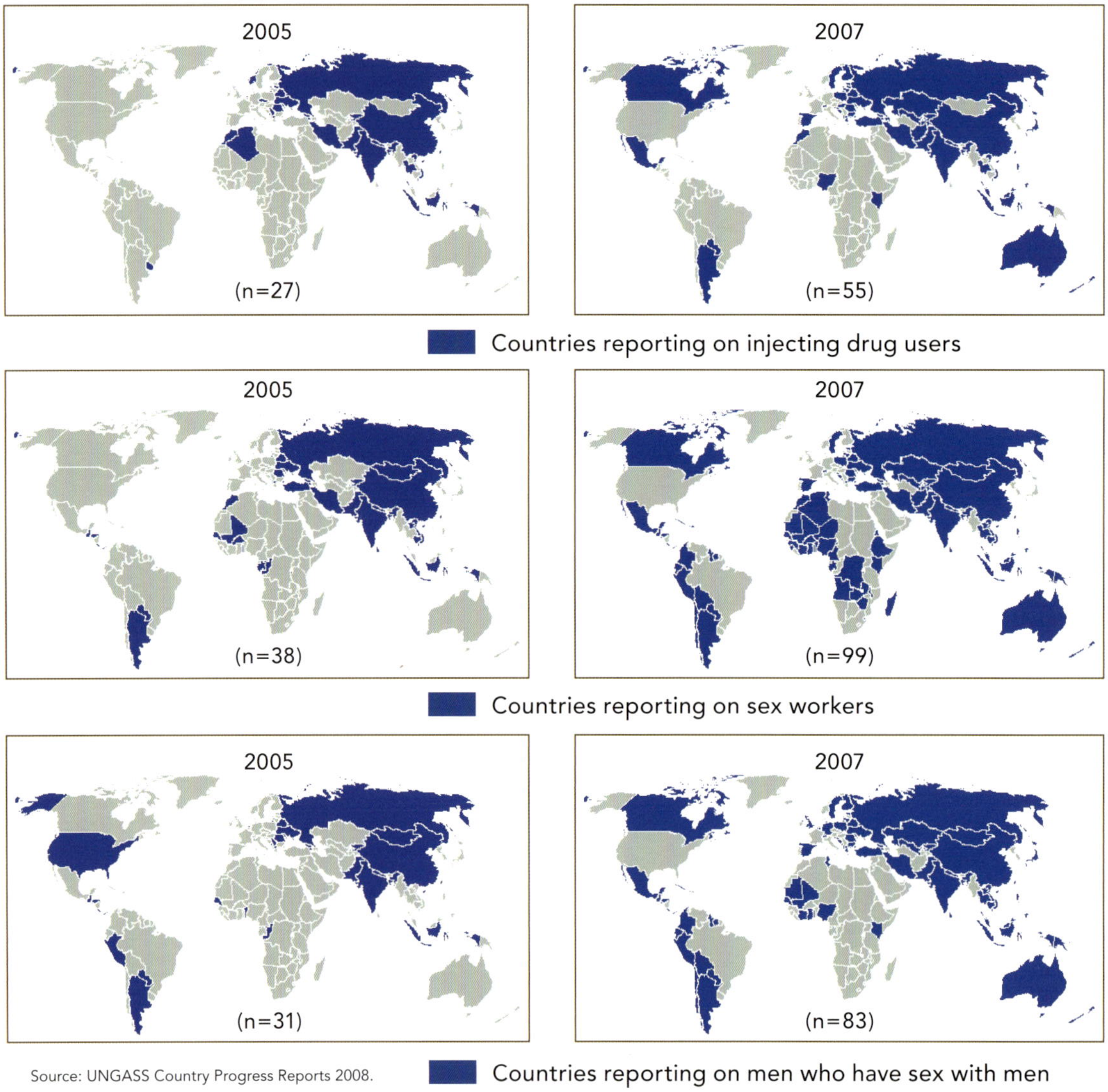

Source: UNGASS Country Progress Reports 2008.

Scaled-up prevention coverage for populations most at risk

Outside sub-Saharan Africa, most epidemics are either low level or concentrated, and are predominantly associated with high-risk behaviours in specific populations. Almost universally, individuals belonging to these populations are exposed to HIV through unprotected sex or through exposure to contaminated injecting equipment. Three populations have been consistently identified as being at higher risk of exposure to HIV: injecting drug users, sex workers, and men who have sex with men.[8]

National reporting on UNGASS indicators indicates that prevention-service delivery for populations most at risk is inconsistent and highly variable within and between regions. Although significant percentages of these populations can correctly identify the means to prevent sexual HIV transmission, many lack access to essential prevention services, such as condoms and sterile needles.

[8] See Chapter 2 for a discussion of the significant role of populations most at risk in epidemics in sub-Saharan Africa.

Of populations most at risk men who have sex with men receive the lowest coverage of HIV prevention services.

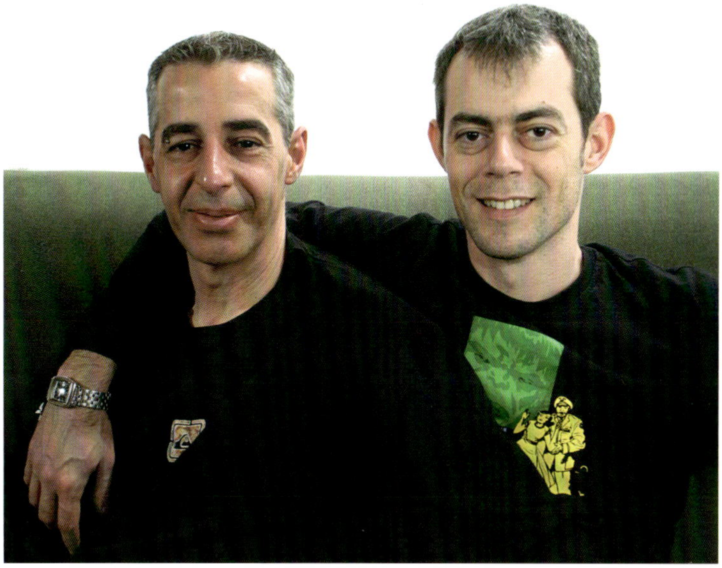

who are older and thus more likely to be HIV-positive (Gregson et al., 2002; Wellings et al., 2006; Bearinger et al., 2007). Yet relatively few scaled-up HIV-prevention programmes aim to alter social norms on intergenerational partnerships.

The breadth of reporting on UNGASS indicators suggests that countries are increasingly recognizing the centrality of HIV prevention efforts that focus on populations most at risk of HIV exposure. As Figure 4.8 illustrates, the number of countries reporting on indicators specifically relating to injecting drug users, men who have sex with men, and sex workers significantly increased between 2005 and 2007 (UNGASS Indicator 9).

Nearly all countries (92%) have a policy or strategy to promote HIV prevention for populations most at risk of HIV exposure (UNGASS Country Progress Reports, 2008), a percentage that has increased over time (e.g. from 81% in 2003). However, prevention services for these populations have been brought to scale in relatively few settings, leaving most people at highest risk of HIV exposure with little or no access to HIV prevention services (Figures 4.9 and 4.10). In addition, nongovernmental informants in nearly two thirds of countries (63%) report having laws, regulations, or policies that present obstacles to effective HIV prevention, treatment, care, and support services for populations most at risk (UNGASS Country Progress Reports 2008). Ultimately, poor coverage for those at greatest risk of exposure to HIV reflects a lack of leadership among political leaders, national ministries, and international donors. The following sections discuss the current coverage of prevention programmes for men who have sex with men, sex workers, and injecting drug users.

Men who have sex with men

As Chapter 2 explained, men who have sex with men face a disproportionate risk of exposure to HIV in diverse settings throughout the world (CDC, 2005). Yet men who have sex with men remain seriously underserved with respect to HIV prevention services. In countries reporting on populations most at risk of HIV exposure, 40% of men who have sex with men report knowing where they can receive an HIV test and having been given a condom in the previous year (UNGASS Indicator 9). Governments from fewer than 20% of countries with generalized epidemics report having implemented focused HIV-prevention programmes for men who have sex with men in most or all of districts with such a need. Nongovernmental respondents from only 10% of these countries report the implementation of such programmes. Nongovernmental respondents from 32% of countries report the existence of laws, regulations, or policies that present obstacles to effective HIV-related services for men who have sex with men (UNGASS Country Progress Reports 2008).

Knowledge that condoms can prevent HIV transmission is widespread among men who have sex with men surveyed in low- and middle-income countries, but many do not have access to condoms. In several countries, (including

FIGURE 4.9 Percentage of countries reporting laws, regulations or policies that present obstacles to effective HIV services for most-at-risk populations

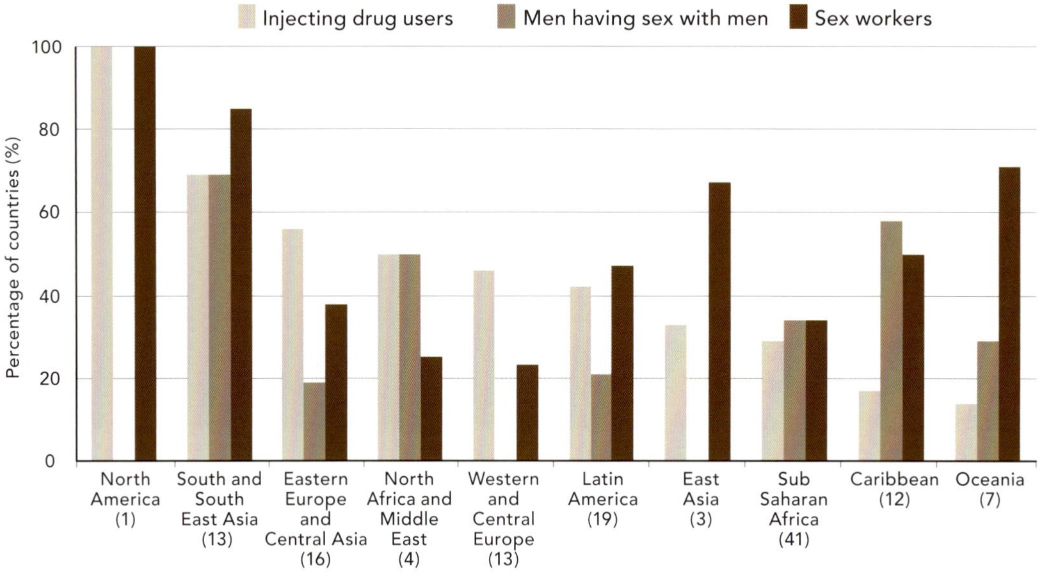

Source: UNGASS Country Progress Reports 2008.

Armenia, Greece, Mexico, Papua New Guinea, and Turkey) fewer than 25% of men who have sex with men have access to condoms. Fewer than 40% of men who have sex with men surveyed in Indonesia, the Philippines, Turkey, and Ukraine said they used a condom the last time they had sex. In Cuba, only slightly more than half of men who have sex with men used a condom at last sex (UNGASS Indicator 9).

Men who have sex with men are as culturally diverse as the world's population, ranging from gay-identified men in major urban settings of high-income countries to "hijra" sex workers in India. Focused programmes for these groups should actively engage local men who have sex with men to ensure that initiatives address the actual needs and circumstances of the intended beneficiaries. Most research on HIV-prevention interventions for men who have sex with men has been done in high-income countries, underscoring the urgent need for greater social science research and intervention studies among men who have sex with men in low- and middle-income countries. Focused ethnographic research studies—such as a recent study that examined the various sexual meanings for male-male relationships in Viet Nam (Vu et al., 2008)—may also aid in the design, tailoring, and implementation of prevention programmes in particular settings. In many cases, however, where sound research focused on men who have sex with men has been undertaken, the findings have not been translated into practice.

A recent trial of a prevention intervention specifically designed for men who have sex with men in Dakar, Senegal, highlights both the potential of evidence-informed HIV-prevention programmes focused on men who have sex with men, and some of the challenges faced by such men in different settings. Developed in collaboration between the health ministry, technical experts and nongovernmental organizations, the project included peer education, increased access to services for HIV and sexually transmitted infections, and media sensitization activities. The intervention led to notable increases in HIV knowledge and use of HIV testing services. However, although knowledge of the

FIGURE 4.10 Percentage of most-at-risk populations reached with HIV prevention programmes, 2005–2007

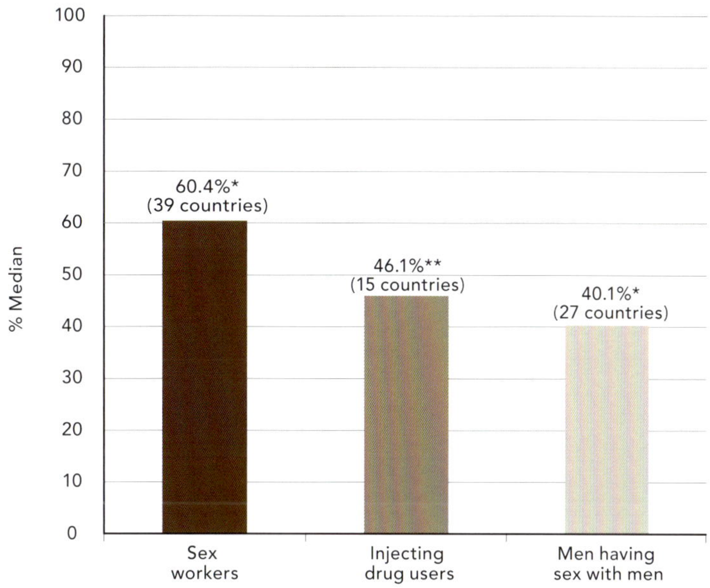

* Percentage of sex workers and men having sex with men reported knowing where they can receive an HIV test and that they were given condoms.

** Percentage of injecting drug users who reported knowing where they could receive an HIV test and be provided with condoms and sterile injecting needles and syringes.

Source: UNGASS Country Progress Reports 2008.

effectiveness of condoms increased, little change was observed in rates of consistent condom use. Consistent use of water-based lubricants was also low, largely because such products are expensive and difficult to use (Population Council & USAID, 2007).

Sex workers

The term "sex workers" constitutes a meaningful single population for epidemiological purposes, but it encompasses broadly diverse groups (women, men, and transgender individuals), and people working in a wide variety of settings (e.g. brothels, informal settings, and on the street). Some sex workers are highly mobile, while some are engaged only in informal exchange of sex for gifts or favours. Many people who engage in sex work do not self-identify as sex workers.

In Kenya, research suggests that prevention projects that result in increased condom use during paid sex could significantly reduce HIV transmission. If condom use increased to 90% during paid sex along the trans-Africa highway that links Mombassa and Kampala, Uganda (where some 8000 female sex workers operate), between 2000–2500 new HIV infections could be prevented annually on that section of the highway, with a decline in HIV incidence from 1.3% to 0.4% (Morris, 2006).

Community empowerment approaches, especially when combined with programmes that address the environment in which sex workers live and work, have consistently proven to be effective in increasing condom use among sex workers and their clients (see Kerrigan et al., 2006). For example, in the Sonagachi district of Calcutta, India, a project to empower sex workers and facilitate their access to essential information and health services lowered HIV incidence among targeted sex workers by two thirds, and increased rates of condom use from 5% to 90% (see Basu et al., 2004; Pardasani, 2005). In the state of Karnataka, India, uptake of HIV prevention services for sex workers was

CHAPTER 4

Stand up for your rights

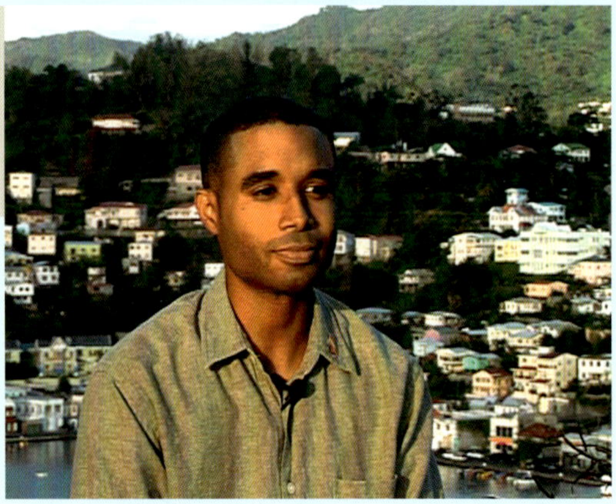

Nigel Mathlin is President of GrenChap, the Caribbean HIV/AIDS partnership

Nigel Mathlin has been active in HIV issues since he attended his first peer education workshop 12 years ago. He recently started a small nongovernmental organization, the Grenada/Caribbean HIV/AIDS Partnership (GrenChap) that concentrates on men who have sex with men and other populations at higher risk of HIV exposure in Grenada.

"It's a continuing journey, it's very challenging, getting the courage to be a public face—standing up, bringing out important issues that are not really very popular", says Mathlin. "People automatically assume that you may be HIV-positive or that you are an MSM, a sex worker, a drug user, or any of the other populations that you advocate for. But the whole point of it is to make all of those things irrelevant. Whether I'm straight or gay it should not affect my access to treatment or my rights."

Stigma against men who have sex with men is a huge obstacle to HIV programming in the eastern Caribbean. Until recently, male–male sex was not even recognized. "It was challenging, nobody really wanted to talk about the issue", explains Mathlin. "People said 'We do not have any gay people in Grenada.' I mean, at present there there is still criminalization of men who have sex with men in many of the Caribbean Islands."

Mathlin tries to take every opportunity to educate people and to give a voice to men who have sex with men. But there is a long way to go. "It is clear that so much work needs and remains to be done", says Mathlin. "Too many people continue to die from AIDS. More people should come for treatment and the attitudes towards gay persons, sex workers ... and injecting drug users must change. Their rights continue to be denied."

Mathlin sees gender as an important cross-cutting issue in the Caribbean. "A lot of Caribbean men want to maintain that ultra-masculine image and if they do not, they're not respected. I call it the rooster scenario." These attitudes make it difficult for people to negotiate safer sex and are the major driver of the epidemic in the region. The situation is compounded by intergenerational sex, poverty, domestic violence, and the breakdown in family structures. Loss of respect for women is another factor that creates vulnerability to HIV.

Mathlin is inspired by progress that is being made across the Caribbean, and is learning from the experience of neighbours like Jamaica, where organizations are challenging the climate of violence towards men who have sex with men with the help of international partners like Human Rights Watch. Other organizations are working hard to change the legal and policy environment that stigmatizes and criminalizes men who have sex with men.

Mathlin has found his role as an HIV advocate challenging. Although he has had encouragement from strangers, those he is close to have not always been as supportive. At times he is even concerned for his safety. He fears that homophobia may force him to leave his beloved home and country, as happened to some of his Jamaican peers.

But work must go on. "I can make a difference", says Mathlin. "No matter of how small the impact is, it is a positive one, and at the end of the day if I can save one or a few lives, or if I can make life easier for people who do not have a voice, I've done my part, that is enough for me."

facilitated by the involvement of sex workers in formative behavioural studies and sexually transmitted infection surveillance studies, mobilization of a peer outreach network, and selection of the location and staff for the project's clinic (Steen et al., 2006). In Africa, peer-based HIV-prevention programmes for sex workers have proven to be highly effective in changing sexual behaviours and reducing the rate of new HIV infections (Wegbreit et al., 2006).

The level of reported access to condoms and HIV testing for sex workers is somewhat higher than for men who have sex with men—across 39 countries, an average of 60% of sex workers reported having access to condoms and HIV testing. Regional variations include 41% in South and South-East Asia, 72.8% in Latin America and the Caribbean, 69% in Eastern Europe and Central Asia (seven countries), and 69.7% in sub-Saharan Africa (UNGASS Indicator 9). Reported rates of condom use with the last client are generally quite high, although there are exceptions; in Lebanon, only about one third of sex workers said they used a condom with their last client.

Injecting drug users

Use of contaminated equipment during injecting drug use represents an especially efficient means of HIV transmission, often leading to the rapid spread of HIV infection in localized networks of drug users. For example, in Karachi, Pakistan, HIV prevalence among injecting drug users rose from less than 1% in early 2004 to 26% in March 2005 (Emmanuel, Archibald & Altaf, 2006).

An estimated 78% of the world's injecting drug users live outside high-income countries (Aceijas et al., 2004). Globally, drug-use rates for opioids and other narcotic substances have stabilized in recent years, if often at elevated levels; increases in opioid use continue to be reported in Central Asia and Eastern Europe (UN Commission on Narcotic Drugs, 2008). National HIV epidemics in these areas are primarily fuelled by transmission among drug users and their sexual partners. A number of countries, most notably in Asia, have also reported an increase in non-opioid drug use in recent years, although the latest data on drug use and manufacture suggest stabilization of these trends (UNODC, 2007).

Effective HIV prevention for injecting drug users involves ready access to substitution treatment[9] for drug dependence and to sterile needles and syringes. In addition, prevention programmes should help injecting drug users to reduce the risks of sexual HIV transmission and link them to other health and social services, including confidential HIV testing, counselling, and antiretroviral therapy (Institute of Medicine, 2006). Together, these programme components are commonly known as "harm reduction". Studies have consistently demonstrated that harm reduction reduces HIV infections and risk behaviours without contributing to increased drug use or increasing other harms in the communities in which such programmes operate (Institute of Medicine, 2006; Fiellin, Green & Heimer, 2007).

Experience in diverse regions has demonstrated the feasibility of bringing harm-reduction programmes to scale, even in the face of official resistance (Physicians for Human Rights, 2007). Common features of high-coverage programmes for injecting drug users include involvement of community organizations, work with law enforcement agencies to minimize harassment, adequate and sustained funding, ease of access for clients, and involvement of injecting drug users in advisory bodies and other appropriate structures (UNAIDS, 2006b).

In 15 countries reporting data on prevention programmes for injecting drug users, median prevention coverage was 46% in 2007 (UNGASS, 2008 Indicator 9).[10] Coverage for injecting drug

[9] Substitution therapy for drug dependence has traditionally involved administration of methadone. Buprenorphine is an alternative to methadone used in a number of countries, and it may be more acceptable to some injectors. A clinical trial (HPTN 058) is under way in China and Thailand to assess the efficacy of buprenorphine in reducing HIV incidence.

[10] With respect to injecting drug users, UNGASS Indicator 9 asked whether individuals knew where to receive an HIV test, had been given a condom in the previous 12 months, and had been given sterile needles and syringes (e.g. by an outreach worker, a peer educator, or a needle exchange project).

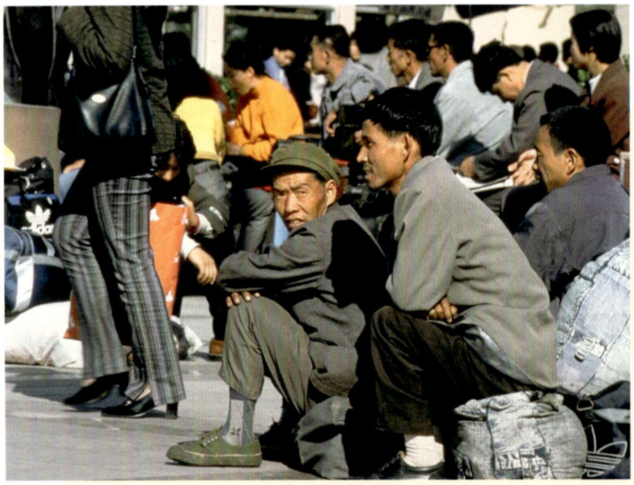

One-tenth or more of China's 1.3 billion people have migrated to urban areas.

HIV prevention for migrant workers

Globally, an estimated 86 million labour migrants were living outside the borders of their country of origin in 2005 (United Nations, 2006). Millions of people worldwide also work in jobs that require constant movement.

The relationship between migration and HIV has been extensively studied, but is still only partially understood. The impact of migration on the spread of HIV may also differ, depending on the circumstances of mobility and a range of other variables (Southern African Migration Project, 2005). Moving for work increases the risk of HIV exposure in several ways. Individuals may move from areas of low HIV prevalence to areas of higher HIV prevalence, increasing the risks associated with sexual risk behaviours. Migrants may engage in higher levels of risk behaviour because they are isolated from their families or social support networks, and migrants often have limited access to prevention services (White, 2003; Khan et al., 2007). In 22% of countries, nongovernmental informants report the existence of laws, regulations, or policies that present obstacles to effective HIV prevention, treatment, care, and support for migrants (UNGASS Country Progress Reports 2008).

Focused peer-education initiatives in work settings that attract large numbers of migrant workers have proven effective in reaching migrants who may be vulnerable to HIV exposure (Population Council, 2003; Clinton Global Initiative, 2007). China has an estimated 200 million migrant workers, and in 2007 announced the launch of HIV-prevention initiatives in workplaces that employ migrants. China also implemented education and behaviour interventions at 420 frontier ports, reaching one million contract workers sent abroad. The All China Trade Union initiated HIV education campaigns in 10 000 evening schools, reaching an estimated three million migrant workers.

Strategic placement of HIV prevention services is especially important for truck drivers and other transport workers. In Brazil, a programme providing prevention counselling, HIV testing, and screening for sexually transmitted infections in customs stations led cross-border truckers to significantly increase their condom use with nonregular partners (Chinaglia et al., 2007). Prevention initiatives for mobile populations must take account of the role of gender in increased risk of exposure to HIV, because women represent half of the world's migrants (Global Commission on International Migration, 2005).

users is lower in Eastern Europe and Central Asia (median 46.8%) than in South and South-East Asia (median 61.5%). An important challenge in expanding access to harm reduction programmes is to ensure gender equity, because most such programmes are designed primarily for men (International Harm Reduction Development Program, 2007; Hankins, 2008).

Lack of official support for harm reduction in many countries, laws that prohibit key components of harm reduction, and onerous regulatory schemes (e.g. strict import limits on opiate maintenance medications) often make it difficult to implement harm reduction initiatives at all, much less bring such programmes to scale (Fiellin, Green & Heimer, 2007). Nongovernmental respondents in 40% of countries report the existence of laws, regulations, or policies that present obstacles to effective HIV services for injecting drug users (UNGASS Country Progress Reports, 2008). Substitution therapy with methadone is available in only 52 countries, and with buprenorphine in only 32 countries. Substitution therapy is largely unavailable in Eastern Europe and Central Asia, where injecting drug use represents the most important mode of HIV transmission (TRC, 2008).

Recent years have seen important but uneven advances in access to harm reduction in various settings. China, for example, has expanded key components of harm reduction, reaching more than 88 000 individuals with methadone maintenance therapy, and nearly 50 000 injecting drug users with needle exchange services as of October 2007. Viet Nam is initiating its first pilot project of methadone substitution therapy in 2008 (Oanh, 2007), and harm reduction programmes in the country distributed 15 million condoms and 7.5 million needles and syringes in the first 10 months of 2007. In 2006, Bulgaria, Estonia, Finland, Latvia, and Lithuania created a regional network to expand and coordinate HIV prevention services for injecting drug users, with financing secured until 2009 from the European Commission. In Thailand, by contrast, a recent report by civil society informants found little expansion of harm reduction programmes, despite

HIV prevention in prison settings

On average, people in prison settings have much higher infection rates than those who live outside prisons (Dolan et al., 2007). In part, this reflects the disproportionate likelihood of incarceration for key populations, such as sex workers and injecting drug users. Within prisons, HIV transmission also occurs, typically through injecting drug use and unprotected sex. In all countries where data on HIV prevalence in prisons is available, women in prisons have higher infection rates than male prisoners.

Comprehensive HIV prevention services are seldom available in prisons. One third (33%) of countries report the existence of laws, regulations, or policies that present obstacles to effective HIV services for prisoners (UNGASS Country Progress Reports 2008). Comprehensive prison-based harm reduction and treatment services for drug users are available only in the Islamic Republic of Iran, Spain, and Switzerland. In 2006, only eight countries had established or piloted needle and syringe exchange programmes in prisons (Lines et al., 2006).

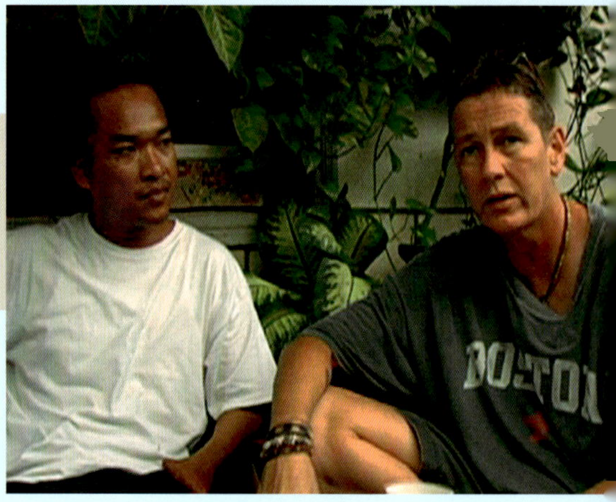

Rebuilding a people: harm reduction in Cambodia

Korsang is Cambodia's first harm reduction project, providing needle and syringe exchange, HIV education, and other services to the drug users of Phnom Penh. Founded in 2003 by Holly Bradshaw, an American grandmother and former drug user, it employs 68 staff members and reaches more than 3000 drug users.

"There was a lot of discrimination against us and it took us a long time [to get off the ground]", says Bradshaw. "The first drop-in centre was in a squat. It was 120 degrees Fahrenheit in the hot season, and we had a table, three chairs, a couple of fans, and a lot of rats."

Many who work at Korsang are young Cambodians who have lived most of their lives as refugees in the United States, before being deported for various crimes. Wicket, who is 27, was one of these young deportees. When he met Bradshaw, he was living with his family in the countryside where he felt out of place and useless. Wicket joined Korsang and was trained to be one of the first volunteers in the programme.

At the heart of Korsang are the peer educators—all of whom are either active or former drug users. "We are picking the ones who are respected, who are from neighbourhoods wwhere the staff cannot enter", says Wicket. "They come into Korsang, they go on outreach to distribute syringes, collect dirty syringes. They educate their peers."

Korsang means to fix or rebuild, and that is exactly what it does for Phnom Penh's drug users. As well as harm reduction and medical services, the project provides food and shelter, and a safe haven for drug users. "Most of the guys are street-based injecting drug users, with nowhere to go", says Wicket. "They're tired, all night long—running from the cops, from the local gangsters, running from the guys who want their money. They have nothing to eat, they have no place to rest, so Korsang is a safe environment for them where they can rest, eat, sleep, talk to their peers, and get whatever medical services that they need."

The attitudes of ordinary Cambodians present the biggest challenge to the project. They have been evicted six times from their premises by angry neighbours. "They do not want to have drug users in their backyard or their building", says Bradshaw. "As soon as we get into a building and get set up we get evicted again. The neighbours sign petitions…and that is a huge problem for Korsang. That is discrimination against drug users."

"What drug users go through is absolutely killing them", says Bradshaw. "The discrimination, the criminalization, the repression…they're being beaten up, hung, starved, denied treatment, but they're not criminals, they're drug users, they've a chronic disease, they need treatment. But it's like they are stigmatized twice…they need their human rights."

Bradshaw is motivated to continue this work by her own experiences as a drug user. She started using drugs at the age of 12 and began injecting heroin in her early twenties. She went through a dozen "detox" programmes, but nothing worked until she found herself facing a 22-year prison sentence. She stopped, and soon began working to provide services for others. She felt that she had to give back what she had taken. "That is all I know, being a drug user, being on treatment, being in jail, working with drug users."

"I do not feel I chose this, I think I was chosen", she says. "That's the reason I'm still alive, you know, to serve the people—that is what I want to do in life. I want to do this until the day I drop."

Safety of the blood supply: a status report

Effective screening of donated blood for HIV before transfusion is a highly cost-effective strategy to prevent HIV transmission. The risk of HIV transmission through a blood transfusion is greater than 90%, because a large volume of virus can be transfused into a patient from an infected unit of blood (Donegan et al., 1994). According to country reports on UNGASS indicators for the *Declaration of Commitment*, 91 countries report having taken steps to ensure that all donated blood is screened for HIV, and that all screening processes are quality assured. However, 34 countries do not screen all donated blood for HIV in accordance with minimum quality standards, and 67 countries failed to provide information on this indicator (UNGASS, 2008 Indicator 3).

More than one million blood units are still not screened for HIV in accordance with minimum quality standards. More than 20 years after sensitive screening testing systems became available, failure to screen all donated blood for HIV in accordance with minimum quality standards is a matter of grave concern. Additional efforts are also needed to reduce unnecessary blood transfusions.

the national government's widely publicized 2004 commitment to increase prevention access for drug users (Thai AIDS Treatment Action Group & Human Rights Watch, 2007).

Aggressive drug control policies often inhibit use of harm-reduction programmes, underscoring the need for interministerial collaboration and sensitization of law enforcement personnel, to avoid approaches that can deter participation in prevention programmes. In most countries in Eastern Europe and Central Asia, for example, police sometimes make arrests for possession of extremely small amounts of narcotics, potentially discouraging drug users from participating in needle exchange projects (Nashkhoev & Sergeyev, 2007). According to Georgia's official report to UNAIDS on UNGASS indicators, the national anti-drug policy climate has inhibited efforts to offer even minimal access to detoxification and drug rehabilitation services. In Thailand in 2003, the alleged extrajudicial killings and associated violence, which resulted in the death of more than 2000 suspected drug dealers and users, continues to reverberate through society. Civil society informants report that injecting drug users are afraid to access harm reduction and other health services. (Thai AIDS treatment Action Group and Human Rights Watch, 2007)

HIV prevention in sexual partnerships

Historically, rigorous evaluation of HIV prevention programmes has primarily concentrated on individuals, rather than couples. This omission is potentially important, because international surveys of young people's sexual behaviour consistently find that sexual partners are a key influence on the particular sexual practices in which young people decide to engage (Marston & King, 2006). At least two types of partnerships appear to justify intensified HIV prevention focus—serodiscordant partnerships and multiple concurrent partnerships. By specifically tailoring programmes to reach people in different kinds of partnerships, HIV prevention efforts may achieve greater impact than programmes that solely aim to affect the behaviours of a single individual.

Serodiscordant partnerships

Where knowledge of HIV status is low and condom use infrequent, the risk of transmission within serodiscordant partnerships can be high, especially when the HIV-infected partner is newly infected but still unaware of the infection. Among serodiscordant heterosexual couples in Uganda, the uninfected partner has an estimated 8% chance of contracting HIV each year (Wawer et al., 2005).

According to Demographic and Health Surveys in five African countries, two thirds of HIV-infected couples are serodiscordant (de Walque, 2007). Similarly, surveys in East Africa indicate that more than 40% of married individuals with HIV have uninfected spouses (Were et al., 2006). The five-country African survey found that the infected partner in a serodiscordant couple was female in 30%–40% of cases. More than half of HIV-positive women surveyed who are married or cohabiting were not infected by their current partner (de Walque, 2007). In Burkina Faso, nearly 90% of cohabiting couples said they did not use a condom the last time they had sex (de Walque, 2007).

HIV prevention focused on people living with HIV

Throughout most of the epidemic, prevention programmes focused primarily on promoting risk reduction among people who were HIV-negative or unaware of their HIV status. Following the advent of combination antiretroviral therapy, which significantly prolongs life and improves quality of life for people living with HIV, there have been increasing calls for enhanced prevention services for people living with HIV (Global HIV Prevention Working Group, 2004). Relatively few studies have examined the effectiveness of prevention programmes specifically focused on people living with HIV, but programmes tailored to the needs of HIV-positive people can reduce risky behaviours (Crepaz et al., 2006).

As this report went to press, WHO was finalizing guidance on HIV prevention and other essential interventions for adults and adolescents living with HIV in resource-limited settings. The WHO guidelines envision counselling and other support for risk reduction, as part of a continuum that includes treatment, care, and support for people living with HIV. Risk-reduction programmes are merely one of many behavioural components of comprehensive HIV prevention and care for people living with HIV, including strategies to promote treatment adherence and to alleviate HIV-related stigma and discrimination. Psychosocial services to promote safe behaviours among HIV-positive people should be sensitive to differences in culture, gender, age, and vulnerabilities. Active engagement of people living with HIV is essential when designing and implementing these services.

In 2008, the Swiss AIDS Commission concluded, following an analysis of four studies, that HIV-positive people with an undetectable viral load following antiretroviral therapy do not risk transmitting HIV to their sexual partners (Vernazza et al., 2008). In response, UNAIDS and WHO emphasized the continuing importance of comprehensive HIV prevention for people living with HIV. UNAIDS and WHO note that the risk of HIV transmission is lower for people with undetectable viral loads, but stress that no study has yet ruled out the risk of HIV transmission.

FIGURE 4.11 Percent change in condom use at last sex, among those with more than one partner in the last 12 months, by sex

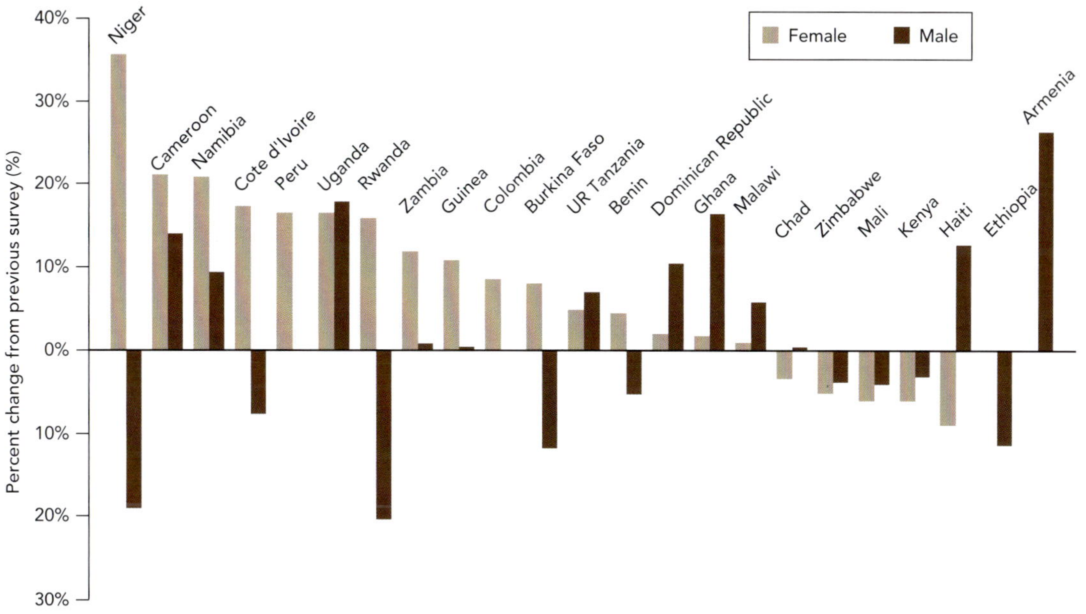

Source: MEASURE DHS 2008.

Providing serodiscordant couples with improved prevention and treatment services, including counselling support, access to male and female condoms, antiretroviral therapy, prompt treatment of sexually transmitted infections, and medical male circumcision can help prevent HIV transmission. Knowledge of HIV status is an important starting point. In sub-Saharan Africa, "couples testing" has reduced HIV transmission among serodiscordant couples (Allen et al., 2003). Voluntary testing of couples is likely to be optimally effective when supported by client-centred counselling. Knowledge of HIV status only boosts prevention if it leads to safer sexual behaviour. Yet the fear of stigma and rejection leads many people to delay or avoid disclosing their status to their regular partner. This underscores the importance of counselling and stigma-reduction initiatives in facilitating timely disclosure between partners. Treatment also has a role to play in reducing the risk of HIV transmission within serodiscordant partnerships, as receipt of antiretroviral therapy is associated with an 80% reduction in transmission among serodiscordant couples (Castilla et al., 2005).

Multiple concurrent partnerships

Although there are only limited data, the potential for concurrent partnerships to accelerate HIV transmission is especially pronounced where there is high background HIV prevalence and/or high rates of population mobility (Cassels, Clark & Morris, 2008). These factors are common in southern Africa, where concurrency has been cited as a potential reason for the subregion's uniquely high levels of HIV infection (see Chapter 2).

According to a national survey of more than 7000 people (ages 15–65) in South Africa, pervasive social norms encourage both concurrency and a rapid turnover in sex partners, with little peer support for commitment to a single partner. Significantly, only 21% of survey respondents said "sticking to one partner and being faithful" could prevent HIV transmission, and only 5% identified reducing the number of sex partners as a sound HIV prevention strategy (CADRE et al., 2007).

Few studies have examined strategies to alter attitudes and practices regarding partnership concurrency. However, the HIV prevention

CHAPTER 4

Increasing condom use among people with multiple partners

Consistent condom use among those who have multiple partners (defined as more than one partner in the preceding 12 months) appears to be increasing, particularly in the areas most affected by the epidemic. In the most recent round of Demographic and Health Surveys, an average of 27% [2%–66%] of women (ages 15–49) and 33% [7%–75%] of men (ages 15–49) who had more than one partner in the last year reported the use of a condom the last time they had sex. In 21 countries where this information has been collected over at least two time points, condom use by women increased in 16 countries, and condom use by men increased in 12 countries (Figure 4.11). However, as Figure 4.12 shows, advances in condom use cannot be taken for granted, because condom use has declined in a number of countries.

FIGURE 4.12 Condom use at last sex, among those with more than one partner in the last 12 months, in three high-burden countries

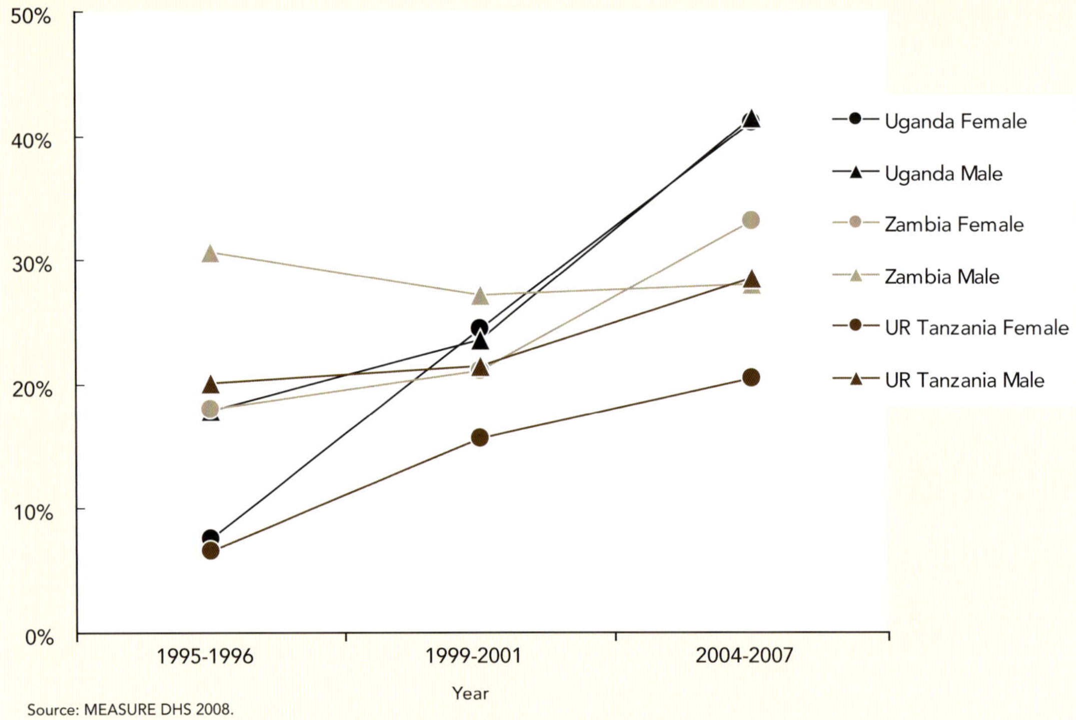

Source: MEASURE DHS 2008.

literature is replete with examples of radical shifts in sexual behaviours and the establishment of new population-based sexual norms (Auerbach, Hayes & Kandathil, 2006). Such dramatic behavioural shifts have often followed high-level campaigns aimed at altering sexual norms and increasing awareness of HIV-related risks. Prevention efforts, especially in hyperendemic settings, should include community-level strategies to educate people regarding the risk of multiple partnerships and to forge new social norms that encourage avoidance of concurrent relationships.

In 2006, the Southern African Development Community's Think Tank on HIV Prevention recommended that addressing multiple and concurrent sexual partnerships should be the top regional HIV prevention priority (SADC, 2006). Regional efforts to better address concurrent partnerships in HIV prevention responses are being accelerated. After reviewing formative research at the end of 2007, the nine countries involved in a regional programme organized by Soul City, a health promotion and social change project, recommended initiation of a regional HIV prevention campaign focused on multiple concurrent partnerships. Soul City participants concluded that the campaign should address communication between children and parents, and between partners; gender disparities (i.e. male domination and women's empowerment); and socialization and peer pressure.

Tailored HIV prevention for heterosexual men

Influencing male sexual behaviour is essential to reduce the number of new HIV infections. Not only do men account for half of HIV infections worldwide, but encouraging men to avoid risky sexual behaviours plays a vital role in preventing new HIV infections in women.

While various prevention models have been developed to provide focused prevention support for men who have sex with men, few HIV prevention programmes have been specifically designed to take into account the values heterosexual men attach to sex, the pleasures they derive from it, and the social pressures associated with sex. A cardinal rule of HIV prevention is that programmes must be culturally relevant to the target population, but this maxim has not been rigorously followed among programmes that ostensibly aim to affect men's behaviours.

Devoting greater attention to the prevention needs of heterosexual men should in no way suggest a diminution of effort with respect to women and girls. On the contrary, effective prevention programmes for men complement initiatives that aim to empower women and girls to prevent HIV transmission. The lack of female-initiated prevention methods underscores the importance of promoting safer, responsible sexual behaviour among men.

HIV prevention efforts for heterosexual men aim to motivate men and women to talk more openly about sex, sexuality, drug use, and HIV. Effective HIV prevention also encourages men to take greater care of themselves, and their partners and families. As early as 2001, UNAIDS documented 12 different "best practice" models of prevention programming for men (UNAIDS, 2001). However, such projects remain localized and have not been brought to scale (ICRW & Instituto Promundo, 2007; WHO & Instituto Promundo, 2007).

Programmes for men and boys that openly address gender power imbalances can help transform gender norms (see Chapter 3). In many countries, prevailing gender norms simultaneously render women vulnerable to male power, while encouraging men to place women at risk. For example, concepts of masculinity that reward multiple partners may place considerable pressure on men to behave in particular ways. As a result of such dynamics, both men and women are at heightened risk of HIV infection.

Global mobilization to eradicate mother-to-child transmission

In the absence of any intervention, the risk of mother-to-child-transmission of HIV is about 15%–30% if the mother does not breastfeed the child. With prolonged breastfeeding, the likelihood of infection can be as high as 45% (De Cock, 2000). Timely administration of a short course of antiretroviral drugs significantly reduces the risk of HIV transmission (Guay et al., 1999).

No validated chemoprophylactic regimen yet exists to reduce the risk of HIV transmission through breastfeeding, although trials are under way to evaluate different experimental approaches. Until a prophylactic regimen is developed, it appears that exclusive breastfeeding and early weaning help minimize the risk of transmission to the newborn in settings where

Integrating medical male circumcision in national HIV prevention efforts

Clinical trials in Kenya, South Africa, and Uganda demonstrate that medical male circumcision reduces the risk (by about 60%) that a woman living with HIV will transmit the virus to her male sexual partner (Auvert et al., 2005; Bailey et al., 2007; Gray et al., 2007). Early results indicating an HIV prevention benefit from circumcision reportedly increased demand for circumcision in some parts of Africa (WHO, 2006a).

Much remains unknown about the potential role of medical male circumcision in slowing the rate of new HIV infections at the population level. Medical male circumcision has other benefits in terms of decreased genital ulcer disease and human papilloma virus (the causative agent of cervical cancer), but male circumcision is unlikely to have a directly protective effect against HIV for women during sexual intercourse. The degree to which the benefits seen under controlled trial conditions can be replicated in everyday life is currently being assessed during programme roll out, particularly at the sites of the three trials. Some observational studies in men who have sex with men have suggested a protective effect from circumcision (see Buchbinder et al., 2005) but other studies have not (Millett & Peterson, 2007; Templeton & Hogben, 2007). Men in the Merck adenovirus vaccine trial were men who have sex with men, and those who were circumcised had the lowest risk of HIV acquisition (Robertson, 2008).

Experts convened by UNAIDS and WHO in March 2007 determined that the research results on the benefits of medical male circumcision for heterosexual men were compelling. The consultation endorsed male circumcision as an efficacious prevention intervention, noting that its impact was likely to be greatest in settings where the prevalence of heterosexually acquired HIV is high, male circumcision levels are low, and the populations at risk of HIV are substantial (UNAIDS & WHO, 2007). A number of countries are implementing male circumcision services as a component of comprehensive HIV prevention, with technical support from UN partners and others through the Second UN Work Plan on Male Circumcision.

Since 2005, a number of modelling and cost-effectiveness studies have estimated the number of infections that could be averted by scaling up adult male circumcision programmes in sub-Saharan Africa (Williams et al., 2006; Hallett et al., 2008). These exercises have determined that male circumcision is a highly cost-effective approach to preventing new HIV infections in high-prevalence settings, with projected savings of future antiretroviral treatment costs greatly exceeding the cost of circumcision programmes (Kahn, Marseille & Auvert, 2006).

A major challenge in bringing circumcision to scale is ensuring that such procedures are performed safely. Historically, many circumcisions in Africa have been performed outside medical settings, often by traditional health practitioners. Infections and other complications from the procedure are common (Schoofs, 2007). There is also the danger that HIV itself could be transmitted through circumcision procedures that lack infection control. However, there is little direct evidence to this effect, and traditional initiation practices are occasions for transmitting norms and values around masculinity. Such practices may therefore be important opportunities for HIV prevention education (Peltzer et al., 2007). Provider training programmes are now under way to ensure acceptable safety and quality of male circumcision procedures (Schoofs, 2007).

Due to the risk that circumcised men and their partners might erroneously conclude that the procedure obviates the need for other protective measures, roll out of medical male circumcision should be accompanied by strengthened HIV prevention efforts. In particular, public education campaigns should emphasize that circumcision offers only partial protection to men and that HIV transmission can still occur during sexual intercourse even following circumcision. In addition, health care providers must carefully counsel men who receive the procedure, and their partners, to refrain from sexual intercourse until circumcision wounds have completely healed.

no safe alternative, infant-feeding methods are available (Kuhn et al., 2007).

In high-income countries, high coverage of services for preventing mother-to-child transmission has maintained HIV transmission rates below 19. In Western Europe, for example, only 191 new HIV diagnoses in children were attributed to mother-to-child transmission in 2006 (EuroHIV, 2007). Similar achievements are feasible in resource-poor settings, as demonstrated by a study in Abidjan, Côte d'Ivoire, which showed that mother-to-child transmission can be limited to below 6% when necessary services were made available (Tonwe-Gold, 2007). In Botswana, where the national government has made prevention of mother-to-child transmission a major priority,

FIGURE 4.13 Number and percentage of HIV-positive pregnant women receiving antiretroviral prophylaxis, 2004–2007

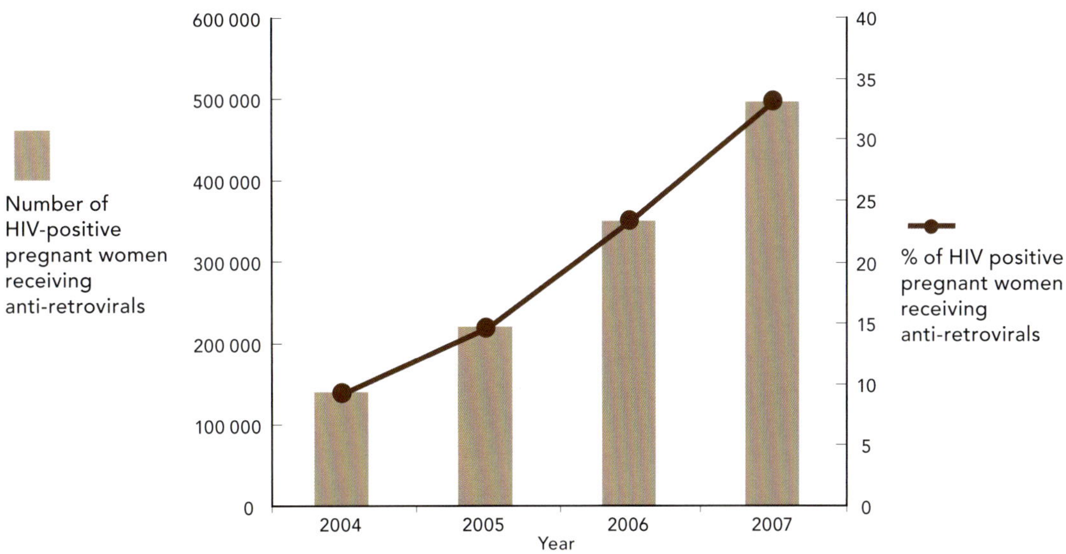

Source: UNAIDS, UNICEF & WHO, 2008; data provided by countries.

FIGURE 4.14 Percentage of HIV-positive pregnant women receiving antiretroviral prophylaxis, 2007

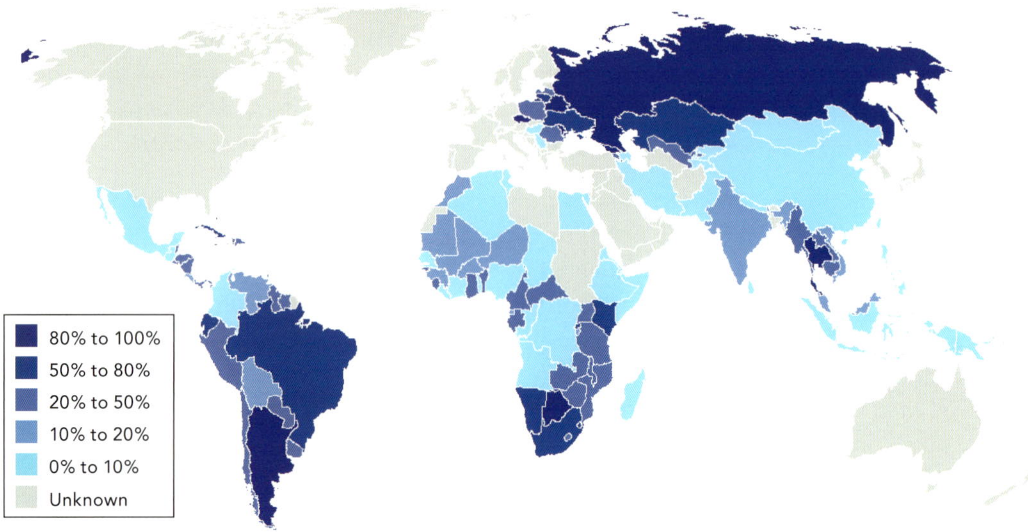

Source: UNAIDS, UNICEF & WHO, 2008; data provided by countries.

the rate at which children born to HIV-positive mothers contract HIV has dropped to 4% (Donnelly, 2007).

Government and nongovernmental informants in 63% of countries with generalized epidemics report having implemented prevention of mother-to-child transmission in most or all districts in need (UNGASS Country Progress Reports 2008), actual programme coverage does not reflect such a high degree of access. Epidemiological estimates suggest that coverage for antiretroviral prophylaxis to HIV-positive pregnant women for prevention of mother-to-child transmission in low- and middle-income countries increased from 9% in 2004 to 33% in 2007(Figure 4.13). These figures are based on revised epidemiological estimates of global and national HIV prevalence (see Chapter 2), and a data reconciliation process between UNAIDS, WHO and UNICEF, and countries reporting on UNGASS indicator 5. Broken links in the continuum of care for prevention of mother-to-child transmission appear to be contributing to reduced coverage. For example, estimates suggest that only 18% of all HIV-positive pregnant women receive testing in antenatal care clinics. However, of women who received testing, 80% of those testing positive received antiretroviral prophylaxis. This suggests that lack of testing may be hindering efforts to increase prevention coverage for pregnant women in need (UNICEF, 2008).

Several countries have made marked progress in expanding coverage for HIV-positive pregnant women in recent years. Between 2004 and 2006, coverage of prevention of mother-to-child transmission increased from 12% to 64% [53%–80%] in Namibia, from 5% to 67% [60%–74%] in Swaziland, and from 15% to 57% [49%–69%] in South Africa. As Figure 4.14 indicates, national progress in scaling up services to prevent mother-to-child transmission is highly variable.

Numerous factors impede expansion of services to prevent mother-to-child transmission. For example, the package of prevention services available to pregnant women is designed for delivery in health-care settings, yet use of antenatal care varies widely within and among countries, and is typically much lower in rural areas (Say & Rain, 2007). In Papua New Guinea, where most women give birth at home, coverage of services to prevent mother-to-child transmission is below 5%. Globally, one in six pregnant women in low- and middle-income countries receive no antenatal care before giving birth (UNICEF, 2008). In the 30 African countries with the lowest human development scores, most births are not attended by a skilled health professional, with the exception of Zimbabwe (UNDP, 2007). Even in antenatal settings where HIV prevention uptake is high, such as Bangkok, surveys indicate that many women fail to use the services because of inconsistent antenatal care, fear of stigmatization, and concerns regarding disclosure of their HIV status (Teeraratkul, 2005).

According to studies in Côte d'Ivoire and South Africa, recommended approaches to breast-feeding are not being widely followed (Becquet, 2005; Doherty, et.al., 2007). In addition, many infants born to HIV-positive mothers do not receive follow-up care, impeding timely diagnosis of HIV infection and prompt initiation of antiretroviral therapy. In Malawi, for example, only 19% of infants born to HIV-positive mothers were tested for HIV within 12 months following delivery (Manzi, et.al., 2005).

In the immediate future, countries, donors, and other partners should build on recent progress to make services that are broadly accessible sufficiently available in low- and middle-income countries to replicate achievements of high-income settings. Such measures will save lives and reduce future treatment costs.

Implementation of provider-initiated HIV testing in antenatal and other settings is already increasing programme uptake. In some clinics, pregnant women who are unlikely to return to the clinic for delivery are provided with doses of nevirapine for themselves and their infants (Stripipatana, 2007). Other clinics are working to engage male partners and fathers. Programmes in Ethiopia and South Africa have mobilized HIV-positive mothers who have experience of services to prevent mother-to-child transmission to provide education, information, and support for pregnant women. A recent study in selected maternity hospitals in St. Petersburg, the Russian Federation, found that the point-of-care offer of rapid HIV testing resulted in identification of a significant number of previously undiagnosed HIV-positive women and the delivery of antiretroviral prophylaxis to 98% of HIV-exposed infants (Kissin et al., 2008).

Sustaining HIV prevention for the long-term

One of the great practical challenges for HIV prevention is to sustain favourable changes in sexual and drug-using behaviours over the long-term. HIV prevention is not a 'one-shot' intervention that confers lifetime immunity against infection. Rather, risk reduction is a lifelong endeavour that requires support, reinforcement, and self-monitoring.

Recent research suggests that, while individuals often significantly reduce sexual risk behaviours in the year following intensive, repeated individual or small-group interventions, they frequently fail to sustain safer behaviours for longer periods. For example, trials of a 10-week individualized counselling intervention for men who have sex with men found that the intervention produced significant short-term behavioural benefits, and reduced HIV incidence. After three years, however, recipients of the intervention did not differ significantly from the control group with respect to HIV incidence, suggesting that the initial favourable impact was not sustained (Coates et al., 2008).

This pattern is also apparent outside trial conditions, where early national prevention success has proven difficult to sustain over the long-term. In Uganda, the African country that has been most successful in lowering HIV prevalence, surveys have documented an increase in risky sexual behaviours in recent years (UNAIDS, 2007b). Likewise, several high-income countries that saw sharp reductions in HIV incidence in the 1980s following heavy investments in focused HIV prevention programmes are now witnessing significant increases in risky sexual behaviour and new HIV infections (EuroHIV, 2007; Osmond et al., 2007).

People find it difficult to sustain behaviour change for a number of reasons. Prevention efforts are often short-term, and individuals may return to early behaviour patterns if prevention initiatives are not maintained or reinforced. Some who adopt safer behaviours may experience 'prevention fatigue' and eventually revert to previous behaviours that are the norm in their community. In addition, environmental changes may alter individual perceptions of risk. In high-income countries, for example, improved treatment prospects have rendered the disease less serious to some, apparently prompting an increase in sexual behaviours that increase risk of exposure to HIV (Suarez et al., 2001).

Like HIV treatment, HIV prevention is for life. To ensure their continued relevance, prevention strategies should be strengthened and revised as the epidemic evolves and underlying circumstances change. Prevention research efforts should specifically concentrate on strategies to prevent environmental changes (e.g. introduction of treatments or new prevention technologies) from undermining existing patterns of adherence to safer behaviours.

To achieve and sustain success, HIV prevention efforts must reach the required intensity and be delivered in a high-quality, evidence-informed manner. Until recently, the issues of quality and intensity seemed somewhat academic in most prevention settings, given that coverage of most essential HIV prevention activities was extremely low. However, as this report demonstrates, that picture is beginning to change, with coverage increasing for both general population initiatives and programmes focused on populations most at risk. With greater coverage of prevention programmes, performance indicators will also have to keep pace by incorporating measures of quality and intensity.

Financing and national political support for HIV prevention has increased, but use of prevention services remains suboptimal, underscoring the need to stimulate greater demand for HIV prevention. The epidemic's history suggests that government programmes or donor policies alone are unlikely to create demand. In diverse countries in various regions, the emergence of mass popular demand for HIV prevention has required the genuine and long-lasting leadership and engagement of effective communities (Piot, 2008). Continued attention is needed to bring critical prevention services to scale, and greater investments are needed in social mobilization strategies. In Ethiopia, for example, the national HIV programme has prioritized mobilizing society from the local level upwards, to accelerate progress towards universal access to HIV prevention, treatment, care, and support.

When greater demand for prevention services is generated, complementary efforts will be required to build the local and national capacities to sustain high-quality prevention efforts into the future. Improved organizational capacity and management skills will be needed at the local level—together with increased analytical capacity at national and subnational levels—to collect, assess, and respond to emerging information on the epidemic. Such measures will ensure sufficient capacity to implement and sustain existing prevention strategies, and enable future prevention approaches and technologies to be rapidly introduced and scaled-up.

As epidemics evolve, policy-makers often find it tempting to short-change prevention efforts, assuming that earlier investments have sufficiently addressed the problem. Experience in the United States is illustrative. At the beginning of the epidemic, in the early 1980s, HIV prevention accounted for 25% of all HIV-related spending. Spending on prevention had fallen to 13% by 1990. By 2006, the 25th year since AIDS was first recognized, only 4 of every 100 dollars the United States Government spent on HIV were directed toward preventing new HIV infections (Henry J Kaiser Family Foundation, 2006).

Sustaining HIV prevention requires national leadership that recognizes both the cost-effectiveness and the humanitarian necessity of investing in prevention, and understands the long-term nature of the threat. Efforts to persuade political leaders to invest in HIV prevention have suffered because there is no natural constituency for prevention. Failure to include people living with HIV and those at high risk of exposure to HIV in the design and implementation of prevention programmes has also weakened such programmes.

In a number of countries, the search for new prevention technologies has generated significant activism and community organization, partly because tens of thousands of people worldwide have been enrolled in prevention trials in recent years. A similar mobilization, but on a much larger scale, is required to demand immediate implementation of the evidence-informed tools that already exist to prevent new infections.

Evidence for action

Are the right actions being taken?

- Nearly all countries (95%) have national policies to provide free access to HIV prevention services.
- Most national governments (89%) report having integrated HIV into secondary school curricula, but far fewer include HIV education in the primary school curriculum (65%) or have an HIV education strategy for out-of-school young people (64%).
- Most national governments (92%) have a policy or strategy for HIV prevention for populations most at risk.

Are the right actions being undertaken in the right manner?

- HIV prevention programmes often fail to provide accurate and comprehensive information to young people. According to nongovernmental informants, 28% of countries have laws, regulations, or policies that present obstacles to effective HIV-related services for young people.
- Nongovernmental informants in 63% of countries have laws, regulations or policies in place that present obstacles to effective HIV-related services for populations most at risk.

Have these actions been sufficiently scaled up to make a difference?

- Survey data from 64 countries indicate that 40% of males and 36% of females (ages 15–24) have accurate and comprehensive knowledge about HIV prevention—far short of the 95% target in the *Declaration of Commitment*.
- The percentage of pregnant women living with HIV who received antiretroviral treatment to prevent mother-to-child transmission increased from 9% in 2004 to 33% in 2007.
- Among the few countries reporting on populations most at risk, 60% of sex workers, 46% of injecting drug users, and 40% of men who have sex with men were reached by HIV prevention programmes in 2007.

Treatment and care: unprecedented progress, remaining challenges

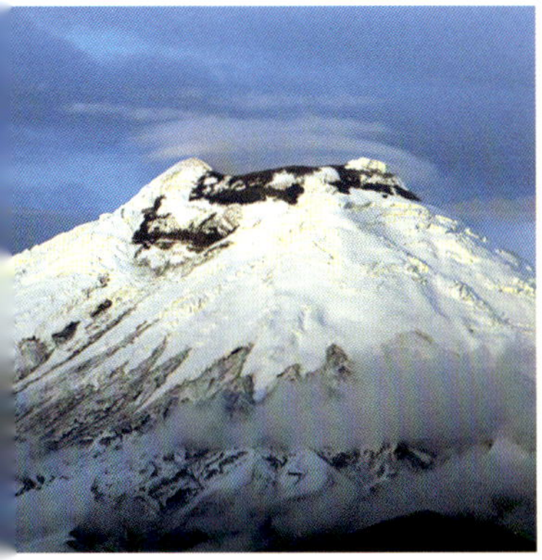

5

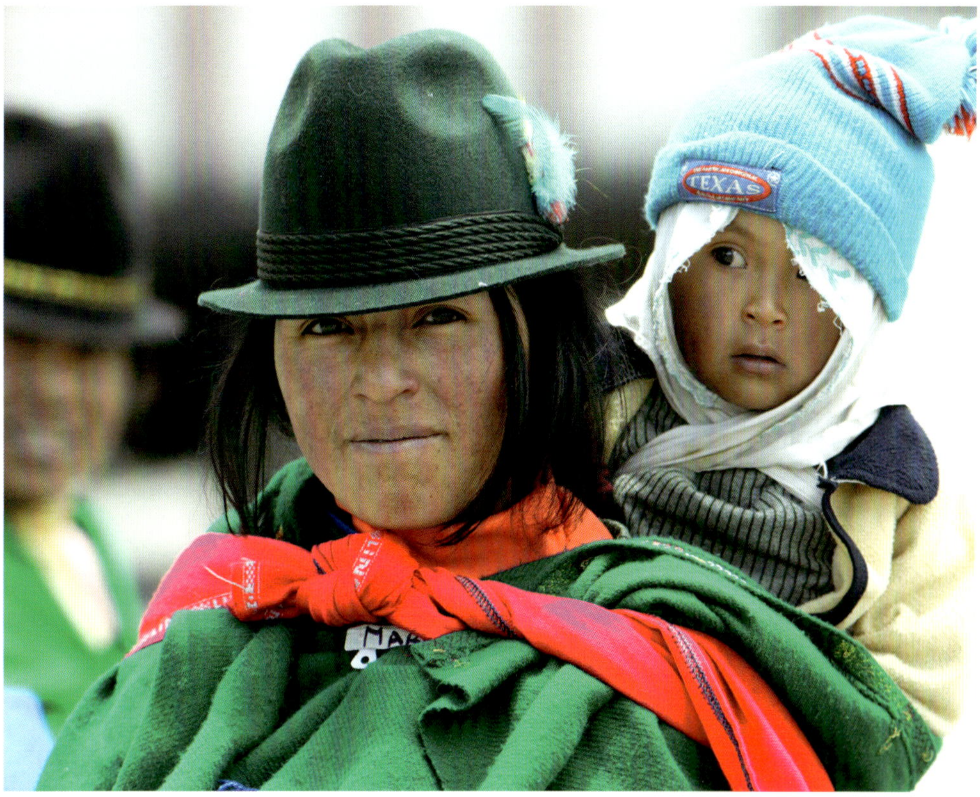

Chapter 5

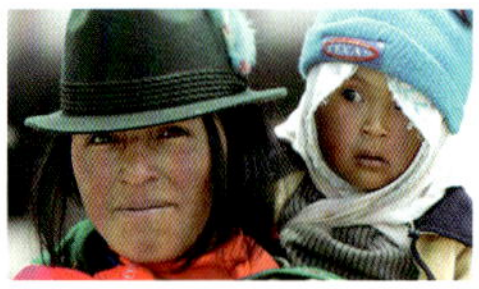

FIGURE 5.1 Selected events related to the treatment of AIDS

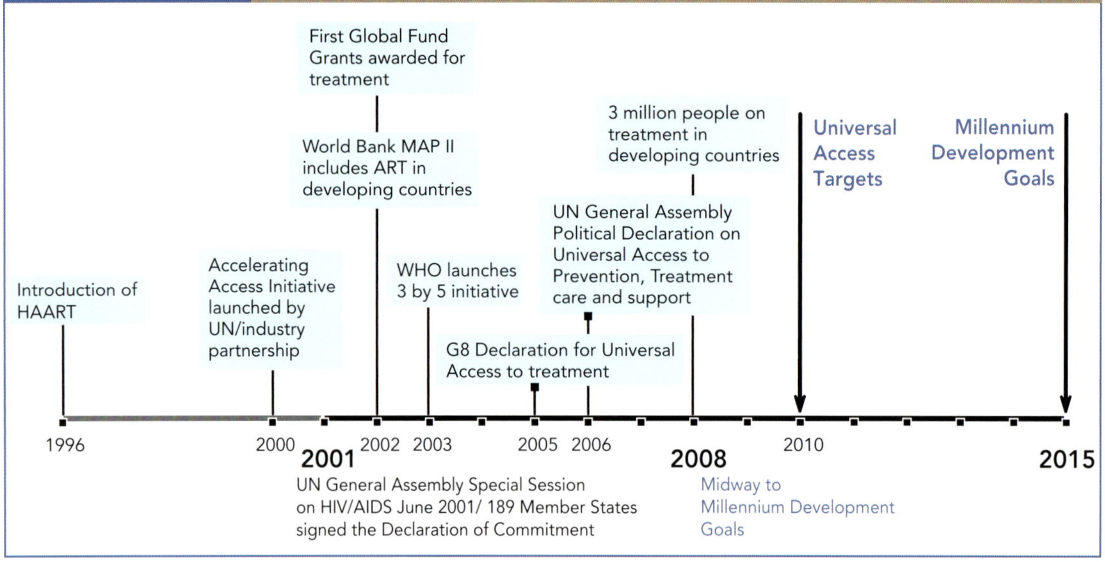

Key findings

- The number of people receiving antiretroviral drugs in low- and middle-income countries has increased 10-fold in only six years, reaching almost 3 million people by the end of 2007.
- The rapid expansion of treatment access in resource-limited settings is saving lives, improving quality of life, and contributing to the rejuvenation of households, communities, and entire societies.
- Intensified action is needed to ensure timely delivery of HIV treatment to children, who are significantly less likely than adults to receive antiretroviral drugs.
- Globally, coverage of antiretroviral treatment for women is higher than or equal to that of men.
- The populations most at risk of HIV exposure, such as injecting drug users, face considerable barriers to HIV treatment access, often as a result of institutionalized discrimination.
- Low testing rates reduce the impact of HIV treatment, because individuals who are diagnosed late in the course of infection have a poorer prognosis. A number of countries, however, are successfully using a range of approaches to increase knowledge of HIV serostatus.
- Despite the existence of affordable medications, too few people living with both HIV and tuberculosis are receiving treatment for both conditions. This situation contributes to substantial, avoidable morbidity and mortality.
- Weaknesses in health-care systems are slowing the scale-up of HIV treatment programmes, underscoring the need for intensified action to strengthen these systems. Antiretroviral therapy scale-up is helping to drive significant improvements in health-care infrastructure in resource-limited settings.
- Among the developments needed to ensure the sustainability of HIV treatment are more affordable second- and third-line therapies, as well as greater success in preventing new HIV infections.

The decision of the global community to push towards universal access to HIV prevention, treatment, care, and support represents a moral commitment of historic proportions. Never before has the world attempted, on such a large scale, to bring broad-based chronic disease management to resource-limited settings. Until this decade, low- and middle-income countries were forced to wait 10–20 years—sometimes for more than a generation—before breakthrough health technologies were broadly available. Slightly more than a decade after the emergence of combination antiretroviral therapy, millions of individuals in resource-limited settings are now benefiting from these medications.

Global commitment to make HIV treatments available in resource-limited settings is bearing fruit. In only six years, the number of people receiving antiretroviral drugs in low- and middle-income countries has increased more than 10-fold (Figure 5.2). In settings where HIV was invariably fatal only a short time ago, introduction of life-preserving therapies has rejuvenated households, revived entire communities, and re-energized the broader response to the epidemic (Sanders, 2008).

Many actors share credit in this achievement, most notably people living with HIV themselves, whose advocacy helped achieve what was once considered impossible.

Notwithstanding these considerable achievements, substantially greater progress will be required to move towards universal access to HIV treatment and care. The number of new HIV infections continues to outstrip the increase each year in the number of people on antiretroviral drugs by 2.5 to 1. Thus, the long-term sustainability of even the current pace of treatment scale-up may be jeopardized.

Children are not benefiting equally from the momentous treatment advances, being less likely than adults to receive antiretroviral drugs. In addition, hundreds of thousands of people who are coinfected with HIV and tuberculosis die needlessly each year due to inadequate tuberculosis diagnostic services, failure to deliver affordable medications to those who need them, and rising rates of tuberculosis drug resistance.

This chapter summarizes the achievements to date in expanding access to HIV treatment

FIGURE 5.2 Number of people receiving antiretroviral drugs in low- and middle-income countries, 2002–2007

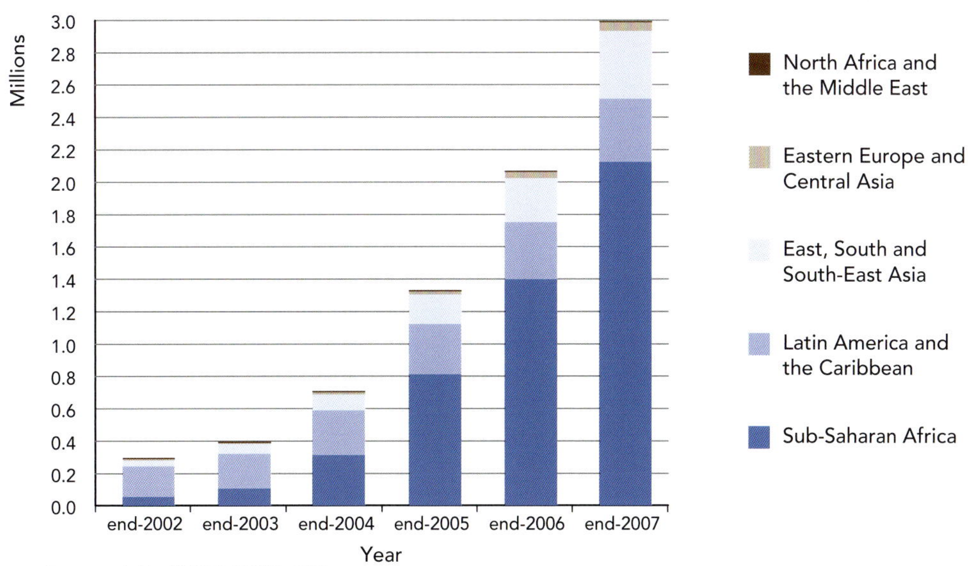

Source: Data provided by UNAIDS & WHO, 2008.

in low- and middle-income countries. It discusses challenges in ensuring equal access to antiretroviral drugs, as well as non-antiretroviral components of HIV treatment and care, including management of opportunistic illnesses and other conditions. Finally, the chapter identifies the impediments to more rapid and broad-based scale-up, and summarizes what is known about how to overcome these obstacles.

Progress in reducing HIV-related illness and death

The impact of antiretroviral drugs on the management of HIV infection has been startling, with improvements in health proving to be far more marked and enduring than anticipated when combination antiretroviral therapy first emerged in the mid-1990s. Recent studies in Denmark suggest that a young man newly diagnosed with HIV is likely to live an additional 35 years with available medications, a tripling of the life expectancy for people with HIV (Lohse et al., 2007). In slightly more than a decade, the introduction of combination antiretroviral therapy has saved an estimated three million years of life in the United States alone (Walensky et al., 2006).

As more is learnt about antiretroviral therapy management through clinical trials and through the accumulation of greater clinical experience, health outcomes as a result of therapy are improving further still. Data derived from national HIV treatment and care monitoring in the United Kingdom, for example, indicates that median time to treatment failure for patients on first-line regimens that include one or more protease inhibitors ranges from 4.3 years to 6.5 years; however, patients started on a regimen containing two nucleoside reverse transcriptase inhibitors (NRTI) and one non-nucleoside reverse transcriptase inhibitor (NNRTI) had a median time before treatment failure of 13.2 years (Beck et al., 2008a). As Chapter 6 explains, increased access to antiretroviral drugs is also improving quality of life for millions of people, benefiting households, communities, and societies.

The growing availability of antiretroviral drugs is lessening the burden of HIV-related mortality

FIGURE 5.3 Estimated number of adult and child deaths due to AIDS globally, 1990–2007

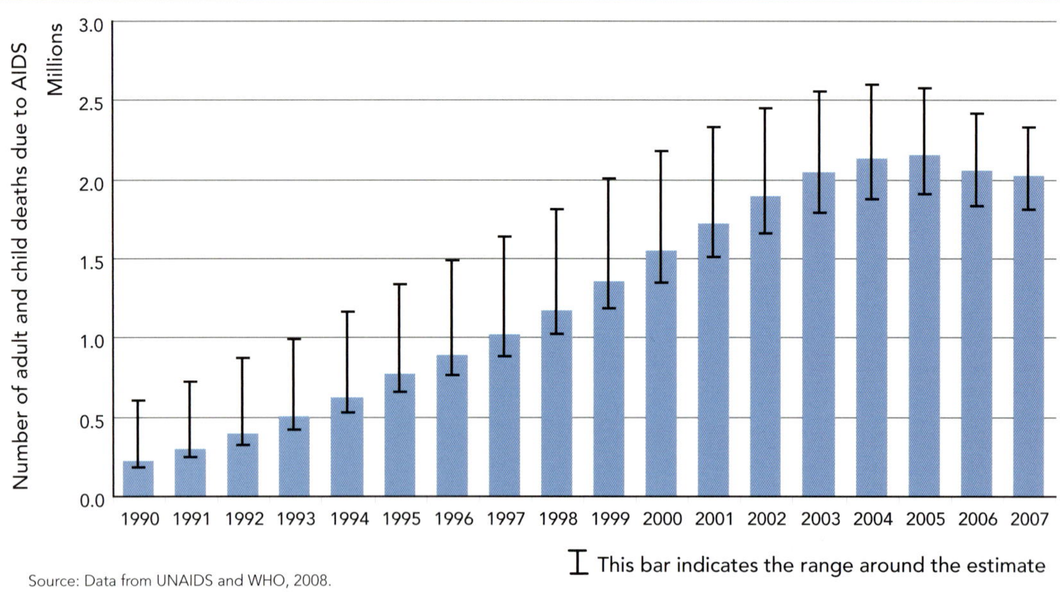

Source: Data from UNAIDS and WHO, 2008.

Becoming courageous, and thriving on antiretroviral drugs

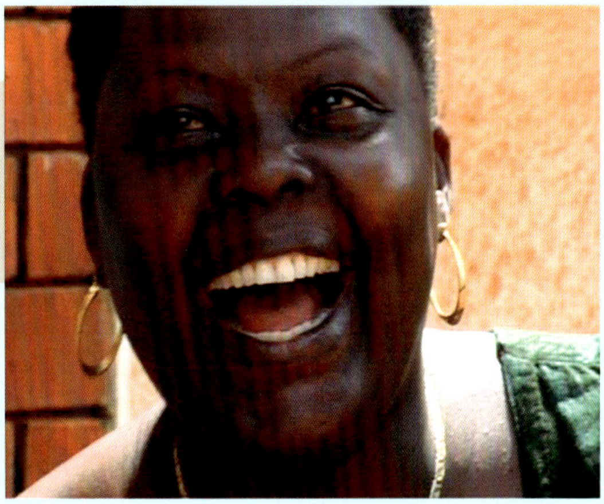

Lillian Mworeko is the Africa regional coordinator for the International Committee of Women Living with HIV and AIDS. She is based in Uganda.

Lillian Mworeko was 29 when she was diagnosed with HIV. It was the day her husband died.

"I was already in shock at the death of my husband, so my results did not bother me so much", she says. "But later on, after the burial, the reality of being HIV-positive came to me. Here I was, a young widow, with a small child, and I was struggling to cope alone."

Alone and having no money, Mworeko sought help from support groups and networks in her hometown in Uganda. She began to learn more about HIV. As she gained confidence she was able to get the support she needed from her family and friends.

"I became courageous, I knew life has to continue," she says.

Her courage stood her in good stead when, some years later, she and her new partner decided to have a child together. She did a lot of reading and research to ensure that she would not transmit the virus to her unborn child. By this time she was already on antiretroviral treatment, but it was not the recommended regimen to prevent mother-to-child transmission. "I had several discussions with my doctors and they had to change my drugs, to conduct tests on my CD4 and viral loads", she says. "I discussed my serostatus with my doctor. He was so supportive. At one time, I thought I was going to need a caesarean, then I changed my mind. I got a lot of support… it is mainly because I shared with them."

Mworeka was also helped by other HIV-positive women who had started a motherhood programme called the Mama's Club. They talked about the challenges they faced and the measures and precautions needed to prevent vertical transmission. The support and interaction with other women was invaluable. But even so, there were shocks in store for Mworeko when she got her new baby home. She had decided to bottle-feed the baby to be absolutely certain that she would not transmit HIV in her breast milk. "I thought it was cheap to be on PMTCT programme", says Mworeko, "but I did not know the price of formula feed. It is expensive and he went through four tins of food a week in the first weeks."

Moworeka considers herself fortunate in having access to antiretroviral therapy and medical support provided by her workplace. "It has given me hope and when I look at life now, it is more positive than before… there were times when I was not sure of the next day, but now, I look at life positively, I've decided to go back to school, to go higher in my career, so that the contribution I make towards the community is higher."

in low- and middle-income countries, as it did in high-income countries a decade ago (Figure 5.3). In rural South Africa, substantial declines in mortality were reported in 2006, as these drugs became increasingly available (Nyirenda et al., 2007). After decades of increasing mortality, the annual number of AIDS deaths globally has declined in the past two years, in part as a result of the substantial increase in HIV treatment access in recent years.

Antiretroviral therapy has been also found to be a cost-effective or cost-saving intervention in high-, middle- and lower-income countries. (Harling, 2005.) Most of the cost-effectiveness studies performed to date, have only included direct costs. If indirect costs are included, Highly Active Antiretroviral Therapy (HAART) in many countries is likely to be a cost-saving intervention as it enables people living with HIV to remain well, and socially and economically active (Badri, 2006).

In spite of promising signs that improved treatment access is yielding results in low- and middle-income countries, treatment success rates may be somewhat lower in resource-limited settings than in high-income settings. At both 6 and 12 months after initiation of antiretroviral therapy, mortality rates for individuals in low- and middle-income countries are at least 28% higher than those for patients in high-income countries (Antiretroviral Therapy in Lower Income Countries Collaboration, 2006). When long-term survival is estimated, although the benefits of antiretroviral therapy in low- and middle-income countries are considerable, they are still less than those enjoyed in high-income countries (Beck, 2008b).

A number of factors are likely to contribute to this, such as more advanced clinical disease in resource-limited settings at the start of therapy and a higher incidence of co-occurring conditions (Beck, 2008b). In the interests of global

FIGURE 5.4 Scale up of antiretroviral coverage over time, select group of generalized and concentrated epidemic countries, 2004 to 2007

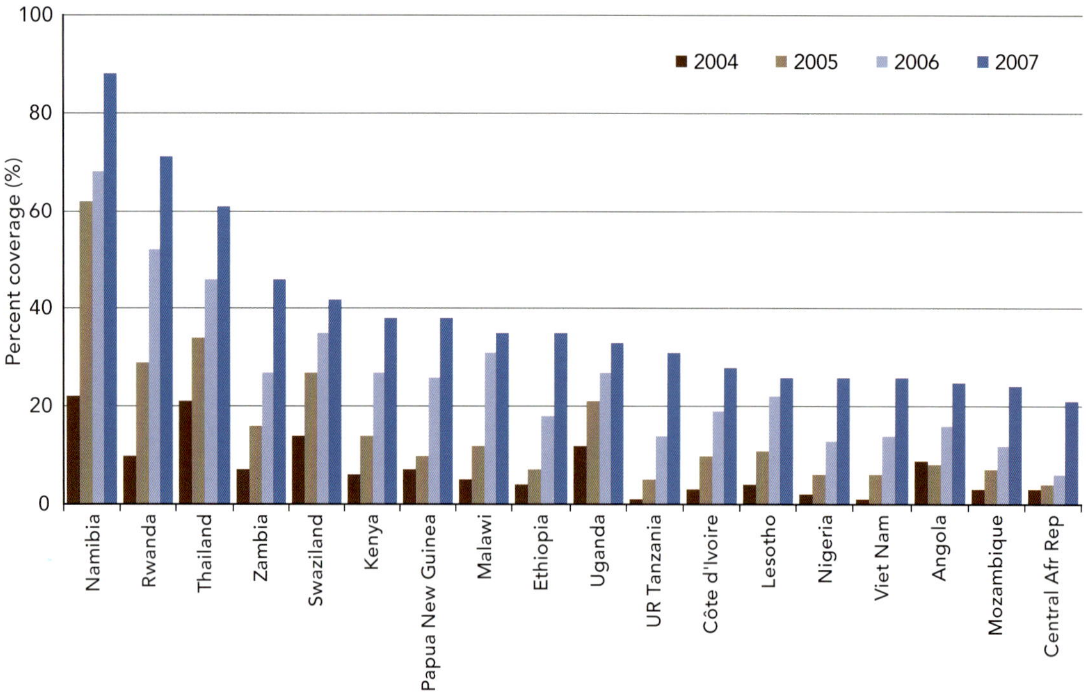

Source: UNGASS Country Progress Reports 2008.

equity, at the same time as efforts focus on the scaling up of antiretroviral drugs in low- and middle-income countries, attention must also be focused on understanding and addressing the sources of suboptimal outcomes for many patients in resource-limited settings.

Antiretroviral management in resource-limited settings

As of December 2007, an estimated 3 million people in low- and middle-income countries were receiving antiretroviral drugs, which represents 31% of those who need the medications, and is a 45% increase over 2006.

Increases in treatment coverage have been extraordinary in many countries (Figure 5.4). For example, in Namibia, where treatment coverage was less than 1% in 2003, 88% of individuals in need were on antiretroviral drugs in 2007. In Rwanda, antiretroviral therapy coverage increased from 1% in 2003 to almost 71% in 2007, aided by a 40-fold growth in the number of antiretroviral treatment sites. Antiretroviral therapy coverage in Thailand rose from 4% in 2003 to 61% in 2007 (UNGASS Indicator 4, 2008).

Figure 5.5 shows percentage coverage of antiretroviral therapy between males and females for generalized and concentrated epidemic countries, based on modelled estimates of male

FIGURE 5.5 Comparison of antiretroviral therapy coverage in 2007 between males and females (for countries with reported data on the number of people on treatment for both sexes separately)

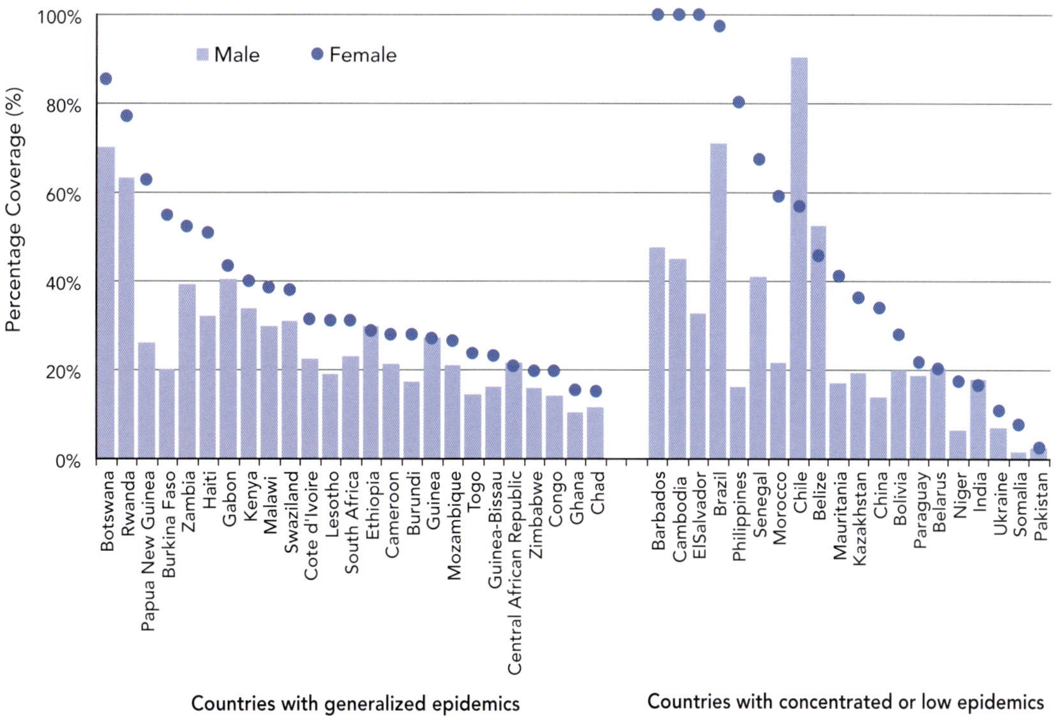

Source: Data from UNAIDS and WHO, 2008.

Note: Coverage estimates are based on applying the ratio of number of males and number of females receiving antiretroviral therapy to the final projected value of all people receiving antiretroviral therapy as of December 2007. This provides December 2007 estimates of number of males and females receiving antiretroviral therapy that are then divided by the estimated number of males and females in need of antiretroviral treatment respectively.

and female need. In most countries, women are receiving more than expected coverage for antiretroviral therapy. This sex disparity is particularly pronounced in generalized epidemics, which may be related to the fact that many HIV-positive women have two portals of entry for treatment—HIV treatment programmes and programmes to prevent mother-to-child transmission. Seven countries have equal coverage for men and women, while in two countries—Belize and Chile—men have much higher coverage than women. Additional research is needed to explore the reasons why women generally receive more coverage than men and to identify more effective strategies for increasing universal access to treatment.

Antiretroviral drugs are being successfully administered in some of the world's most challenging settings. In conflict-affected areas of the Democratic Republic of Congo, for example, an HIV treatment programme by Médecins sans Frontières has achieved treatment adherence rates comparable with those reported in non-conflict settings.

Expanding treatment access: a collective endeavour

The rapid growth in antiretroviral therapy coverage represents one of the great success stories in recent global health history. Less than ten years ago, even as antiretroviral drugs were contributing to sharp declines in HIV-related morbidity and mortality in high-income countries, it was widely assumed that these life-preserving medications would remain unaffordable and thus unavailable in low-income countries, perhaps for decades.

In the case of HIV, alleviating the stark disparities in health-care access that typify global health practice has required the leadership and coordination of diverse stakeholders at global, regional, and national levels. In response to the WHO/UNAIDS "3 by 5" initiative,[1] national governments embraced the push to expand HIV treatment access, establishing ambitious targets and making extensive efforts to build national capacity and address obstacles to scale-up. Civil society has mobilized in support of universal treatment access, with particular leadership provided by people living with HIV. At the global level, the *Political Declaration on HIV/AIDS*, adopted at the UN General Assembly's High Level Meeting on HIV/AIDS in 2006, pledged to move towards universal access to HIV prevention, treatment, care, and support by 2010—a goal that has obtained the strong support of key global and regional bodies, ranging from the G8 industrialized countries to the African Union and the Caribbean Community and Common Market.

Leading donors have helped finance the expansion of access to treatment. PEPFAR aims to reach 2.5 million people with treatment by 2012. As of December 2007, the Global Fund was supporting the delivery of antiretroviral drugs to 1.4 million people, which represents an increase of 88% from the previous year (Global Fund, 2008). UNITAID—a relatively new international mechanism for purchasing drugs that is funded by airline taxes—is playing a major role in scaling up paediatric treatment programmes and services to prevent mother-to-child transmission.

Many private companies are also helping to expand HIV treatment access (Global Business Coalition on HIV/AIDS, 2007). In Botswana, the mining company Debswana entered into a formal partnership with the national government to accelerate treatment scale-up, by covering the delivery of antiretroviral drugs to its HIV-positive workers (UNGASS, 2008a). Ten medium-to-large companies are among the

[1] Launched in December 2003, the "3 by 5" initiative proposed a massive scale-up of antiretroviral therapy, sufficient to ensure that 3 million people would be on antiretroviral drugs by the end of 2005. Although the goal of 3 million people on treatment was not reached until two years after the 2005 deadline, "3 by 5" was critical in catalysing unprecedented action to expand treatment access in resource-limited settings.

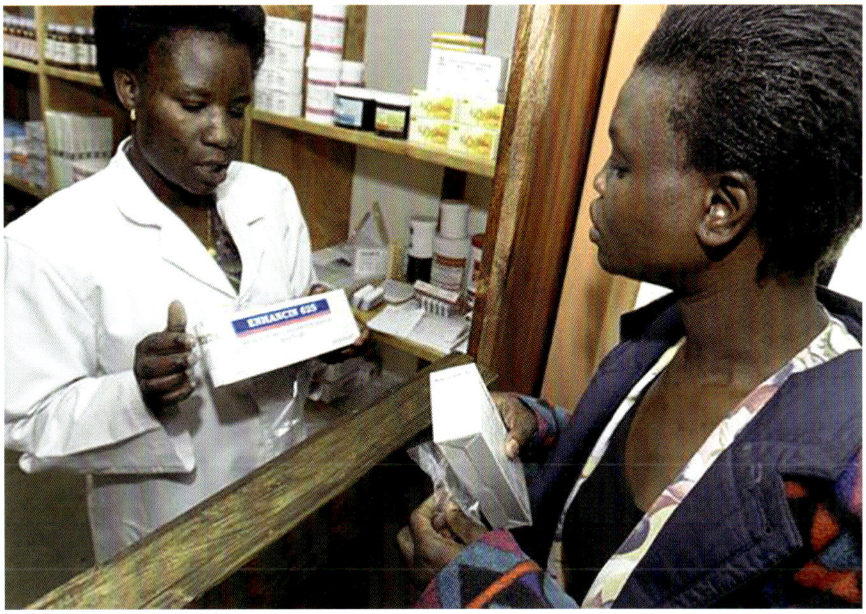

Antiretroviral therapy is for life. Sustaining the supply of life-saving antiretroviral drugs is critical to an effective treatment programme

members of the Suriname Business Coalition Against HIV, which recently implemented a strategic action plan on HIV to increase business involvement in the HIV response (UNGASS, 2008b). However, substantial additional efforts are required to fully engage industry in treatment scale-up, because both government and nongovernmental informants in only 9% of countries with generalized epidemics say that workplace HIV treatment services or treatment referral systems through the workplace have been implemented in all districts in need (UNGASS Country Progress Reports, 2008).

Numerous faith-based organizations are also playing a part in expanding treatment access, providing as much as 40% of all HIV-related health services in some countries (WHO, 2007f). With financial assistance from bodies such as the Global Fund, the Churches Health Association of Zambia will provide antiretroviral drugs to 17 000 individuals by the end of 2008 and is updating more than 100 church health facilities to implement Directly Observed Therapy, Short-course (DOTS) for tuberculosis. According to recent surveys, programmes supported by the Anglican Church were delivering antiretroviral drugs to 10 000 individuals in the United Republic of Tanzania (Anglican United Nations Office, 2007), and Catholic religious orders were supporting delivery of the drugs to more than 90 000 people worldwide (International Union of Superiors General, 2008).

People living with HIV have mobilized in countries throughout the world to support accelerated treatment scale-up and to promote treatment success. In Kenya, a national network of post-test clubs helps newly diagnosed individuals in understanding HIV and becoming active partners in their own health care. After meeting with representatives from 20 pharmaceutical companies, Ashar Alo, a leading network of people living with HIV in Bangladesh, forged an agreement to obtain lower prices for antiretroviral drugs and to establish a drug contribution

Research to improve treatment options

Although available antiretroviral drug regimens markedly improve the health and longevity of HIV-positive patients, a number of uncertainties remain with respect to the medical management of HIV disease. Research continues in an effort to identify the most effective regimens for individuals who have not previously received therapy (Eron et al., 2006; MacArthur et al., 2006; Lazzarin et al., 2007; Delfraissy et al., 2008). Whether to intervene with antiretroviral drugs during acute HIV infection also continues to be a topic of debate, as well as the focus of continuing clinical research (Fidler et al., 2008; Panel on Antiretroviral Guidelines, 2008). Also essential is research to develop new therapeutic options that are simpler to take, less toxic, and more affordable.

A priority that is the subject of urgent research efforts and will continue to grow in importance is the development of optimally effective treatment regimens for individuals in whom one or more antiretroviral drug combinations have failed (Abgrail et al., 2006; Clotet et al., 2007). Researchers are also working to develop new classes of antiretroviral drugs. These include compounds that inhibit the virus from entering cells (Este & Telenti, 2007) or that interfere with the integrase enzyme that plays a role in HIV replication (Grinsztejn et al, 2007).

In addition, extensive research is continuing into the potential for genetic testing to offer eventually the possibility of more precise tailoring of antiretroviral drug regimens to individual patients. Already, in clinical settings where it is available, HLA-B5701 screening permits clinicians to identify hypersensitivity to abacavir and thereby avoid potentially fatal drug toxicities (Phillips & Malial, 2008).

programme. In India, the South India Positive Network (SIP+) provides treatment literacy education for hundreds of transgender individuals living with HIV, and works with local health-care providers to address stigma and other barriers to health-care use by this population.

Introducing and adapting HIV treatment

The process for bringing antiretroviral therapy to scale in resource-limited settings is well characterized (WHO, 2006a). Countries are advised to develop national treatment plans with clear targets, to promote provider-initiated HIV testing and counselling to increase treatment uptake, and to undertake efforts to strengthen health and regulatory systems. All countries report having in place a policy or strategy to promote comprehensive HIV treatment, care, and support. Most (85%) countries with generalized epidemics, and 52% of countries with concentrated epidemics, report having developed national estimates and projected future needs of the number of individuals requiring antiretroviral therapy (UNGASS Country Progress Reports, 2008).

WHO recommends national use and consolidated purchase of standardized antiretroviral drug regimens consisting of fixed-dose combinations. Preferred first-line regimens include two nucleoside reverse transcriptase inhibitors (NRTIs) and one non-nucleoside reverse transcriptase inhibitor (NNRTI). For second-line regimens, preference is given to a combination of two NRTIs (at least one of which is new) and a protease inhibitor boosted with ritonavir (WHO, 2006a).

Most national HIV treatment guidelines are in accord with WHO recommendations on first-line regimens and on routine clinical monitoring (Beck et al., 2006). However, civil society surveys in 16 low- and middle-income countries found that many clinical settings were prescribing regimens that were inconsistent with global treatment guidelines (International Treatment Preparedness Coalition, 2007), highlighting the need for follow-up to ensure adherence to national standards.

The best time to initiate antiretroviral therapy remains a subject of debate. WHO advises clinicians working in settings where CD4 testing is available to consider initiating treatment when a patient's CD4 count falls below 350 cells per mm^3 and to initiate treatment in all patients under 200 CD4 cells per mm^3. Where CD4 testing is unavailable, WHO recommends that antiretroviral therapy be started when patients exhibit clinical signs of advanced or severe immune suppression (WHO, 2006a). The United States Department of Health and Human Services recommends initiation of antiretroviral therapy in patients who have experienced an AIDS-defining opportunistic illness or have a CD4 count less than 350 cells per mm^3 (Panel on Antiretroviral Guidelines, 2008).

Treatment and care for children

Without treatment, approximately half of children with perinatal HIV infection will die by age two (Newell et al., 2004; Marston et al., 2005). Extensive experience in high-income countries has shown that antiretroviral drugs can reduce illness and death in children and adolescents living with HIV (Patel et al., 2008). In Western Europe in 2006, for example, only 10 children infected via mother-to-child transmission died of AIDS (EuroHIV, 2007).

When made accessible in resource-poor settings, treatment for children has proved highly effective. Studies of the effectiveness of antiretroviral treatment have found two-year survival rates exceeding 80% in various settings, including Côte d'Ivoire, Haiti, Malawi, and Zambia (Fassinou et al., 2004; Rouet et al., 2006; Bolton-Moore et al., 2007; Bong et al., 2007; George et al., 2007). Other studies have found survival probability at 12 months ranging from 87% (O'Brien et al., 2006) to more than 95% in settings in sub-Saharan Africa and Asia (Puthanakit et al., 2005 Janssens et al., 2007; Reddi et al., 2007; Arrivé et al., 2008).

Although use of antiretroviral drugs to treat children has increased in recent years in sub-Saharan Africa, children living with HIV are about one third as likely to receive antiretroviral therapy as adults living with HIV as a whole (Prendergast et al., 2007).

According to national governments, paediatric HIV treatment is available in all districts in need in 44% of countries with a concentrated

Redoubling national efforts to achieve universal treatment access in Ethiopia

Ethiopia's initial effort in 2004–2006 to bring antiretroviral therapy to scale reached 65% of its target of 100 000. In November 2006, the Government launched a two-year Millennium AIDS Campaign to generate swifter expansion of treatment access. The campaign relies on decentralization of the response, clear performance targets, coordinated planning, broad-based communications, and improved integration of HIV treatment into health-care settings. In its first seven months the campaign reached almost 1 million people with HIV testing, counselling, and services; it also initiated antiretroviral therapy for more than 31 000 patients (Ethiopia Federal Ministry of Health, 2007).

epidemic and in 36% of countries with a generalized epidemic. Nongovernmental informants suggest that access is in reality even more scarce, affirming the widespread availability of paediatric treatment in only 31% of countries with a concentrated epidemic and 9% of countries with a generalized epidemic (UNGASS Country Progress Reports, 2008).

Several factors threaten treatment access for HIV-infected children. For example, prompt diagnosis of HIV infection in infants is critical, but is often difficult to achieve. HIV-exposed children usually have maternal HIV antibodies in their first months of life, even when they themselves are uninfected; therefore, traditional HIV antibody testing (Enzyme-Linked ImmunoSorbent Assay, or ELISA, or rapid testing) does not reliably detect actual HIV infection in the first 6–18 months. Virological tests—including HIV DNA polymerase chain reaction (PCR), real-time HIV RNA PCR, or use of an ultrasensitive p24 antigen test—are thus required to make an accurate and timely diagnosis. However, access to such technologies is frequently limited and highly variable in resource-limited settings (De Baets et al., 2005; Prendergast et al., 2007). The cost and complexity of these test methods have declined in recent years, making it more feasible to implement such assays in resource-limited settings (WHO, 2006b). Testing of dried blood spots derived from the infant's heelstick avoids difficulties associated with phlebotomy in infants and permits centralization of laboratory capacity (WHO, 2006c). The use of dried blood spots offers the potential to greatly increase early diagnosis and timely treatment of HIV in young children. According to a study in South Africa, use of available, affordable strategies to improve diagnosis of HIV-exposed infants could significantly improve the odds that HIV-infected children will survive (Sherman, Matsebula & Jones 2005).

Clinicians are exploring various strategies to increase treatment uptake for children living with HIV. For example, child health cards that document an infant's status following the child's participation in a programme to prevent mother-to-child transmission enable health workers to respond appropriately at the child's first postnatal visit for immunizations. Just as provider-initiated testing and counselling is helping in the scale-up of services to prevent mother-to-child transmission and HIV treatment generally, this approach is now being used in certain settings where children living with HIV are likely to be found such as paediatric wards in high-prevalence countries.

Available antiretroviral drugs were initially developed for adults; most standard fixed-dose combinations are inappropriate for children. To help clinicians to identify the appropriate dosing of antiretroviral drugs for children, WHO developed updated, user-friendly paediatric dosing tables. In collaboration with the Clinton Foundation, UNITAID has negotiated a 40% decline in the prices of paediatric antiretroviral drugs and, as of December 2007, was supporting HIV diagnostics and treatment for 102 000 children worldwide (UNITAID, 2008).

Monitoring treatment success

In the absence of viral load measurements in resource-limited settings, clinicians are advised to use clinical or immunological monitoring, or both, to decide when to initiate therapy, assess treatment success, and decide when to change from first-line to second-line regimens. Because antiretroviral drugs do not eradicate the virus but rather maintain viral replication at low levels (see Palmer et al., 2008), treatment must be continued without interruption. Antiretroviral treatment failure, as measured by increasing viral load, tends to occur rather slowly in clinical settings, especially now that therapeutic regimens and techniques for clinical management of antiretroviral drug administration have improved (Phillips et al., 2007). Studies in the United Kingdom indicate that nearly 11% of patients will die within five years of extensive failure of the three primary classes of antiretroviral medications (Phillips et al., 2007).

Monitoring for side-effects

Up to half of patients on antiretroviral therapy may experience adverse effects of the medications (Fellay et al., 2001). Common side-effects vary depending on the drug regimen, but can include hypersensitivity, lactic acidosis, increases in blood lipids, bleeding events, anaemia, neuropathy, lipodystrophy, and pancreatitis (NIH, 2008). While most side-effects diminish over time, some can be life-threatening, underscoring the importance of careful patient monitoring (NIH, 2008).

As a leading HIV clinician has advised, "The success of [antiretrovirals] comes at a price" (Lange, 2006). That price is paid by the person taking the drugs. The unpleasant, often painful, and potentially disfiguring side-effects sometimes associated with the drugs may have a significant negative impact on quality of life and on an individual's ability or willingness to adhere to the prescribed regimen.

Management of side-effects constitutes an essential component of antiretroviral drug administration. After more than a decade of clinical experience in administration of antiretroviral drugs, more is known about the side-effect profiles of different antiretroviral drugs. Improvements in the evidence base have made it easier for clinicians to prescribe regimens with a greater likelihood of long-term treatment success and to refine regimens when side-effects emerge. However, management of side-effects can be more difficult in resource-limited settings, where drug substitution may not always be feasible due to limited access to the full array of antiretroviral drugs licensed for use in high-income countries.

The prevalence of HIV drug resistance has grown over time in high-income countries and in Brazil, where antiretroviral drugs have been in use for longer than anywhere else (Weinstock et al., 2004; Barreto et al., 2006). In the low- and lower-middle-income countries where antiretroviral drugs were introduced more recently, much lower rates of resistance prevail, but these may increase as people on therapy live longer.

A high level of treatment adherence is needed to avoid or delay the emergence of drug resistance, which is closely associated with treatment failure (Panel on Antiretroviral Guidelines, 2008). A growing body of data associates treatment interruptions—including those guided by CD4 count—with viral rebound, poorer clinical outcomes, and diminished quality of life (Strategies for Management of Antiretroviral Therapy Study Group, 2006; Burman et al., 2008; UK Collaborative HIV Cohort Study, 2008). Efforts to promote treatment adherence have been helped by the simplification of antiretroviral drug regimens in recent years, including the development of once-daily dosing (Johnson et al., 2006; Niel Malan, 2008).

Although strong treatment adherence can be achieved in resource-limited settings and in various vulnerable populations (see Mills et al., 2006), many people living with HIV find it difficult to adhere to antiretroviral drug regimens. In a clinic setting in Johannesburg, nearly one in six patients who started on treatment dropped out of care over a 15-month period (Dalal et al., 2008). Factors that may contribute to non-adherence are numerous and may vary, depending on the population and setting. Factors include social and economic factors (e.g. poverty, unstable housing, and inadequate transportation to distant treatment centres), and non-HIV-related health conditions (e.g. active chemical dependence or mental illness) (Hicks et al., 2007; Tegger et al., 2008). Ensuring strong treatment adherence for children can be especially difficult due to the shortage of appropriate paediatric formulations, the unpalatability of some paediatric antiretroviral drugs, and the dependence on a caregiver for delivery of the medication.

Although antiretroviral treatment adherence has been the focus of numerous clinical trials, optimal strategies for measuring and improving treatment adherence have yet to be characterized (Panel on Antiretroviral Guidelines, 2008). Patient education, counselling, and use of reminders have shown promise as strategies to support treatment adherence (Wang et al., 2007; Wang & Wu, 2007; Aspeling & van Wyk, 2008).

In rural Uganda, more than 95% of patients were at least 95% adherent (based on pill count) following exposure to various adherence interventions including group education, personal adherence planning, medication companions, and weekly home delivery of the drugs (Weidle et al., 2006). Peer-based programmes that provide continuing aid in adhering to treatment have proven to be effective; for example, in the West Java Province of Indonesia, the programme Pantura Plus Karawang trains and supports volunteers in rural and urban areas to provide adherence assistance to individuals on antiretroviral therapy.

Non-antiretroviral components of comprehensive HIV treatment and care

The medical management of HIV involves much more than treatment of the underlying HIV infection. HIV-related immune suppression increases the risk of a broad range of debilitating, potentially life-threatening conditions;

FIGURE 5.6 Relationship between tuberculosis notification rate and HIV prevalence in Zimbabwe, 1990–2006

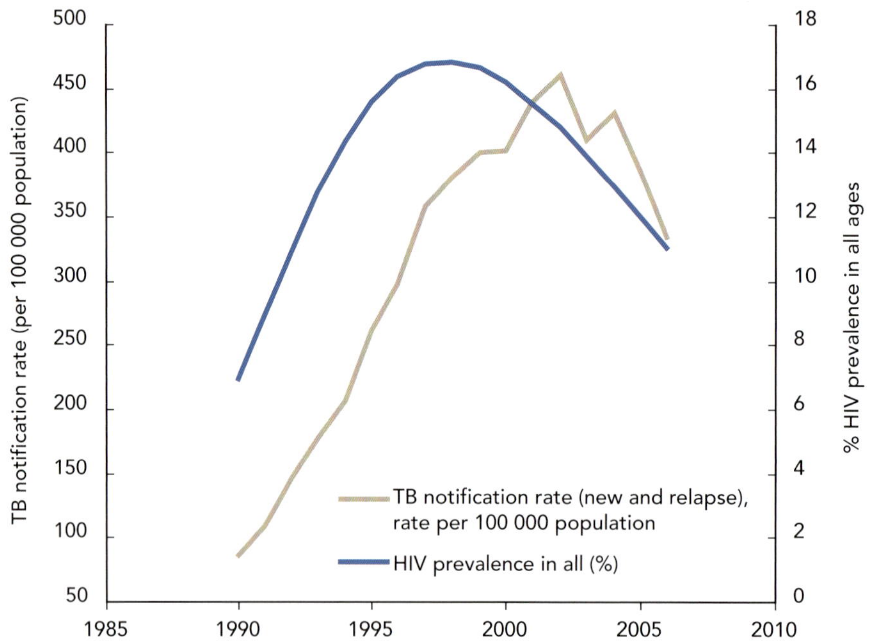

Source: WHO Global TB control report 2008 (WHO, 2008a); UNAIDS HIV prevalence estimates.

therefore, the prevention and treatment of such opportunistic illnesses are central to effective HIV treatment and care. People living with HIV also frequently have other health conditions not directly tied to their HIV infection, and these may be more severe in the presence of HIV, or may complicate antiretroviral therapy. Maximizing the success of HIV treatment also requires attention to nutrition, mental health, and social and economic factors, such as access to transport. Only by ensuring that people living with HIV are actively engaged in their own medical care will clinicians be able to provide prompt and effective treatment for the range of conditions to which HIV-positive people are potentially vulnerable.

Tuberculosis

While the world has rightly focused extraordinary attention on bringing antiretroviral therapy to scale, much less effort has been directed towards an enterprise that could yield comparable reductions in HIV-related morbidity and mortality—timely prevention, diagnosis, and treatment of tuberculosis in people living with HIV.

Tuberculosis remains the most common opportunistic infection for people living with HIV, including those on antiretroviral therapy, and a leading cause of death for people living with HIV in low- and middle-income countries (Egger, 2007). The synergistic relationship between HIV and tuberculosis is illustrated in Figure 5.6, which demonstrates how declines in HIV prevalence in Zimbabwe drove a subsequent drop in tuberculosis cases. Because of the synergistic impact between HIV and tuberculosis, Africa is now experiencing what tuberculosis experts are calling the worst tuberculosis epidemic since the advent of antibiotics (Chaisson, 2008).

An estimated 22% of tuberculosis cases in Africa occur in people living with HIV; in some coun-

FIGURE 5.7 Percentage of incident tuberculosis cases in people living with HIV receiving both antiretroviral and anti-tuberculosis medications, 2007

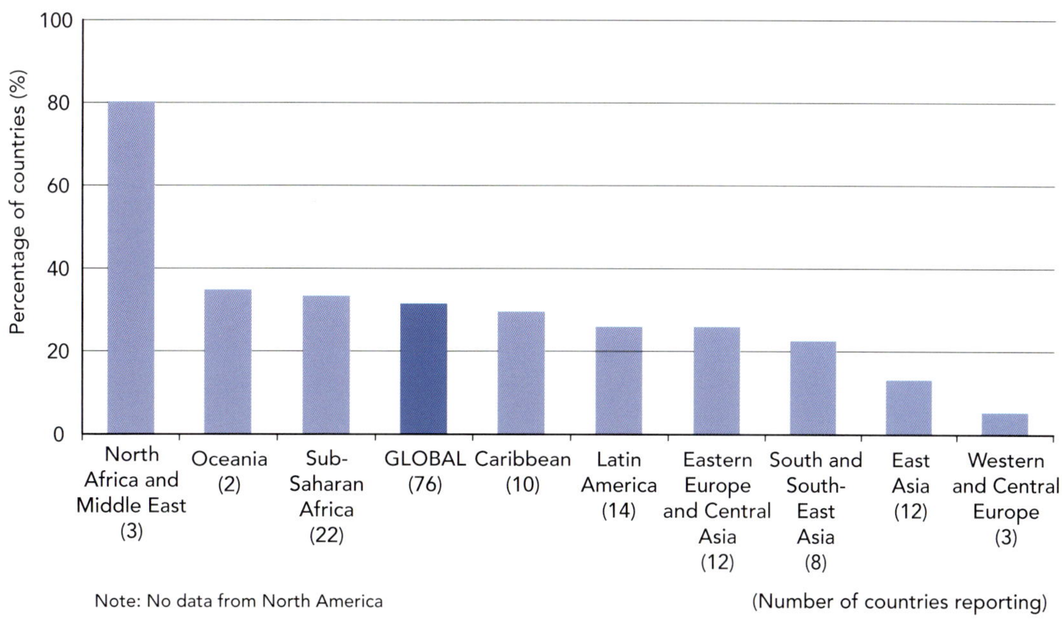

Source: UNGASS data provided by countries, 2008.

FIGURE 5.8 Unmet need for dual treatment of incident tuberculosis cases in people living with HIV, by region, 2007

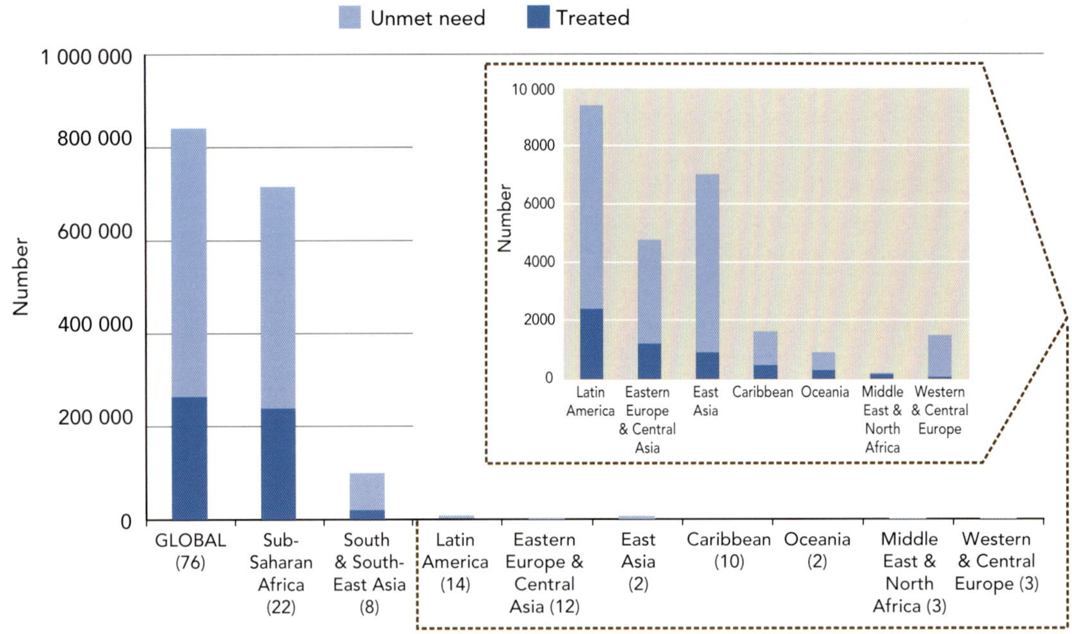

(Number of countries reporting)
Note: No data from North America
Source: UNGASS Country Progress Reports 2008.

tries in the region, this figure is as high as 70% (WHO, 2008a). Up to half of children living with HIV in South Africa are coinfected with tuberculosis (Prendergast et al., 2007). While tuberculosis incidence has declined globally in recent years, the number of cases continues to increase in areas heavily affected by HIV or drug-resistant tuberculosis, such as Africa and Eastern Europe (WHO, 2008a).

Diagnosing and treating active tuberculosis. Tuberculosis is particularly difficult to diagnose in people living with HIV, both with sputum microscopy and clinically (Hopewell et al., 2006; Chaisson & Martinson, 2008). More sensitive diagnostic tools could reduce tuberculosis-related mortality in people living with HIV by 20% (Dowdy et al., 2006), but such technologies are rarely available in resource-limited settings (Chaisson & Martinson, 2008).

Treatment of tuberculosis in individuals living with HIV follows the same basic approach as for patients not infected with HIV. However, despite the existence of affordable, well-understood treatments for tuberculosis, only 32% of tuberculosis cases in people living with HIV received both antiretroviral and anti-tuberculosis drugs (Figure 5.7) (UNGASS data provided by countries, 2008). As measured by the number of patients needing co-treatment, the greatest unmet need for dual HIV and tuberculosis treatment is in sub-Saharan Africa (Figure 5.8). In comparison to tuberculosis patients without HIV infection, tuberculosis patients who are living with HIV have lower treatment success rates, primarily due to an increased risk of death (Figure 5.9) (UNGASS data provided by countries, 2008; WHO, 2008a).

It is recommended that HIV-positive patients routinely receive co-trimoxazole, which can result in a 40% reduction in mortality (WHO,

FIGURE 5.9 Treatment outcomes for HIV-positive and HIV-negative tuberculosis patients, 2005 cohort

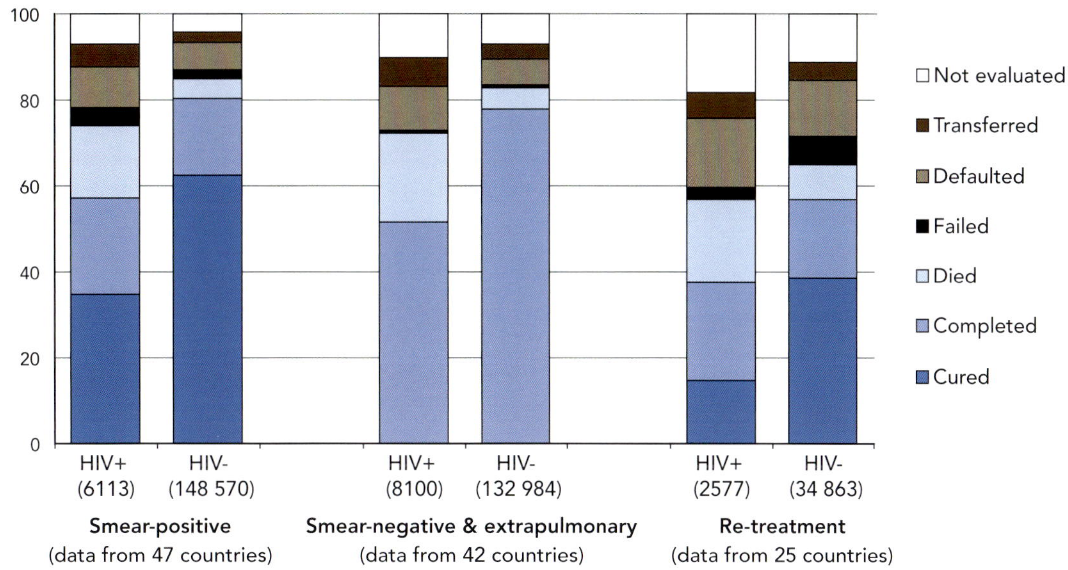

Source: WHO Global tuberculosis control: surveillance, planning, financing. World Health Organization, Geneva.

2007b). In 2006, 78% of HIV-positive tuberculosis patients received co-trimoxazole prophylaxis (WHO, 2008a).

Potential drug–drug interactions, as well as difficulties associated with adhering to multiple regimens, may complicate the simultaneous treatment of tuberculosis and HIV (Hopewell et al., 2006). In 2007, WHO issued a new module for comanagement of tuberculosis and HIV under its Integrated Management of Adolescent and Adult Illness initiative (WHO, 2007b). Careful and continuing education is essential to help patients on HIV and tuberculosis treatment to take a large number of pills appropriately and to adhere to medication changes required by standard co-treatment regimens.

Regardless of HIV status, careful adherence to tuberculosis regimens is essential to avoid the emergence of drug-resistance, which causes treatment failure and can be transmitted to others. People living with HIV have been shown to be twice as likely to have multidrug resistant tuberculosis (MDR-TB) as people who do not have HIV infection (WHO, 2008c). In a rural area of KwaZulu Natal Province in South Africa, an outbreak of extensively drug resistant tuberculosis (XDR-TB), i.e. tuberculosis that is resistant to both first- and second-line anti-tuberculosis drugs), was associated with extremely high mortality among people living with HIV (Gandhi et al., 2006).

Preventing active tuberculosis in people living with HIV. It is recommended that all people living with HIV be screened regularly for active tuberculosis. In the absence of evidence of active disease, individuals should be considered for treatment of latent tuberculosis infection with a 6–9-month course of preventive therapy

(WHO, 2004). According to national governments, only 42% of countries with generalized epidemics have implemented routine tuberculosis screening for HIV-positive patients, and only 27% provide tuberculosis preventive therapy in districts in need for people living with HIV; nongovernmental informants indicate that these two services are widely available in only 24% of countries with generalized epidemics (NCPI data reported from countries, 2008). A WHO survey of 41 countries with moderate-to-high burden of HIV and tuberculosis found that, although 51% of countries had national policies for the provision of preventive tuberculosis therapy to HIV-positive individuals with latent tuberculosis infection, only 15% of countries had implemented the policy at a national scale. Globally, only 27 000 HIV-positive people in low- and middle-income countries were started on isoniazid preventive therapy in 2006, and nearly all of these were in a single country—Botswana (WHO, 2008a).

Preventing further transmission. Health-care settings serve as a potentially important venue for the transmission of tuberculosis—and more worryingly, XDR-TB—to people living with HIV. Mathematical modelling indicates that implementation of available infection control practices in health-care settings could prevent almost half of all XDR-TB cases in South Africa (Basu et al., 2007). According to national reports, more than 60% of countries with generalized epidemics have yet to implement proper infection control procedures to prevent tuberculosis transmission in high-prevalence settings, such as HIV care clinics (UNGASS Country Progress Reports, 2008).

Systemic challenges to address HIV/tuberculosis coinfection. Institutional weaknesses are combining to impede the ability of countries to address the synergistic threat posed by HIV/tuberculosis coinfection. In particular, efforts to reduce tuberculosis-related morbidity and mortality among people living with HIV are undermined by the failure to integrate HIV and tuberculosis service delivery at national and subnational levels, resulting in missed opportunities to deliver optimal prevention, diagnosis, and treatment services.

While financing for tuberculosis control efforts in high-burden countries has more than doubled since 2002, many heavily affected countries have not adequately budgeted for activities to reduce the burden of HIV-related tuberculosis. Health-system barriers, such as inadequate drug supplies and laboratory capacity, remain a constraint to effective management of in people living with HIV (WHO, 2007d).

Of the 63 countries that collectively account for 97% of estimated HIV-positive tuberculosis cases worldwide, 63% have established national plans for integrated delivery of HIV and tuberculosis care. However, many such plans have not been translated into effective delivery systems. Although the Global Plan to Stop TB, 2006–2015 established a global target of testing 1.6 million tuberculosis patients annually for HIV, approximately 700 000 tuberculosis patients were tested for HIV in 2006 (WHO, 2008a) (Figure 5.10).

Technological challenges to improving tuberculosis outcomes in people living with HIV. No new class of tuberculosis drugs has been approved in more than 40 years, and the principal diagnostic test is more than 100 years old. Greatly increased investment in research for new tools to prevent, diagnose, and treat tuberculosis in people living with HIV is needed.

Other HIV-related illnesses

In addition to tuberculosis, individuals living with HIV may be vulnerable to a host of opportunistic illnesses such as *Pneumocystis carinii* pneumonia, cytomegalovirus retinitis, various oral diseases and complications, changes in bone mass and increased risk of bone disease, and cervical cancer. Antiretroviral therapy is often critical to effective management of opportunistic infections because the recovery of immune function usually significantly reduces the risk of suffering an opportunistic illness (Heiden et al.,

FIGURE 5.10 HIV testing for tuberculosis patients, all countries, 2006

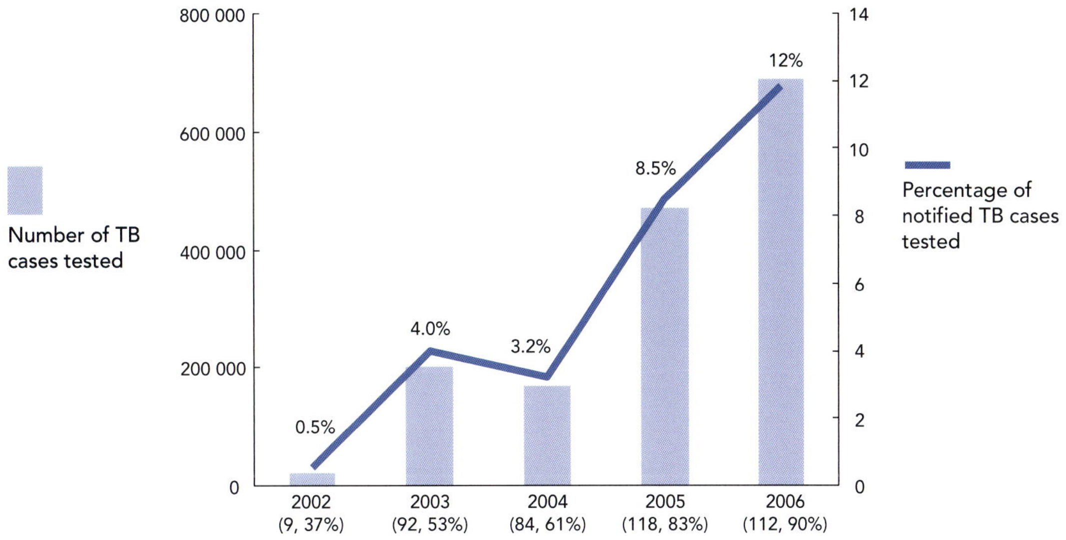

Source: WHO, 2008a.
Note: Numbers under bars represent the number of countries reporting data followed by the percentage of total estimated HIV-positive tuberculosis cases accounted for by reporting countries.

2007). In addition, clinical interventions focus on the opportunistic condition itself, necessitating continuing patient monitoring, accurate diagnostic tools, timely prophylaxis, and targeted treatment.

Access to medications and other health services required for the management of HIV-related opportunistic conditions is often sharply limited in many resource-limited settings. A total of 70% of countries surveyed by WHO cited erratic supplies and frequent stockouts as barriers to national scaling up of co-trimoxazole prophylaxis, which is used in the treatment of tuberculosis and other HIV-related opportunistic infections (Vittoria, 2008).

Hepatitis B is endemic in many countries with high HIV prevalence and is especially concentrated among children. In a study in Côte d'Ivoire, 12% of children living with HIV were coinfected with hepatitis B (Rouet et al., 2008). Adults coinfected with HIV and hepatitis B progress to chronic hepatitis B infection five times faster than adults without HIV infection. Antiretroviral drugs are often difficult to tolerate for individuals coinfected with HIV and hepatitis B, necessitating close and continuing patient monitoring (Hoffman, 2007). Studies have also noted a potential increased risk for antiretroviral drug resistance in children coinfected with HIV and hepatitis B (Rouet et al., 2008). There is no cure for hepatitis B, although the disease can be suppressed with prolonged, sometimes indefinite, therapy. Unfortunately, of the seven drugs currently used to treat chronic hepatitis B infection in high-income countries, only one is widely available in Africa and Asia (Hoffman, 2007).

Treatment needs of injecting drug users

Although it is entirely feasible to obtain excellent medical outcomes through antiretroviral therapy in HIV-positive individuals with chemical dependency, substance addiction may have an important impact on therapeutic approaches. Alcohol consumption, for example, may exacerbate side-effects of the drugs (NIH, 2008), and patients with chemical dependence may find it hard to adhere to prescribed regimens.

Substitution treatment with methadone or buprenorphine is effective for the treatment of opioid dependence. WHO added methadone to the list of essential medications in 2005. However, a major barrier to the successful treatment of HIV-positive people with opioid dependence is the shortage or complete absence of substitution treatment in many parts of the world—the result of government policies that prohibit such services (see Chapter 4). Unmet need for substitution treatment for chemical dependence is especially great in China, India, and the Russian Federation (WHO, 2008b). According to reports by nongovernmental informants, many countries—in Eastern Europe and Central Asia, South and South-East Asia, and North America—have laws, regulations or policies that impede use of HIV services by injecting drug users (UNGASS Country Progress Reports, 2008) (Figure 5.11).

Coinfection with one or more forms of hepatitis is common among people living with HIV in many parts of the world. Studies in the United States suggest that 50%–90% of HIV-positive injecting drug users are also infected with hepatitis C (Centers for Disease Control and Prevention, 2005). HIV infection significantly increases the risk of death from liver disease in individuals infected with hepatitis C (Smit et al., 2008). Although it is possible to achieve excellent clinical outcomes for individuals coinfected with HIV and hepatitis C, simultaneous medical management of both conditions can be complex due to potential drug interactions and toxicities, and uncertainties about the best therapeutic approaches (Sulkowski & Benhamou, 2007).

Diseases of ageing

In settings where antiretroviral drugs have been in widespread use since the mid-1990s, treatment has radically altered the natural course of HIV infection, expanding the spectrum of health problems presented by individuals living with HIV and altering the most common causes of death among HIV-positive people (Smit et al., 2006). In particular, chronic illnesses and co-morbidities cause an increasingly large

FIGURE 5.11 Percentage of countries reporting laws, regulations or policies that present obstacles to services for injecting drug users

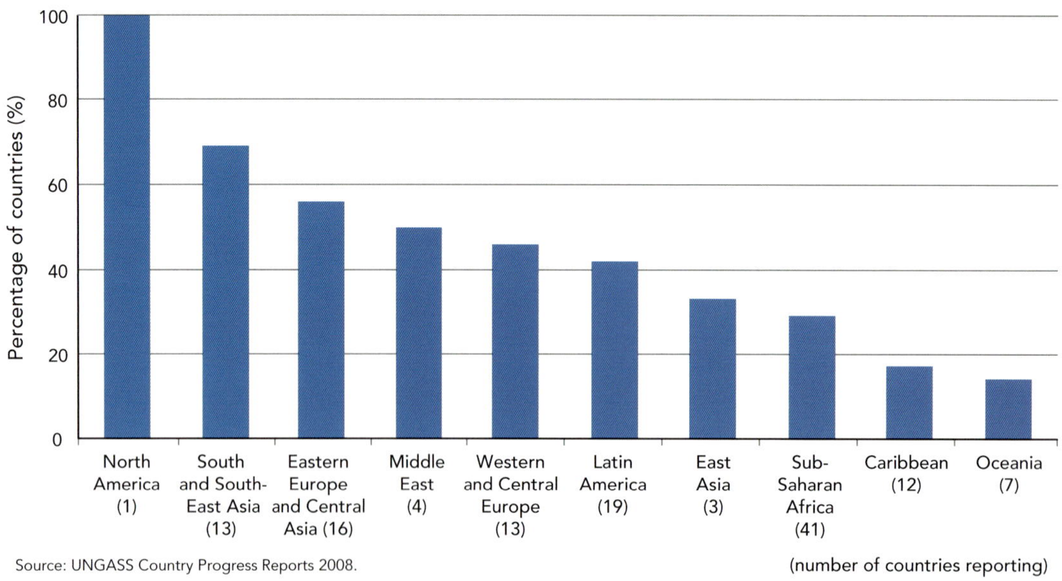

Source: UNGASS Country Progress Reports 2008.

percentage of deaths among people living with HIV in settings where antiretroviral drugs have been used widely for more than a decade. Between 1995 and 2006, the percentage of non-HIV-related deaths among people living with HIV in New York City increased from 8% to 32%, with cardiovascular conditions and non-AIDS-defining cancers accounting for nearly half of all deaths (New York City Department of Health and Mental Hygiene, 2007). In Norway, while the risk of HIV-related death has declined 80% in the era of combination antiretroviral therapy, the mortality rate for individuals living with HIV is still four times higher than in the general population (2007).

As people living with HIV in low- and middle-income countries live longer as a result of increased access to antiretroviral drugs, it is likely that the range and prevalence of HIV-related opportunistic infections will also evolve. For example, based on experience in high-income countries, where the drugs have been widely available since the mid-1990s, various non-AIDS-defining cancers may become increasingly important complications of HIV infection (Grulich et al., 2007; Dhir et al., 2008).

Mental health

As a life-threatening and highly stigmatized illness, HIV infection inevitably has effects on mental health. It is estimated that nearly half of all people living with HIV worldwide will suffer at some point from clinical depression (Miller, 2006). In addition to its psychosocial consequences, HIV infection can have important biological effects on mental health functioning, resulting in cognitive impairment and dementia (Freeman et al., 2005).

Integrating mental health services into antiretroviral treatment programmes is critical to effective care and treatment. On average, patients with a mood, anxiety, or substance abuse disorder have a less robust virological response to antiretroviral therapy than individuals without such a condition (Pence et al., 2007). Depression has also been associated with reduced nutritional intake among people living with HIV (Isaac et al., 2008).

Proven counselling, social support, and psychotherapeutic strategies exist to address the mental health needs of people living with HIV (Catalan et al., 2005). National governments in countries with generalized epidemics report that psychosocial support services are available in all districts in need in 52% of countries, although nongovernmental informants say this is the case in only 27% of such countries (UNGASS Country Progress Reports, 2008.) Professional mental health services are seldom available in low- and middle-income countries. While mental disorders account for more than 11% of the total burden of disease in low- and middle-income countries, many countries invest less than 1% of their health budget in mental health services (Patel, 2007). Expanding mental health capacity in settings where antiretroviral drugs are being administered is an important priority in the push towards universal treatment access.

Nutrition and HIV treatment and care

Nutritional status is one of the best predictors of HIV-related mortality. As HIV disease progresses, nutritional status often declines. HIV infection increases protein, micronutrient, and energy requirements in both adults and children (WHO, 2003; Friis, 2005). At the same time, HIV-related symptoms such as lack of appetite, mouth sores, or nutrient malabsorption may decrease nutritional intake. Lack of access to adequate food is a particular challenge for people who initiate antiretroviral therapy, and has been shown to inhibit uptake of treatment.

HIV exacerbates already severe nutritional deficiencies that are common in many countries that have been heavily affected by the epidemic. Among least-developed countries generally, 35% of the population suffers from inadequate nutrition (UNDP, 2007). Micronutrient deficiencies are one of the most common forms of poor nutrition in low-income countries, and may further compromise the immune systems of people living with HIV, diminishing the body's ability to fight infection (Food and Nutrition Technical Assistance, 2004a; Jones et al., 2006).

In the case of HIV-positive children, poor nutrition accelerates HIV disease progression and increases the risk of death in the early years of life (Walzer et al., 2006). In sub-Saharan Africa and other countries affected by HIV, nutritional deficiencies are common among children (Bryce et al., 2008). It is particularly important to monitor the nutritional intake of breastfed children born to HIV-positive mothers during weaning, this transition often results in under-feeding and a consequent increased risk of mortality or stunting (Becquet et al., 2006).

Timely nutritional support for people living with HIV may help extend the asymptomatic period of relative health for people living with HIV, or, where severe immune deterioration has already occurred, it may reduce the risk of death. (For a summary of available evidence on the impact of nutritional support on health outcomes for people living with HIV, see Gillespie & Kadiyala, 2005) Proven strategies for improving the nutritional status of individuals living with HIV include food rations in food-insecure areas, micronutrient supplementation, and therapeutic foods to address the effects of moderate or severe malnutrition (Gillespie & Kadiyala, 2005). Nutritional care for people living with HIV is available in all districts in only 11% of countries with generalized epidemics, according to nongovernmental reports, although government reports say such services are widely available in 23% of countries (UNGASS Country Progress Reports, 2008).

Nutritional monitoring, along with appropriate and timely intervention, is a critical component of antiretroviral management. At the most basic level, when patients are hungry or undernourished, they find it difficult, sometimes impossible, to adhere to complex regimens (Marston & DeCock, 2004). Depending on the regimen prescribed, taking antiretroviral drugs can require dietary restrictions; some drugs are best taken on an empty stomach, while metabolism of others is optimized when taken at or near mealtime (Food and Nutrition Technical Assistance, 2004b). As with any drug, antiretroviral medicines are likely to be most effective when taken by people who are well nourished. In addition, certain common side-effects of the drugs, such as nausea or loss of appetite, may result in reduced nutritional intake. A recent operational research project by the World Food Programme and the Centre for Infectious Disease Research in Zambia found that patients on antiretroviral therapy who received focused nutritional support experienced better rates of treatment adherence.

Improving access to treatment and care services

Although there has been major progress, treatment scale-up has not kept pace with actual needs. In diverse regions, the quest to bring life-preserving HIV therapies to those who need them has encountered a range of obstacles. To achieve universal access, effective strategies are required to overcome these impediments.

Limited knowledge of HIV serostatus

Affordable technologies exist to diagnose HIV infection, including rapid tests that avoid the need for individuals to return to testing sites to receive their test results. Although diagnosing HIV is fairly straightforward in adults—except soon after exposure to the virus, when more sophisticated technologies are needed to make a definitive diagnosis—it is more complicated in young children, as described above.

Timely diagnosis of HIV infection is critical to effective medical management of HIV infection. Individuals diagnosed late in the course of infection respond less well to antiretroviral therapy and are at increased risk of illness and death (Girardi, Sabin & Monforte 2007). A study of people in New York City found that individuals with an opportunistic illness at the time of their AIDS diagnosis were three times more likely to die within three years than those with fewer than 200

Palliative care in national HIV responses

An issue of emerging importance in the push towards universal access is the role of palliative care as an integral component of national HIV responses. Palliative care includes psychosocial support, access to pain and symptom control, and other measures to address the physical, mental, and spiritual dimensions of coping with HIV and related conditions.

Existing palliative care programmes are under enormous pressure to meet growing demands. For example, in the Motheo District of the Free State, South Africa, there are an estimated 44 000 maternal orphans, 7736 of whom are living with HIV. More than 25 000 children under the age of 10 are thought to be malnourished. The district's one palliative care programme is equipped to serve 1300 children, a fraction of those in need of support (Dippenaar & Marston, 2008).

Legal and regulatory barriers to accessing cheap and simple pain control medication are a major impediment to comprehensive palliative care services. The International Narcotics Control Board has recognized that most countries have low consumption of opioid-based medicines and that seven high-income countries that account for only 12% of the world's population (Austria, Australia, Canada, France, Germany, the United Kingdom and the United States) consume 84% of medical morphine. The Board has urged governments to critically examine and revise the ways they assess domestic needs for opiates (International Narcotics Control Board, 1989).

CD4 cells per mm^3 but no history of an opportunistic infection (New York City Department of Health and Mental Hygiene, 2005).

Many people living with HIV are diagnosed with the virus only after extensive immune deterioration has occurred. For example, in Brazil—despite more than a decade of experience with publicly provided antiretroviral drugs—almost half of people with HIV are diagnosed with infection at the same time they are diagnosed with AIDS (Agence France Presse, 2008). Large population-based surveys in low- and middle-income countries have only recently begun collecting information on respondents' HIV testing history, precluding an analysis of testing trends. Even more recently, serological testing has been incorporated into these surveys, permitting an analysis of both HIV status and testing history. In the 16 countries where this analysis has been possible, most respondents who have tested HIV-positive had never received an HIV test (MEASURE DHS, 2008) In almost 40% of countries with generalized epidemics, governments report that HIV counselling and testing services have not been implemented in all districts in need. Nongovernmental sources report that HIV counselling and testing services are not widely available in 70% of countries (UNGASS Country Progress Reports, 2008). HIV testing and counselling services for tuberculosis patients are not yet universally available: in countries with a generalized epidemic, 46% of government reports indicate these services to be available in all districts in need, but only 27% of nongovernmental reports (UNGASS Country Progress Reports. 2008).

The challenge of ensuring widespread and timely knowledge of HIV serostatus is not unique to low- and middle-income countries. It is estimated that 25% of all HIV-positive people in the United States have yet to be diagnosed (Centers for Disease Control and Prevention, 2002). In New York City, a global financial capital, one in four people who tested HIV-positive received an AIDS diagnosis within one month of their positive test (New York City Department of Health and Mental Hygiene, 2007).

As Chapter 2 describes, the severe stigma attached to HIV in many countries discourages many people from learning their HIV serostatus (Weiser et al., 2006). Yet there is growing evidence that concerted national action to promote testing and tackle HIV stigma can significantly increase testing rates. For example, many countries are implementing provider-initiated HIV testing and counselling in health-care settings (UNAIDS & WHO, 2007), as well as using rapid testing technology, mobile vans, and other outreach methods to increase knowledge of HIV serostatus. In Botswana, the number of people using testing services more than doubled in the year after implementation of provider-initiated testing and counselling (Steen et al., 2007). Social and behavioural science research suggests that the magnitude and nature of services linked to testing are often key determinants of use (Obermeyer & Osborn, 2007).

A national campaign promoting knowledge of HIV serostatus in Malawi culminated in the second 'National HIV Testing and Counseling Week' in July 2007. The 186 631 people tested that week significantly exceeded the campaign's target of 130 000, with more than 80% of these individuals never having been tested previously. The campaign resulted in the diagnosis of HIV infection in 15 667 people, including 6.1% of males tested, 9.7% of non-pregnant females, and 11.3% of pregnant women (Malawi National AIDS Commission, 2007). Likewise, Ethiopia achieved an eight-fold increase in use of HIV testing and counselling services, identifying more than 108 000 new HIV infections, or 6% of all people tested (Ethiopia Federal Ministry of Health, 2007).

As African traditional medicine is often the primary, and sometimes the only, accessible health-care option in some parts of sub-Saharan Africa, involvement of traditional healers in the HIV response is critical. In the KwaZulu Natal Province of South Africa, efforts have focused on building the capacity of traditional healers to discuss HIV and sexuality with those who seek care.

Economic obstacles

Individuals often confront economic impediments to using antiretroviral drugs in the form of user fees, co-payments or other out-of-pocket costs borne by affected households. Most countries (92%, according to nongovernmental reports) have policies providing for free antiretroviral drugs (UNGASS Country Progress Reports, 2008.) However, civil society surveys in 17 countries found that many patients that receive free drugs must cover the sometimes considerable costs of diagnostic tests or treatments for opportunistic infections (International Treatment Preparedness Coalition, 2007). (see Figure 5.12) In recognition of the potential access barriers posed by out-of-pocket costs, the Government of Cameroon began making HIV treatment free in 2007, an approach pursued by numerous other countries.

Treatment may sometimes be much more easily accessible in urban areas than in rural settings. Limited access to transportation can significantly limit treatment access for HIV-positive people in rural areas. Even when a local clinic is able to provide antiretroviral drugs, HIV-positive rural dwellers must sometimes travel hours to obtain CD4 or viral load tests (International Treatment Preparedness Coalition, 2007). In 2008, Indian Railways announced a 50% discount on train fares for HIV-positive individuals travelling to receive HIV treatment.

FIGURE 5.12 Percentage of countries by income status reporting a policy of free services for antiretroviral treatment

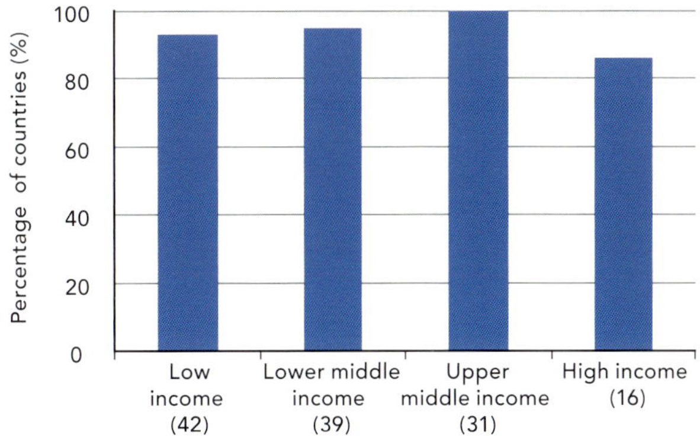

Source: UNGASS Country Progress Reports 2008.

Ensuring equal access

In addition to increasing the overall number of people receiving antiretroviral drugs, focused efforts are required to ensure that all people needing treatment have equal access. Civil society surveys confirm that many people living with HIV, especially those from marginalized groups, often face considerable obstacles to accessing HIV treatment (Human Rights Watch, 2007a; International Treatment Preparedness Coalition, 2007). Nongovernmental respondents report that 74% of countries have policies in place to ensure equal access to HIV prevention, treatment, care, and support for most-at-risk populations; however, they also report that 63% of countries have laws, regulations, or policies that impede service access for such groups (UNGASS Country Progress Reports 2008). For example, several countries stipulate that young people living with HIV must obtain parental consent before receiving antiretroviral drugs. According to the civil society "shadow" report on national progress in the Russian Federation, a national registry of drug users often results in discrimination in service access for HIV-positive people whose names appear on the registry.

Sustaining HIV treatment and care

While considerable progress has been achieved in expanding access to antiretroviral therapy, an exceptional, decades-long collective effort will be needed to sustain access to lifelong HIV treatment. The number of people needing treatment will continue to grow as the HIV disease process continues to advance in the estimated 30 million HIV-positive people worldwide who have never been on treatment. Moreover, per-patient treatment costs are likely to increase over time, as patients on standard fixed-dose combinations move to more costly second- and third-line drugs.

The challenge of sustaining treatment advances is vividly illustrated by the experience of Brazil. The leader of global efforts to expand treatment access, Brazil began offering antiretroviral treatment through its public health system in 1996, then expanded access rapidly while achieving a nearly five-fold reduction in the cost of the medications between 1997 and 2004. Yet recently, budget outlays for HIV treatment have significantly risen (Nunn et al., 2007). It is estimated that the cost of providing the drugs in Brazil in 2008 will be US$ 525 million—more than double the amount spent in 2004 (UNAIDS, 2007b).

To ensure that recent improvements in treatment access are sustained over the long run, focused efforts will be required to address key factors that might jeopardize treatment access in future years.

Human resources

Acute shortages of health-care professionals impede treatment scale-up in many of the countries heavily affected by the epidemic. Home to more than two thirds of all people living with

Global resolve to strengthen health systems in resource-limited settings

Expanding and sustaining treatment access in resource-limited settings will require the creation of strong and durable human capacity to administer antiretroviral therapy. This priority has attracted a broad array of capacity-building efforts. One such initiative led by WHO focuses on ways to "treat, train, and retain" health workers (Samb et al., 2007).

Donors are placing greater emphasis on strengthening health systems to support HIV treatment scale-up. In 2007, PEPFAR spent US$ 638 million to build capacity in public and private health sectors (PEPFAR, 2008). In November 2007, the Global Fund announced that 20% of funding for its 2008 round of competitive grantmaking would focus on system strengthening measures, such as upgrading infrastructure, strengthening supply chain systems, and reinforcing human resources (Global Fund, 2007b).

The push to expand antiretroviral therapy access is helping to support fragile health systems, yielding benefits that extend beyond HIV. For example, 13 PEPFAR-focus countries have exhibited a 36% improvement in meeting safe blood requirements over the last three years (PEPFAR, 2008). Integration of HIV into primary care services can help drive increases in utilization use of health services generally. In Rwanda, for example, the provision of basic HIV care was associated with an increase in non-HIV-related services, such as outpatient consultations, non-HIV-related laboratory tests, syphilis screening, and antenatal care visits (Family Health International, 2007).

At the close of the first-ever conference of the Global Health Workforce Alliance in Kampala, Uganda, in March 2008, more than 1000 participants from 57 countries embraced the Kampala Declaration, which urged increased funding to address health-care worker shortages in Africa. The Alliance estimates that an additional 1.5 million workers must be trained to address the infrastructure crisis in African health systems, at an annual cost of US$ 3.3 billion. Among other things, the declaration calls on high-income countries to pay a fee to countries when recruiting their health workers.

HIV, sub-Saharan Africa has only 3% of the world's health workers and accounts for less than 1% of global health spending (WHO, 2006d). While, for example, 347 physicians are available for every 100 000 people in Norway, there are only two for every 100 000 people in Malawi or the United Republic of Tanzania (UNDP, 2007). Numerous factors contribute to the human resource crisis in health-care systems, including the weakness of national medical education and training programmes, limited implementation of national human resource management policies, and the well-documented "brain drain" of health professionals who migrate from low-paying jobs in their home countries to more remunerative work in high-income or neighbouring countries (Moore & Morrison, 2007; Arah, Ogbu & Okeke, 2008).

The epidemic itself is undermining the capacity of health-care systems to meet the challenge posed by the push towards universal access. While the actual number of health-care workers infected with HIV may appear relatively modest in a given country, these infections can have a major impact on the national HIV response, as a modest number of clinicians are often responsible for delivering antiretroviral drugs, even in high-prevalence countries. The critical need to preserve essential human capacity in

Antiretroviral treatment is enabling millions of people worldwide to live healthy, productive lives. Treatment not only preserves the lives of individuals, but benefits households, communities and entire societies.

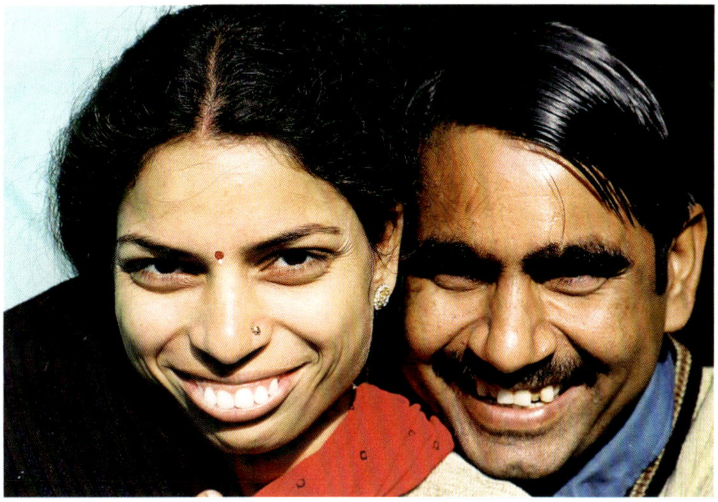

health sectors has prompted some countries to introduce special HIV prevention and treatment services for health workers. For example, in Malawi, more than 1000 health-care workers were receiving antiretroviral drugs in June 2006. The Government of Malawi estimates that improved antiretroviral therapy access saved the lives of 250 health-care workers, generating productivity savings roughly equal to the amount of human resources required to deliver antiretroviral drugs on a national scale (Makombe et al., 2007). Identification of human resource constraints as an impediment to implementation of a Global Fund grant in Malawi prompted the Global Fund to approve allocation of US$ 40 million to support the country's emergency human resource strategy, which has also attracted significant financing from the United Kingdom Department for International Development.

Personnel shortages also impede the functioning of systems that are vital to treatment access. For example, national regulatory authorities are often extremely weak in low- and middle-income countries (Gray, 2004). As a result, many newer and second-line antiretroviral drugs remain unregistered in some high-prevalence countries (International Treatment Preparedness Coalition, 2007). A number of strategies have been proposed to reduce the drug registration bottleneck in low- and middle-income countries, including targeted capacity-building in national regulatory authorities, greater regional collaboration in drug registration, and increased assistance to low-income countries from regulators in high-income countries (Gray, 2004).

Supply management problems may also interfere with the delivery of antiretroviral drugs. Civil society surveys in 17 countries found that antiretroviral drug stockouts (i.e. no stock available) were reported in diverse clinical settings in different regions in 2007 (International Treatment Preparedness Coalition, 2007). While stockouts are a common problem for many health conditions in resource-limited countries, functioning back-up systems are needed to prevent interruption of HIV treatment.

Improving diagnostic capacity

Although a public health approach makes it possible to administer antiretroviral drugs in the absence of sophisticated diagnostic techniques that are standard in high-income settings, improved diagnostic capacity in resource-limited settings will help clinicians to maximize the impact and durability of antiretroviral therapy. The need for virological testing to diagnose HIV in perinatally exposed children has particular implications for local laboratory capacity. Experience indicates the feasibility of implementing CD4 and viral-load testing in resource-limited settings, and the scaling up

Task shifting to increase health system capacity

One of several strategies to address acute health-care worker shortages, task shifting involves the redistribution of clinical tasks within the health team from more to less specialized health workers—for example, from specialist physicians to general practitioners, from physicians to nurses, and from nurses to trained members of the community. Task shifting increases the efficiency of health-care delivery, expands the human resource pool, and facilitates more rapid scale-up of treatment programmes (WHO, 2007e).

Task shifting has emerged in recent years as a major topic of discussion in HIV circles as a result of treatment scale-up, but the approach is common in many resource-limited settings. Non-physician clinicians are prevalent in 25 of 47 African countries surveyed, outnumbering physicians in nine countries (WHO, UNAIDS & PEPFAR, 2008). More than three decades experience with use of community workers for DOTS tuberculosis therapy underscores the capability of such workers to deliver many primary care services (Samb et al., 2007). Although the emphasis on task shifting for antiretroviral therapy scale-up may give rise to concerns about the possibility of second-class care in resource-limited settings, the reality is that task shifting has become common in clinical settings in high-income countries, with increased and satisfactory use of physician's assistants and nurse practitioners (Wilson et al., 2005).

To expedite treatment scale-up and expand human resources, several countries with high HIV prevalence have supplemented the longstanding informal use of non-physicians with more systematic efforts to promote task shifting as a component of their national HIV strategies. These efforts are yielding promising results. In Mozambique, after training medical officers to prescribe antiretroviral drugs in 85% of the country's clinical sites, the number of sites administering the drugs increased more than three-fold in eight months, while treatment coverage increased from 9.4% to 16.4% (Gimbel et al., 2007). Programmes using a nurse-centred approach to HIV service delivery in Haiti and Rwanda report low loss to follow-up, high treatment success rates, and levels of mortality that are comparable with those in more traditional antiretroviral programmes (WHO, UNAIDS & PEPFAR, 2008).

To help guide efforts to extend human resources for HIV, WHO, UNAIDS, and the PEPFAR initiative collaboratively developed detailed guidelines for task shifting; these guidelines address quality-assurance mechanisms and other pertinent issues. Task shifting is not a panacea for infrastructure weaknesses that inhibit treatment scale-up, but instead is one of many approaches that should be pursued, such as increased remuneration for health-care workers in resource-limited settings and improved medical education and training.

of such assays is an important health priority (WHO, 2007a).

Several methods exist for measuring CD4 counts including a new, simple, low-cost assay that may be especially well-suited to small facilities that lack extensive laboratory capacity (Srithanaviboonchai et al., 2008). The Clinton Foundation has negotiated price reductions of up to 80% from the leading makers of technologies for CD4 and viral-load testing.

Ensuring the affordability of antiretroviral drugs

In many countries heavily affected by HIV—including Kenya, Malawi, Nigeria, and Zambia—annual per capita spending on health care of any kind is less than US$ 100 (PPP)

(UNDP, 2007). In settings where health resources are so limited, many medications are deemed too expensive for routine use in resource-limited settings (Steinbrook, 2007). Historically, this has been particularly true for new, patented medications developed by pharmaceutical companies in high-income countries.

As in many other arenas, the HIV response has helped forge new ways of improving access to essential medications in low- and middle-income countries. Due to activist pressure, the emergence of competition from generic manufacturers, and direct negotiations with pharmaceutical companies by UNAIDS and other partners, prices for the leading antiretroviral drugs have fallen sharply during the last ten years. What has emerged is a pricing regime that has long been advocated by global health experts but seldom put into practice; that is, "tiered" pricing, whereby companies charge different prices depending on a country's ability to pay. The new approach to drug pricing has freed up substantial resources for health services in low- and middle-income countries. For example, it is estimated that Brazil saved approximately US$ 1 billion between 2001 and 2005 as a result of its domestic generic manufacture of eight antiretroviral drugs and its negotiation of price reductions from manufacturers (Nunn et al., 2007). National governments in 94% of countries with generalized epidemics, as well as in 61% of countries with concentrated epidemics, report having national policies for using generic drugs or parallel importation of medications to promote antiretroviral access (UNGASS Country Progress Reports 2008).

Prices have been reduced under the adoption of international trade rules that provide for flexible application of intellectual property provisions with respect to medications needed to address serious public health problems. Under prevailing rules, countries may issue compulsory licenses for patented medications where access is necessary to protect public health.

In addition, the existence of a flourishing generic pharmaceutical industry in countries such as Brazil, India, South Africa, and Thailand has exerted a downward pressure on prices and increased the range of affordable options for national treatment programmes. India, the largest supplier of medications to low- and middle-income countries, exports two thirds of the drugs it manufactures (Steinbrook, 2007).

The existing global intellectual property framework has not precluded the emergence of controversies and uncertainties. In 2007, for example, a public dispute arose between Thailand and Abbott Laboratories after the country announced plans to issue a compulsory license for the noncommercial use of the company's lopinavir-ritonavir antiretroviral drug. This decision by Thailand followed the government's unsuccessful negotiations with Abbott to agree on an affordable price for the medication. In addition, since 2005, India has been issuing patents, as required by the World Trade Organization. Whether this change might ultimately drive prices upward by impeding the ability of India's generics industry to produce key antiretroviral drugs is a source of concern.

Despite the pricing breakthroughs of recent years, further declines in the cost of purchasing antiretroviral drugs are needed to accelerate treatment scale-up. This is especially true with regard to second- and third-line antiretroviral drugs, which typically cost significantly more than first-line drugs in low- and middle-income countries. Although only 4% of patients on antiretroviral therapy in 23 countries surveyed by WHO were on second-line regimens in 2006 (WHO, 2007a), the need for second-line therapies will grow over time. An estimated 3% of patients on first-line antiretroviral drugs—or approximately 180 000 individuals in 2008—will need to switch to second-line regimens each year (WHO, 2006b). Following negotiations with leading manufacturers of generic medications, in May 2007 the Clinton Foundation and UNITAID announced steep price reductions on 16 different formulations of eight second-line antiretroviral drugs. WHO has issued guidance to countries on criteria to use in selecting second-line regimens for use in national treatment guidelines (WHO, 2007a).

While major progress has been achieved, daunting challenges lie ahead if the world is to move towards universal access. Yet experience during this decade underscores that such challenges can be overcome. As Chapter 7 explains, sustaining the long-term response will demand strong political commitment, even greater resources, expanded national capacity, and the active involvement of all stakeholders, especially people living with HIV.

Evidence for action

Are the right actions being taken?

- All countries have a national policy or strategy to promote comprehensive HIV treatment, care, and support.
- Nearly all (85%) countries with generalized epidemics and 52% with concentrated epidemics report having reliable estimates and having projected future needs of the number of individuals requiring antiretroviral therapy.
- National governments in 92% of low- and middle-income countries report that current policies provide for delivery of antiretroviral drugs free of charge.

Are the right actions being undertaken in the right manner?

- Globally, women are receiving higher coverage of antiretroviral therapy than men, although children have sharply lower coverage of antiretroviral drugs than adults and adolescents in generalized epidemic countries where burden is highest.
- Nongovernmental informants report that many countries (40%), including most in Eastern Europe and Central Asia, South and South-East Asia, and North America, have laws, regulations or policies that impede access to HIV-related services among injecting drug users.
- HIV and tuberculosis treatment services have not been effectively integrated in most countries in which there are large numbers of individuals with coinfection with HIV and tuberculosis. National governments indicate that only 42% of countries with generalized epidemics have implemented routine tuberculosis screening for HIV-positive patients, and only 27% provide tuberculosis preventive therapy in all districts in need; nongovernment responses indicate that these two services are widely available in only 24% of countries with generalized epidemics.

Have these actions been sufficiently scaled up to make a difference?

- By the end of 2007, antiretroviral drugs reached 3 million people in low- and middle-income countries, representing 31% of estimated global need and a 45% improvement over 2006.
- AIDS deaths have started to decline, in part as a result of improved treatment access. Expanded antiretroviral access is also improving quality of life for people living with HIV.
- Only 32% of incident tuberculosis cases in people living with HIV received dual treatment for their HIV and tuberculosis in 2007.

Mitigating the epidemic's impact on households, communities and societies

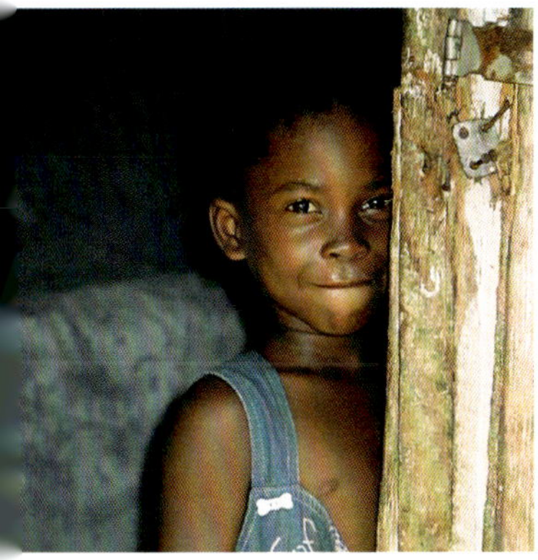

6

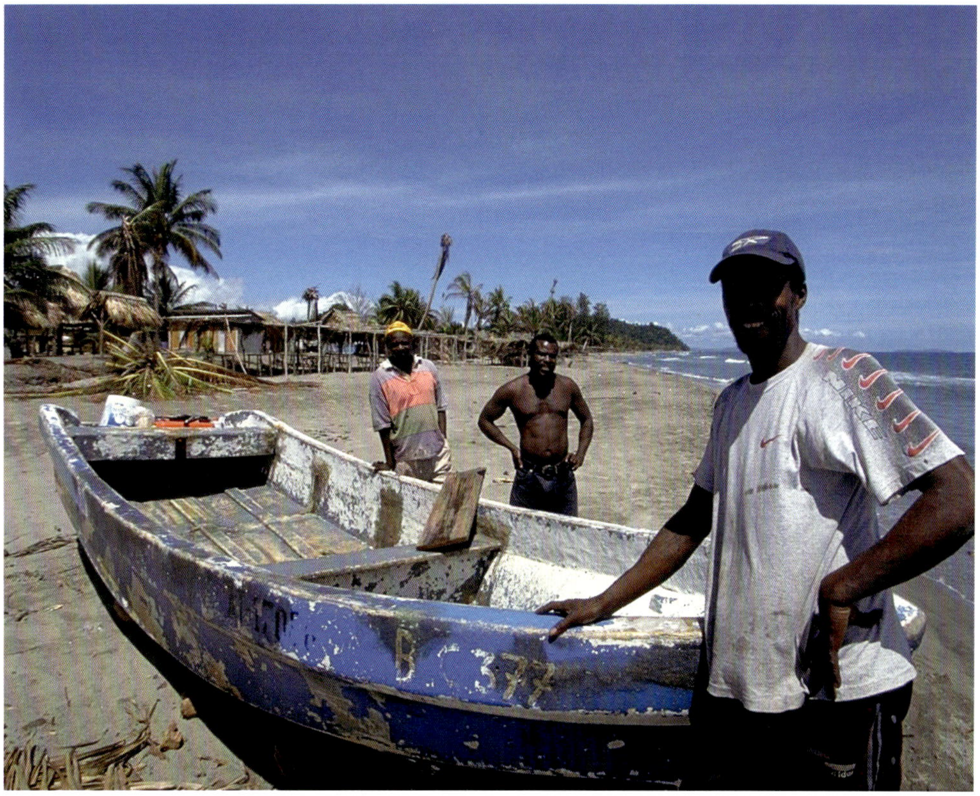

Chapter 6

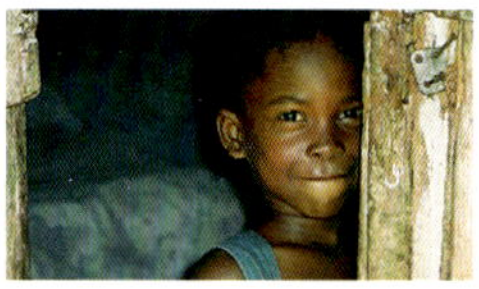

FIGURE 6.1 Selected events related to mitigating the impact of AIDS

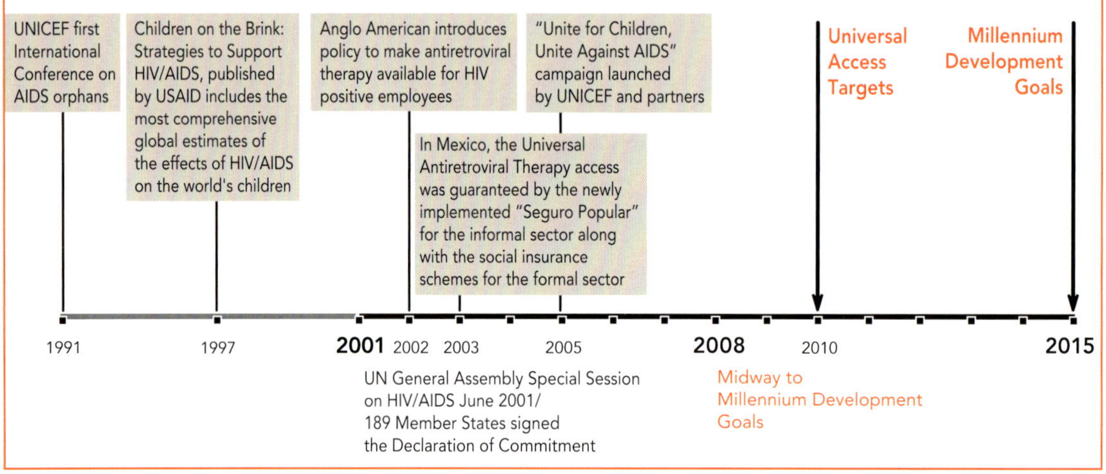

Key findings

- The HIV epidemic continues to inflict significant damage on affected households, particularly on women and children.
- Social protection programmes that provide cash assistance to HIV-affected households have the proven potential to alleviate the epidemic's impact and should immediately be brought to scale in the most heavily-affected countries.
- Legal reform, coupled with community awareness campaigns, legal aid, and support for law enforcement, can strengthen protection for widows and children orphaned through HIV.
- Although most high-prevalence countries have strategies in place to support children orphaned or made vulnerable by HIV, few national programmes reach more than a small minority of such children.
- The epidemic is having particularly harsh effects on women, and scaled-up measures to increase women's independent income-generating potential should be implemented.
- Although the epidemic's macroeconomic effects are less severe than earlier feared, HIV is nevertheless having profound negative effects in certain industries and agricultural sectors of high-prevalence countries.
- To address the continuing deterioration of government capacity in high-prevalence countries, strategic, scaled-up approaches are needed to preserve and build capacity in the public sector; such approaches should include innovative strategies to extend limited capacity as far as possible.
- Antiretroviral treatment programmes are critical to mitigating the epidemic's impact but should be complemented by initiatives that specifically address the households, communities, and sectors most heavily affected by HIV.

The HIV epidemic has resulted in history's single sharpest reversal in human development (UNDP, 2005). In the most heavily affected countries, HIV has reduced life expectancy, deepened poverty among vulnerable households and communities, skewed the size of populations, undermined national systems, and weakened institutional structures.

The epidemic's effects have been more muted, although still considerable, in regions where HIV prevalence is lower than in sub-Saharan Africa. In Asia, for example, HIV has lowered life expectancy by 3 years in Cambodia and by 1.7 years in Myanmar (Commission on AIDS in Asia, 2008).

Understanding the impact of the AIDS epidemic and how to mitigate it has proven to be far more complicated and nuanced than first believed, as is the case with most other aspects of the epidemic. A modest but important body of research has focused on the epidemic's impact; however, there has been comparatively little rigorous study and documentation of the most promising strategies for mitigating the epidemic's detrimental effects. This chapter summarizes the latest evidence regarding what is known, and still unknown, about the epidemic's multi-faceted impact, with a particular focus on high-burden settings. A comprehensive discussion of the many different impacts of HIV is beyond the scope of a single chapter; the discussion here is thus limited to the epidemic's effects on households (with particular attention to the needs of women and children), on national economies and their subsidiary components, and on public sectors and national institutions.

This chapter pays particular attention to potential avenues for minimizing the epidemic's impact, often highlighting areas where additional research is urgently required. As the chapter explains, the introduction in recent years of antiretroviral drugs in resource-limited settings often offers the greatest promise for curtailing the epidemic's most harmful effects. However, just as antiretroviral drugs are not a cure for HIV itself, treatment access alone will not resolve the social and economic damage caused by the epidemic. Improving the scale and scope of prevention programmes is absolutely critical to long-term efforts to minimize the epidemic's impact. In addition, policy and programmatic initiatives are needed that specifically address the epidemic's impact on households, women and children, and national sectors and institutions.

Assessing the epidemic's impact: challenges and obstacles

Efforts to characterize the impact of HIV often seek to compare the situation now with projections of how households, communities, and societies would be faring had the epidemic never occurred. However, as HIV infection has expanded and its impact deepened, the communities and countries most heavily affected by the epidemic have also undergone profound changes unrelated to HIV, making it difficult to isolate the epidemic's precise effects (Bhorat & Kanbur, 2005). In many countries—for example, South Africa and Zimbabwe—it is difficult to disentangle the epidemic's effects from other major social and economic changes that have occurred over the last two to three decades.

The epidemic has revealed a high degree of resourcefulness and resilience in the societies most heavily affected by HIV, thereby avoiding or muting certain anticipated consequences of the epidemic. Yet such resilience can also mask profound individual or collective trauma, the effects of which are poorly understood.

HIV is sometimes referred to as a "long-wave" event, with many of its ramifications occurring far into the future, at uncertain intervals (Gillespie et al., 2007). Conventional economic and social science tools are poorly equipped to project the potential future of the epidemic. Thus, while it is possible to measure school attendance and other physical attributes of well-being among children orphaned by HIV, it is more difficult to quantify the cost of losing one or both parents, or to project the future societal impact of such a large cohort of young adults having come of age without parental anchors. It has been suggested that the epidemic, by causing the premature death of millions of mothers and fathers, is severing traditional mechanisms for transferring knowledge and values (Bell, Devarajan & Gersbach, 2004), yet the available tools do not adequately assess this phenomenon or its likely impact.

Certain initial assumptions about the epidemic's macro-level impacts have not been borne out. The epidemic has not shattered national economies or threatened the viability of any national government. However, the appearance of societies functioning 'normally' may conceal severe social stresses and strains because the modest nature of macro-level effects masks both severe burdens in subpopulations, and sharp increases in inequality caused by the epidemic.

Mitigating the impact on households, women, and children

While poor individuals and households are not necessarily more likely to become infected with HIV (Dinkelman, Lam & Leibbrandt, 2007; Mishra et al., 2007), the impact of HIV infection is often magnified in conditions of poverty. For example, the financial burden associated with HIV for the poorest households in India represents 82% of annual income, while the comparable burden for the wealthiest families is slightly more than 20% (Asia Development Bank & UNAIDS, 2004a). Studies in the United Republic of Tanzania found that people living with HIV typically experience more than a dozen episodes of illness before dying, with an average of 12 months of deteriorating health in the year before death (Bollinger, Stover & Riwa, 1999; Beegle, 2003). An analysis of data from Botswana found that HIV results in a decline in per capita household income of 10%, with average income losses almost twice as high for households in the lowest income level (Greener, 2005).

HIV infection also results in significant additional expenses, which poor households are least capable of bearing. Even where HIV treatment services are ostensibly free, patients often remain liable for considerable out-of-pocket costs in the form of co-payments, user fees, transport costs, and uncovered items (e.g. medications for opportunistic infections) (International Treatment Preparedness Coalition, 2007). In South Africa, where funerals can cost up to 7 months of income, 61% of households lack funeral insurance (Collins & Leibbrandt, 2007). To cover these costs, affected households are often required to reduce spending on other items, such as food or education.

Scaling up antiretroviral drugs and the effect on productivity

In addition to prolonging life and alleviating suffering due to illness, antiretroviral therapy represents a critical means of alleviating the epidemic's economic effects on households. Among tea workers in Kenya, rapid improvements in productivity were seen in the first year after starting antiretroviral therapy (Simon et al., 2007). However, recovery of health and productivity are not certain nor immediate, which has led some employers to permit workers to delay returning to work until 3–6 months after initiation of antiretroviral drugs.

Social protection

Studies of public sector cash assistance schemes in southern Africa found that 50% of households in South Africa were reached by such programmes, and that 70% of local households reached by district-level pilot schemes in Malawi and Zambia were HIV-affected. UNICEF estimates that well-designed social cash transfer programmes[1] could reach 80% of HIV-affected households in need of assistance in low- and middle-income countries with high HIV prevalence (UNICEF, 2007a).

[1] In industrialized countries, "social cash transfer programmes" might be referred to as welfare or social insurance, i.e., cash payments to needy households.

FIGURE 6.2 Estimated number of children under 18 orphaned by AIDS in sub-Saharan Africa (1990–2007)

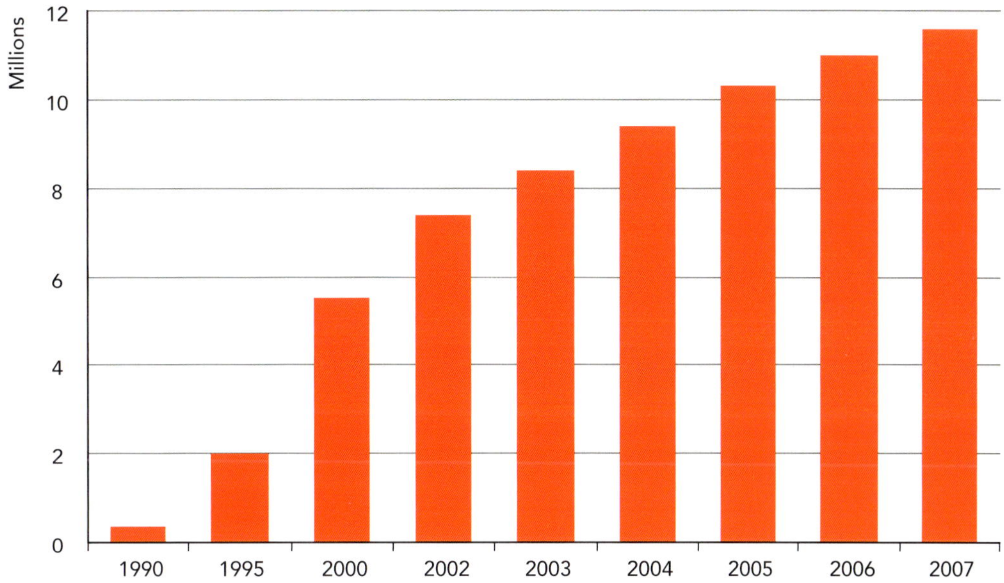

Source: UNAIDS/WHO, 2008.

With the exception of households in which one or more members are on antiretroviral drugs, it is not recommended that HIV serostatus serve as an eligibility criterion for social cash transfer schemes, due to the possibility of stigmatizing recipient households (UNICEF, 2007a). Schemes gearing eligibility to a low income level reach a large share of HIV-affected households, which tend to be poorer than non-affected households due to the economic consequences of infection. Similarly, eligibility criteria targeting households that include one or more orphans, or are labour-constrained, also reach many HIV-affected households (UNICEF, 2007a).

Minimizing administrative hurdles is essential for maximizing uptake of social cash transfer programmes. In South Africa, comparatively slow uptake of social cash transfer programmes appeared to stem from the administrative complexity of application procedures, as well as delays associated with the country's overburdened welfare administration (UNICEF, 2007a). It is also important to improve ease of access in both urban and rural settings.

While cash transfer schemes represent a rational policy response to the challenge that HIV poses to poor households, some have asked whether this approach is affordable in the low-income countries most heavily affected by HIV. According to a costing exercise undertaken by the International Labour Organization, a national poverty-targeted cash transfer scheme need cost no more than 0.5% of gross domestic product (Pal et al., 2005)—a finding supported by a similar UNICEF analysis in Mozambique (Webb, 2007).

Orphans and other children made vulnerable by HIV

The needs of HIV-affected households include those of the children living in these households. In sub-Saharan Africa, nearly 12 million children under age 18 have lost one or both parents to HIV (UNAIDS & WHO 2008). In Botswana and Zambia, an estimated 20% of children under 17 are orphans, with most orphaned as a result of HIV (Haacker, 2004a). Zimbabwe reports that 24% of its children (ages 0–17) have lost one or both parents to HIV (Figure 6.2).

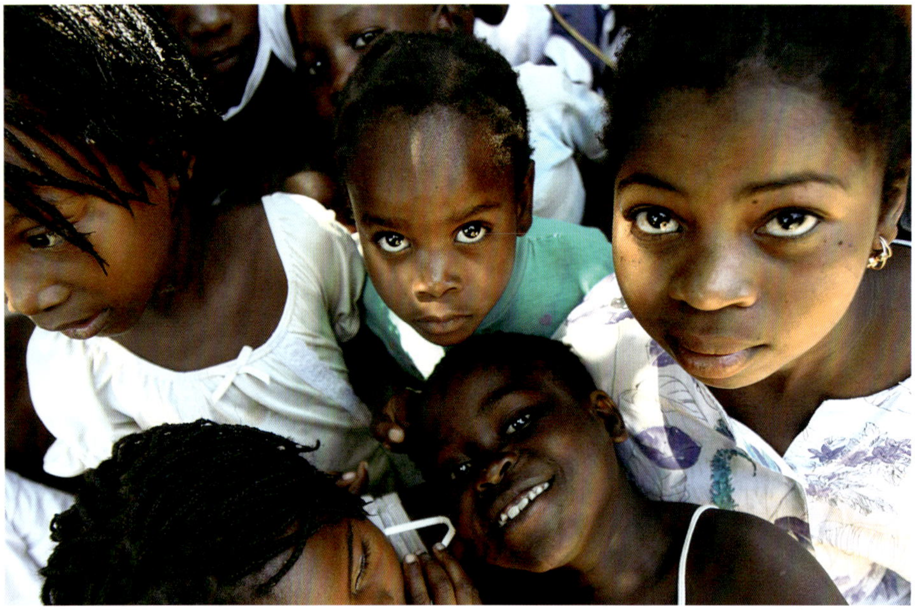

Achieving universal access to HIV treatment would prevent up to 5 million children from becoming orphans.

In addition to the trauma of losing one or both parents, being orphaned as a result of HIV can increase vulnerability in many ways. Loss of a parent may result in a significant decline in standard of living; it also potentially increases the likelihood of exploitation. Especially where both parents have died, a child may become head of the household, assuming enormous burdens at an early age. The impact of orphanhood may be especially severe for girls, who are generally more likely than boys not to be in school (see UNDP, 2007).

Much of the burden of caring for children orphaned as a result of HIV falls on the elderly, especially grandmothers who step in when one or both parents have died. Surveys in rural South Africa have detected an increase in the number of households headed by individuals over 50 (Preston-Whyte et al., 2007). In Namibia, the United Republic of Tanzania, and Zimbabwe, 40%–60% of orphaned children are cared for by grandmothers (UNICEF, 2007b).

Mitigating the impact on orphans and vulnerable children

The policy response to children orphaned and made vulnerable by HIV has significantly expanded since 1991, when UNICEF hosted the first international meeting on the issue (Webb, 2007). From the early focus on "AIDS orphans", programme responses have increasingly recognized the many different ways that HIV may increase the vulnerability of children, including parental illness and loss of household income. Rights-based programming has increased the sensitivities of policy-makers and programme implementers to discrimination against HIV-affected children, and thus helped them to avoid such discrimination.

Among 33 countries with generalized epidemics reporting these data, 91% of national governments report having a specific policy or strategy to address the HIV-related needs of children orphaned or made vulnerable by HIV (UNGASS Country Progress Reports 2008). The 15 countries with the highest HIV prevalence have operational definitions for this population, an operational plan, and estimates of the number of children currently being reached by support programmes. The degree to which such plans have been costed, budgeted, and implemented cannot currently be gauged, although national governments in nearly 73% of countries with generalized epidemics regarded their national efforts to address the needs of orphans and vulnerable children as above average. Government reports on these policy

FIGURE 6.3 Ratio of school attendance among orphans to non-orphans in countries with HIV prevalence greater than 5%

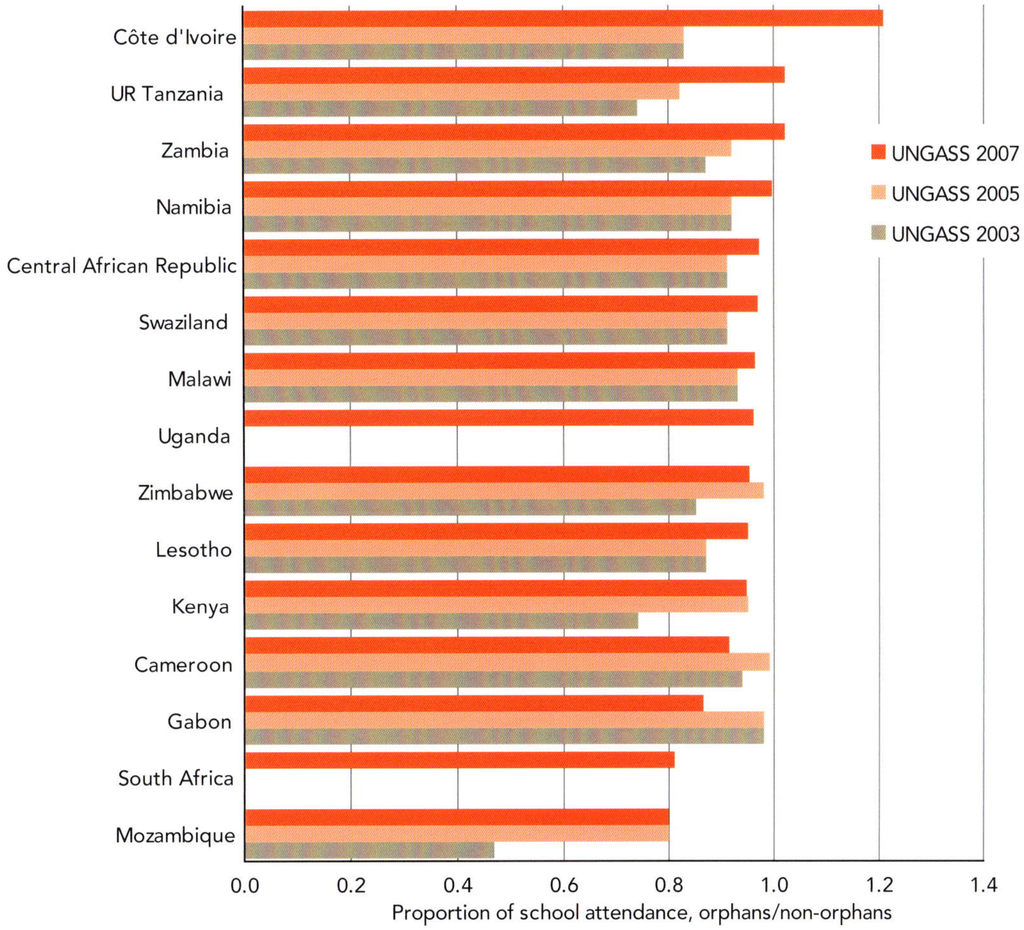

Source: UNGASS Country Progress Reports 2008.

issues were largely confirmed by reports from nongovernmental sources in these countries (UNGASS Country Progress Reports 2008).

In recent years, donor support for children-focused care and support initiatives has increased. As of September 2007, PEPFAR had provided care and support to 2.7 million children orphaned or made vulnerable by HIV; the programme had also provided training or re-training for 143 000 caregivers (PEPFAR, 2007). In Swaziland, the Global Fund is financing care and support services for 100 000 children orphaned as a result of HIV (Global Fund, 2008).

Education

Education is critical to children's future potential and sense of self-esteem, and to the generational transmission of knowledge and values within societies. Studies present conflicting findings on the impact of HIV-related orphanhood on rates of schooling, with some indication that effects may be specific to context and findings subject to methodological variations. In 56 countries where recent household survey data are available, orphans who had lost both parents were, on average, 12% less likely to attend school than non-orphans. In countries with HIV prevalence greater than 5%, orphans were only 4% less likely to be in school than non-orphans, suggesting that heavily affected countries are closing some of the educational disparities seen earlier in the epidemic.[2]

School attendance by orphans was consistently higher in 2007 than in 2005 in high-prevalence countries, except in Cameroon and Zimbabwe (Figure 6.3). Several of these countries have benefited from orphan-focused external assistance from the PEPFAR initiative or other sources. Of particular note are the efforts of such countries as Côte d'Ivoire, Gabon, the United Republic of Tanzania, and Zambia, where school attendance rates are actually higher among orphans than among non-orphans.

Some experts have suggested that monitoring whether children are in school at a particular time is a less useful measure of HIV's impact on children than studying eventual educational attainment. In Uganda and Zambia, for example, while educational attainment progressively rose for five-year birth cohorts until 1977, educational levels began falling as the epidemic began reducing life expectancy (Birdsall & Hamoudi, 2004). As a result of the epidemic, children as a whole are becoming less educated in the most heavily affected countries, potentially diminishing national capacity to accumulate human capital for future growth, prosperity, and development (Birdsall & Hamoudi, 2004).

Social protection

In eastern and southern Africa, national governments, civil society, and other stakeholders are increasingly focused on the provision of a minimum package of social protection to vulnerable children, including those affected by HIV (Webb, 2007). Such minimum packages vary considerably among countries. In Botswana, the country's Orphan Care Programme was supporting more than 53 000 children orphaned by HIV as of December 2007, providing food baskets, psychological counselling, and educational assistance (e.g. waiver of school fees). Zimbabwe's National Orphan Care Policy takes a sectoral approach, working to strengthen community care capacity through extended families. Namibian's Ministry of Gender Equality and Child Welfare administers foster-care grants that were supporting 65 000 children in 2007, while South Africa has reached more than one million orphans and vulnerable children with support services, mostly in the form of child support grants.

Among 10 countries in which 5% or more of adults are HIV-infected and where recent household surveys have been conducted, a population-adjusted average of 15% of orphans live in households receiving some form of assistance, such as medical care, school assistance, financial support, or psychosocial services. In some high-burden countries, programme utilization data suggest somewhat higher coverage than has been found in household surveys. South Africa and the United Republic of Tanzania, for example, report reaching 67% and 50%, respectively, of households that include one or more children orphaned or made vulnerable by HIV (Table 6.1).[3]

Targeting cash support to HIV-affected households would significantly increase assistance to children, who represent a significant share of households. In a pilot project in the Kalomo district of Zambia, 68% of children reached by social cash transfers were orphans, including 35% who had lost both parents (UNICEF, 2007a).

CHAPTER 6

[2] This indicator pertains to orphans generally, rather than just to children orphaned specifically as a result of HIV.

[3] Programme data should be interpreted with caution due to the possibility of duplicative counting as a result of reporting by multiple organizations in the same locality, or receipt by the same household of multiple services.

TABLE 6.1 Support to orphans and vulnerable children as reported by countries with adult HIV prevalence ≥5 % (2005 estimates)

Country	OVC supported	OVC total[1]	Coverage in 2007 (n=10)
Population based survey data			
Botswana	Not reported	Not reported	**Not reported**
Cameroon	412	4,431	**9%**
Central African Republic	Not reported	Not reported	**7%**
Gabon	259	2,637	**10%**
Kenya	Not reported	Not reported	**17%[2]**
Lesotho	Not reported	Not reported	**Not reported**
Malawi	Not reported	Not reported	**19%**
Namibia	882	5,343	**17%**
Swaziland	1,472	3,576	**41%**
Uganda	569	5,321	**11%**
Zambia	578	3,671	**16%**
Zimbabwe	1,972	6,322	**31%**
Population adjusted average	***34,161***	***4,970***	***15%***
Programme based data			
Côte d'Ivoire	37,250	420,943	**9%**
South Africa	1,057,900	1,577,200	**67%**
United Republic of Tanzania	471,315	930,000	**51%**
Population adjusted average	***2,928,143***	***1,566,465***	***53%***

[1] Total number of OVC as reported by countries.
[2] Information based on survey implemented by PEPFAR in Kenya on OVC support in 2007, source: Kenya UNGASS country report 2008.

Source: UNGASS Country Progress Reports 2008.

Orphan-support initiatives confront a host of challenges in high-prevalence countries. In 2007, the percentage of children orphaned or made vulnerable by HIV who were reached by orphan support services declined in Zimbabwe due to the impact of hyperinflation on national budgets, according to the country's report to UNAIDS on core indicators. Coverage for orphan support services is sometimes markedly higher in urban areas than in rural communities. Stigma may discourage households from registering affected children in national support programmes. In some countries, support for children affected by the epidemic is largely shouldered by underfinanced civil society groups, with little government support.

Scaling up antiretroviral drugs and the impact on children in the household

Antiretroviral treatment for HIV-infected adults also yields clear benefits for children living in affected households. Longitudinal household data from Kenya indicate that the number of hours children are in school each week increases by 20% within six months of initiation of antiretroviral drugs for an adult household member. Similarly, children living in such households experience sharp improvements in their nutritional status—as measured by quantitative assessments—once an adult household member starts on antiretroviral drugs (Thirumurthy, Zivin & Goldstein, 2007). A recent study in Uganda

FIGURE 6.4 Orphans due to AIDS in sub-Saharan Africa, from 2006 projected to 2015

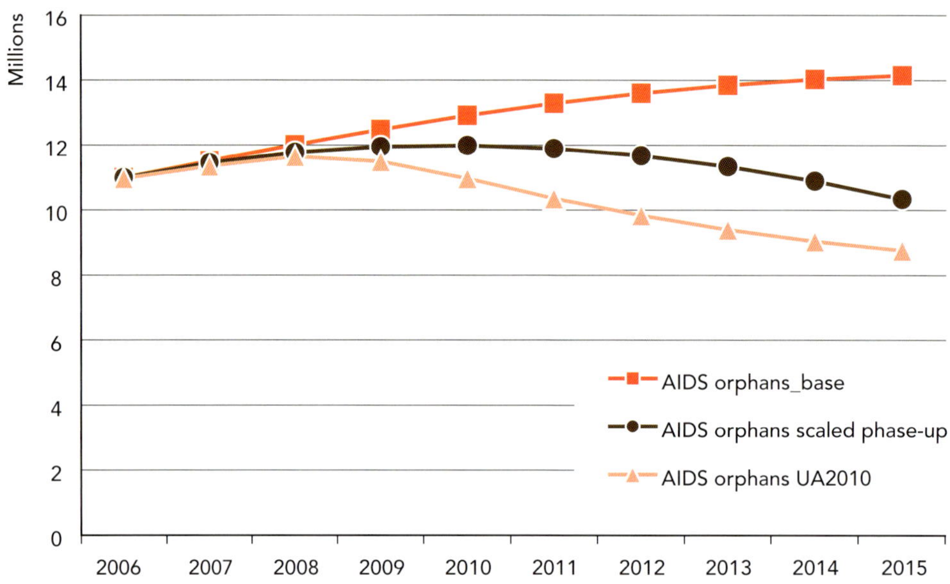

Source: UNICEF, UNAIDS, WHO, 2008.

found an 81% reduction in child mortality among uninfected children of adults on antiretroviral drugs, as well as a 93% reduction in orphanhood (Mermin, 2008).

Improved antiretroviral access also offers the prospect of significantly reducing the number of children who will be orphaned as a result of HIV in the future. As Figure 6.4 indicates, the number of children under age 18 orphaned as a result of HIV is expected to grow to more than 14 million by 2015 if the current pace of antiretroviral scale-up continues. Achieving universal treatment access by 2010, however, would reduce the number of orphans in 2015 by more than five million. A scaled phase-up to universal access by 2015 would result in a number of orphans that is approximately four million below current projections.

Addressing the epidemic's disproportionate impact on women

In addition to being more physiologically and socially vulnerable to infection, women also disproportionately suffer the epidemic's negative effects. As the primary caregivers in Africa and other regions, women have seen their household and community burdens grow as a result of HIV, often compromising their health, their ability to generate income, and other markers of well-being. Women account for two thirds of all caregivers for people living with HIV in Africa (Secretary-General's Task Force, 2004).

Women who are widowed as a result of HIV are at high risk of becoming destitute as a result of legal regimes that fail to recognize or protect women's right to inherit property. In Zambia, one study found that the amount of land under the control of a widow-headed household fell by 35% within three years of the death of the husband (Chapoto, Jayne & Mason, 2007).

Measures to expand women's economic opportunities

Among low-income women in Africa, those having some type of formal or informal work are less likely to die than those who lack work (Chapoto & Jayne, 2005). Accordingly, increasing women's financial options helps to mitigate some of the epidemic's most harmful effects. Microfinance initiatives are frequently cited as a possible means to empower women by increasing their economic independence. A randomized controlled trial of a microfinance initiative in the Philippines recently found that access to a microsavings account improved women's decision-making within the household, enhanced their self-perception of savings behaviour, and positively affected actual consumption of durable goods (Karlan, Ashraf & Yin, 2007). In another study, 90% of women participating in microfinance initiatives reported significant improvement in their lives, including improved sense of community solidarity in crises and reductions in partner violence (Pronyk, 2006).

In one of the most extensive studies of women-focused microfinance initiatives, researchers examined the impact of an intervention that combined microfinance with participatory training on HIV infection, gender norms, domestic violence, and sexuality. Although no impact on HIV incidence was observed, the combined microfinance initiative was associated with a reduction of more than half of physical and sexual violence by an intimate partner. The study also found significant improvements across a broad range of qualitative indicators of empowerment (Kim et al., 2007).

To make microfinance feasible, initiatives should address transport and literacy barriers that many women confront in accessing financial assistance. In addition, microfinance programmes should include community-based work with men, to address traditional gender norms and the resistance of some men to women-focused financial assistance.

Support for caregivers

In Kenya, Mozambique, Viet Nam, and other countries, community networks ease caregivers' burdens and provide emotional and practical support for those caring for people living with HIV (Global Coalition on Women and AIDS, 2006). Swaziland provides a small allowance to HIV caregivers (IRIN News, 2006), while a Global Fund-supported project in South Africa trains caregivers and provides financial and other support to households that include children orphaned by HIV (Global Fund Partnership Forum, 2006). In Kenya, Grassroots Organizations Operating Together in Sisterhood (GROOTS) is a network of self-help groups that aid women responsible for home-based care and supporting community capacity to address HIV-related care needs (International Center for Research on Women, 2007).

Legal reform

As Chapter 3 explained, enactment of laws protecting women's property and inheritance rights would increase women's economic independence. In addition to reducing women's risk and vulnerability to HIV, such laws would also help mitigate the epidemic's impact on women by expanding their economic opportunities. Although progress has been slow in the implementation and enforcement of such laws in many countries, civil society groups are mobilizing to promote such legal reforms. In Zambia, for example, the Justice for Widows and Orphans Project serves as a referral point for widows who need assistance with inheritance and property rights (ICRW, 2007). Positive Women's Network—based in Chennai, India—and other south Asian organizations provide legal assistance to help women to secure their property rights (Swaminathan, Bhatla & Chakraborty, 2007).

Mitigating the macroeconomic impact of the epidemic

The epidemic continues to exact a toll on national and subnational economies, and on individual economic sectors. As the discussion below indicates, the long-term ramifications of the epidemic in different regions remain somewhat uncertain and subject to debate among economists.

The epidemic's economic impact

Estimating the epidemic's macroeconomic effects is complicated by the fact that high-burden countries have been undergoing important changes at the same time that they have been experiencing HIV. These changes include globalization, fluctuations in prices for commodities, political upheaval, civil and international conflict, and other humanitarian crises. As both national epidemics and the many ancillary factors that may affect economic growth often differ sharply from one setting to the next, it is challenging to reach generalized conclusions about HIV's impact on economic growth.

With one of the highest HIV burdens in the world, Botswana nevertheless experienced average economic growth of 4.8% between 1990 and 2005 (UNDP, 2007). Likewise, economic growth in heavily affected Uganda in 1990–2005 actually increased over rates reported for 1975–1990, even as HIV was responsible for more than 100 000 deaths per year (WHO, UNICEF & UNAIDS, 2006). South Africa, home to the largest population of people living with HIV, has enjoyed robust economic growth since 1999 (Gillespie et al., 2007). Certain heavily affected countries—including Kenya, Zambia, and Zimbabwe—experienced negative economic growth in 1990–2005, but it is difficult to link this weak negative performance to HIV.

Using standard economic models, the best available evidence suggests that HIV is likely to reduce economic growth in high-prevalence countries by 0.5% to 1.5% over 10–20 years (Piot, Greener & Russell, 2007)—an impact that is notable but not catastrophic.[4] However, while the macroeconomic impact may be manageable, it is clear that the epidemic is deepening poverty, even in less-affected countries outside Africa. Even within economies that are steadily growing, HIV can create a "poverty trap" that ensnares the most vulnerable (Bell, 2004). Given the heavier burdens borne by poor households, HIV also widens inequality within societies, which may increase vulnerability to HIV in the future, as discussed in Chapter 2. Ironically, the sickness and death of skilled workers may also increase inequality by reducing overall labour demand and leading to a fall in the wages of unskilled workers (Dorward & Mwale, 2004).

In Botswana, modelling indicates that HIV has increased the share of households below the poverty line by 6%, and increased the percentage of individuals living in poor households by 4%. As a result of HIV, every income earner in the lowest income level can expect to support an additional eight dependents (Greener, 2004). Outside Africa, economic analyses by the Asia Development Bank and UNAIDS indicate that HIV will slow the annual rate of poverty reduction by 60% in Cambodia, 38% in Thailand, and 23% in India between 2003 and 2015 (ADB & UNAIDS, 2004). It is estimated that HIV imposes an additional US$ 2 billion in costs each year on affected households in Asia (Commission on AIDS in Asia, 2008).

[4] Such estimates are notably lower than projections developed earlier in the epidemic. In 2001, for example, economists estimated that HIV was likely to cause economic growth in Botswana to plummet from roughly 5.5% per year to between 1.5% and 2.5% (MacFarlan, 2001). In the intervening years, however, economic growth in Botswana has remained robust, notwithstanding extremely high levels of HIV infection.

Recent suggestions that the epidemic's long-term impact on national economies will not be as severe as previously predicted are not universally shared. A 2006 economic analysis suggested that the lower projections of macroeconomic impact are based on assumptions that heavily-affected countries have excess supplies of unskilled labour. Questioning the validity of such assumptions in light of the long-term mortality toll from HIV, this analysis argued that a "broader and longer-term perspective" suggests that "AIDS could cause the outright collapse of many economies, particularly in sub-Saharan Africa" (TD Bank Financial Group, 2006).

TABLE 6.2 HIV-Related Labour Costs

Sector	Country	Number of Workers in Sector	Estimated HIV Prevalence *(% of Adult Population)*	Cost per AIDS Death or Retirement *(Multiple of Annual Compensation)*	Aggregate Annual Costs *(% of Labour Cost*
Retail	South Africa	500	10.50	0.7	0.50
Agribusiness	South Africa	700	23.70	1.1	0.70
	Uganda	500	5.60	1.9	1.20
	Kenya	22,000	10.00	1.1	1.00
	Zambia	1,200	28.50	0.9	1.30
Manufacturing	South Africa	1,300	14.00	1.2	1.10
	Uganda	300	14.40	1.2	1.90
	Ethiopia	1,500	5.30	0.9	0.60
	Ethiopia	1,300	6.20	0.8	0.60
Media	South Africa	3,600	10.20	1.3	1.30
Utility	South Africa	>25,000	11.70	4.7	2.20
Mining	South Africa	600	23.60	1.4	2.40
	Botswana	500	29.00	4.4	8.40
Tourism	Zambia	350	36.80	3.6	10.80

Source: Piot P et al. (2007). Squaring the Circle: AIDS, Poverty, and Human Development.

The epidemic's relatively modest macro-economic impact also obscures much more severe effects on individual industries. Costs to companies as a result of HIV include lost productivity (due to absenteeism or death of a worker), medical costs, and death-related benefits (Haacker, 2004b). In Africa, company costs associated with HIV vary from 0.5% to 10% of total labour costs (Simon, unpublished data, in Piot, Greener & Russell, 2007) (Table 6.2). At the upper reaches of this range, the impact on profits is likely to be considerable. For example, among mining companies in southern Africa, future costs associated with HIV are projected to equal 8% (gold mining) and 3.6% (platinum mining) of total labour costs, reflecting a notable loss of company profits (Fourie, 2005).

A number of potential strategies are available to mitigate the epidemic's impact on economic growth, poverty, and inequality. As noted, increased access to antiretroviral therapy may help preserve the labour productivity and viability of HIV-infected households, although minimization or elimination of out-of-pocket costs associated with treatment is necessary to avert potential increases in economic inequality.

Workplace programmes

Workplace HIV prevention programmes have been effective, and a growing (although still insufficient) number of companies are now offering their employees coverage for antiretroviral drugs (see Chapter 5). When asked to state whether workplace services were available in all or most districts in need, fewer than one in four (24%) governments (and nongovernmental informants in only 12% of countries) said that prevention services are widely available, but only 9% of countries with generalized epidemics indicate widespread availability of treatment or treatment referrals through the workplace (UNGASS Country Progress Reports 2008). In addition, because many people in sub-Saharan Africa work

FIGURE 6.5 Percentage of countries with sectors included in the national AIDS strategy and earmarked budgets

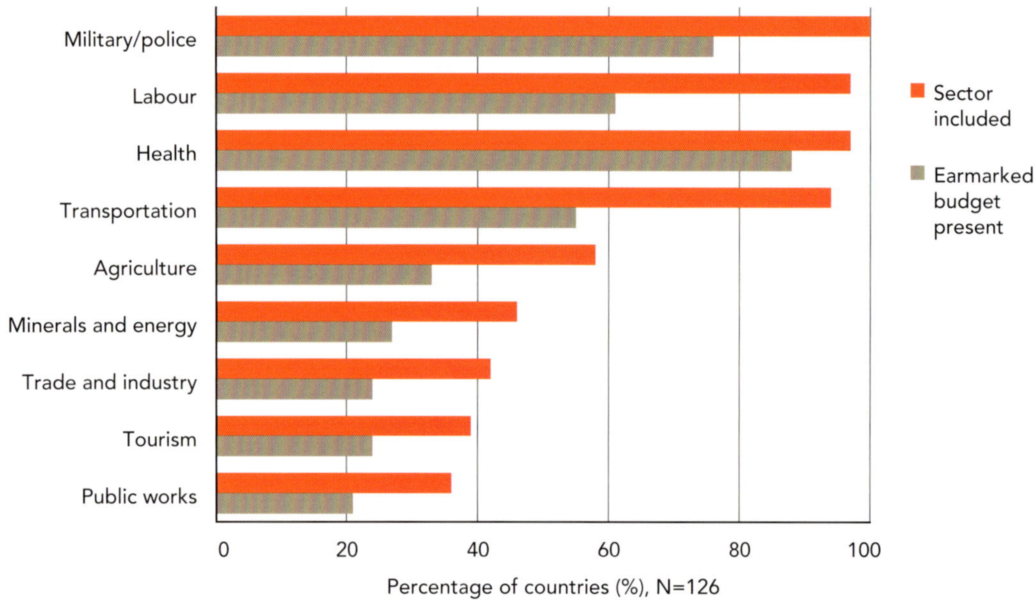

Source: UNGASS Country Progress Reports 2008.

in agriculture or the informal sector, traditional workplace programmes fail to reach a sizeable share of the workforce.

The 33 countries with generalized epidemics reporting these data generally include labour (97%), military and police (100%), and transport (94%) in their national HIV strategies. Other areas are included less frequently in national HIV strategies; agriculture is addressed in 58% of strategic plans in countries with generalized epidemics, trade and industry in 42%, minerals and energy in 46%, tourism in 39%, and public works in 36%. Even when they are included in national HIV strategies, many non-health sectors do not receive budget support to address the epidemic's sectoral impact, according to government reports (UNGASS Country Progress Reports 2008) (Figure 6.7).

Poverty-sensitive macroeconomic policies

Poverty-sensitive pro-growth strategies can potentially help to ensure sufficiently high economic growth to compensate for the epidemic's drag on the economy. Yet certain kinds of economic growth—for example, those that encourage population mobility or contribute to greater away-from-home work—may potentially worsen national epidemics. Access to a trading centre and a higher proportion of short-term residents were among the factors found to be highly associated with HIV risk in a study in Limpopo, South Africa (Pronyk, 2007).

Workers against HIV

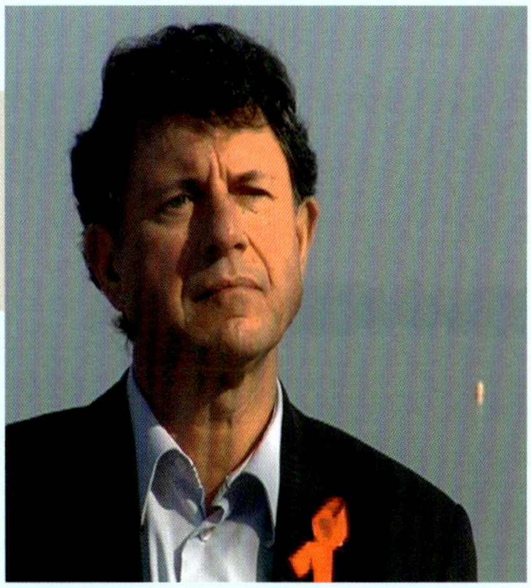

Alan Leather is Deputy General Secretary of Public Services International, the global public sector union federation, and chairs the management committee of the Global Unions AIDS Programme.

"The majority of people who are HIV-positive are at work, so the workplace is the ideal place to respond to HIV and AIDS", says veteran trade unionist Alan Leather. "Throughout their history, trade unions have campaigned for the rights of workers to live and work in decent conditions. Trade unions realize that this is something their members wish them to be active in."

Leather chairs the Global Unions AIDS Programme (GUAP), which aims to make HIV a priority for all trade unions and workers. GUAP represents the 12 major global trade union organizations, which in turn represent 200 million workers.

Many trade unions around the world have been able to negotiate HIV workplace policies with employers. Tackling stigma and discrimination against HIV-positive workers has been particularly important, and has challenged trade unionists themselves. "We have to get leaders to openly address HIV and AIDS, to talk about it as something normal for a trade union to address", says Leather. "If we're going to really challenge stigma and discrimination in the workplace, we have to talk about the normality of this disease."

Leather says that although employers are now much more responsive to HIV issues than previously, workplace policies are not always implemented. "Some employers are responding, but others are not", says Leather. "They believe it is not their responsibility, they believe it is the responsibility of the health system or somebody else."

GUAP has two major areas of work: advocacy at the international level and project work, mainly in the high-prevalence countries of sub-Saharan Africa. Some of their projects have been innovative and successful. For example, the International Transport Federation has been active in Africa and other parts of the world, implementing programmes to protect long-distance drivers in transport corridors. They have concentrated on setting up education and treatment centres on transport routes to make sure that transport workers are aware of their vulnerability. Another example is the work of Education International, the global union federation that represents 30 million teachers worldwide, which runs HIV awareness programmes in schools and colleges throughout the world. Last World AIDS Day, they campaigned for all teachers to give one hour to teaching about HIV and AIDS.

Although there has been progress in strengthening the response to HIV in work settings, Leather feels that there is still a long way to go. "From my side, I'd like to see more involvement from labour so that I could have more of a back seat role to young trade unionists, who are going to take responsibilities in the future."

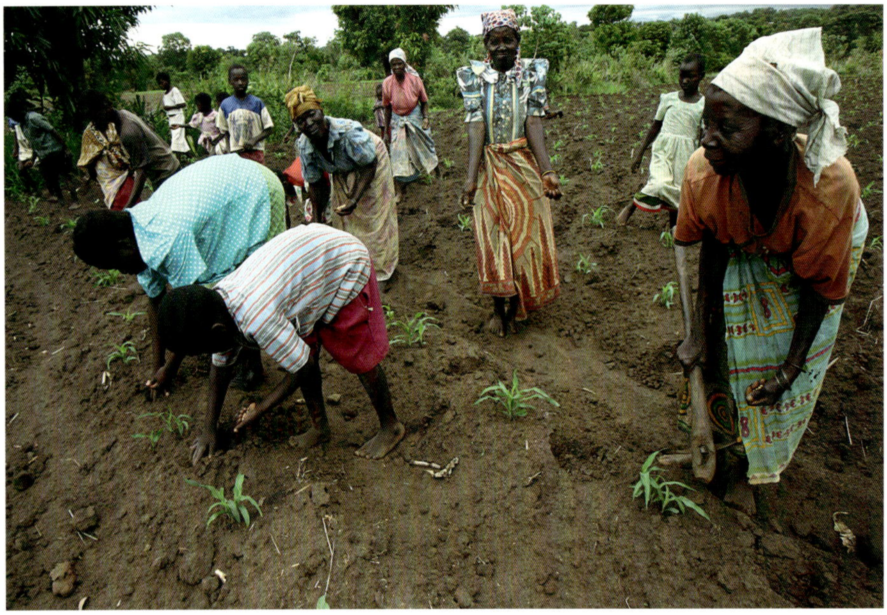

Many HIV-affected households depend on agriculture for their livelihood. Especially in the most affected countries, HIV often reduces agricultural productivity and threatens food security.

The epidemic's impact on agricultural sectors

As agriculture is a primary livelihood base for many people living with, or affected by, HIV, the epidemic has had major effects on food security in high-prevalence countries. The weight of the limited but growing body of evidence indicates that HIV-affected households experience a loss of agricultural production, although some of the radical HIV-related effects feared earlier in the epidemic, such as a widespread shift toward subsistence crops, have not been documented in the few rigorous studies that have been undertaken in rural African settings (Jayne et al., 2004). Average bean production in death-affected households in Rwanda, for example, is 18% lower than the national average (Donovan, 2004). The tendency of urban-dwelling, underemployed household members to return to rural communities when the household becomes affected by HIV sometimes compensates for productivity losses. However, it is unclear how long the surplus of workers in the informal sector will persist if the epidemic's burden continues to mount (Jayne et al., 2004).

Mitigating the impact on agriculture

Few scaled-up interventions have been implemented, much less evaluated, to mitigate the epidemic's impact on agricultural sectors and food security (Barnett, 2004). A four-pronged approach is recommended to mitigate the epidemic's effects on agriculture and food security. The approach consists of: initiatives to protect and improve the livelihoods of rural households (through both farm and non-farm avenues); social protection policies to provide financial and nutritional assistance where appropriate; focused nutrition programmes for key populations at higher risk (e.g. girls and women); and improvements in the development, implementation, and accountability of policy-making in the agricultural sector (Gillespie & Kadiyala, 2005).

Of the 33 countries with generalized epidemics reporting these data, 58% report including the agricultural sector in national HIV strategies, although one in three (33%) governments report that there is no earmarked budget to address HIV in the agricultural sector (UNGASS Country Progress Reports 2008).

Mitigating the epidemic's impact on national systems and institutions

The responsibilities of governments to act on their nation's behalf, include formulating and implementing an effective strategic response to HIV. The epidemic itself, however, is undermining public sectors in many countries, impeding governments' abilities to lead efforts to address HIV. Not only does the epidemic often erode government finances—reducing tax receipts while generating new revenue needs—it also robs the public sector of essential human resources (Haacker, 2004b).

Impact on the capacity to govern

Preliminary evidence from a study of the epidemic's impact on governance in seven African countries indicates that the epidemic is undermining parliamentary capacity, resulting in substantial additional governmental expense. In Zimbabwe, the number of by-elections in national parliaments more than doubled between 2000 and 2007, with more than two thirds of by-elections resulting from the death of parliament members due to undisclosed illness. In addition to the potential impact on the quality of representation provided to the constituents of deceased representatives, such vacancies take a toll on the public purse, e.g. each by-election in Malawi costs an average of almost US$ 79 000 (Chirambo, 2007).

HIV has additional, less direct effects on governance. The same seven-country study in Africa found that the stigma associated with HIV deters candidates for public office or elected parliamentary members from leading a strong national AIDS response. The perceived HIV status of candidates is frequently used as a political weapon to cast doubt on the suitability of another party's candidate. In the seven African countries studied, including some with HIV prevalence exceeding 20%, researchers identified no member of parliament or cabinet minister who was openly living with HIV (Chirambo, 2007).

Impact on health and other social sectors

A few years ago studies in Africa documented substantial human resource losses to public health sectors due to HIV-related absenteeism and death. (Zambia Central Board of Health & Center for International Health and Development, 2004). More recently, a sero-survey in two public hospitals in South Africa found that 11.5% of health-care workers were HIV-positive, including nearly 14% of nurses. Almost one in five infected health-care workers had a CD4 count below 200, with almost half having CD4 counts under 350 (Connelly et al., 2007), suggesting a high likelihood of additional deaths among workers in the near future.

The epidemic's impact on the public sector extends well beyond health systems. For example, the damage inflicted by the epidemic on national education systems—primarily through the absenteeism and premature mortality of teachers living with HIV—has been well documented (Birdsall & Hamoudi, 2004). In 2005, HIV-related mortality reduced the service delivery capacity of the Zambian Wildlife Authority by 6.2% and increased labour costs almost 10%, constraining the government's ability to protect the country's wildlife and parks (Rosen et al., 2006).

Improving government capacity by scaling up antiretroviral drugs

A number of strategies have been tried or suggested to mitigate the epidemic's impact on governance. As noted with respect to other working contexts, increasing access to antiretroviral drugs can significantly improve productivity, reduce absenteeism, prolong life, and improve quality of life. Because of the critical need for health-care workers and other public servants, it has sometimes been suggested that key workers should be prioritized for HIV prevention and treatment services, although concerns have been raised regarding the potential inequities of such an approach. In January 2008, the government of Malawi announced plans to offer income

Impact of HIV on national militaries and global security

At a landmark meeting in 2000, AIDS became the first health issue ever formally discussed by the United Nations Security Council, which subsequently enacted a series of resolutions acknowledging the epidemic's global security dimensions. There are a number of ways the epidemic might affect global security; for example, by causing state failure or by weakening national militaries, thereby inviting aggressive action by a neighbouring country or weakening national readiness to contribute troops for international peacekeeping missions.

There is little evidence that HIV is likely to lead to state failure. However, many national militaries, especially in the most heavily-affected countries, are struggling to manage the administrative, practical and operational issues associated with high levels of HIV infection among military personnel. Although it is often difficult to obtain reliable information on the health status of national militaries, international data indicate that HIV prevalence in national militaries is typically equal to or greater than infection levels in the general population (Garrett, 2005).

A total of 85% of countries said that their national HIV strategic frameworks in 2007 address the needs of national militaries. Of countries with such policies, 66% earmarked budget allocations to support HIV activities in the military, according to national governments (UNGASS Country Progress Reports 2008). International donors have stepped in to provide financial and technical support for these efforts, including the United States Department of Defense HIV/AIDS Prevention Programme.

Many countries have demonstrated the feasibility of implementing HIV prevention services throughout military structures, including peer education, condom promotion, treatment for sexually transmitted infections, and antiretroviral treatments. In Kenya, for example, the national armed forces provided antiretroviral drugs in 2007 to an estimated 90% of military personnel in need and has provided voluntary counselling and testing to thousands of civilians who live near the military's 17 designated testing sites. Of the 109 countries reporting the existence of a national strategy for HIV among national uniformed services, most reported reaching a significant proportion of this population with condom provision (86%), services for sexually transmitted infections (89%), HIV voluntary testing and counselling (89%), and HIV treatment (77%) (UNGASS Country Progress Reports, 2008). The United Nations Department of Peacekeeping Operations, which oversees more than 100 000 personnel serving in 18 UN peacekeeping missions, provides HIV orientation and basic prevention services for all peacekeepers.

supplements of US$ 35 per month (over and above the average monthly salary of US$ 200) to HIV-positive public servants, with the aim of improving their nutritional intake and quality of life (Reuters, 2008).

Enhancing HIV prevention in the public sector

Especially in high-prevalence settings, workplaces should be regarded as high-priority venues for HIV prevention activities. In the case of health-care workers, all employees should be trained and monitored with respect to effective infection control and the implementation of universal precautions, and health-care facilities should ensure ready access to essential prevention technologies including gloves, gowns, and other protective gear, as well as kits to facilitate the timely initiation of antiretroviral prophylaxis in the event of a significant blood exposure.

Innovative measures to expand human resource capacity

As described in Chapter 5, countries are innovating, to expand limited human resource capacity to address the HIV epidemic. An example is the "Treat, Train, Retain" strategy, which aims to shore up human capacity in health sectors, and to task-shift from more to less specialized staff members, to stretch available capacity as far as possible. While most such innovation has focused on health systems, such approaches have potential applicability to other public sectors affected by HIV.

Moving forward: action to mitigate impact

National governments, donors, and other stakeholders should prioritize impact mitigation as a key component of the HIV response and strengthen efforts to mitigate the epidemic's impact on households and communities. Understanding the epidemic's effects in individual countries and subnational units is a necessary step toward greater strategic action to mitigate impact. As of December 2007, 60% of countries with generalized epidemics said they had evaluated the epidemic's socioeconomic impact, although only 6 of 33 countries with HIV prevalence greater than 1% indicated that such estimates had effectively informed decisions on resource allocations.

Mainstreaming HIV in development instruments and processes—in poverty reduction strategy papers, planning for the Millennium Development Goals, and mid-term expenditure frameworks—provides a potentially important means of increasing attention to the many ways that the epidemic may deepen poverty, increase inequality, and undermine economic growth and social development. All low-income countries and all countries with generalized epidemics report having integrated HIV into their general development plans by the end of 2007. Addressing the epidemic's impact should also be prioritized in sectoral planning processes.

International donors should devote increased financial and technical resources to efforts to mitigate the epidemic's impact. In addition to project-specific activities, such as food distribution or psychosocial support to HIV-affected families, donors should deliver the budgetary support required to implement strong social cash transfer regimes. Governments, donors and nongovernmental organizations should pay increased attention to strategies focused on supporting kinship and community networks that are struggling to care for the large and growing number of children orphaned or made vulnerable by HIV.

Strong national capacity for data collection and analysis, and multidisciplinary policy development is required to ensure the soundness of national approaches to impact mitigation. As noted, many of the policy reforms proposed to alleviate the epidemic's effects may inadvertently exacerbate other problems, such as HIV risk and vulnerability, economic inequality, and HIV stigma. The traditional "silo" approach to decision-making—whereby decision-making jurisdiction for individual ministries is sharply delineated and ministerial 'turf' is carefully guarded—does not promote the long-term effectiveness and sustainability of impact mitigation strategies. Agriculture ministries, for example, may have impressive expertise on crop distribution, agricultural productivity and the like, but they may lack an understanding of the ramifications of particular policies on rural wages, population migration, or subgroups of HIV-affected households. Similarly, finance ministries, while rightly focused on balancing budgets in the short term, may be poorly equipped to assess the long-term financial wisdom of immediate investments in impact mitigation.

Evidence for action

Are the right actions being taken?

- Among 33 countries with generalized epidemics, government respondents in 91% report having policies or strategies to address the needs of children orphaned or made vulnerable by HIV.
- All national governments in countries with generalized epidemics reporting having national strategies to address HIV among workers and uniformed service personnel, and most have policies to address HIV in the transportation (94%) and agricultural (58%) sectors.
- Governments in 60% of countries with generalized epidemics report having evaluated the epidemic's socioeconomic impact.

Are the right actions being undertaken in the right manner?

- In countries with HIV prevalence greater than 5%, orphans were only 4% less likely to attend school than non-orphans.
- Where non-health sectors are addressed in national HIV strategies, they often do not receive budget support to address the epidemic's sectoral impact.
- National governments in only 6 of 33 countries with generalized epidemics say that an evaluation of the epidemic's socioeconomic impact has influenced budget allocations.

Have these actions been sufficiently scaled up to make a difference?

- In 11 countries with HIV prevalence of 5% or greater, only 15% of households with orphans received any form of assistance in 2007.
- HIV treatment or referral for treatment is available in workplaces in all districts in need in only 9% of countries with generalized epidemics.

Mobilizing sufficient financial resources for the HIV response

Financial resources for the HIV response have significantly increased in recent years. The US$ 10 billion made available for HIV programmes in 2007 from all sources, including domestic public funds and out-of-pocket spending, represented a 12% increase over expenditures in 2006 and a seven-fold increase in this decade (Figure A). However, substantial additional resources will be required to support a robust and sustainable HIV response in the coming years.

Mobilizing domestic resources

Increased domestic spending on HIV is not only important to help finance essential HIV activities in low- and middle-income countries, but it also serves as a concrete sign of national commitment in the HIV response. To meet future global resource needs for the HIV response, UNAIDS projects that low- and middle-income countries collectively will need to cover roughly one third of HIV-related costs in the coming years. However, the domestic financial burden for the HIV response will vary considerably among countries, depending in large measure on national financial capacity. While it is anticipated that upper-middle-income countries should cover domestic HIV-related costs on their own, external support will be required for the bulk of future HIV-related costs on least-developed countries.

Too often, national HIV expenditures do not match national needs. This is especially the case with many countries with low-level or concentrated epidemics. Within the category of HIV prevention spending in concentrated epidemics, countries often opt for broad prevention programmes for the general population rather than for the more cost-effective interventions focused on populations most at risk.

FIGURE A Estimated total annual resources available for HIV, 2000–2007, and projected financial resources required by 2010 if current scale up continues (US$ billion)*

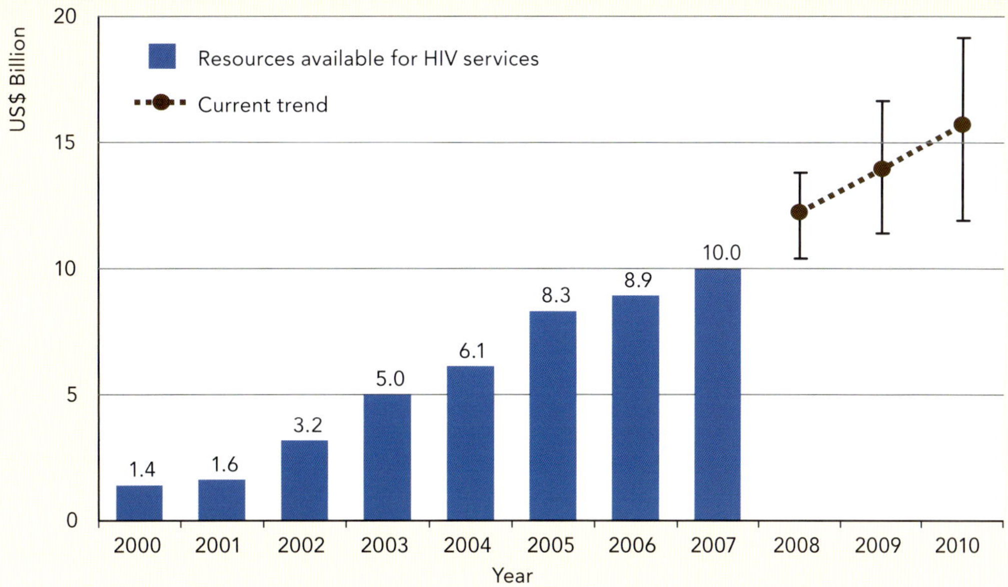

* This represents the projected trend in resource needs if the current rate of scale-up of services is maintained constant

FIGURE B Spending in programmes specifically directed to the populations most at risk for HIV as a percentage of total prevention spending by type of epidemic—public and international Funds, 2006

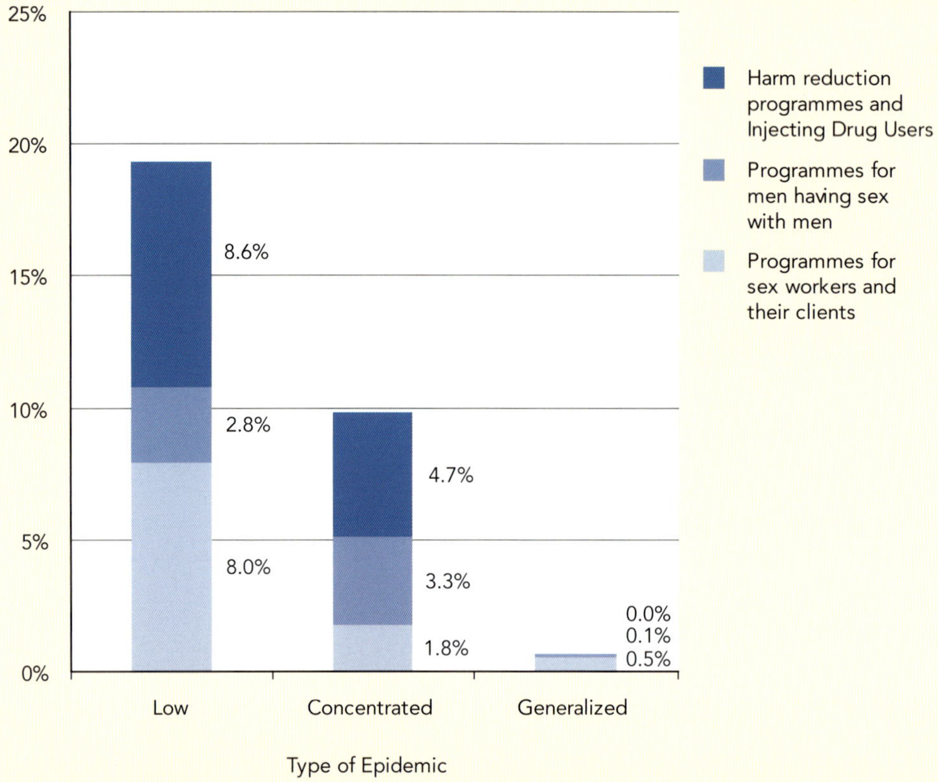

Source: UNGASS Country Progress Reports, 2008

FIGURE C Per capita HIV expenditures from domestic public sources in low- and middle-income countries, 2004-2007

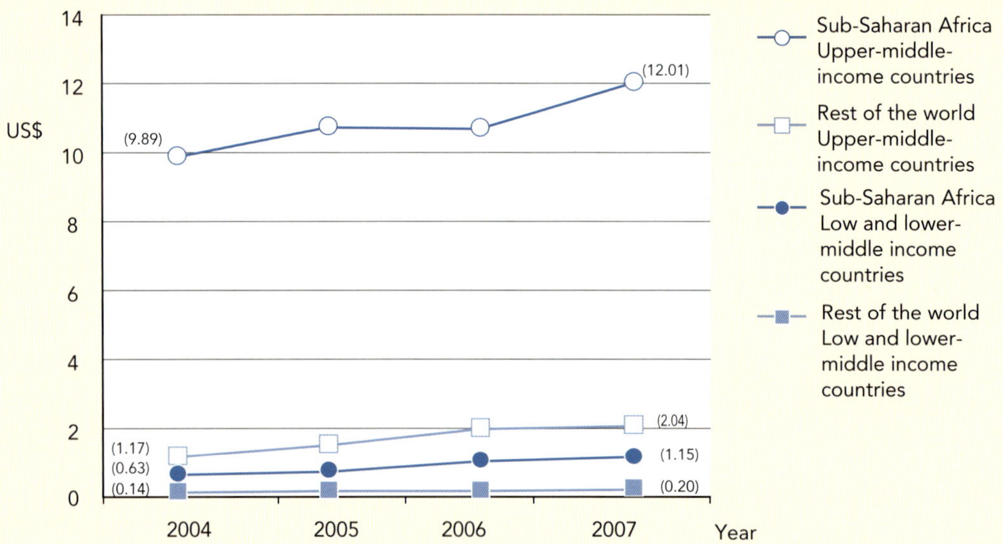

Source: UNGASS Country Progress Reports, 2008

FIGURE D Public domestic expenditures, Malawi (US$ millions)

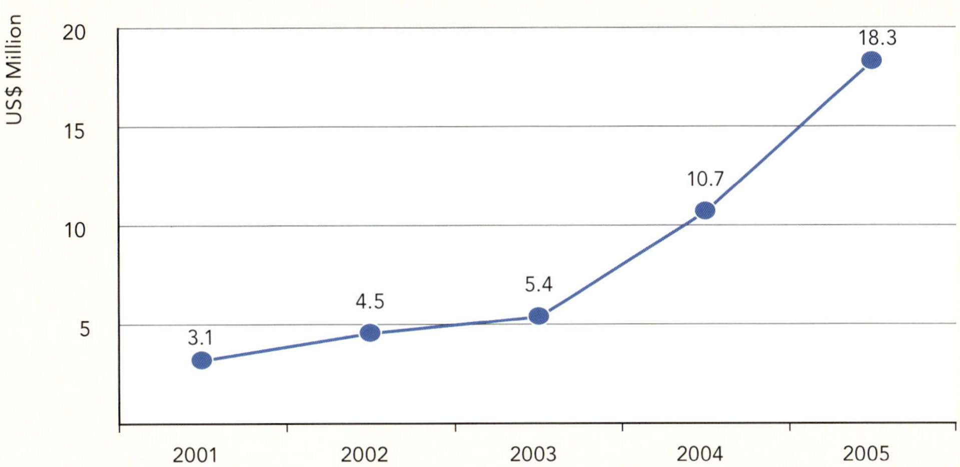

For concentrated epidemics generally, risk-reduction programmes focused on populations most at risk represent only 10% of overall HIV-prevention spending (Figure B).

In low-income and lower-middle income countries, per capita domestic spending on HIV more than doubled between 2005 and 2007(Figure C). Per capita government expenditure in five sub-Saharan African upper-middle income countries is the highest among low- and middle-income countries, and it increased by more than 10% in 2007 to reach an estimated US$ 12 per capita in 2007.

A number of low- and middle-income countries have exhibited great HIV leadership this decade, significantly increasing domestic HIV outlays while redoubling efforts to mobilize greater external support. They are achieving these increases through various strategies to place the HIV response on a sound, long-term financial footing. By moving in the late 1990s to provide antiretrovirals through the country's social security programme, Mexico helped ensure the sustainability of its national response; more recently by the expansion of a financial protection system that protects the previously uninsured population against the catastrophic financial impact of selected diseases including HIV. Malawi has enacted legislation requiring all ministries to spend at least 2% of their budgets on HIV activities and has increased nearly six-fold its domestic expenditures for HIV between 2001 and 2005 (Figure D).

The magnitude of domestic HIV spending—as well as the balance between external and domestic sources for HIV financing—varies considerably among countries. As Figure E illustrates, among 20 low- and middle-income countries with the largest amounts of domestic expenditures devoted to HIV, Brazil spends the most in absolute terms, while Botswana has by far the highest per capita domestic spending on HIV.

FIGURE E Annual domestic spending: top 20 countries (US$ 2.73 billion). UNGASS reports (US$ million)

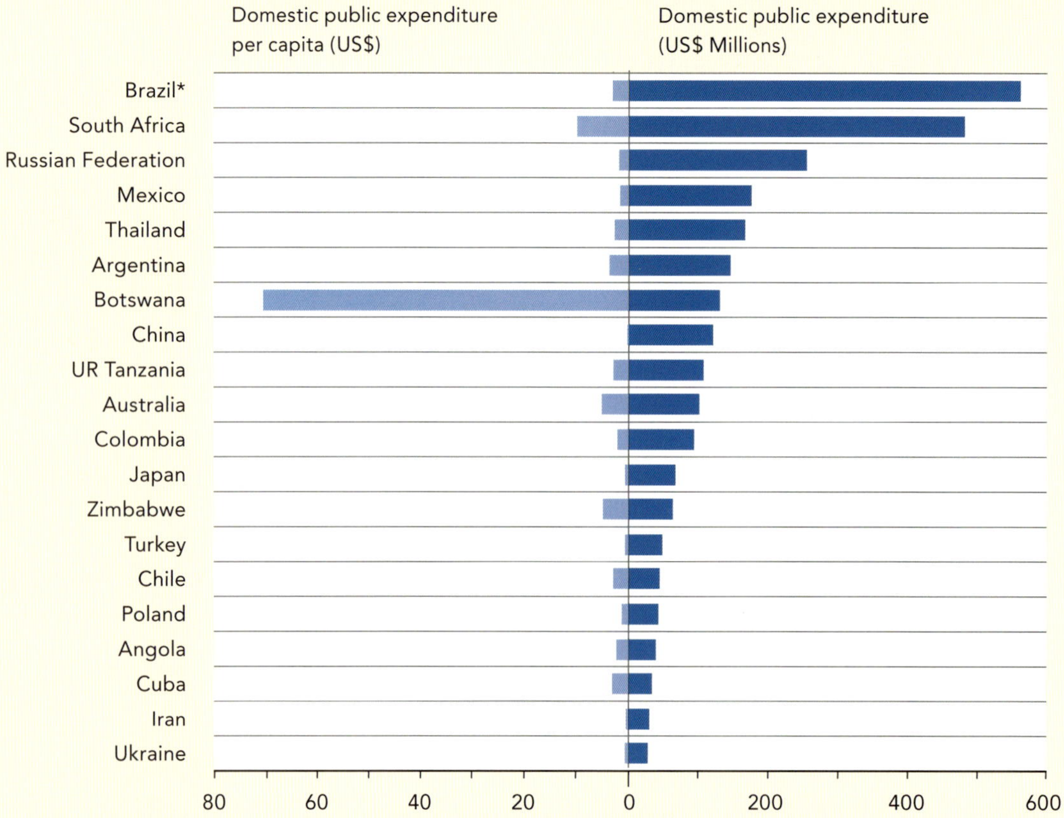

*Partial data

National spending on HIV by income level

In Figure F, the per capita spending on HIV includes both domestic and international sources. The Figure demonstrates that in the countries with more elevated income brackets, an increasing proportion of overall funding comes from domestic public resources.

Mobilizing international resources

To finance the push towards universal access to HIV prevention, treatment, care, and support, even greater support will be required from the international community. The Global Fund alone anticipates needing US$ 6.7 billion in 2008, with annual funding requirements growing to US$ 7.7 billion by 2010 (Global Fund, 2007). UNAIDS projects that international donors will need to mobilize roughly two thirds of the total amount required in future years to finance a strong HIV response in low- and middle-income countries.

Contributors to the growth in funding for HIV programmes in low- and middle-income countries have been numerous. While the US accounts for the largest share in financing, other countries provide a larger proportion of their gross domestic product (Figures G and H).

FIGURE F HIV expenditures by finance sources and income level 2007, or latest data available

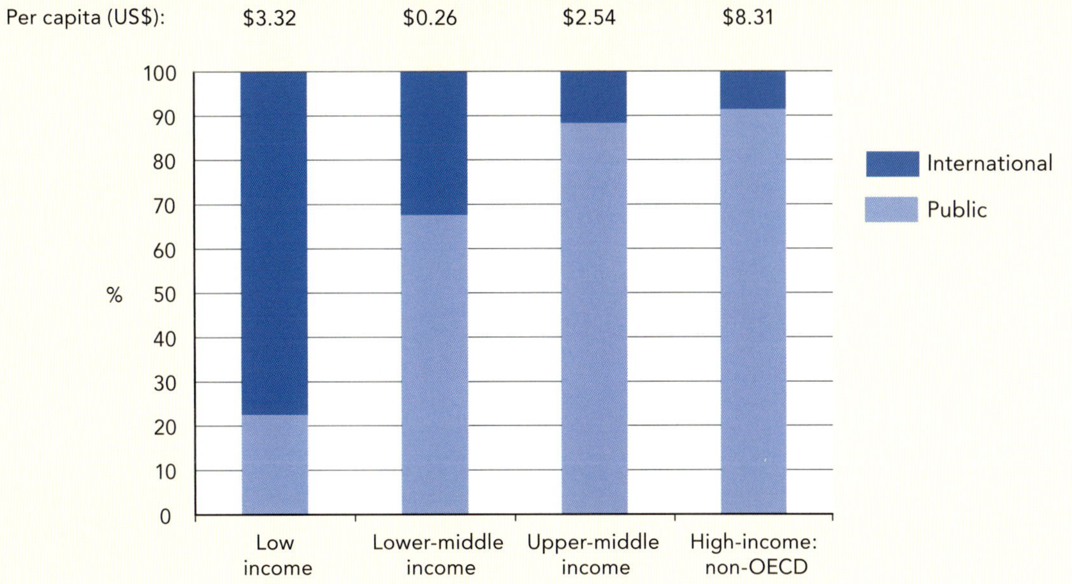

FIGURE G Resources available to HIV-related programmes by source and bilateral disbursements, 2006

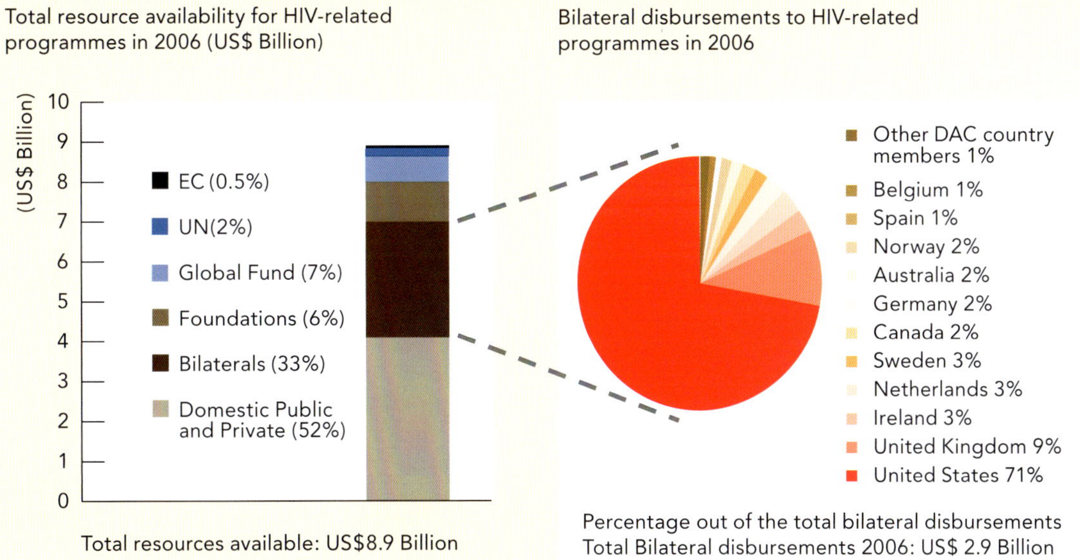

The organizational disbursements are different than commitments or obligations, as well as different from in-country expenditures

Source: UNAIDS analysis based on OECD/DAC online database (last visited on May 6, 2008), Resource availability UNAIDS 2005, Funders Concerned About AIDS (FCAA), European HIV/AIDS Funders Group (EFG) for Philanthropic sector.

FIGURE H Disbursements for HIV per US$ 1 Million GDP, 2006

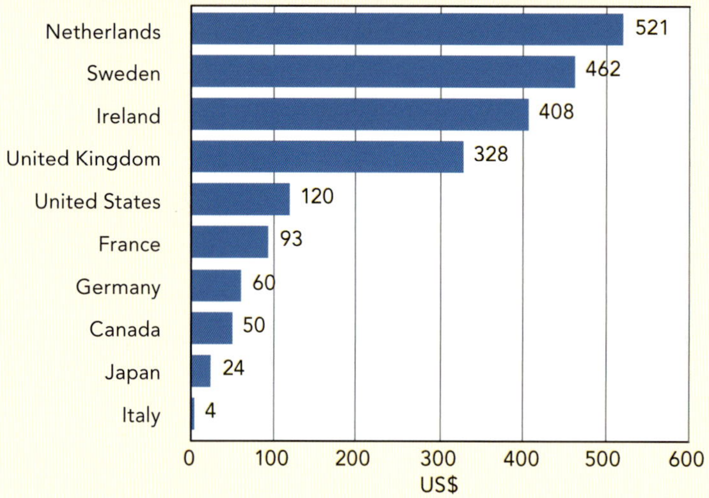

Sources: UNAIDS and Kaiser Family Foundation analysis, June 2007; Global Fund to Fight AIDS, Tuberculosis and Malaria online data query May 2007; International Monetary Fund, World Economic Outlook Database, April 2007.

International donors take various approaches to HIV assistance. With respect to amounts actually disbursed in 2006, more than 80% of HIV assistance from Canada, Ireland, Italy, the Netherlands, the US and the UK was channelled through bilateral programmes, while France directed more than 80% of its HIV assistance through the Global Fund.

Created in direct response to the 2001 *Declaration of Commitment,* the Global Fund had by March 2008 committed US$ 10.1 billion in multiyear funding for health programmes in 136 countries, with the majority of such funding dedicated to HIV initiatives. Country-level disbursements by the Global Fund rose from US$ 430 000 in 2002 to US$ 641 million in 2006, reflecting a rapid escalation of financial support for national efforts on HIV, tuberculosis and malaria. The US, the UK and France had by March 2008 pledged the largest amounts to the Global Fund.

Support for HIV activities in low- and middle-income countries from US-based philanthropic foundations nearly doubled between 2004 and 2006, reaching US$ 979 million. According to Funders Concerned about AIDS, research dwarfed other purposes for foundation spending on HIV in 2006. In 2004, the last year for which data are available, European foundations spent US$ 101 million on HIV in low- and middle-income countries, a tripling over amounts spent in 2002-2003 (European HIV/AIDS Funders, 2006).

FIGURE I Annual resources available 2000–2007 and funding gap between projected financial resources if current scale-up continues and a phased scale-up scenario to reach universal access between 2010 and 2015 (US$ billion)

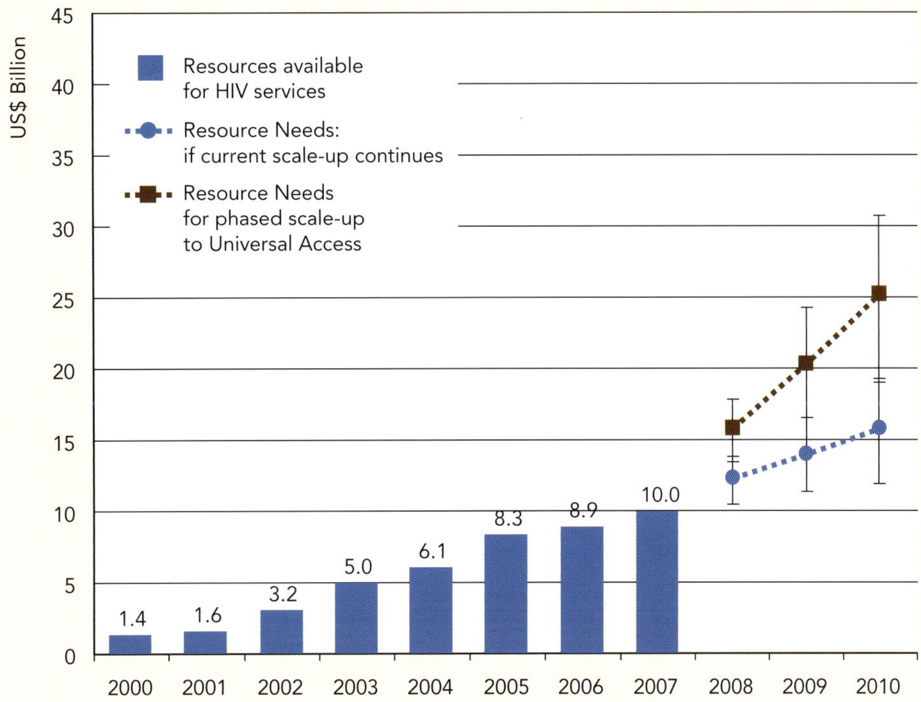

A growing resource gap

Simply to maintain the current pace of scale-up in service provision, funding levels will need to increase by more than 50% by the end of this decade (Figure I). However, this trajectory would leave the world falling short of universal access to HIV prevention, treatment, care, and support—even by 2015, five years after the globally agreed deadline for achieving this result (UNAIDS, 2007c).

To achieve and sustain universal access to HIV prevention, treatment, care, and support, substantially greater resources will be required. As Figure I illustrates, the gap between available resources and amounts needed to move towards universal access is increasing from year to year.

Funding shortfalls for HIV are part of a broader pattern in the development arena. Reiterating a commitment articulated in other international agreements, donor countries pledged in the *Declaration of Commitment on HIV/AIDS* to devote 0.7% of their gross domestic product to development assistance. As of 2005, few countries had achieved this target—Denmark (0.81%), Luxembourg (0.82%), the Netherlands (0.82%), Norway (0.94%). Among OECD countries as a whole, an average of 0.33% of gross national income were devoted to official development assistance in 2005—a percentage that had not increased since 1990, notwithstanding numerous international agreements to increase development aid.

(For a discussion of the challenges countries face in translating resources into high-impact programmes, as well as strategies for sustaining robust HIV financing over the coming years and decades, see Chapter 7.)

Where do we go from here? Sustaining an effective, robust HIV response for the long-term

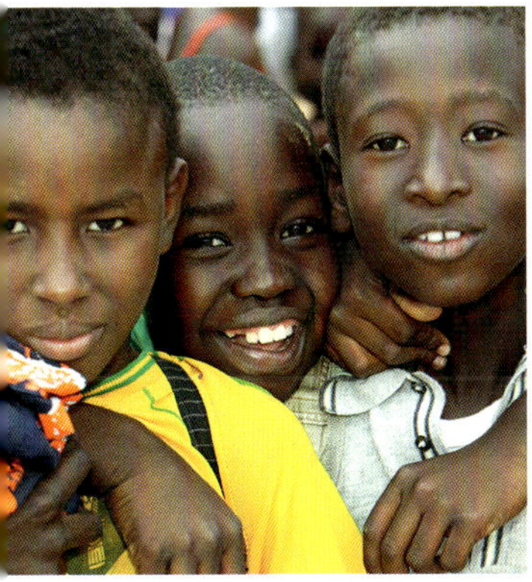

7

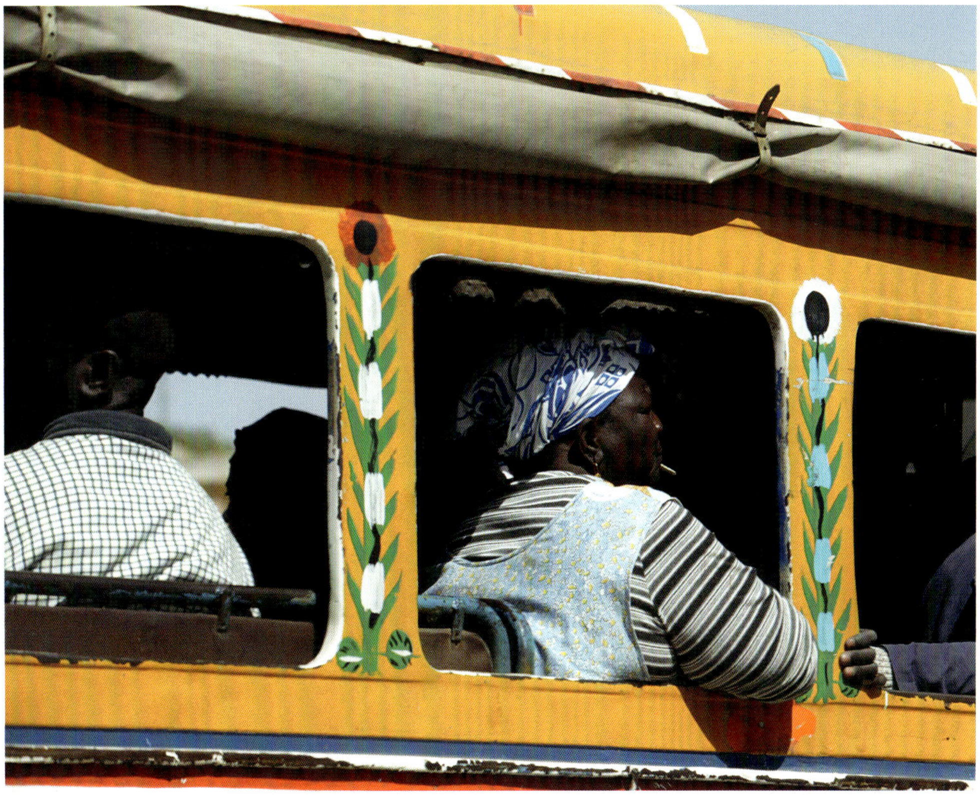

Chapter 7

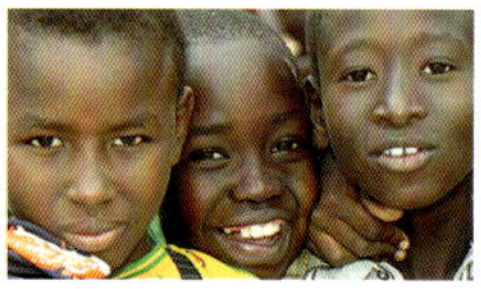

FIGURE 7.1 Total annual resources available for AIDS, 1986–2007

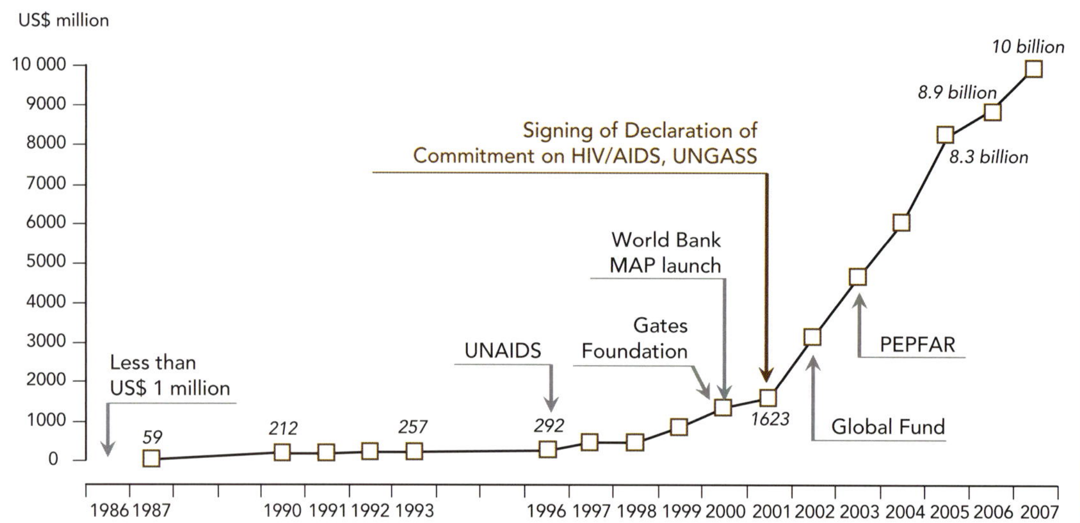

Notes: [1] 1986–2000 figures are for international funds only
[2] Domestic funds are included from 2001 onwards
[i] 1996-2005 data: Extracted from 2006 Report on the Global AIDS Epidemic (UNAIDS, 2006)
[ii] 1986-1993 data: Mann.&. Tarantola, 1996
Source: UNAIDS & WHO unpublished estimates, 2007.

As discussed in previous chapters, the world currently possesses the means to prevent new HIV infections, reduce HIV-related illness and death, and mitigate the epidemic's harmful effects on households, communities, and societies.

Moving towards universal access to HIV prevention, treatment, care, and support is an important step toward an effective, sustainable HIV response. Substantial, although variable, progress has been made in scaling up towards universal access. As Tables 7.1 and 7.2 show, several countries have already achieved their national universal access targets for prevention of mother-to-child transmission and antiretroviral treatment.

The countries that have significantly expanded the scale of these services have demonstrated strong national and decentralised leadership and coordination of the HIV response, including alignment of funding and partners with national AIDS strategies. In countries where services have rapidly expanded, it is evident that there is clear political will from the very highest levels of government for undertaking inclusive processes that emphasize all aspects of the response and involve all relevant stakeholders. The enthusiasm and transparency with which some governments are responding to the epidemic are encouraging more development partners to support nationally owned and determined HIV strategies.

However, movement towards universal access to HIV prevention, treatment, care, and support has not occurred equally throughout the world. As Figure 7.2 indicates, certain regions lag behind in bringing critical prevention and treatment services to scale. Progress between 2005 and 2007 in expanding access to antiretroviral treatments and preventing mother-to-child transmission was most apparent in sub-Saharan Africa. However, continued success in the region will be essential if universal access is to be achieved, as coverage levels before 2005 in Africa were extremely low.

Countries that have made notable progress towards universal access have worked to increase human-resource capacity for service delivery, improve access to commodities and equipment, and strengthen health systems more generally. Significant civil society engagement has also been essential to successful scaling up of services. An active, vocal, and engaged civil society promotes realization of human rights, expands implementation capacity in countries, and improves service access for marginalised groups and those most in need.

This chapter focuses on the steps that must now be taken, to extend the recent successes outlined in this report to all countries and regions and across the full breadth of the HIV response. This chapter looks beyond the 2015 deadline for the Millennium Development Goals, examining the actions and architecture that will be needed at national and global levels to sustain a robust response to HIV over the long-term.

In particular, this chapter explores the pressing challenges that individual countries, and the global community as a whole, will face in the coming years, in the quest to mount an effective, sustainable response. These challenges can be summarized as follows:

- ensuring strong and multisectoral leadership in the coming years and decades, even when other priorities emerge and improved access to antiretroviral drugs makes the epidemic seem less severe;
- implementing innovative, durable mechanisms to adequately fund the HIV response over time;
- avoiding the temptation to de-prioritize HIV prevention as the epidemic evolves,

FIGURE 7.2 Comparison of 2005 and 2007 percentage coverage of antiretroviral therapy for people with advanced HIV and percentage coverage of antiretroviral drugs for HIV positive pregnant women by region

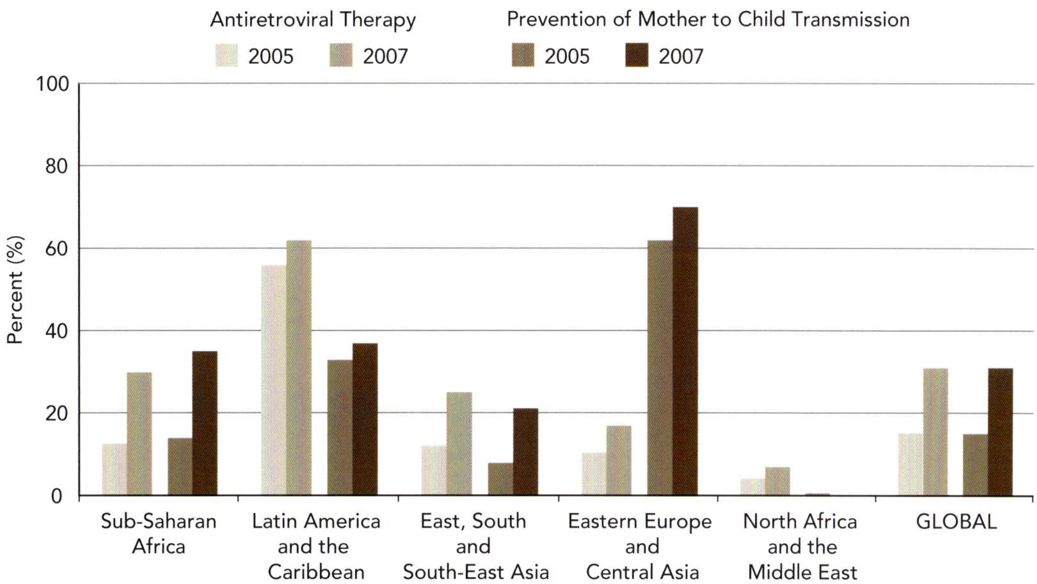

Source: UNAIDS/UNICEF/WHO.

TABLE 7.1 **Percent Coverage of Antiretrovirals for Prevention of Mother-to-Child Transmission** Breakdown by Quartiles (N=63)

Less than 25% Coverage (36 Countries)	25% to 49% Coverage (16 Countries)	50% to 75% Coverage (7 Countries)	Greater than 75% Coverage (4 Countries)
Angola	Benin	Brazil	Argentina
Burkina Faso	Cambodia	Kenya	Botswana
Burundi	Central African Republic	Namibia	Russian Federation
Cameroon	Dominican Republic	Rwanda	Thailand
Chad	Gambia	South Africa	
China	Honduras	Swaziland	
Colombia	Lesotho	Ukraine	
Congo, Republic of the	Malawi		
Côte d'Ivoire	Mozambique		
Democratic Republic of the Congo	Myanmar		
El Salvador	Niger		
Eritrea	Peru		
Ethiopia	Uganda		
Gabon	United Republic of Tanzania		
Ghana	Zambia		
Guatemala	Zimbabwe		
Guinea			
Guinea-Bissau			
Haiti			
India			
Indonesia			
Iran, Islamic Republic of			
Liberia			
Madagascar			
Malaysia			
Mali			
Nepal			
Nigeria			
Pakistan			
Papua New Guinea			
Senegal			
Sierra Leone			
Somalia			
Togo			
Venezuela			
Viet Nam			

All values are based on need estimates using UNAIDS/WHO methodology. Includes all countries for which number of pregnant women receiving antiretroviral therapy was reported for 2007, except countries for which UNAIDS/WHO need estimates are not available, or with need estimates less than 500.

TABLE 7.2 Percent Coverage of Antiretroviral Therapy for Adults and Children with Advanced HIV Breakdown by Quartiles (N=106)

Less than 25% Coverage (45 Countries)	25% to 49% Coverage (40 Countries)	50% to 75% Coverage (14 Countries)	Greater than 75% Coverage (7 Countries)
Algeria	Angola	Argentina	Botswana
Armenia	Bahamas	Barbados	Brazil
Azerbaijan	Belize	Cambodia	Chile
Bangladesh	Benin	Czech Republic	Costa Rica
Belarus	Burkina Faso	El Salvador	Cuba
Bolivia	Cameroon	Moldova	Lao People's Democratic Republic
Burundi	Cote d'Ivoire	Netherlands	Namibia
Central African Republic	Dominican Republic	Panama	
Chad	Ecuador	Romania	
China	Equatorial Guinea	Rwanda	
Congo, Republic of the	Estonia	Senegal	
Democratic Republic of the Congo	Ethiopia	Thailand	
Djibouti	Gabon	Trinidad and Tobago	
Egypt	Guatemala	Uruguay	
Eritrea	Guinea		
Gambia	Guyana		
Ghana	Haiti		
Guinea-Bissau	Honduras		
Hungary	Jamaica		
Indonesia	Kenya		
Iran, Islamic Republic of	Lebanon		
Kazakhstan	Lesotho		
Kyrgyzstan	Malawi		
Liberia	Malaysia		
Lithuania	Mali		
Madagascar	Morocco		
Mauritania	Nicaragua		
Mauritius	Nigeria		
Mozambique	Papua New Guinea		
Myanmar	Peru		
Nepal	Philippines		
Niger	Poland		
Pakistan	South Africa		
Paraguay	Suriname		
Russian Federation	Swaziland		
Serbia	Uganda		
Sierra Leone	United Republic of Tanzania		
Somalia	Venezuela		
Sri Lanka	Viet Nam		
Sudan	Zambia		
Tajikistan			
Togo			
Ukraine			
Uzbekistan			
Zimbabwe			

All values are based on need estimates using UNAIDS/WHO methodology. Includes all countries for which number of adults and children on antiretroviral therapy was reported for 2007, except countries for which UNAIDS/WHO need estimates are not available, or with need estimates less than 500.

CHAPTER 7

and ensuring that effective prevention interventions focus on populations and risk behaviours that are truly driving the local epidemics;

- putting in place the architecture needed to support robust, adaptable treatment and care programmes;
- mitigating the epidemic's short- and long-term impact on households, communities, and societies;
- implementing national responses with governance characteristics that increase effectiveness and sustainability; and
- recognizing that technocratic solutions alone will not effectively manage the epidemic, but that an effective long-term response must be grounded in human rights.

The need for a stronger, more comprehensive response is clear. Continuing at the current pace of scale-up—rather than accelerating service expansion to achieve universal access to prevention, treatment, care, and support—would result in more than one million additional AIDS deaths each year by 2015 (Figure 7.3). If HIV prevention is not brought to scale, more than twice as many new HIV infections will occur in the coming years than if a comprehensive response was implemented (Stover et al., 2006).

Leadership in the response

HIV presents special challenges for leadership. As Nobel laureate Amartya Sen has observed, collective action is typically easier to mobilize for visible crises such as famines, natural disasters, or the outbreak of highly infectious diseases. Yet even a "hidden" problem will eventually become apparent when its breadth and ramifications are as profound as HIV. However, almost without exception, action to address HIV has occurred too late. The epidemic's history underscores that delaying effective action will not make HIV disappear, but will instead ensure that the problems posed by the epidemic become even more acute in the future.

The "hidden" challenge posed by HIV could further intensify in the coming years, as antiretroviral therapy is brought to scale in resource-limited

FIGURE 7.3 Annual AIDS deaths comparing projected current rate of scale up and the phased scale-up strategy to reach universal access between 2010 and 2015

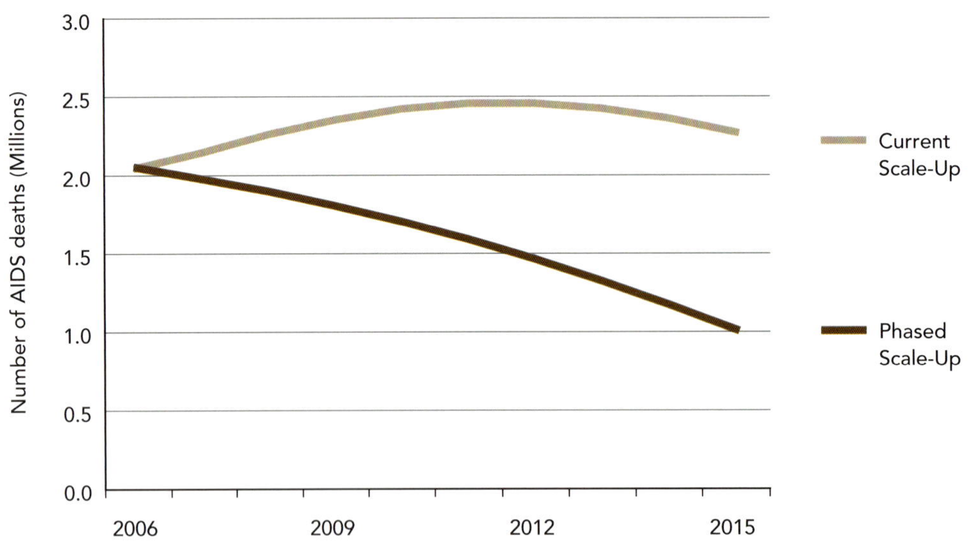

Source: UNAIDS, 2008.

CHAPTER 7

settings. As high-income countries have learnt over the last decade, reductions in illness and death due to treatment advances can mask continuing high HIV prevalence and incidence, potentially encouraging policy-makers and affected communities to become complacent about the epidemic's enduring threat. True leaders will avoid being lulled into complacency and instead will pursue evidence-informed policies and programmes to reduce the epidemic's long-term toll.

National leadership in the HIV response

Recent years have provided examples of admirable leadership on HIV in a growing number of countries.

- Nine different ministries in the Government of Barbados have core HIV working groups with budgetary allocations for HIV-related activities.
- Botswana has achieved among the world's highest coverage for HIV treatment, delivering antiretroviral drugs in 2007 to more than 90% of those who need the medications.
- In 2008, concerned about the continuing high rate of new HIV infections among men who have sex with men, Brazil embarked on a major intensification of national prevention efforts focused on this population.
- In China, after years of inadequate attention to the country's growing HIV epidemic, the national government has taken important steps to respond, including establishment of almost 400 methadone maintenance clinics that were providing drug treatment services to nearly 90 000 drug users by October 2007.
- In Europe, several countries (including Ireland, the Netherlands, Sweden, and the United Kingdom) contribute a share of international HIV financing that exceeds their respective proportions of the global economy (see section on "Mobilizing sufficient financial resources for the HIV response").
- With the aim of building sufficient capacity for an effective, sustainable response, India had, by March 2007, trained more than 794 000 individuals in the delivery of essential HIV services.
- In Papua New Guinea, implementation of provider-initiated HIV testing and counselling in health-care settings resulted in a nine-fold increase in the use of testing in health-sector sites between 2006 and 2007.
- Ranking 161st out of 177 countries in the Human Development Index (UNDP, 2007), and challenged by recovering from the 1994 genocide, Rwanda achieved the highest coverage of any low-income country in 2007 for both antiretroviral therapy (71%) and prevention of mother-to-child transmission (55%).
- Beginning in 2003, the United States Government greatly increased its financial and technical assistance to low- and middle-income countries, providing an unprecedented US$ 18.8 billion in funding for HIV prevention, treatment, care, and support initiatives (Office of US Global AIDS Coordinator et al., 2008).

Strong leadership on HIV requires a focus on long-term objectives, refusing to permit intervening challenges to undermine the national HIV response. After Brazil committed in 1996 to make antiretroviral drugs available through its public sector, the country experienced serious financial difficulties, including the collapse of the real, the national currency. Notwithstanding considerable pressure from the International Monetary Fund to sharply lower public spending, Brazilian President Fernando Henrique Cardoso remained firm on the country's commitment to providing HIV treatments. The result is the survival today of tens of thousands of people who might otherwise have died from HIV-related illness.

Leadership means avoiding the temptation to 'wish the epidemic away' once progress in the response begins to be reported. Leaders on HIV recognize that the epidemic is a generations-long challenge that requires persistence, vision, and flexibility; in short, HIV leadership means planning for the long-term. While three- and five-year planning will continue to play a key role in national responses, these processes must increasingly be situated within longer-term planning efforts. Namibia provides an example of this approach; its current five-year plan for HIV, which runs through 2009, is specifically linked to the goals and strategies of a longer-term development planning process that extends through 2030.

Leaders look to evidence for guidance. Thus, while some may be tempted to address the epidemic by placing travel restrictions on people living with HIV or by limiting prevention for young people to lessons on remaining sexually abstinent, leaders on HIV will be persuaded by public health evidence that such strategies are ineffective and counterproductive.

Leadership from heads of government and national ministries is critical, but effective national responses depend on commitment and action from different groups. Leadership on HIV is needed from all walks of life (especially in countries where HIV is hyperendemic) including community groups, faith-based organizations, private businesses, and young and old. Above all, people living with HIV must be empowered to help lead national responses.

By providing essential services, promoting tolerance and compassion, and advocating for stronger action, faith-based groups in all regions are essential partners in the response. Faith-based groups that are helping lead the HIV response include Caritas Internationalis, Ecumenical Advocacy Alliance, Tear Fund, Islamic Relief, the Sangha Metta Project, and the Art of Living foundation. Likewise, parliamentarians have a vital role to play in leading and strengthening national responses. This was reflected in the First Global Parliamentary Meeting on HIV/AIDS in November 2007, hosted by the Philippines Senate, where nearly 200 parliamentarians from countries in all regions agreed to take bold steps to increase treatment access, reduce stigma and discrimination, strengthen evidence-informed HIV prevention, and improve the effectiveness of national responses.

Engaging nongovernmental actors in the HIV response may sometimes require innovative approaches. For example, to encourage greater business involvement in the national response, the Chinese Government launched a new policy in 2007 that permits tax deductions for business donations to HIV prevention and care activities. At the global level, the Global Business Coalition on HIV/AIDS and the World Economic Forum continue to generate greater action and commitment on HIV from private industry.

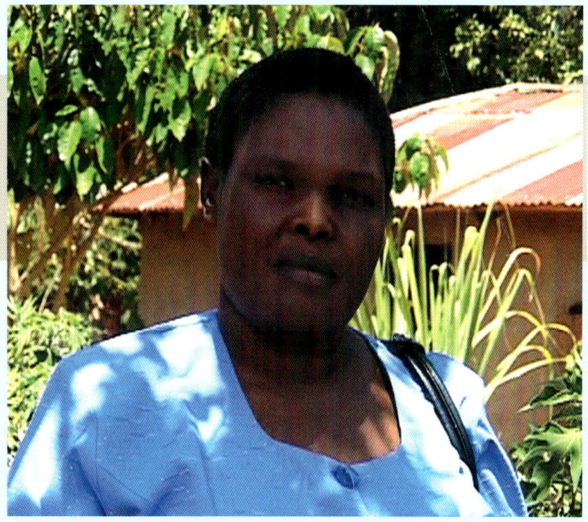

Discover and recover

Reverend Patricia Sawo is Regional Coordinator for ANERELA+, Eastern Africa

One morning in September 1999, Patricia Sawo awoke in terrible pain and discovered that her body was covered in shingles, a common opportunistic disease in people living with HIV. At the time, she was a church leader in Kenya and was training as a Christian counsellor. Her fear that this indicated HIV infection threw her into turmoil.

"I had been one of those preachers who believed that HIV was a curse and a punishment from God", she says. Later, she confided in two colleagues, who advised her that seven days of fasting and prayer would bring healing from God. But she continued to test HIV-positive.

When church leaders began discussing strategies to identify and isolate all HIV-positive people, Sawo decided to go public about her status. But her courage had disastrous repercussions: in two weeks Sawo lost her position of leadership in the church, and was forced to end her studies. Her husband lost his job, and the family lost their home, because of HIV-related stigma. All but two of Sawo's friends deserted her. Without any form of support, the children were forced to leave their schools.

"For two years I lived in loneliness and isolation", says Sawo. "But I could see that I was not going to die. I walked into an NGO and asked them if they could train me as a church leader." Through them, she made contact with other HIV-positive clergy, and in 2002 she attended a meeting of HIV-positive church leaders in Uganda. There she met Canon Gideon Byagumisaha who had been living with HIV for 10 years. "I heard three very powerful words and my life changed. He said HIV is preventable and manageable, and death is avoidable."

At this meeting, ANERELA+, the African network of religious leaders, was established. The network has three main objectives:

- to establish a network of religious leaders living with or affected by HIV;
- to empower church leaders to become agents of change; and
- to empower church leaders to stimulate discussion and action on HIV and AIDS in their home congregations.

"ANERELA+ gave me a family", Sawo says. She began working on ANERELA+'s behalf to establish a religious network in Kenya. Her job with ANERELA+ helped the family financially, enabling her children to return to school. Her daughter, who would have become a maid, is now at university.

When Sawo first began speaking about HIV, people started coming for help in such numbers that her house became like a clinic. This led her and other church members to establish a centre where people could get care and support. Their first visitor was a man suffering from acute meningitis who had been dumped in the road outside the hospital. After treatment, he was brought to the centre where his care continued. This man has now fully recovered and is back at work after two years of incapacitating illness. Called "Discover and Recover", the centre helps prevent many unnecessary deaths from AIDS. Initially it was a day-care centre, but has grown to include a nursery school for 28 children affected by HIV.

Engaging people living with HIV as essential partners in the national response

At the 1994 Paris AIDS Summit, 42 countries declared the greater involvement of people living with HIV (GIPA) to be critical to national HIV responses. Engagement of people living with HIV in the development, implementation, and monitoring of national efforts is not solely a question of fairness. The effectiveness of national HIV initiatives depends on their resonance with those most affected by the epidemic. Therefore, the perspectives and insights of people living with HIV are invaluable assets, which can help ensure that national efforts achieve maximum impact.

To date, there have been few tools to measure the engagement of people living with HIV in national responses. In 2005, a global "think tank" meeting of people living with HIV resulted in agreement to develop a "GIPA report card", to permit country-level assessments of GIPA engagement. This effort was subsequently spearheaded by the Global Network of People living with HIV/AIDS (GNP+). In early 2008, the report card was being piloted in India, Kenya, Lesotho, and Trinidad and Tobago, with expectations for wider implementation in coming years.

Sustaining long-term financing for HIV

While money alone will not ensure long-term success, a robust HIV response cannot be sustained without adequate funding. Even in low-income countries, domestic public sector budgets have a critical role to play in financing the long-term response. Nevertheless, the global community, having committed to reversing the epidemic, must recognize the limited ability of low-income countries to fund essential HIV services. In low- and middle-income countries, international donors will need to provide most of the financing for HIV in the coming years.

It is unrealistic to expect HIV-dedicated funding to fully support the broad array of economic and social actions that will strengthen the HIV response. These actions include universal primary and secondary education, meaningful economic opportunities for women, comprehensive and well-functioning social protection systems, and support for agricultural sectors and rural communities. International donors should generate the financing needed to achieve universal access to HIV prevention, treatment, care, and support, but they should also substantially increase funding for official development assistance of all kinds. Broad-based progress on non-HIV-specific indicators in health, economic, and social aspects are urgently needed to maximize the impact of national HIV responses. It is disheartening to note that most high-income countries have failed to honour promises to devote at least 0.7% of their gross national product to official development assistance. As of 2005, only five country members of the Organization for Economic Cooperation and Development (Denmark, Luxembourg, Sweden, the Netherlands, and Norway) were investing at least 0.7% of gross national income towards development assistance (UNDP, 2007a).

The quest for sustainable financing for HIV response has led to a number of imaginative initiatives. For example, Product RED, the brainchild of Bono and Bobby Shriver, chair of DATA (Debt AIDS Trade Africa), devotes a percentage of each product sold towards the Global Fund. Participating companies include clothing retailers (such as Gap, and Emporio Armani), American Express, leading computer makers (such as Apple, Dell, and Microsoft),

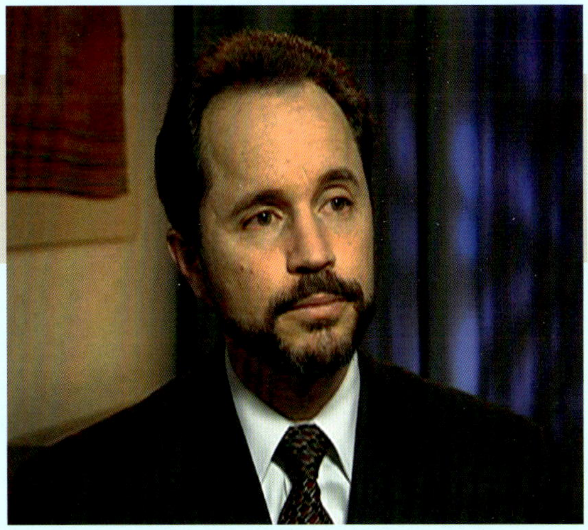

It concerns everyone

Gary M. Cohen is Executive Vice_President of Becton Dickinson

"My involvement in HIV/AIDS really was an outgrowth of travels in the developing world", says business leader Gary Cohen. "I became involved, not only on a professional level, but also on a very personal level, following personal exposure to the impact of HIV/AIDS in sub-Saharan Africa."

On his many journeys in the region with UNICEF, Red Cross, and other agencies, Cohen found that every family had lost loved ones and been touched by the epidemic in many ways. This led him to an understanding of HIV as the most important health threat of our time; a health threat with a direct impact on the business community. "I personally think it would be extremely short-sighted for any global organizations—even for small or middle sized companies—to regard this as an issue that does not concern them", says Cohen.

Cohen is executive vice president of Becton Dickinson (BD), a leading medical technology company with annual revenues of approximately US$ 6.5 billion and 28 000 people worldwide. Cohen's personal commitment to the response has led him to actively pursue ways in which his company can address the HIV epidemic. In addition to strong workplace programmes, BD supports the AIDS response through careful collaborations with existing organizations and agencies. For example, BD has worked with PEPFAR to strengthen laboratory systems throughout sub-Saharan Africa. The company has committed half of the US$ 18 million budget, as well as providing technical assistance.

BD is also collaborating with the Clinton Foundation to ensure sustainable access to CD4 testing, and with the FIND foundation to improve tuberculosis diagnosis. Other collaborations provide training and support for health workers and health systems in high-prevalence countries. For example, BD has trained more than 2500 laboratory technicians, and supported the establishment of Wellness Centres for Nurses affected by HIV.

Cohen believes that all companies have a contribution to make, according to their core competencies. "With HIV/AIDS, it is easy to get caught up in big numbers and almost become numbed to it", he says. "What I encourage people to do is reduce it to a single number ... go and meet one person who is living with this disease or who's been affected by this disease."

In 2004, Cohen met a 14-year-old Kenyan orphan who had been diagnosed as HIV-positive. He took responsibility for her and now she is in a top-quality school, performing near the top of her class, and dreams of one day becoming a lawyer.

hoteliers, newspapers, and the Hallmark greeting card company. In its first two years, Product RED raised more than US$ 100 million to support essential health programmes in low- and middle-income countries.

Another creative financing vehicle for HIV is UNITAID, launched in 2006 with leadership from the governments of France, Brazil, Chile, Norway, and the United Kingdom. UNITAID is an international drug purchase facility funded through an international airline tax, which ensures a continuous flow of revenue. As of March 2008, more than 24 countries had either implemented the airline tax or were planning to do so. As Chapter 5 explained, UNITAID in its brief existence has already come to play an important role in the expansion of HIV treatment access for children.

In February 2008, UN Secretary-General Ban Ki-moon appointed former French Foreign Minister Philippe Douste-Blazy as a special adviser on innovative financing for the Millennium Development Goals. Douste-Blazy has argued for the development of a worldwide citizen movement to generate sustainable financing for international development aid.

Making the money work

Additional efforts are also needed to ensure that increased financing can be rapidly translated into sound, high-impact programmes in low- and middle-income countries. In addition to maximizing the coordination of different funders and providers, technical support will be needed to build national capacity to mount and sustain strong HIV responses that focus on those most at risk and vulnerable. Donor policies should also support, rather than impede, the engagement of civil society and affected communities in national HIV responses.

Harmonization and alignment

Greater progress is needed to bring the efforts of all country-level players into alignment with nationally owned and determined strategies. Nearly half (45%) of governments report that not all external partners align their efforts with national HIV strategies (UNGASS Country Progress Reports, 2008). Where national stakeholders pursue their own individual agendas, the strategic impact of HIV efforts is often muted.

Reducing uncertainty of financing.

The uncertainty of external financing inhibits the ability of countries to plan for the future, a particular impediment for national efforts to ensure the long-term sustainability of the HIV response. While the global trend of in-country disbursement from bilateral donors has steadily increased, the availability and magnitude of funding from specific donors continues to change from year to year. One possible response to this problem is "basket funding", whereby multiple donors pool their financing in multiyear grants to support national responses.

Engaging and funding civil society.

The HIV response has placed people at the centre of development practice. For example, the World Bank's Multi-Country HIV/AIDS Program mobilized more than 66 000 civil society organizations to participate in the HIV response in Africa (World Bank, 2007). Similarly, the Global Fund has pursued a novel approach, relying on broadly inclusive country bodies to assess needs, formulate programmes, and submit applications for multiyear funding. These and other innovations will continue to be needed in the coming years, to ensure broad participation and engagement in national HIV responses.

Overcoming implementation bottlenecks

Coordinating the efforts of funders and technical agencies is critical to early identification of implementation bottlenecks, timely delivery of technical assistance to expedite implementation and scale-up, and capacity-building to ensure the sustainability of national responses. Supporting countries to successfully implement grants from the Global Fund represents one of UNAIDS' highest priorities.

Improving the relevance and impact of UN technical support to countries

To increase the coherence and effectiveness of UN efforts on HIV, the UNAIDS Cosponsors and Secretariat have agreed to a division of labour for the provision of technical support. This division of labour identifies lead and collaborating agencies in particular thematic areas, taking advantage of each agency's expertise and comparative advantage with respect to specific issues. The implementation of these recommendations was independently evaluated, and the evaluation found that UN agencies have adopted the division of labour, adapting it as appropriate in national settings. Several agencies have adjusted their staffing levels in direct response to their revised responsibilities (Attawell & Dickinson, 2007).

The UN has taken other steps to improve the quality, timeliness, and impact of its support to countries. Technical support facilities will have been established in seven regions by the end of 2008, and WHO has established regional "knowledge hubs" to help countries translate strategic information into programmes and policies.

Technical support facilities provide timely, high-quality technical support to country partners in priority areas (strategic and operational planning, costing and budgeting, monitoring and evaluation, programme and financial management) and in regionally defined thematic areas. The facilities have established pools of local and regional consultants, and provide professional development services to increase the capacity of locally provided technical support. They work in partnership with UNAIDS Cosponsors to ensure that policies, methodologies, and tools used by their consultants are state-of-the-art, and promote shared values and understanding of UN and global agreements. Particular attention is given to increasing access to Global Fund grants, by providing technical support to Global Fund recipients to develop proposals and implement grants.

In 2008, UNAIDS and the Global Fund entered into a comprehensive framework to improve the coordination and effectiveness of their respective efforts to aid countries in moving towards universal access to HIV prevention, treatment, care, and support. Under the agreed division of responsibilities, UNAIDS helps countries to develop evidence-informed funding proposals, supports the Global Fund's technical review process, and provides countries with focused technical assistance to accelerate implementation of programmes approved by the Global Fund.

The Global Implementation Support Team (GIST)—a novel collaboration between the Global Fund, UNAIDS, UNFPA, UNICEF, WHO, the World Bank, UNDP, GTZ, the United States Government, the AIDS Alliance, ICASO, ICAD, and ICTC of Brazil—work together in a collaborative and coordinated way to solve major bottlenecks inhibiting the provision of universal access to HIV prevention, treatment, care, and support services. An independent evaluation found that the GIST mechanism has improved coordination among multilateral funders and technical agencies, and has helped drive reforms at the global level to increase the efficiency and impact of multilateral support to countries (Attawell & Dickinson, 2007).

Maintaining a strong focus on HIV prevention

As emphasized in Chapter 4, long-term success in the HIV response demands sharp and sustained reductions in the rate of new HIV infections. Yet HIV prevention is consistently under-prioritized in many national responses. Nearly three decades into the epidemic, most young people in heavily-affected countries lack basic knowledge about HIV; about two out of three HIV-positive pregnant women do not receive antiretroviral drugs and other services to prevent mother-to-child transmission; and in countries with concentrated epidemics, most populations at greatest risk of exposure to HIV do not receive even basic HIV prevention services.

Unfortunately, preventing new HIV infections may not become easier as the epidemic evolves. As treatment access increases, the disability and death associated with HIV could become less visible, encouraging communities to become complacent, and tempting leaders to reduce investments in prevention programmes. Success in lowering the epidemic's human toll may cause some countries to declare premature victory in the HIV response. And as difficult budget decisions inevitably arise, some decision-makers may find it simpler to reduce funding for prevention services that, by definition, lack clear, demonstrable outcomes because they are intended to prevent negative consequences from occurring.

In many respects, prioritizing HIV prevention represents the ultimate manifestation of HIV leadership. Supporting evidence-informed prevention efforts requires countries to address difficult issues, invest wisely in the future, and address the societal factors that increase HIV risk and vulnerability. Until sufficient political will exists to put in place the HIV prevention strategies demonstrated to be effective, the epidemic will continue to expand, undermining the sustainability of the HIV response.

Availability of prevention services will not automatically ensure their widespread uptake. Where HIV prevention has succeeded, a popular movement has endeavoured to make risk reduction a societal norm, generating strong demand for prevention services. This also requires strong leadership. Much has been learnt about how to generate and support strong community mobilization, but encouraging such a popular movement requires the courage to invest in strategies that increase the HIV accountability of national governments and other stakeholders. Some may resist being held accountable, but true HIV leaders will welcome the development of a genuine social movement as a critical ingredient of success.

Tailoring national responses to documented needs

Countries need sound, timely information on their epidemic and on the status of the response, to permit rational selection of priority programmes, most effective allocation of limited funds, and implementation of the policies calculated to best address the underlying dynamics that increase HIV risk and vulnerability. This is true for all aspects of the epidemic, but it is particularly critical to the success of HIV prevention efforts. For example, understanding the transmission dynamics of the last 1000 new HIV infections would help countries to implement prevention measures focused on the groups at greatest risk of HIV exposure, and on the factors that appear to be driving the epidemic's spread. Epidemiological assays have emerged in recent years that improve the ability to assess the rate and characteristics of new HIV infections in selected low-level and concentrated epidemics (McDougal et al., 2006), although these have not been validated for use in generalized epidemics. However, modelling techniques are available to enable countries to make short-term estimates of new HIV infections, including identifying the modes of transmission (Gouws et al., 2006).

Information on new HIV infections should be complemented by reliable data on relevant behaviours. Both UNICEF and the United

CHAPTER 7

FIGURE 7.4 HIV spending on prevention, treatment, and care, Mexico, 1995–2005 (US$ millions)

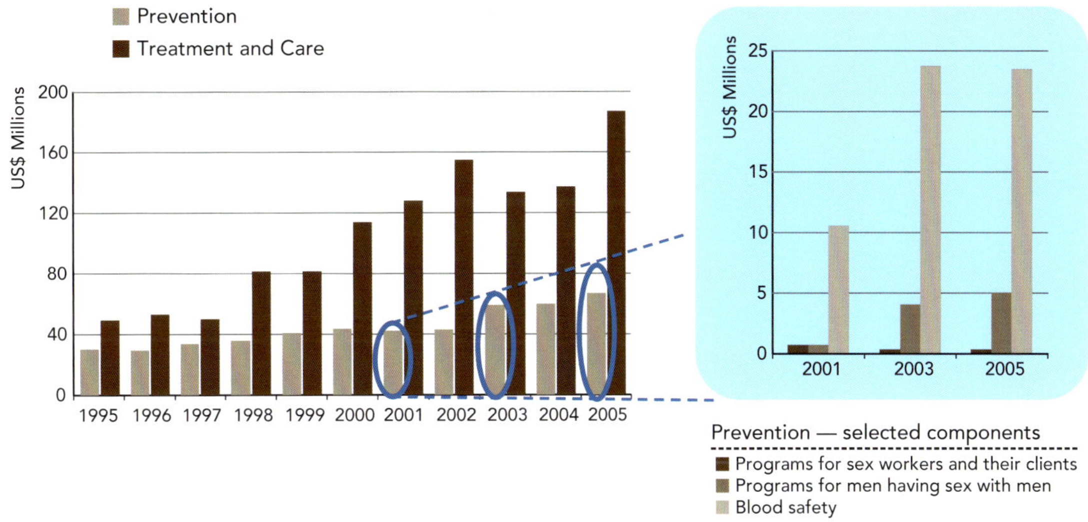

Source: Personal communication with Centro Nacional para la Prevención y control del SIDA (CENSIDA), Ministry of Health, Mexico (2008).

States Agency for International Development (USAID) have made critical contributions to behavioural epidemiology, by sponsoring household surveys that collect information on sexual debut, number of sex partners, HIV status, and other relevant issues. In some settings, however, such surveys may need to be tailored to elicit the range of information needed to support rational development of prevention strategies. For example, questions regarding the number of sex partners may shed little light on the frequency and duration of partnership concurrency, a potentially important factor in the rate of HIV spread. Countries should take particular efforts to ensure that national information systems generate data pertinent to the populations most at risk of infection.

Countries should use improved HIV information to increase the strategic impact of prevention efforts. In recent years, numerous countries have developed or devised national strategies on the basis of emerging information. In both Madagascar and Morocco, evidence documenting the practice of injecting drug use persuaded national authorities to allocate resources towards initiatives aimed at reducing the risk of drug-related transmission of HIV. As Figure 7.4 shows, earlier this decade Mexico heeded evidence documenting the high rate of HIV infections among men who have sex with men and increased expenditures for HIV prevention, after years of static funding.

Too often, however, national HIV expenditures do not match national needs. This is especially the case in many countries with low-level or concentrated epidemics, where rational funding would focus primarily on HIV prevention services for populations most at risk of HIV exposure. In countries with generalized epidemics, more resources are required for treatment, care, and social mitigation (Figure 7.5). Most countries in Latin America have low-level epidemics (HIV prevalence is well below 1%) but HIV prevention accounted for just 15% of HIV spending in 2007. Countries with concentrated epidemics often opt for broad prevention programmes for the general population rather than for more cost-

FIGURE 7.5 Resources needed in 2010 using a phased scale-up strategy towards universal access*

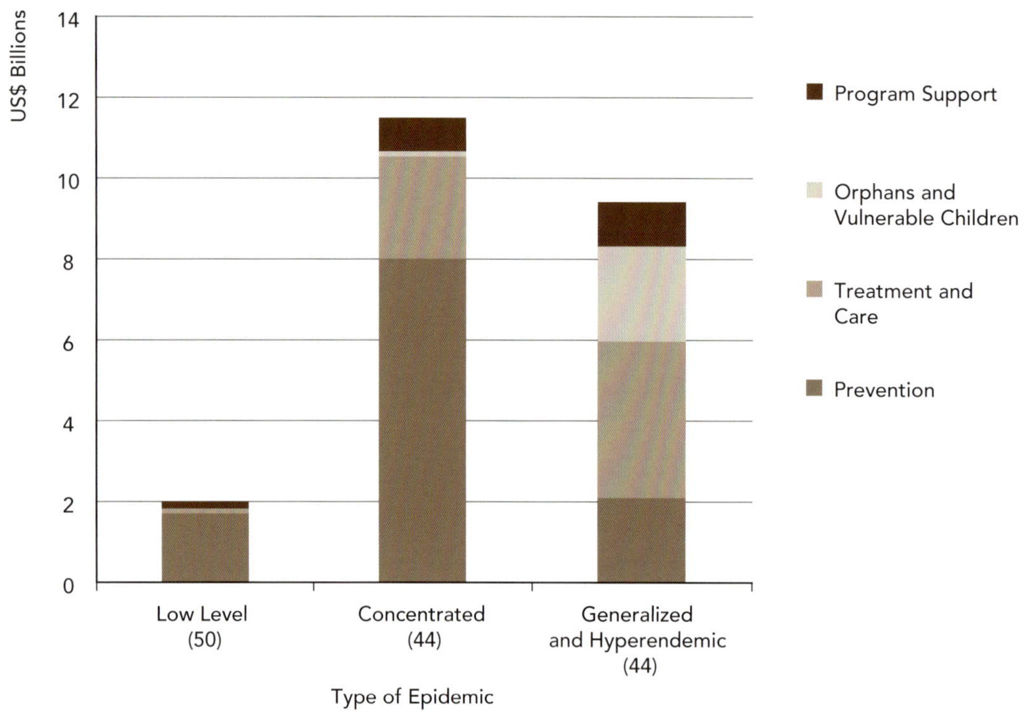

* Estimates in 138 low- and middle-income countries for implementing the most effective programmatic services as determined by data derived from national efforts to "know and act on your epidemic"
Source: UNAIDS, 2008.

effective interventions focused on populations most at risk. Data from countries with concentrated epidemics suggest that risk-reduction programmes focused on populations most at risk represent only 10% of overall HIV prevention spending.

Recognizing the long-term nature of investing in treatment and care

Chapter 5 examined recent successes in expanding treatment access, and potential obstacles to the sustainability of treatment programmes. Antiretroviral treatment is for life, underscoring the imperative of ensuring the continuity of HIV treatment programmes.

Improved prevention of new HIV infections is critical to the continued viability of HIV treatment programmes. Future treatment challenges are already daunting, with 30 million people living with HIV but not yet receiving treatment. Unless the epidemic's expansion is halted, future prospects for ensuring universal access to antiretroviral drugs will be uncertain, at best.

Ensuring sufficient human resources to implement and monitor HIV prevention, treatment, care, and support programmes will require both ingenuity and long-term commitment. Sustained investments in education and training initiatives, task-shifting and other innovative strategies to extend existing capacity as far as possible, and continued national commitment to antiretroviral treatment programmes, will be needed to build the long-term capacity required to maintain national responses at a high level in the future (see Samb et al., 2007).

Allowing evidence to drive the national response in Mozambique

Infection rates in Mozambique are increasing but infection rates in neighbouring countries are stabilizing. HIV prevention accounted for a decreasing share of Mozambique's HIV expenditures between 2004 and 2006 (Figure 7.6) and the main component of the increasing care and treatment expenditure is for antiretroviral drugs.

FIGURE 7.6 Prevention, care and treatment expenditures from public and international funding sources—Mozambique, 2004–2006, US$ millions

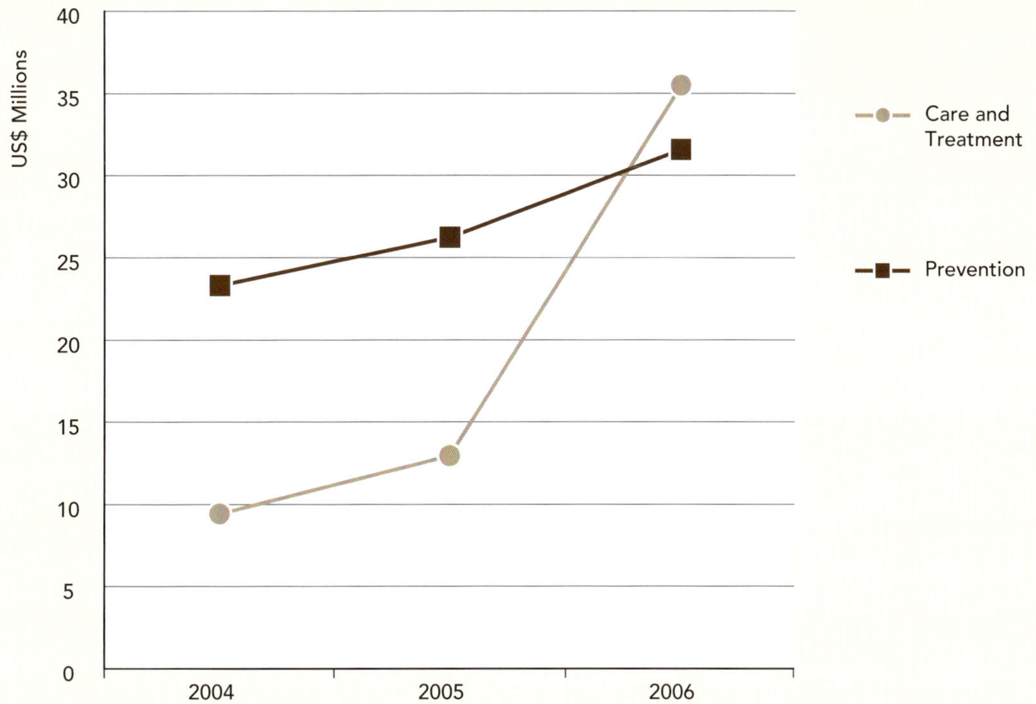

Source: UNGASS Country Progress Reports 2008.

In light of evidence of increasing infections, Mozambique recognized the need to strengthen HIV prevention. The country established a multistakeholder Prevention Reference Group in October 2007, which aimed to build the evidence base needed to intensify HIV prevention. With participation of various national ministries, the National AIDS Council, international technical agencies, and civil society, the reference group is assembling evidence to identify and characterize the key drivers of the epidemic. Rapid behavioural and epidemiological surveys in key populations are being undertaken, and relevant HIV activities are being mapped. This collective body of data will enable Mozambique to establish evidence-informed policies, prioritize programmes, and appropriately allocate available HIV prevention resources.

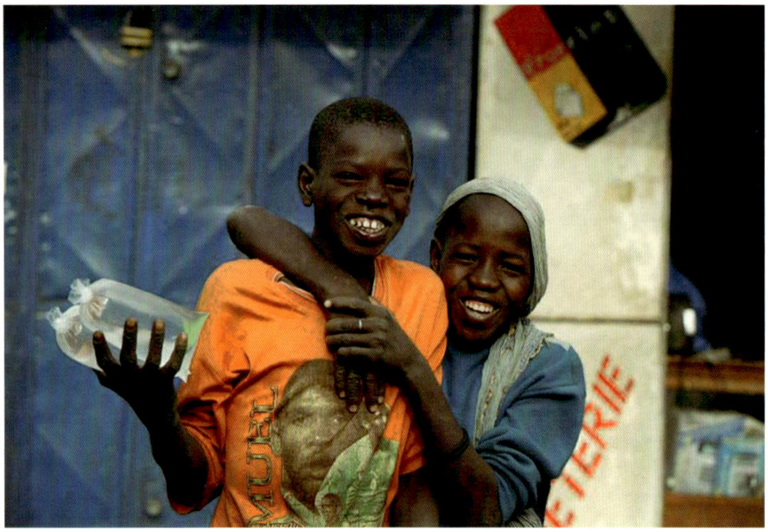

Reducing the epidemic's burden is critical to achievement of the full array of Millennium Development Goals.

In the process of establishing national targets, many countries have come to recognize specific obstacles to the rapid scale-up of services. A "phased scale-up" approach to moving towards universal access, which assumes different rates of scale-up for each country, based on current service coverage and capacity, will require approximately US$ 970 million annually in human resource initiatives by 2010 (UNAIDS, 2007c). This scenario envisages that each country will reach universal access for specific interventions at different times, with essentially all countries achieving universal access by 2015. While limited capacity sometimes impedes treatment scale-up, the global commitment to expand treatment access is also driving major improvements in health systems, and a robust HIV response has the potential to overcome barriers to service delivery.

In 2001, African leaders committed to prioritize improvements to the health sector in national budget allocations (Abuja Declaration Organization of African Unity, 2001). Government health spending in low-income countries generally has risen modestly since the late 1990s, but a number of African countries spend a substantially smaller share of national resources on health than neighbouring countries and most countries in other regions (UNDP, 2007a). India, home to an estimated 2.5 million people living with HIV, spends only 0.9% of its national GDP on health (UNDP, 2007a). Development economists suggest current spending levels on health in low-income countries are only one quarter to one third of the amount needed to ensure delivery of basic health services (Center for Global Development, 2007). To sustain the long-term HIV response, substantially greater health spending—from both domestic and external sources—will be required.

Cheaper second- and third-line drugs are urgently required for treatment programmes to be sustainable. This imperative is already attracting the efforts of stakeholders at global and national levels, and these efforts should be intensified and broadened to maximize treatment success in future years. Similar attention is needed to make the full range of HIV diagnostic technologies more accessible. Importantly, global and national flexibility will be needed to adapt to new developments in therapeutic and diagnostic tools for HIV. In particular, greater financial and technical support, and improved regional cooperation, should be focused on building the capacity of national regulatory bodies to introduce safe and effective medical products needed for the clinical management of HIV infection.

The HIV response in high income countries

Twenty-three high-income countries reported their progress towards the implementation of the *Declaration of Commitment on HIV/AIDS* in 2008, which was an increase from 15 countries in 2006. The 2008 responses comprised 49% of all high-income countries, which remains well below the 84% response rates from low- and middle-income countries. The high-income countries on average reported on 10 indicators compared with an average 16 out of 25 indicators on which the 124 low- and middle-income countries reported.

Coverage of antiretroviral combination therapy was on average greater in high-income countries compared with levels reported by low- and middle-income countries. Although most high-income countries have either concentrated or low-level HIV epidemics, only 17 of 23 high-income countries reported information on populations most at risk of HIV exposure. Response rates were higher for HIV testing indicators compared with HIV prevention and knowledge indicators. Access to HIV services for documented and undocumented migrants is not uniform among high income countries, even those within the European Union. While members of these groups have free access to HIV services at point of delivery in some European countries, in others access to HIV services for these populations are only on a fee-for-service basis.

In some high-income and low- and middle income countries, changes in young people's sexual behaviour were observed between 1995 and 2002 For example, national school-based behavioural surveillance in the United States demonstrated that the proportion of young males having sex before the age of 15 declined from 21% in 1995 to 15% in 2002. A similar decline was seen among young women from 19% to 13%[1]. This compares with a reduction from 15% to 12% in young men and from 12% to 11% in young women in 23 low- and middle-income countries surveyed over the same time period[2].

It is unclear why reporting rates are substantially lower in high-income countries. This may be partly due to the fact that the relevant data are not held in a central location and are administered by different institutions. Although there are notable exceptions, this under-reporting raises questions about the progress of high-income countries in implementing a single, integrated HIV monitoring and evaluation framework, or "Third One".

1 Abma JC et al., Teenagers in the United States: sexual activity, contraceptive use, and childbearing, 2002, Vital and Health Statistics, 2004, Series 23, No. 24.

2 DHS www.measuredhs.com

Ensuring coordination and coherence of national efforts

In line with international efforts to improve the harmonization and alignment of international development aid with country-owned strategies and plans, country-level action on HIV aims to promote the "Three Ones"—one national AIDS authority, one national strategic framework, and one national monitoring and evaluation system.

Multisectoral, costed, and prioritized strategies for national responses are in place in most countries. A total of 97% of countries have a multisectoral HIV strategy, 92% have a national HIV coordinating body, 92% have a national monitoring and evaluation plan in place or in development, and all low- and middle-income countries have integrated HIV into national development plans.

However, when country-level efforts are evaluated according to quality criteria developed by UNAIDS, the weaknesses of many national approaches become apparent. In only 69% of countries—far fewer than the 97% that report having a national strategy—have national strategies been translated into costed operational plans with programme goals, detailed programme costing, and identified funding sources. In sub-Saharan Africa, only about half of national HIV strategies meet UNAIDS quality criteria (Figure 7.7).

FIGURE 7.7 Countries reporting quality implementation of the national AIDS strategy

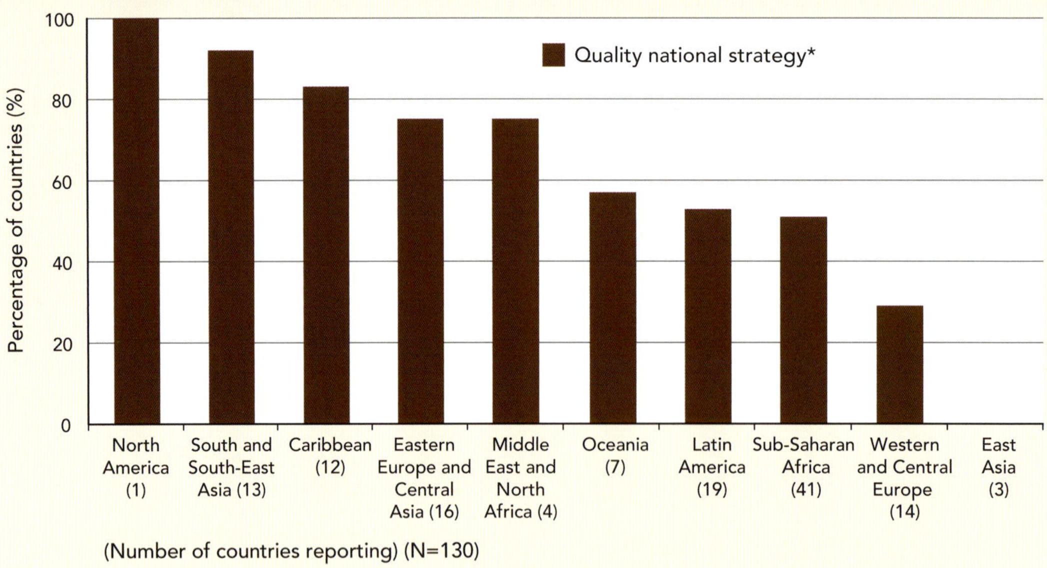

* One national multisectoral strategy and operational plan with goals, targets, costing, and identified funding per programmatic area, and a monitoring and evaluation framework.
Source: UNGASS Country Progress Reports 2008.

Despite continuing weaknesses, country-level efforts under the "Three Ones" exhibit important improvement over time (Figure 7.8). Indeed, many countries have used the "Three Ones" principles to drive improvements in national preparedness. In 2007, for example, Tajikistan developed its first national plan for HIV monitoring and evaluation, supported by a detailed budget and focused on national indicators agreed to by all national partners. In Indonesia, a presidential decree in 2006 clearly established the National AIDS Commission as the sole body responsible for leading and coordinating the country's HIV response.

FIGURE 7.8 Country progress in improving the implementation quality of the "Three Ones": one national strategic framework, one national AIDS authority, and one national monitoring and evaluation system*

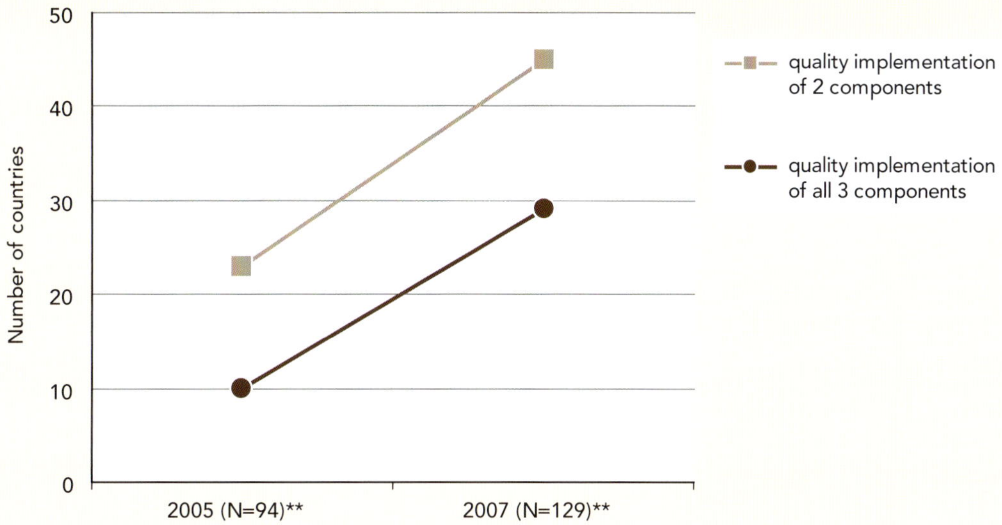

* Quality implementation refers to:

1 One national multisectoral strategy and operational plan with goals, targets, costing, and identified funding per programmatic area, and a monitoring and evaluation framework;
2 One national coordinating body with terms of reference, a defined membership, an action plan, a functional secretariat, and regular meetings;
3 One national M&E plan which is costed and for which funding is secured, a functional national monitoring and evaluation unit or technical working group, and central national database with AIDS data.

** Only countries that have all three or two of the three components in place are displayed; other countries have only one or none of the components in place, or did not report.

Source: UNGASS Country Progress Reports 2008.

National governments are increasingly partnering with civil society in the development, implementation, and monitoring of national HIV strategies. According to government reports, 83% of national HIV coordinating bodies include civil society representatives (UNGASS Country Progress Reports, 2008). In most cases, governments report that the national strategy or framework was developed with active participation from civil society (ranging from 62% in South and South-East Asia to 100% in North America). Civil society members have been involved in the review of national HIV strategies in 78% of countries, and rated their contribution as good or very good with respect to national planning and budgeting in 58% of countries.

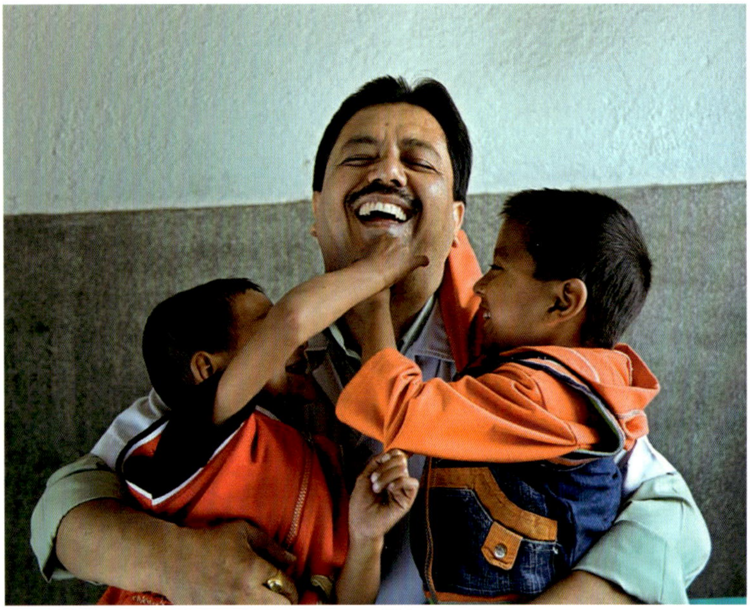

Achieving universal access to HIV prevention, treatment, care and support is as critical step towards a sustainable, long-term response to HIV.

Mitigating the epidemic's long-term impact

Treatment scale-up will help to contain and minimize some of the epidemic's most severe ramifications, but will not make either HIV or its harmful consequences disappear. Substantially less attention has been directed towards intervention research and scale-up of programmes relating to impact mitigation than for other aspects of the HIV response. For example, access to HIV treatment, prevention of mother-to-child transmission, and other essential HIV services has significantly expanded in recent years, but little progress has been made in delivering essential care and support to children orphaned or made vulnerable by the epidemic.

Working to minimize the epidemic's impact is not only a humanitarian imperative, it is also part of the long-term response to the epidemic. The millions of children affected by HIV represent the future; providing proper care and support to such children and the households in which they live is critical to the long-term health and well-being of entire societies and communities. Likewise, households that slip deeper into poverty as a result of HIV illness will find it even more difficult in future years to prosper and contribute to society.

As Chapter 6 emphasized, a "silo" approach to impact mitigation will not be optimally effective. Instead, countries need cross-cutting planning and oversight mechanisms to address the multiple, complex ways in which HIV affects societies, communities, and households. It is therefore essential to mainstream HIV impact mitigation efforts into broader development strategies.

Governance of the response

Countries confront a host of governance challenges in their efforts to respond effectively to HIV. Throughout the epidemic, countries have struggled to achieve a response that is genuinely multisectoral and actively owned and led by national stakeholders. Coordination of diverse actors at country-level also remains an ongoing challenge.

Significant progress has been achieved on each of the "Three Ones" principles—a single multisectoral action framework, a single national HIV coordinating authority, and a unified monitoring and evaluation system (see box "Ensuring coordination and coherence of national efforts"). In too many countries, however, these achievements are more evident on paper than in practice.

Although national HIV strategic frameworks almost uniformly articulate an approach to HIV that is multisectoral, the response in many countries remains heavily concentrated in health ministries. While non-health ministries often participate in national coordinating bodies, which is an important achievement, many lack budgetary support to undertake HIV-related activities. For example, although 98% of countries have a national HIV strategy that includes the education sector, only 65% provide budgetary support for HIV programming in educational settings (UNGASS Country Progress Reports, 2008). Malawi's mandate to diverse ministries to earmark budgetary support for HIV activities (see section on "Mobilizing sufficient financial resources for the HIV response") offers an example of how countries can facilitate the active engagement of multiple sectors in the national HIV response.

Decentralizing the response

Effective governance of the response ensures that national strategies and mandates are translated into meaningful action in districts and communities. Decentralization of the response helps empower subnational units to implement programmes that meet local needs.

In Ethiopia, service expansion under the country's Millennium AIDS Campaign has been accelerated through decentralization of service delivery. Building on local leadership and community involvement, 24 000 health "extension" workers were trained to aid households and promote community-health initiatives, including antiretroviral treatment delivery. This focus on decentralized service delivery has been associated with a dramatic increase in the number of individuals receiving antiretroviral drugs—from 8276 in 2005 to 122243 in 2007.

Although many local governments have taken important action to address HIV over the years, the primary focus of donors on support for national governments has sometimes impeded the ability to implement strong, decentralized HIV responses.[3] District-level planning that addressed capacity-building initiatives and resource mobilization for local entities may help overcome some of the historical challenges to an effective decentralized HIV response. (UNDP, 2005.) In the Mbeya region of the United Republic of Tanzania, for example, sustained action and donor support at the subnational level has enabled the region to reach more than 80% of the population with basic prevention services, and to reduce HIV prevalence over the last decade (UNAIDS, 2007b). At the same time as increasing funding to support local governments in the implementation of HIV strategies that address local needs, greater donor assistance

CHAPTER 7

[3] Through its Multi-Country HIV/AIDS Program in Africa, the World Bank directed 38% of its HIV-related assistance to support local responses in countries (World Bank, 2007).

is also needed for local communities that are organizing to increase the reach, impact, and accountability of local HIV initiatives.

Grounding the response in human rights

True leaders must often face up to issues that others prefer to ignore. Confronting HIV means addressing issues that make many people uncomfortable, such as human sexuality and drug use. It also requires compassion and effective action with respect to groups that society often prefers to ignore.

While action to address the needs of marginalized populations most at risk remains limited, recent years have nevertheless provided important examples of such leadership, including the launching of a national anti-homophobia campaign in Mexico and the repeal of sodomy laws in the Bahamas. Likewise, the evidence-informed support for needle exchange projects in countries such as the Islamic Republic of Iran, Malaysia and Viet Nam serve as clear examples of courageous, visionary leadership in the response to HIV.

As the epidemic evolves and the number and range of HIV-related technologies grows, it will be tempting to think of the response solely in technocratic terms. This would be a mistake. Given the realities of HIV—its concentration in marginalized populations, the ways in which it is entwined with human sexuality, and the ways in which its transmission depends on how humans relate to one another—the epidemic is unlikely ever to lend itself to a purely technological solution.

In every country that has achieved major progress in reducing the rate of new HIV infections, the national HIV response has been grounded in the promotion of human rights. Compassion and inclusion remain touchstones for an effective response to the epidemic.

Achieving and sustaining an effective response: a long-term action agenda

- Address documented national needs, and base national action on sound evidence of what works, ensuring full implementation of evidence-informed policies and programmes.
- Plan for the future, by implementing strategic planning and evaluation mechanisms that extend beyond three- and five-year cycles.
- Invest in a truly effective response to HIV, with particular attention to evidence-informed HIV prevention strategies that help contain national epidemics.
- Couple scale-up of programmes with multisectoral leadership to reduce the societal factors that increase HIV risk and vulnerability, including gender inequities, stigma and discrimination, and social marginalization.
- Empower people living with HIV to help lead national HIV responses and involve civil society in the development, implementation, and evaluation of national HIV strategies.
- Harmonize and align the efforts of all stakeholders with nationally driven HIV strategies and priorities, strengthening the quality and flexibility of technical support to build durable national capacity—not only in health systems, but throughout other key sectors, and in both public and private sectors—to sustain a robust and effective HIV response for the coming years.
- Mobilize sufficient financial resources to reach the global target of universal access, putting in place innovative mechanisms to sustain financing for the long-term.

Annex

HIV and AIDS estimates and data, 2007 and 2001

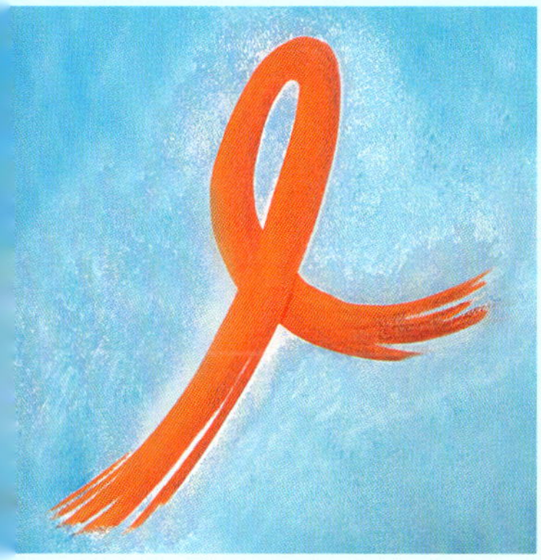

1

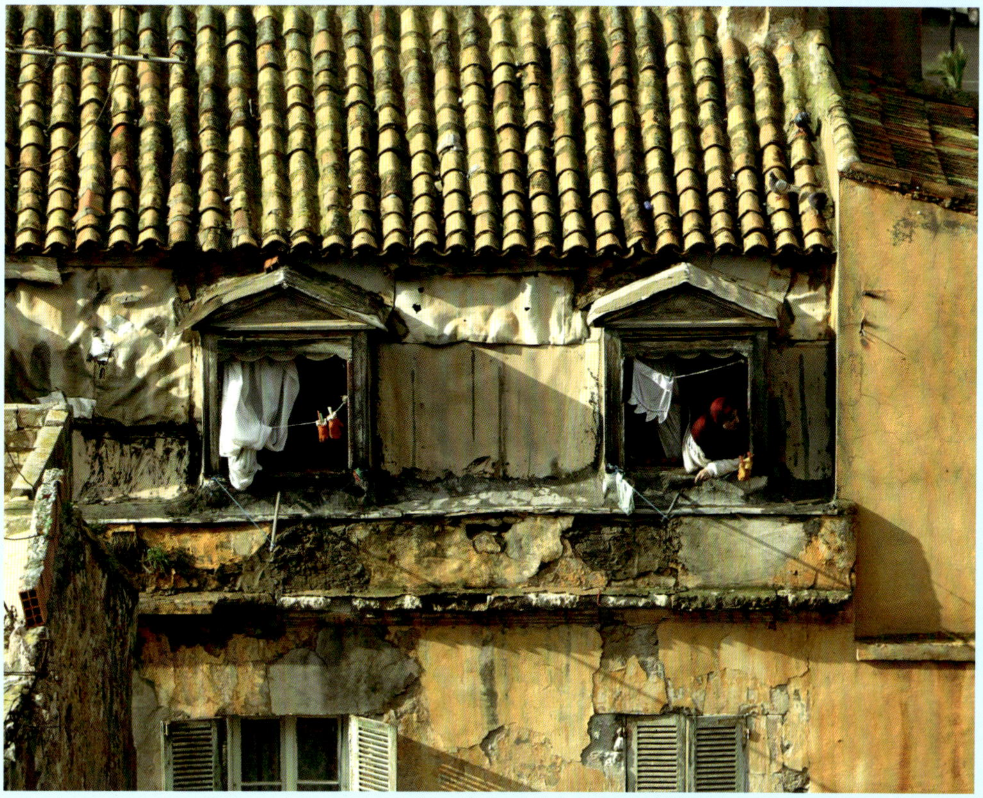

HIV and AIDS estimates and data, 2007 and 2001

The estimates and data provided in this Annex relate to 2007 and 2001, unless stated otherwise. These estimates have been produced and compiled by UNAIDS/ WHO. They have been shared with national AIDS programmes for review and comments, but are not necessarily the official estimates used by national governments. For countries where no recent data were available, country-specific estimates have not been listed in the tables. In order to calculate regional totals, older data or regional models were used to produce estimates for these countries.

The estimates are given in rounded numbers. However, unrounded numbers were used in the calculation of rates and regional totals, so there may be minor discrepancies between the regional and global totals and the sum of the country figures.

The general methodology and tools used to produce the country-specific estimates in the table have been described in a series of papers in *Sexually Transmitted Infections* 2008; 84(Suppl 1) "Improved data, methods and tools for the 2007 HIV and AIDS estimates and projections", and in *Sexually Transmitted Infections* 2006; 82(Suppl 1). The estimates produced by UNAIDS/WHO are based on methods and on parameters that are informed by the UNAIDS Reference Group on HIV/AIDS Estimates, Modelling and Projections, available at http://www.epidem.org/

This group is made up of leading researchers in AIDS, epidemiology, demography and related areas. The Reference Group assesses the most recent published and unpublished work drawn from research studies in different countries. It also reviews advances in the understanding of HIV epidemics, and suggests methods to improve the quality and accuracy of the estimates.

Based on suggestions from the Reference Group, software has been developed to model the course of HIV epidemics and their impact. Country analysts were trained in the use of these tools during a series of workshops in 2007. These changes in procedures and assumptions and improved coordination with countries have resulted in improved estimates of HIV and AIDS for 2007. To allow readers to assess recent trends in the epidemic, we also present 2001 estimates developed using the same methodology and data as for the 2007 estimates.

The new estimates in this report are presented together with ranges, called 'plausibility bounds'. These bounds reflect the certainty associated with each of the estimates. The wider the bounds, the greater the uncertainty surrounding an estimate. The extent of uncertainty depends mainly on the type of epidemic, and the quality, coverage and consistency of a country's surveillance system and, in generalized epidemics, whether or not a population-based survey with HIV testing was conducted. A full description of the methods used to develop plausibility bounds can be found in *Sexually Transmitted Infections* 2008, 84(Suppl 1).

Adults in this report are defined as men and women aged 15+ years. This is different from previous reports where the estimates for adults were restricted to 15–49-year-olds. Since the burden of disease extends beyond the age of 49 and to better assess that need, the UNAIDS Reference Group on Estimates, Modelling and Projections has recommended changing the reporting to all ages. The HIV prevalence proportion rate however continues to be for adults 15–49 to allow comparisons across countries.

Notes on specific indicators listed in Annex 1

1. Estimated number of people living with HIV, 2007 and 2001

These estimates include all people with HIV infection, whether or not they have developed symptoms of AIDS, in 2007 and 2001. For some countries where sufficient data from the last six years were not available, no estimates have been made.

Adults and children
Estimated number of adults and children living with HIV in 2007 and 2001.
Adults are 15 years and over. Children are defined as those aged 0–14 years.

Adults (15+ years)
Estimated number of adults living with HIV, 2007 and 2001.

Adult (15–49 years) prevalence proportion (%)
To calculate the adult HIV prevalence proportion, the estimated number of adults (15–49 years) living with HIV in 2007 was divided by the 2007 adult population (aged 15–49) and similarly for 2001.

Women (15+ years)
Estimated number of women (aged 15+) living with HIV in 2007 and 2001.

Children (0–14 years)
Estimated number of children under aged 15 living with HIV in 2007 and 2001.

Young women (15–24) prevalence proportion (%) 2007
Estimated percent of young women aged 15–24 who are living with HIV in 2007.

Young men (15–24) prevalence proportion (%) 2007
Estimated percent of young men aged 15–24 who are living with HIV in 2007.

2. AIDS deaths adults and children

Estimated number of adults and children who died of AIDS during 2007 and 2001.

3. Orphans due to AIDS

Orphans (0–17 years) currently living

Estimated number of children aged 0–17 years in 2007 and 2001 who have lost one or both parents to AIDS.

Plausibility bounds for the above indicators

Depending on the reliability of the data available, there may be more or less uncertainty surrounding each estimate. While a measure of uncertainty applies to all estimates, in this report the plausibility bounds are presented for the following estimates:

- estimated number of adults (15+ years) and children (0–14 years) living with HIV in 2007 and 2001;
- estimated number of adults (15+ years) living with HIV in 2007 and 2001;
- estimated number of women (15+ years) living with HIV in 2007 and 2001;
- estimated number of children (0–14 years) living with HIV in 2007 and 2001;
- estimated HIV prevalence among young women and men (15–24 years) in 2007;
- estimated number of AIDS deaths in adults (15+ years) and children (0–14 years) during 2007 and 2001; and
- orphans (0–17 years) due to AIDS in 2007 and 2001.

4. Trends of HIV prevalence in most-at-risk groups in capital city

These indicators are recommended for reporting against the goals of the 2001 United Nations General Assembly Special Session on HIV/AIDS in countries with low-level epidemics or concentrated HIV epidemics. In theory, assessing progress in reducing the occurrence of new infections is best done through monitoring changes in incidence over time. However, in practice, prevalence data, rather than incidence data, are what are actually available. In analysing prevalence data of most-at-risk populations, it is desirable to report on those persons who are newly initiated to behaviours that put them at risk for infection. In this round of UNGASS reporting, guidance was provided to encourage this type of reporting, though whether or not this restricted analysis was used for reporting is not represented in this table.

The specific populations at higher risk of HIV exposure in the tables include:

- injecting drug users;
- female sex workers; and
- men who have sex with men.

1. Estimated number of people living with HIV						
	Adults and children 2007		Adults and children 2001		Adults (15+) 2007	
Country	Estimate	[low estimate – high estimate]	Estimate	[low estimate – high estimate]	Estimate	[low estimate – high estimate]
Global	33 000 000	[30 000 000 – 36 000 000]	29 500 000	[27 000 000 – 33 700 000]	30 800 000	[28 200 000 – 34 000 000]
Sub-Saharan Africa	22 000 000	[20 500 000 – 23 600 000]	20 400 000	[19 200 000 – 23 200 000]	20 300 000	[18 700 000 – 21 700 000]
Angola	190 000	[150 000 – 240 000]	120 000	[84 000 – 360 000]	180 000	[140 000 – 210 000]
Benin	64 000	[58 000 – 73 000]	53 000	[46 000 – 61 000]	59 000	[53 000 – 67 000]
Botswana	300 000	[280 000 – 310 000]	280 000	[270 000 – 290 000]	280 000	[270 000 – 300 000]
Burkina Faso	130 000	[110 000 – 160 000]	140 000	[120 000 – 160 000]	120 000	[100 000 – 140 000]
Burundi	110 000	[78 000 – 130 000]	150 000	[120 000 – 170 000]	90 000	[66 000 – 120 000]
Cameroon	540 000	[430 000 – 640 000]	530 000	[460 000 – 590 000]	500 000	[390 000 – 590 000]
Central African Republic	160 000	[150 000 – 170 000]	130 000	[120 000 – 140 000]	140 000	[130 000 – 150 000]
Chad	200 000	[130 000 – 240 000]	150 000	[100 000 – 260 000]	180 000	[110 000 – 220 000]
Comoros	<200	[<1000]	<100	[<500]	<200	[<1000]
Congo	79 000	[65 000 – 94 000]	84 000	[73 000 – 100 000]	73 000	[59 000 – 86 000]
Côte d'Ivoire	480 000	[400 000 – 550 000]	590 000	[540 000 – 670 000]	420 000	[350 000 – 490 000]
Democratic Republic of Congo	...	[400 000 – 500 000]	...	[320 000 – 410 000]	...	[360 000 – 450 000]
Djibouti	16 000	[12 000 – 19 000]	13 000	[9300 – 17 000]	15 000	[11 000 – 18 000]
Equatorial Guinea	11 000	[8200 – 14 000]	9500	[7600 – 12 000]	9800	[7400 – 13 000]
Eritrea	38 000	[25 000 – 58 000]	27 000	[19 000 – 42 000]	35 000	[22 000 – 54 000]
Ethiopia	980 000	[880 000 – 1 100 000]	920 000	[830 000 – 1 000 000]	890 000	[800 000 – 970 000]
Gabon	49 000	[37 000 – 68 000]	38 000	[26 000 – 51 000]	46 000	[35 000 – 65 000]
Gambia	8200	[3700 – 13 000]	6400	[3100 – 11 000]	7500	[3400 – 12 000]
Ghana	260 000	[230 000 – 290 000]	260 000	[230 000 – 290 000]	250 000	[220 000 – 280 000]
Guinea	87 000	[73 000 – 110 000]	55 000	[40 000 – 72 000]	81 000	[67 000 – 110 000]
Guinea-Bissau	16 000	[11 000 – 23 000]	13 000	[9000 – 18 000]	15 000	[10 000 – 21 000]
Kenya[2]	...	[1 500 000 – 2 000 000	...	[1 300 000 – 1 700 000]	...	[1 400 000 – 1 800 000]
Lesotho	270 000	[260 000 – 290 000]	250 000	[240 000 – 270 000]	260 000	[250 000 – 270 000]
Liberia	35 000	[29 000 – 41 000]	24 000	[17 000 – 58 000]	32 000	[26 000 – 37 000]
Madagascar	14 000	[9100 – 23 000]	8100	[5800 – 13 000]	13 000	[8800 – 22 000]
Malawi	930 000	[860 000 – 1 000 000]	850 000	[790 000 – 910 000]	840 000	[780 000 – 900 000]
Mali	100 000	[88 000 – 120 000]	82 000	[70 000 – 96 000]	93 000	[79 000 – 110 000]
Mauritania	14 000	[8300 – 26 000]	9400	[5400 – 16 000]	14 000	[8100 – 25 000]
Mauritius	13 000	[7500 – 28 000]	1800	[<1000 – 3900]	13 000	[7400 – 28 000]
Mozambique	1 500 000	[1 300 000 – 1 700 000]	1 000 000	[880 000 – 1 200 000]	1 400 000	[1 200 000 – 1 600 000]
Namibia	200 000	[160 000 – 230 000]	150 000	[130 000 – 180 000]	180 000	[150 000 – 220 000]
Niger	60 000	[44 000 – 85 000]	43 000	[33 000 – 57 000]	56 000	[42 000 – 81 000]
Nigeria	2 600 000	[2 000 000 – 3 200 000]	2 200 000	[1 700 000 – 4 200 000]	2 400 000	[1 600 000 – 2 900 000]
Rwanda	150 000	[130 000 – 170 000]	190 000	[170 000 – 210 000]	130 000	[120 000 – 150 000]
Senegal	67 000	[47 000 – 96 000]	24 000	[17 000 – 31 000]	64 000	[45 000 – 92 000]
Sierra Leone	55 000	[42 000 – 76 000]	34 000	[18 000 – 56 000]	51 000	[38 000 – 72 000]
Somalia	24 000	[13 000 – 45 000]	17 000	[11 000 – 30 000]	24 000	[13 000 – 43 000]
South Africa	5 700 000	[4 900 000 – 6 600 000]	4 700 000	[4 000 000 – 5 500 000]	5 400 000	[4 700 000 – 6 200 000]
Swaziland	190 000	[180 000 – 200 000]	160 000	[150 000 – 170 000]	170 000	[160 000 – 180 000]
Togo	130 000	[110 000 – 150 000]	110 000	[92 000 – 130 000]	120 000	[97 000 – 140 000]
Uganda	940 000	[870 000 – 1 000 000]	1 100 000	[990 000 – 1 300 000]	810 000	[740 000 – 910 000]
United Republic of Tanzania	1 400 000	[1 300 000 – 1 500 000]	1 400 000	[1 300 000 – 1 500 000]	1 300 000	[1 200 000 – 1 400 000]
Zambia	1 100 000	[1 000 000 – 1 200 000]	940 000	[870 000 – 1 000 000]	980 000	[920 000 – 1 100 000]
Zimbabwe	1 300 000	[1 200 000 – 1 400 000]	1 900 000	[1 800 000 – 2 000 000]	1 200 000	[1 100 000 – 1 300 000]

1. Estimated number of people living with HIV

	Adults (15+) 2001		Adult (15–49) prevalence percent 2007		Adult (15–49) prevalence percent 2001		Women (15+) 2007	
Country	Estimate	[low estimate – high estimate]	Estimate	[low estimate – high estimate]	Estimate	[low estimate – high estimate]	Estimate	[low estimate – high estimate]
Global	27 900 000	[25 500 000 – 31 700 000]	0.8	[0.7 – 0.9]	0.8	[0.7 – 0.9]	15 500 000	[14 200 000 – 16 900 000]
Sub-Saharan Africa	19 100 000	[17 900 000 – 21 400 000]	5.0	[4.6 – 5.4]	5.7	[5.3 – 6.4]	12 000 000	[11 100 000 – 12 900 000]
Angola	110 000	[80 000 – 310 000]	2.1	[1.7 – 2.5]	1.6	[1.1 – 4.3]	110 000	[82 000 – 130 000]
Benin	49 000	[43 000 – 57 000]	1.2	[1.1 – 1.4]	1.3	[1.2 – 1.5]	37 000	[33 000 – 42 000]
Botswana	270 000	[250 000 – 280 000]	23.9	[22.5 – 24.9]	26.5	[25.6 – 27.8]	170 000	[160 000 – 180 000]
Burkina Faso	130 000	[110 000 – 150 000]	1.6	[1.4 – 1.9]	2.1	[1.8 – 2.4]	61 000	[52 000 – 73 000]
Burundi	130 000	[100 000 – 160 000]	2.0	[1.3 – 2.5]	3.5	[2.7 – 4.2]	53 000	[39 000 – 69 000]
Cameroon	490 000	[430 000 – 550 000]	5.1	[3.9 – 6.2]	6.0	[5.3 – 6.8]	300 000	[240 000 – 360 000]
Central African Republic	120 000	[110 000 – 130 000]	6.3	[5.9 – 6.7]	6.4	[5.9 – 6.9]	91 000	[85 000 – 97 000]
Chad	140 000	[97 000 – 220 000]	3.5	[2.4 – 4.3]	3.4	[2.4 – 6.0]	110 000	[66 000 – 130 000]
Comoros	<100	[<500]	<0.1	[0.1]	<0.1	[0.1]	<100	[<200]
Congo	77 000	[67 000 – 92 000]	3.5	[2.8 – 4.2]	4.4	[3.8 – 5.3]	43 000	[36 000 – 51 000]
Côte d'Ivoire	550 000	[500 000 – 630 000]	3.9	[3.2 – 4.5]	6.0	[5.5 – 6.8]	250 000	[210 000 – 290 000]
Democratic Republic of Congo	...	[290 000 – 370 000]	...	[1.2 – 1.5]	...	[1.2 – 1.5]	...	[210 000 – 270 000]
Djibouti	12 000	[9000 – 15 000]	3.1	[2.3 – 3.8]	3.1	[2.2 – 3.9]	8700	[6500 – 11 000]
Equatorial Guinea	8900	[7100 – 12 000]	3.4	[2.6 – 4.6]	3.7	[2.9 – 4.7]	5900	[4400 – 7900]
Eritrea	25 000	[17 000 – 39 000]	1.3	[0.8 – 2.0]	1.2	[0.8 – 1.8]	21 000	[13 000 – 33 000]
Ethiopia	840 000	[760 000 – 930 000]	2.1	[1.8 – 2.2]	2.4	[2.1 – 2.6]	530 000	[470 000 – 580 000]
Gabon	36 000	[25 000 – 49 000]	5.9	[4.4 – 8.3]	5.6	[3.9 – 7.6]	27 000	[20 000 – 38 000]
Gambia	6100	[3000 – 10 000]	0.9	[0.4 – 1.3]	0.9	[0.4 – 1.4]	4500	[2000 – 7200]
Ghana	240 000	[220 000 – 270 000]	1.9	[1.7 – 2.2]	2.3	[2.1 – 2.6]	150 000	[130 000 – 160 000]
Guinea	52 000	[38 000 – 68 000]	1.6	[1.3 – 2.2]	1.2	[0.9 – 1.6]	48 000	[40 000 – 64 000]
Guinea-Bissau	12 000	[8400 – 16 000]	1.8	[1.3 – 2.6]	1.8	[1.3 – 2.5]	8700	[6100 – 12 000]
Kenya[2]	...	[1 200 000 – 1 600 000]	...	[7.1 – 8.5]	...	[7.4 – 9.8]	...	[800 000 – 1 100 000]
Lesotho	240 000	[230 000 – 260 000]	23.2	[21.9 – 24.5]	23.9	[22.8 – 25.2]	150 000	[140 000 – 160 000]
Liberia	22 000	[16 000 – 48 000]	1.7	[1.4 – 2.0]	1.4	[1.0 – 3.1]	19 000	[16 000 – 22 000]
Madagascar	8000	[5700 – 13 000]	0.1	[<0.1 – 0.2]	0.1	[<0.1 – 0.2]	3400	[2200 – 5800]
Malawi	780 000	[730 000 – 840 000]	11.9	[11.0 – 12.9]	13.3	[12.4 – 14.3]	490 000	[450 000 – 530 000]
Mali	76 000	[66 000 – 90 000]	1.5	[1.2 – 1.8]	1.5	[1.3 – 1.8]	56 000	[47 000 – 67 000]
Mauritania	9300	[5300 – 16 000]	0.8	[0.5 – 1.5]	0.7	[0.4 – 1.2]	3900	[2300 – 7400]
Mauritius	1800	[<1000 – 3900]	1.7	[1.0 – 3.6]	0.3	[0.1 – 0.5]	3800	[2100 – 8100]
Mozambique	960 000	[840 000 – 1 100 000]	12.5	[10.9 – 14.7]	10.3	[8.8 – 11.9]	810 000	[690 000 – 960 000]
Namibia	140 000	[120 000 – 170 000]	15.3	[12.4 – 18.1]	14.6	[12.2 – 17.1]	110 000	[88 000 – 130 000]
Niger	41 000	[31 000 – 55 000]	0.8	[0.6 – 1.1]	0.7	[0.6 – 1.0]	17 000	[12 000 – 26 000]
Nigeria	2 000 000	[1 600 000 – 3 500 000]	3.1	[2.3 – 3.8]	3.2	[2.5 – 5.7]	1 400 000	[980 000 – 1 700 000]
Rwanda	160 000	[140 000 – 180 000]	2.8	[2.4 – 3.2]	4.3	[3.9 – 4.7]	78 000	[69 000 – 88 000]
Senegal	23 000	[16 000 – 30 000]	1.0	[0.7 – 1.4]	0.4	[0.3 – 0.5]	38 000	[27 000 – 54 000]
Sierra Leone	32 000	[17 000 – 53 000]	1.7	[1.3 – 2.4]	1.3	[0.7 – 2.1]	30 000	[23 000 – 43 000]
Somalia	17 000	[10 000 – 30 000]	0.5	[0.3 – 1.0]	0.5	[0.3 – 0.8]	6700	[3600 – 13 000]
South Africa	4 600 000	[3 900 000 – 5 300 000]	18.1	[15.4 – 20.9]	16.9	[14.3 – 19.9]	3 200 000	[2 800 000 – 3 700 000]
Swaziland	150 000	[140 000 – 160 000]	26.1	[25.1 – 27.1]	26.3	[25.0 – 27.4]	100 000	[99 000 – 110 000]
Togo	100 000	[86 000 – 120 000]	3.3	[2.7 – 4.1]	3.6	[3.0 – 4.3]	69 000	[57 000 – 84 000]
Uganda	950 000	[840 000 – 1 100 000]	5.4	[5.0 – 6.1]	7.9	[7.5 – 9.2]	480 000	[440 000 – 540 000]
United Republic of Tanzania	1 200 000	[1 100 000 – 1 300 000]	6.2	[5.8 – 6.6]	7.0	[6.5 – 7.4]	760 000	[710 000 – 810 000]
Zambia	860 000	[790 000 – 940 000]	15.2	[14.3 – 16.4]	15.4	[14.4 – 16.7]	560 000	[520 000 – 610 000]
Zimbabwe	1 700 000	[1 600 000 – 1 900 000]	15.3	[14.6 – 16.1]	26.0	[25.2 – 27.6]	680 000	[650 000 – 720 000]

1. Estimated number of people living with HIV						
	Women (15+) 2001		Children (0–14) 2007		Children (0–14) 2001	
Country	Estimate	[low estimate – high estimate]	Estimate	[low estimate – high estimate]	Estimate	[low estimate – high estimate]
Global	14 100 000	[13 000 000 – 15 900 000]	2 000 000	[1 900 000 – 2 300 000]	1 600 000	[1 400 000 – 2 100 000]
Sub-Saharan Africa	11 200 000	[10 500 000 – 12 600 000]	1 800 000	[1 700 000 – 2 000 000]	1 400 000	[1 300 000 – 1 900 000]
Angola	67 000	[48 000 – 190 000]	17 000	[12 000 – 35 000]	7700	[3700 – 41 000]
Benin	31 000	[27 000 – 36 000]	5400	[4700 – 6300]	3500	[2800 – 4600]
Botswana	160 000	[150 000 – 170 000]	15 000	[13 000 – 16 000]	13 000	[12 000 – 14 000]
Burkina Faso	59 000	[52 000 – 69 000]	10 000	[8400 – 12 000]	10 000	[6600 – 13 000]
Burundi	77 000	[61 000 – 92 000]	15 000	[12 000 – 19 000]	15 000	[12 000 – 18 000]
Cameroon	300 000	[260 000 – 340 000]	45 000	[38 000 – 51 000]	36 000	[28 000 – 44 000]
Central African Republic	80 000	[74 000 – 86 000]	14 000	[12 000 – 16 000]	9800	[8200 – 11 000]
Chad	85 000	[60 000 – 130 000]	19 000	[14 000 – 27 000]	11 000	[5300 – 36 000]
Comoros	...	[<100]	...	[<100]	...	[<100]
Congo	45 000	[39 000 – 54 000]	6600	[5600 – 7700]	7600	[6500 – 9200]
Côte d'Ivoire	320 000	[290 000 – 360 000]	52 000	[44 000 – 58 000]	47 000	[36 000 – 58 000]
Democratic Republic of Congo	...	[170 000 – 220 000]	...	[37 000 – 52 000]	...	[31 000 – 43 000]
Djibouti	7200	[5300 – 9100]	1100	[<1000 – 1400]	<1000	[<500 – 1200]
Equatorial Guinea	5300	[4200 – 6900]	<1000	[<1100]	...	[<1000]
Eritrea	15 000	[10 000 – 23 000]	3100	[2300 – 4400]	1900	[1200 – 3300]
Ethiopia	500 000	[450 000 – 550 000]	92 000	[80 000 – 100 000]	75 000	[66 000 – 85 000]
Gabon	21 000	[15 000 – 29 000]	2300	[1600 – 3200]	1500	[1000 – 2200]
Gambia	3600	[1800 – 6000]	...	[<1000]	<500	[<1000]
Ghana	140 000	[130 000 – 150 000]	17 000	[15 000 – 19 000]	12 000	[10 000 – 14 000]
Guinea	31 000	[23 000 – 41 000]	6300	[5000 – 7900]	3100	[1900 – 5000]
Guinea-Bissau	7100	[5000 – 9800]	1500	[1100 – 2200]	<1000	[1200]
Kenya[2]	...	[800 000 – 1 000 000]	...	[130 000 – 180 000]	...	[110 000 – 160 000]
Lesotho	140 000	[130 000 – 150 000]	12 000	[11 000 – 13 000]	8000	[7300 – 8800]
Liberia	13 000	[9300 – 28 000]	3100	[2300 – 6300]	2000	[1300 – 10 000]
Madagascar	1900	[1200 – 3200]	<500	[<1000]	<200	[<500]
Malawi	440 000	[410 000 – 480 000]	91 000	[80 000 – 100 000]	65 000	[57 000 – 74 000]
Mali	46 000	[39 000 – 54 000]	9400	[7800 – 11 000]	5600	[3600 – 6800]
Mauritania	2400	[1400 – 4200]	<500	[<1000]	<200	[<500]
Mauritius	<500	[<200 – 1100]	<100	[<200]	...	[<100]
Mozambique	570 000	[500 000 – 660 000]	100 000	[87 000 – 120 000]	53 000	[41 000 – 81 000]
Namibia	85 000	[70 000 – 99 000]	14 000	[12 000 – 16 000]	7500	[6100 – 9100]
Niger	12 000	[8900 – 17 000]	3200	[2500 – 4200]	1600	[1200 – 2400]
Nigeria	1 200 000	[970 000 – 2 100 000]	220 000	[170 000 – 370 000]	150 000	[83 000 – 580 000]
Rwanda	97 000	[87 000 – 110 000]	19 000	[17 000 – 21 000]	26 000	[23 000 – 30 000]
Senegal	14 000	[9800 – 18 000]	3100	[2500 – 3700]	1200	[<1000 – 1700]
Sierra Leone	19 000	[10 000 – 31 000]	4000	[3000 – 5300]	2100	[<1000 – 3600]
Somalia	4500	[2500 – 7900]	<1000	[<1600]	<500	[<1000]
South Africa	2 700 000	[2 300 000 – 3 200 000]	280 000	[230 000 – 320 000]	150 000	[120 000 – 190 000]
Swaziland	91 000	[86 000 – 96 000]	15 000	[14 000 – 17 000]	10 000	[9000 – 11 000]
Togo	61 000	[51 000 – 73 000]	10 000	[8400 – 12 000]	7600	[6100 – 10 000]
Uganda	560 000	[500 000 – 660 000]	130 000	[120 000 – 150 000]	150 000	[140 000 – 170 000]
United Republic of Tanzania	740 000	[680 000 – 790 000]	140 000	[130 000 – 150 000]	120 000	[100 000 – 130 000]
Zambia	470 000	[430 000 – 520 000]	95 000	[86 000 – 110 000]	80 000	[71 000 – 91 000]
Zimbabwe	1 000 000	[970 000 – 1 100 000]	120 000	[110 000 – 140 000]	130 000	[120 000 – 140 000]

1. Estimated number of people living with HIV					2. AIDS deaths			
	Young women (15–24) rate (%) 2007		Young men (15–24) rate (%) 2007		Deaths in adults and children 2007		Deaths in adults and children 2001	
Country	Estimate	[low estimate – high estimate]	Estimate	[low estimate – high estimate]	Estimate	[low estimate – high estimate]	Estimate	[low estimate – high estimate]
Global	0.6	[0.5 – 0.8]	0.4	[0.3 – 0.5]	2 000 000	[1 800 000 – 2 300 000]	1 700 000	[1 500 000 – 2 300 000]
Sub-Saharan Africa	3.2	[2.6 – 3.8]	1.1	[0.8 – 1.4]	1 500 000	[1 300 000 – 1 700 000]	1 300 000	[1 200 000 – 1 900 000]
Angola	0.3	[0.1 – 0.5]	0.2	[0.1 – 0.4]	11 000	[7100 – 28 000]	5900	[2400 – 36 000]
Benin	0.9	[0.6 – 1.2]	0.3	[0.1 – 0.5]	3300	[2700 – 4400]	2900	[2100 – 3900]
Botswana	15.3	[10.0 – 20.8]	5.1	[2.1 – 7.9]	11 000	[6600 – 17 000]	16 000	[13 000 – 19 000]
Burkina Faso	0.9	[0.5 – 1.3]	0.5	[0.2 – 0.8]	9200	[7400 – 11 000]	10 000	[6100 – 13 000]
Burundi	1.3	[0.6 – 2.0]	0.4	[0.2 – 0.7]	11 000	[8600 – 14 000]	14 000	[12 000 – 17 000]
Cameroon	4.3	[1.0 – 5.9]	1.2	[0.5 – 2.2]	39 000	[33 000 – 45 000]	29 000	[22 000 – 39 000]
Central African Republic	5.5	[4.1 – 7.0]	1.1	[0.5 – 1.5]	11 000	[9500 – 12 000]	8800	[6900 – 11 000]
Chad	2.8	[1.3 – 4.1]	2.0	[0.9 – 2.9]	14 000	[11 000 – 20 000]	8600	[3900 – 30 000]
Comoros	<0.1	[0.1]	0.1	[<0.1 – 0.2]	...	[<100]	...	[<100]
Congo	2.3	[1.3 – 3.3]	0.8	[0.3 – 1.1]	6400	[3000 – 10 000]	8300	[6900 – 10 000]
Côte d'Ivoire	2.4	[1.0 – 3.4]	0.8	[0.3 – 1.3]	38 000	[33 000 – 43 000]	43 000	[30 000 – 57 000]
Democratic Republic of Congo	...	[0.7 – 1.2]	...	[0.1 – 0.4]	...	[24 000 – 34 000]	...	[26 000 – 35 000]
Djibouti	2.1	[1.4 – 3.0]	0.7	[0.3 – 1.1]	1100	[<1000 – 1300]	<1000	[<200 – 1100]
Equatorial Guinea	2.5	[1.7 – 3.7]	0.8	[0.4 – 1.4]	...	[<1000]	...	[<1000]
Eritrea	0.9	[0.4 – 1.6]	0.3	[0.1 – 0.6]	2600	[1800 – 3900]	1700	[1100 – 3300]
Ethiopia	1.5	[1.1 – 1.9]	0.5	[0.2 – 0.7]	67 000	[57 000 – 77 000]	70 000	[57 000 – 84 000]
Gabon	3.9	[2.0 – 6.3]	1.3	[0.6 – 2.4]	2300	[1400 – 3700]	1800	[1100 – 2700]
Gambia	0.6	[0.3 – 1.0]	0.2	[0.1 – 0.4]	...	[<1000]	...	[<500]
Ghana	1.3	[0.9 – 1.7]	0.4	[0.2 – 0.6]	21 000	[18 000 – 24 000]	15 000	[12 000 – 20 000]
Guinea	1.2	[0.9 – 1.8]	0.4	[0.2 – 0.6]	4500	[3300 – 5900]	2600	[1500 – 4300]
Guinea-Bissau	1.2	[0.3 – 2.5]	0.4	[0.2 – 0.8]	1100	[<1000 – 1500]	...	[<1000]
Kenya[2]	...	[4.6 – 8.4]	...	[0.8 – 2.5]	...	[85 000 – 130 000]	...	[100 000 – 160 000]
Lesotho	14.9	[10.6 – 18.4]	5.9	[2.5 – 9.6]	18 000	[16 000 – 20 000]	13 000	[9900 – 16 000]
Liberia	1.3	[0.8 – 1.7]	0.4	[0.2 – 0.6]	2300	[1700 – 4700]	1700	[1100 – 10 000]
Madagascar	0.1	[<0.1 – 0.2]	0.2	[0.1 – 0.3]	<1000	[1300]	<200	[<500]
Malawi	8.4	[6.7 – 10.4]	2.4	[0.9 – 3.8]	68 000	[59 000 – 77 000]	60 000	[49 000 – 71 000]
Mali	1.1	[0.7 – 1.5]	0.4	[0.2 – 0.5]	5800	[4600 – 7300]	4300	[2500 – 5400]
Mauritania	0.5	[0.2 – 1.0]	0.9	[0.4 – 1.9]	<1000	[<500 – 1300]	<200	[<500]
Mauritius	1.0	[0.5 – 2.2]	1.8	[0.8 – 4.5]	...	[<500]	...	[<100]
Mozambique	8.5	[5.9 – 11.1]	2.9	[1.2 – 4.2]	81 000	[67 000 – 98 000]	47 000	[33 000 – 77 000]
Namibia	10.3	[6.2 – 14.5]	3.4	[1.4 – 5.3]	5100	[3100 – 7100]	6700	[5000 – 9000]
Niger	0.5	[0.3 – 0.8]	0.9	[0.4 – 1.5]	4000	[3000 – 5600]	1800	[1300 – 2900]
Nigeria	2.3	[1.2 – 3.3]	0.8	[0.3 – 1.2]	170 000	[130 000 – 270 000]	130 000	[67 000 – 540 000]
Rwanda	1.4	[0.9 – 1.9]	0.5	[0.3 – 0.7]	7800	[5700 – 10 000]	22 000	[20 000 – 25 000]
Senegal	0.8	[0.5 – 1.2]	0.3	[0.1 – 0.5]	1800	[1200 – 2600]	<1000	[1400]
Sierra Leone	1.3	[0.7 – 1.9]	0.4	[0.2 – 0.7]	3300	[2300 – 4700]	2100	[<1000 – 3400]
Somalia	0.3	[0.1 – 0.6]	0.6	[0.3 – 1.4]	1600	[<1000 – 3000]	<1000	[<500 – 1300]
South Africa	12.7	[9.1 – 17.0]	4.0	[1.7 – 6.0]	350 000	[270 000 – 420 000]	180 000	[130 000 – 250 000]
Swaziland	22.6	[17.7 – 27.2]	5.8	[2.2 – 9.3]	10 000	[8600 – 12 000]	7700	[6300 – 9700]
Togo	2.4	[1.4 – 3.3]	0.8	[0.4 – 1.2]	9100	[6900 – 12 000]	7200	[5400 – 9500]
Uganda	3.9	[2.7 – 5.2]	1.3	[0.6 – 1.9]	77 000	[68 000 – 89 000]	120 000	[110 000 – 150 000]
United Republic of Tanzania	0.9	[0.5 – 1.3]	0.5	[0.4 – 0.7]	96 000	[86 000 – 110 000]	110 000	[99 000 – 130 000]
Zambia	11.3	[8.5 – 14.2]	3.6	[1.6 – 5.2]	56 000	[47 000 – 66 000]	78 000	[68 000 – 89 000]
Zimbabwe	7.7	[3.8 – 11.7]	2.9	[1.2 – 4.4]	140 000	[130 000 – 150 000]	150 000	[130 000 – 170 000]

	3. Orphans due to AIDS				4. HIV prevalence (%) in most-at-risk groups in capital city					
	Orphans (0–17) currently living 2007		Orphans (0–17) living in 2001		Injecting drug users		Female sex workers		Men who have sex with men	
Country	Estimate	[low estimate – high estimate]	Estimate	[low estimate – high estimate]	Year	HIV (%)	Year	HIV (%)	Year	HIV (%)
Global	15 000 000	[13 000 000 – 19 000 000]	8 000 000	[6 900 000 – 12 000 000]	...	...	...	...	...	...
Sub-Saharan Africa	11 600 000	[10 600 000 – 15 300 000]	6 500 000	[5 600 000 – 10 000 000]	...	...	...	...	...	...
Angola	50 000	[20 000 – 260 000]	23 000	[5900 – 200 000]	...	...	2007	23.1	...	...
Benin	29 000	[22 000 – 40 000]	11 000	[6800 – 25 000]	...	...	2006	25.5	...	...
Botswana	95 000	[81 000 – 110 000]	57 000	[45 000 – 74 000]	...	...	...	...	...	...
Burkina Faso	100 000	[62 000 – 130 000]	77 000	[23 000 – 120 000]	...	...	2005	8.9	...	...
Burundi	120 000	[100 000 – 150 000]	72 000	[53 000 – 93 000]	...	...	2002	16.8	...	...
Cameroon	300 000	[230 000 – 390 000]	110 000	[74 000 – 170 000]	...	...	2004	26.4	...	...
Central African Republic	72 000	[58 000 – 86 000]	32 000	[22 000 – 46 000]	...	...	...	...	...	...
Chad	85 000	[42 000 – 270 000]	31 000	[7000 – 170 000]	...	...	...	...	...	...
Comoros	<100	[<200]	...	[<100]	...	...	2007	0.0	...	...
Congo	69 000	[57 000 – 84 000]	55 000	[42 000 – 70 000]	...	...	...	...	...	...
Côte d'Ivoire	420 000	[320 000 – 530 000]	220 000	[100 000 – 370 000]	...	...	...	...	...	...
Democratic Republic of Congo	...	[270 000 – 380 000]	...	[210 000 – 310 000]	...	...	2007[1]	14.7	...	...
Djibouti	5200	[1900 – 9600]	1500	[<200 – 4600]	...	...	...	...	...	...
Equatorial Guinea	4800	[3800 – 6100]	1900	[<1000 – 2700]	...	...	...	...	...	...
Eritrea	18 000	[12 000 – 32 000]	5700	[2800 – 16 000]	...	...	2006	9.7	...	...
Ethiopia	650 000	[540 000 – 780 000]	310 000	[220 000 – 430 000]	...	...	...	...	...	...
Gabon	18 000	[11 000 – 28 000]	8000	[4700 – 13 000]	...	...	2007	20.0	...	...
Gambia	2700	[1300 – 4700]	<1000	[<500 – 1000]	...	...	...	...	...	...
Ghana	160 000	[130 000 – 200 000]	45 000	[29 000 – 74 000]	...	...	2006	38.0	2006	25.0
Guinea	25 000	[15 000 – 39 000]	10 000	[5000 – 26 000]	...	...	2007	34.5	...	...
Guinea-Bissau	5900	[4200 – 8300]	1900	[<1000 – 2900]	...	...	...	...	...	...
Kenya[2]	...	[990 000 – 1 400 000]	...	[510 000 – 870 000]]	2007	50.0	...	...	2007	43.0
Lesotho	110 000	[93 000 – 120 000]	37 000	[26 000 – 49 000]	...	...	...	...	...	...
Liberia	15 000	[10 000 – 87 000]	6200	[2600 – 55 000]	...	...	...	...	...	...
Madagascar	3400	[2100 – 6000]	<500	[<1000]	...	...	2007	0.5	...	...
Malawi	550 000	[470 000 – 640 000]	240 000	[150 000 – 340 000]	...	...	2006	69.1	...	...
Mali	44 000	[27 000 – 56 000]	16 000	[3600 – 22 000]	...	...	2006	35.3	...	...
Mauritania	3000	[1500 – 5900]	<500	[<200 – 1300]	...	...	...	...	2007	19.1
Mauritius	<500	[<1000]	<100	[<500]	...	...	...	...	...	...
Mozambique	400 000	[280 000 – 590 000]	120 000	[53 000 – 350 000]	...	...	...	...	...	...
Namibia	66 000	[50 000 – 85 000]	23 000	[16 000 – 34 000]	...	...	...	...	...	...
Niger	25 000	[18 000 – 39 000]	7300	[4800 – 11 000]	...	...	2006	38.4	...	...
Nigeria	1 200 000	[640 000 – 4 100 000]	460 000	[110 000 – 3 400 000]	2007	5.6	2007	32.7	2007	13.5
Rwanda	220 000	[190 000 – 250 000]	230 000	[180 000 – 270 000]	...	...	...	...	...	...
Senegal	8400	[4600 – 14 000]	3800	[1900 – 7100]	...	...	2006	19.8	2004	21.5
Sierra Leone	16 000	[6400 – 26 000]	6000	[1300 – 10 000]	...	...	2005	8.5	...	...
Somalia	8800	[4900 – 16 000]	2000	[<1000 – 5700]	...	...	...	...	...	...
South Africa	1 400 000	[1 100 000 – 1 800 000]	400 000	[260 000 – 590 000]	...	...	...	...	...	...
Swaziland	56 000	[48 000 – 65 000]	19 000	[13 000 – 26 000]	...	...	...	...	...	...
Togo	68 000	[50 000 – 91 000]	31 000	[18 000 – 53 000]	...	...	2005	29.3	...	...
Uganda	1 200 000	[1 100 000 – 1 400 000]	1 100 000	[910 000 – 1 300 000]	...	...	...	...	...	...
United Republic of Tanzania	970 000	[850 000 – 1 100 000]	610 000	[500 000 – 740 000]	...	...	...	...	...	...
Zambia	600 000	[530 000 – 660 000]	390 000	[290 000 – 490 000]	...	...	2004	65.4	...	...
Zimbabwe	1 000 000	[920 000 – 1 100 000]	720 000	[610 000 – 830 000]	...	...	...	...	...	...

[1] This data was reported in the 2007 UNGASS report.

[2] At the time of production of the current report, analyses incorporating new data from a population based survey with data from other sources were ongoing. This is why only ranges are published based on preliminary analysis. As soon as updated final estimates are available, they will be published on the UNAIDS website.

1. Estimated number of people living with HIV						
	Adults and children 2007		Adults and children 2001		Adults (15+) 2007	
Country	Estimate	[low estimate – high estimate]	Estimate	[low estimate – high estimate]	Estimate	[low estimate – high estimate]
East Asia	**740 000**	**[480 000 – 1 100 000]**	**490 000**	**[330 000 – 750 000]**	**730 000**	**[480 000 – 1 100 000]**
China	700 000	[450 000 – 1 000 000]	470 000	[320 000 – 730 000]	690 000	[450 000 – 1 000 000]
Democratic People's Republic of Korea	...	...	...	...	...	...
Japan	9600	[7900 – 10 000]	8100	[7600 – 8500]	9600	[7900 – 10 000]
Mongolia	<1000	[1500]	...	...	<1000	[<500 – 1500]
Republic of Korea	13 000	[7500 – 42 000]	6800	[3400 – 13 000]	13 000	[7500 – 42 000]
Oceania	**74 000**	**[66 000 – 93 000]**	**25 000**	**[19 000 – 41 000]**	**73 000**	**[65 000 – 91 000]**
Australia	18 000	[11 000 – 36 000]	14 000	[8100 – 29 000]	18 000	[11 000 – 36 000]
Fiji	...	[<500]	...	[<500]	...	[<500]
New Zealand	1400	[<1000 – 2600]	1200	[<1000 – 2000]	1400	[<1000 – 2600]
Papua New Guinea	54 000	[53 000 – 55 000]	10 000	[9800 – 11 000]	53 000	[52 000 – 54 000]
South and South-East Asia	**4 200 000**	**[3 500 000 – 5 300 000]**	**4 200 000**	**[3 100 000 – 5 500 000]**	**4 100 000**	**[3 400 000 – 5 200 000]**
Afghanistan	...	...	...	...	...	...
Bangladesh	12 000	[7700 – 19 000]	7500	[4800 – 12 000]	12 000	[7600 – 19 000]
Bhutan	<500	[<1000]	...	[<100]	<500	[<1000]
Brunei Darussalam	...	...	...	...	...	...
Cambodia	75 000	[67 000 – 84 000]	120 000	[110 000 – 140 000]	70 000	[63 000 – 80 000]
India	2 400 000	[1 800 000 – 3 200 000]	2 700 000	[1 700 000 – 3 800 000]	2 300 000	[1 700 000 – 3 100 000]
Indonesia	270 000	[190 000 – 400 000]	93 000	[37 000 – 140 000]	270 000	[190 000 – 400 000]
Iran (Islamic Republic of)	86 000	[68 000 – 110 000]	46 000	[36 000 – 58 000]	85 000	[67 000 – 110 000]
Lao People's Democratic Republic	5500	[3300 – 13 000]	1200	[<100 – 2500]	5400	[3300 – 13 000]
Malaysia	80 000	[52 000 – 120 000]	44 000	[33 000 – 65 000]	79 000	[51 000 – 120 000]
Maldives	...	[<100]	...	[<100]	...	[<100]
Myanmar	240 000	[160 000 – 370 000]	300 000	[230 000 – 380 000]	240 000	[150 000 – 360 000]
Nepal	70 000	[50 000 – 99 000]	56 000	[41 000 – 80 000]	68 000	[49 000 – 97 000]
Pakistan	96 000	[69 000 – 150 000]	51 000	[37 000 – 79 000]	94 000	[68 000 – 150 000]
Philippines	8300	[6000 – 11 000]	<1000	[1200]	8200	[5900 – 11 000]
Singapore	4200	[2600 – 7300]	2900	[1800 – 5300]	4100	[2500 – 7200]
Sri Lanka	3800	[2800 – 5100]	3000	[2200 – 4000]	3700	[2800 – 5000]
Thailand	610 000	[410 000 – 880 000]	660 000	[490 000 – 850 000]	600 000	[400 000 – 860 000]
Timor-Leste	...	...	...	...	...	...
Viet Nam	290 000	[180 000 – 470 000]	160 000	[97 000 – 250 000]	280 000	[170 000 – 470 000]
Eastern Europe and Central Asia	**1 500 000**	**[1 100 000 – 1 900 000]**	**650 000**	**[510 000 – 1 100 000]**	**1 500 000**	**[1 100 000 – 1 900 000]**
Armenia	2400	[1800 – 3500]	1800	[1300 – 2600]	2400	[1700 – 3500]
Azerbaijan	7800	[4700 – 16 000]	...	[<500]	7800	[4700 – 16 000]
Belarus	13 000	[10 000 – 19 000]	13 000	[9600 – 18 000]	13 000	[10 000 – 18 000]
Bosnia and Herzegovina	<500	[<1000]	...	...	...	...
Bulgaria	...	...	...	...	...	...
Croatia	<500	[<1000]	...	...	...	...
Estonia	9900	[5400 – 19 000]	3500	[1400 – 10 000]	9900	[5300 – 18 000]
Georgia	2700	[1500 – 6100]	...	[<500]	2700	[1500 – 6100]
Kazakhstan	12 000	[7000 – 29 000]	3500	[<500 – 6500]	12 000	[6900 – 29 000]
Kyrgyzstan	4200	[2300 – 7700]	1000	[<1000 – 1800]	4200	[2200 – 7600]
Latvia	10 000	[7400 – 15 000]	4200	[2900 – 9700]	10 000	[7300 – 15 000]
Lithuania	2200	[1200 – 4600]	1400	[<1000 – 3200]	2200	[1200 – 4600]

1. Estimated number of people living with HIV								
	Adults (15+) 2001		Adult (15–49) prevalence percent 2007		Adult (15–49) prevalence percent 2001		Women (15+) 2007	
Country	Estimate	[low estimate – high estimate]	Estimate	[low estimate – high estimate]	Estimate	[low estimate – high estimate]	Estimate	[low estimate – high estimate]
East Asia	490 000	[330 000 – 740 000]	0.1	[<0.1 – 0.2]	0.1	[<0.1 – 0.2]	200 000	[130 000 – 320 000]
China	470 000	[320 000 – 730 000]	0.1	[<0.1 – 0.2]	0.1	[<0.1 – 0.2]	200 000	[120 000 – 310 000]
Democratic People's Republic of Korea	...	...	...	...	...	...	...	...
Japan	8100	[7600 – 8500]	...	[<0.1]	...	[<0.1]	2300	[2000 – 2500]
Mongolia	...	[<100]	0.1	[<0.1 – 0.2]	...	[<0.1]	<200	[<500]
Republic of Korea	6800	[3400 – 13 000]	<0.1	[0.1]	<0.1	[0.1]	3600	[2000 – 12 000]
Oceania	25 000	[19 000 – 40 000]	0.4	[0.3 – 0.5]	0.2	[0.1 – 0.3]	22 000	[21 000 – 24 000]
Australia	14 000	[8100 – 29 000]	0.2	[0.1 – 0.3]	0.1	[<0.1 – 0.3]	1200	[<1000 – 2400]
Fiji	...	[<500]	0.1	[<0.1 – <0.2]	0.1	[<0.1 – <0.2]	...	[<200]
New Zealand	1200	[<1000 – 1900]	0.1	[<0.1 – 0.2]	0.1	[<0.1 – 0.2]	...	[<500]
Papua New Guinea	9800	[9600 – 9900]	1.5	[1.4 – 1.6]	0.3	[0.2 – 0.4]	21 000	[20 000 – 22 000]
South and South-East Asia	4 100 000	[3 000 000 – 5 400 000]	0.3	[0.2 – 0.4]	0.4	[0.3 – 0.5]	1 500 000	[1 200 000 – 1 900 000]
Afghanistan	...	...	...	...	...	...	...	...
Bangladesh	7500	[4800 – 12 000]	...	[<0.1]	...	[<0.1]	2000	[1200 – 3400]
Bhutan	...	[<100]	0.1	[<0.1 – 0.2]	...	[<0.1]	<100	[<200]
Brunei Darussalam	...	...	...	...	...	...	...	...
Cambodia	120 000	[110 000 – 130 000]	0.8	[0.7 – 0.9]	1.5	[1.5 – 2.0]	20 000	[17 000 – 23 000]
India	2 600 000	[1 600 000 – 3 700 000]	0.3	[0.2 – 0.5]	0.5	[0.3 – 0.7]	880 000	[670 000 – 1 200 000]
Indonesia	93 000	[37 000 – 140 000]	0.2	[0.1 – 0.3]	0.1	[<0.1 – 0.2]	54 000	[36 000 – 87 000]
Iran (Islamic Republic of)	45 000	[36 000 – 58 000]	0.2	[0.1 – 0.3]	0.1	[<0.1 – 0.2]	24 000	[18 000 – 32 000]
Lao People's Democratic Republic	1100	[<100 – 2500]	0.2	[0.1 – 0.4]	<0.1	[0.1]	1300	[<1000 – 3100]
Malaysia	43 000	[33 000 – 64 000]	0.5	[0.3 – 0.8]	0.3	[0.2 – 0.5]	21 000	[13 000 – 34 000]
Maldives	...	[<100]	...	[<0.1]	...	[<0.1]	...	[<100]
Myanmar	290 000	[220 000 – 370 000]	0.7	[0.4 – 1.1]	0.9	[0.7 – 1.2]	100 000	[63 000 – 150 000]
Nepal	55 000	[41 000 – 78 000]	0.5	[0.4 – 0.7]	0.5	[0.3 – 0.7]	17 000	[12 000 – 25 000]
Pakistan	50 000	[36 000 – 77 000]	0.1	[<0.1 – 0.2]	<0.1	[0.1]	27 000	[19 000 – 42 000]
Philippines	<1000	[1200]	...	[<0.1]	...	...	2200	[1600 – 3100]
Singapore	2900	[1700 – 5200]	0.2	[0.1 – 0.3]	0.1	[<0.1 – 0.2]	1200	[<1000 – 2100]
Sri Lanka	3000	[2200 – 4000]	...	[<0.1]	...	[<0.1]	1400	[<1000 – 1800]
Thailand	650 000	[480 000 – 830 000]	1.4	[0.9 – 2.1]	1.7	[1.2 – 2.1]	250 000	[170 000 – 360 000]
Timor-Leste	...	...	...	...	...	...	...	...
Viet Nam	150 000	[96 000 – 240 000]	0.5	[0.3 – 0.9]	0.3	[0.2 – 0.5]	76 000	[46 000 – 120 000]
Eastern Europe and Central Asia	650 000	[500 000 – 1 100 000]	0.8	[0.6 – 1.1]	0.4	[0.3 – 0.7]	460 000	[350 000 – 590 000]
Armenia	1800	[1300 – 2600]	0.1	[<0.1 – 0.2]	0.1	[<0.1 – 0.2]	...	[<1000]
Azerbaijan	<500	[<1000]	0.2	[0.1 – 0.3]	...	<0.1	1300	[<1000 – 2900]
Belarus	12 000	[9600 – 17 000]	0.2	[0.1 – 0.3]	0.2	[0.1 – 0.3]	3900	[2800 – 5500]
Bosnia and Herzegovina	...	...	<0.1	[<0.2]	...	...	...	...
Bulgaria	...	...	...	...	...	...	...	...
Croatia	...	...	<0.1	[<0.2]	...	...	...	...
Estonia	3500	[1400 – 10 000]	1.3	[0.7 – 2.5]	0.5	[0.2 – 1.4]	2400	[1300 – 4800]
Georgia	<500	[<1000]	0.1	[<0.1 – 0.3]	...	[<0.1]	<1000	[<500 – 1500]
Kazakhstan	3400	[<500 – 6400]	0.1	[<0.1 – 0.3]	<0.1	[0.1]	3300	[1800 – 7700]
Kyrgyzstan	1000	[<1000 – 1800]	0.1	[<0.1 – 0.3]	<0.1	[0.1]	1100	[<1000 – 2000]
Latvia	4200	[2800 – 9700]	0.8	[0.6 – 1.2]	0.3	[0.2 – 0.8]	2700	[1800 – 4000]
Lithuania	1400	[<1000 – 3200]	0.1	[<0.1 – 0.2]	0.1	[<0.1-0.2]	<1000	[<500 – 1200]

1. Estimated number of people living with HIV						
	Women (15+) 2001		Children (0–14) 2007		Children (0–14) 2001	
Country	Estimate	[low estimate – high estimate]	Estimate	[low estimate – high estimate]	Estimate	[low estimate – high estimate]
East Asia	**130 000**	**[83 000 – 200 000]**	**7800**	**[5300 – 11 000]**	**3500**	**[2500 – 5100]**
China	120 000	[80 000 – 200 000]	...	...	...	...
Democratic People's Republic of Korea	...	...	...	...	...	...
Japan	1800	[1700 – 2000]	...	...	...	...
Mongolia	...	[<100]	...	...	...	...
Republic of Korea	1800	[<1000 – 3300]	...	...	...	...
Oceania	**4600**	**[4000 – 5900]**	**1100**	**[1200]**	**<500**	**...**
Australia	<1000	[<500 – 2100]	...	...	...	...
Fiji	...	[<100]	...	...	...	...
New Zealand	<200	[<500]	...	...	...	...
Papua New Guinea	3400	[3300 – 3600]	1100	[<1000 – 1200]	<200	[<500]
South and South-East Asia	**1 500 000**	**[1 100 000 – 2 000 000]**	**140 000**	**[110 000 – 180 000]**	**98 000**	**[50 000 – 150 000]**
Afghanistan	...	...	...	...	...	...
Bangladesh	<100	[<500]	...	...	...	...
Bhutan	...	[<100]	...	...	...	...
Brunei Darussalam	...	...	...	...	...	...
Cambodia	31 000	[26 000 – 37 000]	4400	[4000 – 5000]	3600	[2900 – 4600]
India	1 000 000	[630 000 – 1 500 000]	...	...	...	...
Indonesia	10 000	[2600 – 20 000]	...	...	...	...
Iran (Islamic Republic of)	12 000	[8700 – 16 000]	...	...	...	...
Lao People's Democratic Republic	<500	[<100 – <1000]	...	...	...	...
Malaysia	10 000	[6900 – 16 000]	...	...	...	...
Maldives	...	[<100]	...	...	...	...
Myanmar	97 000	[72 000 – 130 000]	...	...	...	...
Nepal	12 000	[8200 – 18 000]	...	...	...	...
Pakistan	13 000	[9100 – 21 000]	...	...	...	...
Philippines	<500	[<1000]	...	...	...	...
Singapore	<1000	[<500 – 1500]	...	...	...	...
Sri Lanka	<1000	[1100]	...	...	...	...
Thailand	240 000	[170 000 – 310 000]	14 000	[12 000 – 17 000]	10 000	[7500 – 14 000]
Timor-Leste	...	...	...	...	...	...
Viet Nam	37 000	[22 000 – 61 000]	...	...	...	...
Eastern Europe and Central Asia	**180 000**	**[130 000 – 300 000]**	**12 000**	**[9100 – 15 000]**	**2800**	**[2200 – 4800]**
Armenia	<500	[<1000]	...	...	...	...
Azerbaijan	...	[<100]	...	...	...	...
Belarus	3300	[2400 – 4700]	...	...	...	...
Bosnia and Herzegovina	...	...	...	...	...	...
Bulgaria	...	...	...	...	...	...
Croatia	...	...	...	...	...	...
Estonia	<1000	[<500 – 2100]	...	...	...	...
Georgia	<100	[<200]	...	...	...	...
Kazakhstan	<1000	[<200 – 1600]	...	...	...	...
Kyrgyzstan	...	[<500]	...	...	...	...
Latvia	<1000	[2200]	...	...	...	...
Lithuania	<500	[<200 – <1000]	...	...	...	...

	1. Estimated number of people living with HIV				2. AIDS deaths			
	Young women (15–24) rate (%) 2007		Young men (15–24) rate (%) 2007		Deaths in adults and children 2007		Deaths in adults and children 2001	
Country	Estimate	[low estimate – high estimate]	Estimate	[low estimate – high estimate]	Estimate	[low estimate – high estimate]	Estimate	[low estimate – high estimate]
East Asia	<0.1	[0.1]	<0.1	[0.1]	40 000	[24 000 – 63 000]	15 000	[8200 – 24 000]
China	0.1	[<0.1 – 0.2]	0.1	[<0.1 – 0.2]	39 000	[23 000 – 62 000]	15 000	[8100 – 24 000]
Democratic People's Republic of Korea	...	...	...	...	...	...	...	...
Japan	...	[<0.1]	...	[<0.1]	<100	[<500]	...	[<100]
Mongolia	...	[<0.1]	0.1	[<0.1 – 0.2]	...	[<100]	...	...
Republic of Korea	<0.1	[0.1]	<0.1	[0.2]	<500	[<1000]	<200	[<500]
Oceania	0.2	[0.1 – 0.3]	0.3	[0.1 – 0.4]	1000	[<1000 – 1400]	...	[<500]
Australia	<0.1	[0.1]	0.2	[0.1 – 0.4]	<100	[<500]	<100	[<200]
Fiji	...	[0.1]	0.1	[<0.1 – 0.2]	...	[<100]	...	[<100]
New Zealand	...	[<0.1]	0.1	[<0.1 – 0.2]	...	[<100]	...	[<100]
Papua New Guinea	0.7	[0.5 – 0.9]	0.6	[0.2 – 0.8]	<1000	[1100]	...	[<500]
South and South-East Asia	0.5	[0.3 – 0.7]	0.3	[0.1 – 0.5]	340 000	[230 000 – 450 000]	250 000	[140 000 – 370 000]
Afghanistan	...	...	...	...	...	[<100]	...	...
Bangladesh	...	[<0.1]	...	[<0.1]	<500	[<1000]	...	[<100]
Bhutan	<0.1	[0.1]	0.1	[<0.1 – 0.3]	...	[<100]	...	...
Brunei Darussalam	...	...	...	...	...	...	...	...
Cambodia	0.3	[0.1 – 0.6]	0.8	[0.3 – 1.2]	6900	[4300 – 8100]	14 000	[11 000 – 16 000]
India	0.3	[<0.1 – 0.5]	0.3	[<0.1 – 0.5]	...	...	...	...
Indonesia	0.1	[<0.1 – 0.2]	0.3	[0.1 – 0.5]	8700	[4900 – 13 000]	<100	[<200]
Iran (Islamic Republic of)	0.1	[<0.1 – 0.2]	0.2	[0.1 – 0.3]	4300	[3100 – 6100]	1000	[<1000 – 1500]
Lao People's Democratic Republic	0.1	[<0.1 – 0.2]	0.2	[0.1 – 0.5]	<100	[<200]	<100	[<200]
Malaysia	0.3	[0.2 – 0.5]	0.6	[0.3 – 1.0]	3900	[2600 – 5600]	<1000	[<500 – 1400]
Maldives	...	[<0.1]	...	[<0.1]	...	[<100]	...	...
Myanmar	0.6	[0.3 – 1.0]	0.7	[0.3 – 1.2]	25 000	[19 000 – 34 000]	24 000	[17 000 – 34 000]
Nepal	0.3	[0.2 – 0.4]	0.5	[0.3 – 0.9]	5000	[3500 – 7500]	2600	[1800 – 4100]
Pakistan	0.1	[<0.1 – 0.2]	0.1	[<0.1 – 0.2]	5100	[3500 – 8200]	1900	[1200 – 3100]
Philippines	...	[<0.1]	...	[<0.1]	<200	[<500]	...	[<100]
Singapore	0.1	[<0.1 – 0.2]	0.2	[0.1 – 0.3]	<200	[<500]	<100	[<200]
Sri Lanka	...	[<0.1]	<0.1	[0.1]	...	[<500]	<200	[<500]
Thailand	1.2	[0.4 – 2.0]	1.2	[0.5 – 2.1]	30 000	[16 000 – 47 000]	66 000	[46 000 – 92 000]
Timor-Leste	...	...	...	...	...	...	...	...
Viet Nam	0.3	[0.1 – 0.5]	0.6	[0.3 – 1.1]	24 000	[14 000 – 39 000]	5500	[1700 – 17 000]
Eastern Europe and Central Asia	0.1	[<0.1 – 0.2]	0.9	[0.5 – 1.3]	58 000	[41 000 – 88 000]	6700	[4700 – 12 000]
Armenia	0.1	[<0.1 – 0.2]	0.2	[0.1 – 0.3]	<200	[<500]	...	[<100]
Azerbaijan	0.1	[<0.1 – 0.2]	0.3	[0.1 – 0.6]	<100	[<200]	...	...
Belarus	0.1	[<0.1 – 0.2]	0.3	[0.1 – 0.4]	1100	[1500]	<500	[<1000]
Bosnia and Herzegovina	...	...	...	...	...	...	...	...
Bulgaria	...	...	...	...	...	[<100]	...	[<100]
Croatia	...	...	...	...	...	...	...	...
Estonia	0.7	[0.3 – 1.6]	1.6	[0.7 – 3.7]	<500	[<1000]	...	[<100]
Georgia	0.1	[<0.1- 0.2]	0.1	[<0.1 – 0.4]	...	[<100]	...	[<100]
Kazakhstan	0.1	[<0.1- 0.2]	0.2	[0.1 – 0.4]	<500	[<1000]	<100	[<200]
Kyrgyzstan	0.1	[<0.1 – 0.2]	0.2	[0.1 – 0.3]	<200	[<500]	...	[<100]
Latvia	0.5	[0.2 – 0.7]	0.9	[0.4 – 1.6]	<500	[<1000]	...	[<100]
Lithuania	0.1	[<0.1 – 0.2]	0.1	[<0.1 – 0.3]	<200	[<500]	...	[<100]

	3. Orphans due to AIDS				4. HIV prevalence (%) in most-at-risk groups in capital city					
	Orphans (0–17) currently living 2007		Orphans (0–17) living in 2001		Injecting drug users		Female sex workers		Men who have sex with men	
Country	Estimate	[low estimate – high estimate]	Estimate	[low estimate – high estimate]	Year	HIV (%)	Year	HIV (%)	Year	HIV (%)
East Asia	...	...	...	...	...	...	...	...	...	...
China	...	...	...	...	2007	8.1	2007	0.3	2007	2.1
Democratic People's Republic of Korea	...	...	...	...	...	...	...	...	...	...
Japan	...	...	...	...	...	...	...	...	2005	5.3
Mongolia	...	...	...	...	...	...	...	...	2005	0.0
Republic of Korea	...	...	...	...	...	...	...	...	...	...
Oceania	...	...	...	...	...	...	...	...	...	...
Australia	...	...	...	...	2007	1.5	2006	0.0	...	...
Fiji	...	...	...	...	...	...	...	...	...	...
New Zealand	...	...	...	...	2007[1]	0.0	2007[1]	0.0	2007[1]	0.9
Papua New Guinea	...	...	...	...	...	...	...	...	...	...
South and South-East Asia	...	...	...	...	...	...	...	...	...	...
Afghanistan	...	...	...	...	2006	3.0	2007	0.0	...	...
Bangladesh	...	...	...	...	2006	6.4	2006	0.2	2006	0.2
Bhutan	...	...	...	...	...	...	...	...	...	...
Brunei Darussalam	...	...	...	...	...	...	...	...	...	...
Cambodia	...	...	...	...	...	...	2007	12.7	2005	4.5
India	...	...	...	...	2006	6.9	...	...	2006	6.4
Indonesia	...	...	...	...	2007	52.4	2007	9.5	2007	5.2
Iran (Islamic Republic of)	...	...	...	...	2007	18.8	...	...	...	...
Lao People's Democratic Republic	...	...	...	...	...	...	...	...	2007	5.6
Malaysia	...	...	...	...	2007	4.5	...	...	2007	7.1
Maldives	...	...	...	...	...	...	...	...	...	...
Myanmar	...	...	...	...	...	...	...	...	...	...
Nepal	...	...	...	...	2007	34.7	2007	1.7	2007	3.3
Pakistan	...	...	...	...	...	...	2007	0.9	...	...
Philippines	...	...	...	...	2007	0.1	2007	0.1	2007	0.3
Singapore	...	...	...	...	...	...	...	...	...	...
Sri Lanka	...	...	...	...	...	...	2006	0.2	...	...
Thailand	...	...	...	...	2007	28.8	2007	5.0	2007	24.6
Timor-Leste	...	...	...	...	...	...	...	...	...	...
Viet Nam	...	...	...	...	2006	23.1	2006	4.2	2006	9.0
Eastern Europe and Central Asia	...	...	...	...	...	...	...	...	...	...
Armenia	...	...	...	...	2007	6.8	2007	0.4	2007	2.0
Azerbaijan	...	...	...	...	2003	13.0	...	...	...	...
Belarus	...	...	...	...	2006	16.6	2006	1.0	2006	0.2
Bosnia and Herzegovina	...	...	...	...	2006	0.1	...	...	...	...
Bulgaria	...	...	...	...	2006	3.4	2006	0.2	2006	0.0
Croatia	...	...	...	...	2006	0.6	2006	1.4	2006	3.0
Estonia	...	...	...	...	2005	62.1	2006	7.7	2007	1.7
Georgia	...	...	...	...	2006	0.0	2006	0.6	2007	3.6
Kazakhstan	...	...	...	...	2006	7.4	2006	1.4	2006	1.0
Kyrgyzstan	...	...	...	...	...	...	...	...	...	...
Latvia	...	...	...	...	2007	22.5	...	...	...	...
Lithuania	...	...	...	...	2007	9.7	2007	0.0	2007	1.2

[1] This data were reported in the 2007 UNGASS report.

1. Estimated number of people living with HIV						
	Adults and children 2007		Adults and children 2001		Adults (15+) 2007	
Country	Estimate	[low estimate – high estimate]	Estimate	[low estimate – high estimate]	Estimate	[low estimate – high estimate]
Republic of Moldova	8900	[6000 – 15 000]	<1000	[<200 – 1400]	8800	[6000 – 15 000]
Romania	15 000	[12 000 – 16 000]	15 000	[14 000 – 16 000]	14 000	[11 000 – 16 000]
Russian Federation	940 000	[630 000 – 1 300 000]	390 000	[260 000 – 860 000]	940 000	[630 000 – 1 300 000]
Tajikistan	10 000	[5000 – 23 000]	2500	[<100 – 5300]	10 000	[4900 – 23 000]
Turkmenistan	<500	[<1000]	...	...	<500	[<1000]
Ukraine	440 000	[340 000 – 540 000]	210 000	[180 000 – 260 000]	430 000	[330 000 – 530 000]
Uzbekistan	16 000	[8100 – 45 000]	1400	[<1000 – 3800]	16 000	[8000 – 44 000]
Western and Central Europe	730 000	[580 000 – 1 000 000]	610 000	[490 000 – 810 000]	730 000	[580 000 – 990 000]
Albania	...	[<1000]	...	...	...	...
Austria	9800	[7600 – 13 000]	5500	[4700 – 6400]	9800	[7600 – 13 000]
Belgium	15 000	[8900 – 29 000]	13 000	[7500 – 23 000]	15 000	[8900 – 29 000]
Czech Republic	1500	[<1000 – 2800]	1300	[<1000 – 2400]	1500	[<1000 – 2800]
Denmark	4800	[3700 – 6900]	3300	[2700 – 4000]	4800	[3700 – 6900]
Finland	2400	[1400 – 4400]	2000	[1200 – 3700]	2400	[1400 – 4400]
France	140 000	[78 000 – 240 000]	120 000	[66 000 – 200 000]	140 000	[78 000 – 240 000]
Germany	53 000	[31 000 – 97 000]	44 000	[27 000 – 80 000]	52 000	[31 000 – 97 000]
Greece	11 000	[6100 – 19 000]	8400	[4900 – 15 000]	11 000	[6100 – 19 000]
Hungary	3300	[2000 – 5900]	2800	[1700 – 4900]	3300	[2000 – 5900]
Iceland	<500	[<1000]	...	<500	<500	[<1000]
Ireland	5500	[4100 – 7700]	4600	[3100 – 6400]	5500	[4100 – 7700]
Israel	5100	[2500 – 12 000]	3600	[1800 – 9400]	4900	[2500 – 12 000]
Italy	150 000	[110 000 – 210 000]	140 000	[100 000 – 190 000]	150 000	[110 000 – 210 000]
Luxembourg	...	[<1000]	<500	[<1000]	...	[<1000]
Malta	<500	[<1000]	<200	[<500]	200	[<500]
Montenegro	...	...	...	...	...	...
Netherlands	18 000	[10 000 – 32 000]	16 000	[9300 – 27 000]	18 000	[10 000 – 32 000]
Norway	3000	[1700 – 5000]	2400	[1500 – 4000]	3000	[1700 – 5000]
Poland	20 000	[11 000 – 34 000]	15 000	[8600 – 25 000]	19 000	[11 000 – 34 000]
Portugal	34 000	[20 000 – 63 000]	29 000	[18 000 – 51 000]	34 000	[20 000 – 63 000]
Serbia	6400	[3900 – 12 000]	5100	[3100 – 11 000]	6400	[3900 – 12 000]
Slovakia	<500	[<1000]	...	...	<500	[<1000]
Slovenia	<500	[<1000]	...	...	<500	[<1000]
Spain	140 000	[80 000 – 230 000]	120 000	[70 000 – 200 000]	140 000	[80 000 – 230 000]
Sweden	6200	[3500 – 11 000]	5300	[3100 – 9100]	6200	[3500 – 11 000]
Switzerland	25 000	[14 000 – 43 000]	22 000	[13 000 – 38 000]	25 000	[14 000 – 43 000]
The former Yugoslav Republic of Macedonia	<500	[<1000]	...	...	<500	[<1000]
United Kingdom of Great Britain & Northern Ireland	77 000	[37 000 – 160 000]	47 000	[27 000 – 82 000]	77 000	[37 000 – 160 000]
North Africa and Middle East	380 000	[280 000 – 510 000]	300 000	[210 000 – 400 000]	350 000	[250 000 – 490 000]
Algeria	21 000	[11 000 – 43 000]	12 000	[7000 – 28 000]	21 000	[11 000 – 43 000]
Bahrain	<1000	[<2000]	...	...	...	...
Cyprus	<500	[<1000]	...	...	...	...
Egypt	9200	[7200 – 13 000]	5700	[4500 – 7800]	9000	[7100 – 12 000]
Iraq	...	...	...	...	...	...
Jordan	<1000	[<2000]	...	...	...	...
Kuwait	<1000	[<2000]	...	...	...	...

ANNEX 1

1. Estimated number of people living with HIV

	Adults (15+) 2001		Adult (15–49) prevalence percent 2007		Adult (15–49) prevalence percent 2001		Women (15+) 2007	
Country	Estimate	[low estimate – high estimate]	Estimate	[low estimate – high estimate]	Estimate	[low estimate – high estimate]	Estimate	[low estimate – high estimate]
Republic of Moldova	<1000	[<200 – 1400]	0.4	[0.3 – 0.7]	<0.1	[0.1]	2600	[1700 – 4400]
Romania	14 000	[13 000 – 15 000]	0.1	[<0.1 – 0.2]	0.1	[<0.1 – 0.2]	7000	[5500 – 7700]
Russian Federation	390 000	[260 000 – 850 000]	1.1	[0.8 – 1.6]	0.5	[0.3 – 1.0]	240 000	[150 000 – 350 000]
Tajikistan	2400	[<100 – 5200]	0.3	[0.1 – 0.6]	0.1	[<0.1 – 0.2]	2100	[<1000 – 5000]
Turkmenistan	...	...	<0.1	[<0.2]	...	...	...	...
Ukraine	210 000	[180 000 – 250 000]	1.6	[1.2 – 2.0]	0.8	[0.7 – 1.0]	190 000	[140 000 – 230 000]
Uzbekistan	1400	[<1000 – 3700]	0.1	[<0.1 – 0.3]	...	[<0.1]	4600	[2100 – 12 000]
Western and Central Europe	**610 000**	**[490 000 – 810 000]**	**0.3**	**[0.2 – 0.4]**	**0.2**	**[0.1 – 0.3]**	**200 000**	**[160 000 – 270 000]**
Albania	...	...	...	[<0.2]	...	...	...	...
Austria	5500	[4700 – 6400]	0.2	[0.1 – 0.3]	0.1	[<0.1 – 0.2]	2900	[2100 – 3900]
Belgium	13 000	[7500 – 23 000]	0.2	[0.1 – 0.5]	0.2	[0.1 – 0.4]	4100	[2400 – 8400]
Czech Republic	1300	[<1000 – 2400]	...	[<0.1]	...	[<0.1]	<500	[<1000]
Denmark	3300	[2700 – 4000]	0.2	[0.1 – 0.3]	0.1	[<0.1 – 0.2]	1100	[<1000 – 1600]
Finland	2000	[1200 – 3700]	0.1	[<0.1 – 0.2]	0.1	[<0.1 – 0.2]	<1000	[<500 – 1300]
France	120 000	[66 000 – 200 000]	0.4	[0.2 – 0.7]	0.4	[0.2 – 0.6]	38 000	[21 000 – 68 000]
Germany	44 000	[27 000 – 79 000]	0.1	[<0.1 – 0.2]	0.1	[<0.1 – 0.2]	15 000	[8500 – 27 000]
Greece	8300	[4900 – 15 000]	0.2	[0.1 – 0.3]	0.1	[<0.1 – 0.2]	3000	[1700 – 5400]
Hungary	2800	[1700 – 4900]	0.1	[<0.1 – 0.2]	0.1	[<0.1 – 0.2]	<1000	[1600]
Iceland	<500	[<1000]	0.2	[0.1 – 0.4]	0.2	[0.1 – 0.3]	<200	[<500]
Ireland	4600	[3100 – 6300]	0.2	[0.1 – 0.3]	0.2	[0.1 – 0.3]	1500	[1100 – 2100]
Israel	3500	[1800 – 9100]	0.1	[<0.1 – 0.3]	0.1	[<0.1 – 0.3]	2900	[1500 – 6700]
Italy	140 000	[100 000 – 190 000]	0.4	[0.3 – 0.6]	0.4	[0.3 – 0.6]	41 000	[30 000 – 58 000]
Luxembourg	<500	[<1000]	0.2	[0.1 – 0.4]	0.2	[0.1 – 0.3]	<200	[<500]
Malta	<200	[<500]	0.1	[<0.1 – 0.2]	0.1	[<0.1 – 0.2]	...	[<100]
Montenegro	...	...	...	...	...	...	...	...
Netherlands	16 000	[9200 – 27 000]	0.2	[0.1 – 0.3]	0.2	[0.1 – 0.3]	4900	[2800 – 8600]
Norway	2400	[1500 – 4000]	0.1	[<0.1 – 0.2]	0.1	[<0.1 – 0.2]	<1000	[<500 – 1400]
Poland	15 000	[8600 – 25 000]	0.1	[<0.1 – 0.2]	0.1	[<0.1 – 0.2]	5500	[3000 – 9700]
Portugal	29 000	[17 000 – 50 000]	0.5	[0.3 – 0.9]	0.5	[0.3 – 0.8]	9400	[5500 – 18 000]
Serbia	5100	[3100 – 11 000]	0.1	[<0.1 – 0.2]	0.1	[<0.1 – 0.2]	1800	[1100 – 3500]
Slovakia	...	...	<0.1	[<0.2]	...	...	...	...
Slovenia	...	...	<0.1	[<0.2]	...	...	...	...
Spain	120 000	[70 000 – 200 000]	0.5	[0.3 – 0.8]	0.5	[0.3 – 0.8]	28 000	[16 000 – 47 000]
Sweden	5300	[3000 – 9100]	0.1	[<0.1 – 0.2]	0.1	[<0.1 – 0.2]	2900	[1600 – 4800]
Switzerland	22 000	[13 000 – 38 000]	0.6	[0.3 – 1.0]	0.6	[0.3 – 1.0]	9200	[5100 – 16 000]
The former Yugoslav Republic of Macedonia	...	...	<0.1	[<0.2]	...	...	...	...
United Kingdom of Great Britain & Northern Ireland	47 000	[27 000 – 82 000]	0.2	[0.1 – 0.5]	0.2	[0.1 – 0.3]	22 000	[11 000 – 48 000]
North Africa and Middle East	**280 000**	**[200 000 – 360 000]**	**0.3**	**[0.2 – 0.4]**	**0.3**	**[0.2 – 0.4]**	**190 000**	**[130 000 – 260 000]**
Algeria	12 000	[6900 – 27 000]	0.1	[<0.1 – 0.2]	0.1	[<0.1 – 0.2]	6000	[3100 – 12 000]
Bahrain	...	...	...	[<0.2]	...	...	...	...
Cyprus	...	...	...	[<0.2]	...	...	...	...
Egypt	5600	[4500 – 7700]	...	[<0.1]	...	[<0.1]	2600	[1900 – 3600]
Iraq	...	...	...	[<0.2]	...	...	...	...
Jordan	...	...	...	[<0.2]	...	...	...	...
Kuwait	...	...	...	[<0.2]	...	...	...	...

1. Estimated number of people living with HIV						
	Women (15+) 2001		Children (0–14) 2007		Children (0–14) 2001	
Country	Estimate	[low estimate – high estimate]	Estimate	[low estimate – high estimate]	Estimate	[low estimate – high estimate]
Republic of Moldova	...	[<500]	...	[<100]	...	[<100]
Romania	7100	[6600 – 7400]	...	[<500]	...	[<1000]
Russian Federation	86 000	[50 000 – 200 000]	5200	[3500 – 7500]	<1000	[2800]
Tajikistan	<500	[<100 – <1000]	<100	[<200]	...	[<100]
Turkmenistan	...	...	...	...	...	...
Ukraine	75 000	[62 000 – 95 000]	5100	[3900 – 6400]	1100	[<1000 – 1500]
Uzbekistan	<500	[<200 – <1000]	<200	[<100 – <500]	...	[<100]
Western and Central Europe	160 000	[120 000 – 210 000]	1300	[<1000 – 1800]	2100	[1600 – 3000]
Albania	...	...	...	...	...	...
Austria	1500	[1200 – 1800]	...	...	...	...
Belgium	3400	[2000 – 6100]	...	...	...	...
Czech Republic	<500	[<1000]	...	...	...	...
Denmark	...	[<100]	...	...	...	...
Finland	...	[<1000]	...	...	...	...
France	30 000	[17 000 – 52 000]	...	...	...	...
Germany	12 000	[6800 – 21 000]	...	...	...	...
Greece	2200	[1300 – 4000]	...	...	...	...
Hungary	<1000	[<500 – 1300]	...	...	...	...
Iceland	<100	[<200]	...	...	...	...
Ireland	1200	[<1000 – 1700]	...	...	...	...
Israel	2100	[1000 – 5300]	...	...	...	...
Italy	36 000	[26 000 – 51 000]	...	...	...	...
Luxembourg	<200	[<500]	...	...	...	...
Malta	...	[<100]	...	...	...	...
Montenegro	...	...	...	...	...	...
Netherlands	4100	[2300 – 7100]	...	...	...	...
Norway	<1000	[<500 – 1100]	...	...	...	...
Poland	3900	[2300 – 6700]	...	...	...	...
Portugal	7700	[4600 – 14 000]	...	...	...	...
Serbia	1300	[<1000 – 2900]	...	...	...	...
Slovakia	...	...	...	...	...	...
Slovenia	...	...	...	...	...	...
Spain	25 000	[14 000 – 42 000]	...	...	...	...
Sweden	2300	[1300 – 3900]	...	...	...	...
Switzerland	7300	[4200 – 13 000]	...	...	...	...
The former Yugoslav Republic of Macedonia	...	...	...	...	...	...
United Kingdom of Great Britain & Northern Ireland	12 000	[6900 – 22 000]	...	...	...	...
North Africa and Middle East	150 000	[110 000 – 200 000]	26 000	[18 000 – 34 000]	20 000	[8800 – 34 000]
Algeria	3000	[1700 – 7400]	...	...	...	...
Bahrain	...	...	...	...	...	...
Cyprus	...	...	...	...	...	...
Egypt	1500	[1100 – 2100]	...	...	...	...
Iraq	...	...	...	...	...	...
Jordan	...	...	...	...	...	...
Kuwait	...	...	...	...	...	...

ANNEX 1

1. Estimated number of people living with HIV					2. AIDS deaths			
	Young women (15–24) rate (%) 2007		Young men (15–24) rate (%) 2007		Deaths in adults and children 2007		Deaths in adults and children 2001	
Country	Estimate	[low estimate – high estimate]	Estimate	[low estimate – high estimate]	Estimate	[low estimate – high estimate]	Estimate	[low estimate – high estimate]
Republic of Moldova	0.2	[0.1 – 0.4]	0.4	[0.2 – 0.9]	<100	[<200]	...	[<100]
Romania	0.2	[0.1 – 0.3]	0.2	[0.1 – 0.3]	...	[<1000]	...	[<500]
Russian Federation	0.6	[0.3 – 1.0]	1.3	[0.6 – 2.3]	40 000	[23 000 – 71 000]	1900	[1100 – 6400]
Tajikistan	0.1	[<0.1 – 0.4]	0.4	[0.2 – 1.2]	<500	[<1000]	<100	[<200]
Turkmenistan	...	...	...	...	...	...	...	...
Ukraine	1.5	[1.0 – 2.0]	1.5	[0.6 – 2.2]	19 000	[14 000 – 25 000]	4000	[2400 – 6100]
Uzbekistan	0.1	[<0.1 – 0.2]	0.1	[<0.1 – 0.3]	<500	[<1000]	...	[<100]
Western and Central Europe	**0.2**	**[0.1 – 0.3]**	**0.2**	**[0.1 – 0.3]**	**8000**	**[4800 – 17 000]**	**9600**	**[6800 – 16 000]**
Albania	...	...	...	...	...	...	...	...
Austria	0.1	[<0.1 – 0.2]	0.2	[0.1 – 0.4]	...	[<100]	...	[<100]
Belgium	0.1	[<0.1 – 0.3]	0.2	[0.1 – 0.5]	<100	[<500]	<100	[<200]
Czech Republic	...	[<0.1]	<0.1	[0.1]	...	[<100]	...	[<100]
Denmark	0.1	[<0.1 – 0.2]	0.2	[0.1 – 0.3]	...	[<100]	...	[<100]
Finland	<0.1	[0.1]	0.1	[<0.1 – 0.2]	...	[<100]	...	[<100]
France	0.2	[0.1 – 0.5]	0.4	[0.2 – 0.8]	1600	[<1000 – 4100]	<1000	[<500 – 1700]
Germany	0.1	[<0.1 – 0.2]	0.1	[<0.1 – 0.2]	<500	[<100 – 1300]	<200	[<1000]
Greece	0.1	[<0.1 – 0.2]	0.2	[0.1 – 0.3]	<100	[<500]	<100	[<200]
Hungary	<0.1	[0.1]	0.1	[<0.1 – 0.2]	...	[<100]	...	[<100]
Iceland	0.1	[<0.1 – 0.2]	0.2	[0.1 – 0.4]	...	[<100]	...	[<100]
Ireland	0.1	[<0.1 – 0.2]	0.2	[0.1 – 0.3]	<100	[<200]	...	[<100]
Israel	0.1	[<0.1 – 0.2]	<0.1	[0.1]	<200	[<500]	<100	[<200]
Italy	0.2	[0.1 – 0.4]	0.4	[0.2 – 0.7]	1900	[<1000 – 5000]	3100	[1900 – 5200]
Luxembourg	0.1	[<0.1 – 0.3]	0.2	[0.1 – 0.5]	...	[<100]	...	[<100]
Malta	0.1	[<0.1 – 0.2]	0.1	[<0.1 – 0.2]	...	[<100]	...	[<100]
Montenegro	...	...	...	...	...	...	...	...
Netherlands	0.1	[<0.1 – 0.2]	0.2	[0.1 – 0.4]	<200	[<500]	<100	[<500]
Norway	0.1	[<0.1 – 0.2]	0.1	[<0.1 – 0.2]	...	[<100]	...	[<100]
Poland	0.1	[<0.1 – 0.2]	0.1	[<0.1 – 0.2]	<200	[<500]	...	[<100]
Portugal	0.3	[0.1 – 0.7]	0.5	[0.2 – 1.1]	<500	[<200 – 1100]	<1000	[<500 – 1200]
Serbia	0.1	[<0.1 – 0.2]	0.1	[<0.1 – 0.2]	<100	[<200]	...	[<100]
Slovakia	...	...	...	...	...	...	...	...
Slovenia	...	...	...	...	<100	[<200]	...	...
Spain	0.2	[<0.1 – 0.4]	0.6	[0.2 – 1.1]	2300	[<1000 – 6600]	3000	[1500 – 5700]
Sweden	0.1	[<0.1 – 0.2]	0.1	[<0.1 – 0.2]	<100	[<200]	...	[<100]
Switzerland	0.5	[0.2 – 1.0]	0.4	[0.1 – 0.9]	<500	[<1000]	<500	[<1000]
The former Yugoslav Republic of Macedonia	...	...	...	...	...	...	...	...
United Kingdom of Great Britain & Northern Ireland	0.1	[<0.1 – 0.3]	0.3	[0.1 – 0.6]	<500	[<100 – 1200]	<200	[<500]
North Africa and Middle East	**0.3**	**[0.1 – 0.5]**	**0.1**	**[<0.1 – 0.2]**	**27 000**	**[20 000 – 35 000]**	**22 000**	**[10 000 – 37 000]**
Algeria	0.1	[<0.1 – 0.2]	0.1	[<0.1 – 0.3]	<1000	[<500 – 1600]	<200	[<500]
Bahrain	...	...	...	...	...	...	...	...
Cyprus	...	...	...	...	...	...	...	...
Egypt	...	[<0.1]	...	[<0.1]	[<500]	<1000	...	<500
Iraq	...	...	...	...	...	...	...	...
Jordan	...	...	...	...	...	...	...	...
Kuwait	...	...	...	...	...	...	...	...

	3. Orphans due to AIDS				4. HIV prevalence (%) in most-at-risk groups in capital city					
	Orphans (0–17) currently living 2007		Orphans (0–17) living in 2001		Injecting drug users		Female sex workers		Men who have sex with men	
Country	Estimate	[low estimate – high estimate]	Estimate	[low estimate – high estimate]	Year	HIV (%)	Year	HIV (%)	Year	HIV (%)
Republic of Moldova	...	...	...	...	2007	17.5	2007	2.9	2007	4.8
Romania	...	...	...	...	...	...	...	...	...	...
Russian Federation	...	...	...	...	2006	10.3	...	...	2006	0.9
Tajikistan	...	...	...	...	2006	23.5	2006	3.7	...	...
Turkmenistan	...	...	...	...	...	...	...	...	...	...
Ukraine	...	...	...	...	2006	61.2	2006	4.0	2007	4.4
Uzbekistan	...	...	...	...	2005	17.9	2005	4.7	2005	10.8
Western and Central Europe	...	...	...	...	...	...	...	...	...	...
Albania	...	...	...	...	...	...	...	...	2005	0.8
Austria	...	...	...	...	...	...	...	...	...	...
Belgium	...	...	...	...	...	...	...	...	...	...
Czech Republic	...	...	...	...	...	...	...	...	...	...
Denmark	...	...	...	...	...	...	...	...	...	...
Finland	...	...	...	...	2007[1]	1.4	...	...	2007[1]	4.5
France	...	...	...	...	...	...	...	...	...	...
Germany	...	...	...	...	...	...	...	...	2007	10.7
Greece	...	...	...	...	2006	0.7	...	...	...	...
Hungary	...	...	...	...	2006	0.0	...	...	...	...
Iceland	...	...	...	...	...	...	...	...	...	...
Ireland	...	...	...	...	...	...	...	...	...	...
Israel	...	...	...	...	...	...	...	...	...	...
Italy	...	...	...	...	...	...	...	...	...	...
Luxembourg	...	...	...	...	...	...	...	...	...	...
Malta	...	...	...	...	...	...	...	...	...	...
Montenegro	...	...	...	...	...	...	...	...	...	...
Netherlands	...	...	...	...	...	...	...	...	...	...
Norway	...	...	...	...	...	...	...	...	...	...
Poland	...	...	...	...	...	...	...	...	...	...
Portugal	...	...	...	...	...	...	...	...	...	...
Serbia	...	...	...	...	...	...	...	...	...	...
Slovakia	...	...	...	...	...	...	...	...	...	...
Slovenia	...	...	...	...	2006	0.0	...	...	2006	2.1
Spain	...	...	...	...	2005	17.8	2005	2.2	2005	9.2
Sweden	...	...	...	...	2007	5.1	...	...	...	...
Switzerland	...	...	...	...	2006	10.9	...	...	2007	8.1
The former Yugoslav Republic of Macedonia	...	...	...	...	2006	0.8	2006	0.0	2006	2.8
United Kingdom of Great Britain & Northern Ireland	...	...	...	...	...	...	...	...	...	...
North Africa and Middle East	...	...	...	...	...	...	...	...	...	...
Algeria	...	...	...	...	...	...	2007	4.0	...	...
Bahrain	...	...	...	...	...	...	...	...	...	...
Cyprus	...	...	...	...	...	...	...	...	...	...
Egypt	...	...	...	...	...	...	...	...	...	...
Iraq	...	...	...	...	...	...	...	...	...	...
Jordan	...	...	...	...	...	...	...	...	...	...
Kuwait	...	...	...	...	...	...	...	...	...	...

[1] This data was reported in the 2007 UNGASS report.

1. Estimated number of people living with HIV						
	Adults and children 2007		Adults and children 2001		Adults (15+) 2007	
Country	Estimate	[low estimate – high estimate]	Estimate	[low estimate – high estimate]	Estimate	[low estimate – high estimate]
Lebanon	3000	[1700 – 7200]	2200	[1100 – 5600]	3000	[1600 – 7100]
Libyan Arab Jamahiriya	...	...	...	...	...	...
Morocco	21 000	[15 000 – 31 000]	13 000	[8800 – 19 000]	21 000	[15 000 – 31 000]
Oman	...	...	...	...	...	...
Qatar	...	...	...	...	...	...
Saudi Arabia	...	...	...	...	...	...
Sudan	320 000	[220 000 – 440 000]	270 000	[180 000 – 350 000]	290 000	[190 000 – 420 000]
Syrian Arab Republic	...	...	...	...	...	...
Tunisia	3700	[2700 – 5400]	2200	[1600 – 3300]	3600	[2600 – 5400]
Turkey	<2000	[<5000]	...	...	...	...
United Arab Emirates	...	...	...	...	...	...
Yemen	...	...	...	...	...	...
North America	1 200 000	[760 000 – 2 000 000]	1 100 000	[670 000 – 1 700 000]	1 200 000	[750 000 – 2 000 000]
Canada	73 000	[43 000 – 110 000]	49 000	[29 000 – 75 000]	73 000	[43 000 – 110 000]
United States of America	1 200 000	[690 000 – 1 900 000]	1 000 000	[620 000 – 1 600 000]	1 100 000	[690 000 – 1 900 000]
Caribbean	230 000	[210 000 – 270 000]	210 000	[180 000 – 240 000]	220 000	[200 000 – 250 000]
Bahamas	6200	[4000 – 8700]	5700	[4400 – 7500]	6100	[3900 – 8600]
Barbados	2200	[1500 – 3200]	2100	[1600 – 2800]	2200	[1500 – 3200]
Cuba	6200	[3600 – 12 000]	2400	[3900]	6200	[3600 – 12 000]
Dominican Republic	62 000	[52 000 – 71 000]	65 000	[53 000 – 76 000]	59 000	[50 000 – 69 000]
Haiti	120 000	[100 000 – 140 000]	98 000	[83 000 – 110 000]	110 000	[95 000 – 130 000]
Jamaica	27 000	[19 000 – 36 000]	23 000	[16 000 – 29 000]	26 000	[19 000 – 35 000]
Trinidad and Tobago	14 000	[9500 – 19 000]	12 000	[8200 – 17 000]	13 000	[9200 – 19 000]
Latin America	1 700 000	[1 500 000 – 2 100 000]	1 400 000	[1 200 000 – 1 900 000]	1 700 000	[1 400 000 – 2 000 000]
Argentina	120 000	[90 000 – 150 000]	100 000	[77 000 – 130 000]	120 000	[88 000 – 150 000]
Belize	3600	[2200 – 5300]	2900	[1700 – 4400]	3400	[2100 – 5000]
Bolivia	8100	[6500 – 11 000]	6200	[4900 – 8300]	7900	[6300 – 10 000]
Brazil	730 000	[600 000 – 890 000]	660 000	[520 000 – 810 000]	710 000	[580 000 – 870 000]
Chile	31 000	[23 000 – 39 000]	25 000	[20 000 – 32 000]	31 000	[23 000 – 39 000]
Colombia	170 000	[110 000 – 230 000]	140 000	[96 000 – 190 000]	160 000	[110 000 – 230 000]
Costa Rica	9700	[6100 – 15 000]	5200	[3200 – 8200]	9600	[6000 – 15 000]
Ecuador	26 000	[15 000 – 40 000]	19 000	[12 000 – 32 000]	25 000	[14 000 – 39 000]
El Salvador	35 000	[24 000 – 72 000]	28 000	[17 000 – 220 000]	34 000	[23 000 – 67 000]
Guatemala	59 000	[41 000 – 84 000]	52 000	[38 000 – 68 000]	53 000	[35 000 – 77 000]
Guyana	13 000	[7600 – 18 000]	12 000	[9500 – 17 000]	12 000	[7200 – 17 000]
Honduras	28 000	[18 000 – 44 000]	31 000	[18 000 – 61 000]	26 000	[17 000 – 42 000]
Mexico	200 000	[150 000 – 310 000]	180 000	[130 000 – 260 000]	200 000	[140 000 – 300 000]
Nicaragua	7700	[5300 – 15 000]	4400	[3200 – 15 000]	7500	[5200 – 15 000]
Panama	20 000	[16 000 – 26 000]	17 000	[13 000 – 21 000]	19 000	[15 000 – 26 000]
Paraguay	21 000	[12 000 – 38 000]	11 000	[7000 – 22 000]	20 000	[12 000 – 37 000]
Peru	76 000	[57 000 – 97 000]	57 000	[45 000 – 74 000]	74 000	[55 000 – 96 000]
Suriname	6800	[4200 – 12 000]	3500	[1700 – 5600]	6700	[4200 – 12 000]
Uruguay	10 000	[5900 – 19 000]	6300	[3400 – 25 000]	10 000	[5800 – 19 000]
Venezuela	...	...	...	...	...	...

1. Estimated number of people living with HIV

	Adults (15+) 2001		Adult (15–49) prevalence percent 2007		Adult (15–49) prevalence percent 2001		Women (15+) 2007	
Country	Estimate	[low estimate – high estimate]	Estimate	[low estimate – high estimate]	Estimate	[low estimate – high estimate]	Estimate	[low estimate – high estimate]
Lebanon	2200	[1100 – 5500]	0.1	[<0.1 – 0.3]	0.1	[<0.1 – 0.3]	<1000	[<500 – 2000]
Libyan Arab Jamahiriya	...	...	...	[<0.2]	...	...	...	...
Morocco	12 000	[8700 – 19 000]	0.1	[<0.1 – 0.2]	0.1	[<0.1 – 0.2]	5900	[4100 – 9100]
Oman	...	...	...	[<0.2]	...	...	...	...
Qatar	...	...	...	[<0.2]	...	...	...	...
Saudi Arabia	...	...	...	[<0.2]	...	...	...	...
Sudan	250 000	[170 000 – 320 000]	1.4	[1.0 – 2.0]	1.4	[1.0 – 1.8]	170 000	[120 000 – 250 000]
Syrian Arab Republic	...	...	...	[<0.2]	...	...	...	...
Tunisia	2200	[1600 – 3300]	0.1	[<0.1 – 0.2]	<0.1	[0.1]	1000	[<1000 – 1600]
Turkey	...	...	...	[<0.2]	...	...	...	...
United Arab Emirates	...	...	...	[<0.2]	...	...	...	...
Yemen	...	...	...	[<0.2]	...	...	...	...
North America	**1 100 000**	**[660 000 – 1 700 000]**	**0.6**	**[0.4 – 1.0]**	**0.6**	**[0.4 – 0.9]**	**250 000**	**[150 000 – 420 000]**
Canada	49 000	[28 000 – 74 000]	0.4	[0.2 – 0.6]	0.3	[0.2 – 0.4]	20 000	[11 000 – 32 000]
United States of America	1 000 000	[620 000 – 1 600 000]	0.6	[0.4 – 1.0]	0.6	[0.4 – 1.0]	230 000	[140 000 – 400 000]
Caribbean	**200 000**	**[170 000 – 230 000]**	**1.1**	**[1.0 – 1.2]**	**1.1**	**[0.9 – 1.2]**	**110 000**	**[95 000 – 120 000]**
Bahamas	5600	[4300 – 7300]	3.0	[1.9 – 4.2]	3.1	[2.3 – 4.1]	1600	[1000 – 2400]
Barbados	2100	[1600 – 2800]	1.2	[0.8 – 1.7]	1.2	[0.9 – 1.6]	...	[<1000]
Cuba	2300	[<100 – 3900]	0.1	[<0.1 – 0.2]	<0.1	[0.1]	1800	[1000 – 3600]
Dominican Republic	63 000	[50 000 – 73 000]	1.1	[0.9 – 1.2]	1.3	[1.0 – 1.5]	30 000	[25 000 – 35 000]
Haiti	94 000	[79 000 – 110 000]	2.2	[1.9 – 2.5]	2.2	[1.9 – 2.6]	58 000	[50 000 – 68 000]
Jamaica	22 000	[16 000 – 29 000]	1.6	[1.1 – 2.1]	1.4	[1.0 – 1.9]	7600	[5200 – 10 000]
Trinidad and Tobago	12 000	[8000 – 17 000]	1.5	[1.0 – 2.1]	1.4	[1.0 – 2.0]	7700	[5400 – 11 000]
Latin America	**1 400 000**	**[1 200 000 – 1 800 000]**	**0.5**	**[0.4 – 0.6]**	**0.5**	**[0.4 – 0.7]**	**550 000**	**[470 000 – 680 000]**
Argentina	100 000	[76 000 – 130 000]	0.5	[0.4 – 0.7]	0.5	[0.4 – 0.6]	32 000	[23 000 – 43 000]
Belize	2800	[1600 – 4100]	2.1	[1.2 – 3.1]	2.1	[1.2 – 3.1]	2000	[1200 – 3000]
Bolivia	6100	[4800 – 8100]	0.2	[0.1 – 0.3]	0.1	[<0.1 – 0.2]	2200	[1700 – 2900]
Brazil	640 000	[510 000 – 790 000]	0.6	[0.5 – 0.8]	0.6	[0.5 – 0.8]	240 000	[200 000 – 310 000]
Chile	25 000	[20 000 – 31 000]	0.3	[0.2 – 0.4]	0.3	[0.2 – 0.4]	8700	[6400 – 11 000]
Colombia	130 000	[95 000 – 190 000]	0.6	[0.4 – 0.8]	0.5	[0.4 – 0.8]	47 000	[32 000 – 66 000]
Costa Rica	5100	[3200 – 8100]	0.4	[0.2 – 0.6]	0.2	[0.1 – 0.4]	2700	[1600 – 4500]
Ecuador	19 000	[12 000 – 31 000]	0.3	[0.2 – 0.5]	0.3	[0.2 – 0.4]	7100	[3900 – 12 000]
El Salvador	28 000	[17 000 – 220 000]	0.8	[0.6 – 1.5]	0.8	[0.5 – 5.9]	9700	[6500 – 20 000]
Guatemala	48 000	[35 000 – 62 000]	0.8	[0.5 – 1.1]	0.8	[0.6 – 1.1]	52 000	[35 000 – 76 000]
Guyana	12 000	[9100 – 17 000]	2.5	[1.4 – 3.7]	2.5	[1.9 – 3.4]	7100	[4300 – 10 000]
Honduras	30 000	[18 000 – 56 000]	0.7	[0.4 – 1.1]	0.9	[0.5 – 1.6]	7400	[4600 – 12 000]
Mexico	170 000	[120 000 – 250 000]	0.3	[0.2 – 0.5]	0.3	[0.2 – 0.4]	57 000	[39 000 – 87 000]
Nicaragua	4300	[3100 – 15 000]	0.2	[0.1 – 0.4]	0.2	[0.1 – 0.5]	2100	[1400 – 3900]
Panama	16 000	[13 000 – 21 000]	1.0	[0.8 – 1.3]	1.0	[0.8 – 1.2]	5500	[4100 – 7600]
Paraguay	11 000	[6800 – 21 000]	0.6	[0.4 – 1.1]	0.4	[0.2 – 0.7]	5800	[3400 – 10 000]
Peru	56 000	[44 000 – 73 000]	0.5	[0.3 – 0.6]	0.4	[0.3 – 0.5]	21 000	[15 000 – 29 000]
Suriname	3400	[1700 – 5500]	2.4	[1.5 – 4.3]	1.3	[0.7 – 2.2]	1900	[1200 – 3500]
Uruguay	6300	[3400 – 25 000]	0.6	[0.3 – 1.1]	0.4	[0.2 – 1.4]	2800	[1600 – 5500]
Venezuela	...	...	...	...	...	...	...	...

1. Estimated number of people living with HIV

	Women (15+) 2001		Children (0–14) 2007		Children (0–14) 2001	
Country	Estimate	[low estimate – high estimate]	Estimate	[low estimate – high estimate]	Estimate	[low estimate – high estimate]
Lebanon	<1000	[<500 – 1500]	...	...	...	...
Libyan Arab Jamahiriya	...	...	...	...	...	...
Morocco	3300	[2200 – 5100]	...	...	...	...
Oman	...	...	...	...	...	...
Qatar	...	...	...	...	...	...
Saudi Arabia	...	...	...	...	...	...
Sudan	140 000	[100 000 – 180 000]	25 000	[18 000 – 33 000]	20 000	[8400 – 33 000]
Syrian Arab Republic	...	...	...	...	...	...
Tunisia	...	[<1000]	...	...	...	...
Turkey	...	...	...	...	...	...
United Arab Emirates	...	...	...	...	...	...
Yemen	...	...	...	...	...	...
North America	190 000	[120 000 – 320 000]	4400	[2600 – 7300]	5400	[3400 – 8900]
Canada	13 000	[7200 – 20 000]	...	...	...	...
United States of America	180 000	[110 000 – 300 000]	...	...	...	...
Caribbean	92 000	[79 000 – 100 000]	11 000	[9400 – 12 000]	8200	[6800 – 10 000]
Bahamas	1300	[<1000 – 1800]	...	[<200]	...	[<200]
Barbados	...	[<1000]	...	[<100]	...	[<100]
Cuba	<1000	[<100 – 1200]	...	...	...	...
Dominican Republic	34 000	[27 000 – 39 000]	2700	[2200 – 3300]	2700	[2200 – 3500]
Haiti	43 000	[36 000 – 51 000]	6800	[5800 – 8100]	4700	[3600 – 6200]
Jamaica	5800	[4000 – 7900]	...	[<1000]	<500	[<1000]
Trinidad and Tobago	6900	[4800 – 9700]	...	[<500]	...	[<500]
Latin America	450 000	[380 000 – 590 000]	44 000	[37 000 – 58 000]	36 000	[29 000 – 56 000]
Argentina	25 000	[18 000 – 34 000]	...	...	...	...
Belize	1600	[<1000 – 2400]	<200	[<500]	<200	[<500]
Bolivia	1500	[1100 – 2000]	...	...	...	...
Brazil	220 000	[170 000 – 270 000]	...	...	...	...
Chile	6500	[5000 – 8600]	...	...	...	...
Colombia	35 000	[24 000 – 51 000]	...	...	...	...
Costa Rica	1400	[<1000 – 2300]	...	...	...	...
Ecuador	4900	[2900 – 8500]	...	...	...	...
El Salvador	7200	[3900 – 52 000]	...	...	...	...
Guatemala	47 000	[35 000 – 62 000]	...	...	...	...
Guyana	7000	[5300 – 9600]	...	[<1000]	...	[<1000]
Honduras	7700	[4500 – 15 000]	1600	[1000 – 3000]	1500	[<1000 – 4000]
Mexico	46 000	[31 000 – 68 000]	...	...	...	...
Nicaragua	1100	[<1000 – 3900]	...	...	...	...
Panama	4300	[3200 – 5600]	...	...	...	...
Paraguay	2900	[1700 – 5700]	...	...	...	...
Peru	15 000	[11 000 – 20 000]	...	...	...	...
Suriname	<1000	[<500 – 1600]	<200	[<500]	<100	[<200]
Uruguay	1600	[<1000 – 6800]	...	...	...	...
Venezuela	...	...	...	...	...	...

1. Estimated number of people living with HIV					2. AIDS deaths			
	Young women (15–24) rate (%) 2007		Young men (15–24) rate (%) 2007		Deaths in adults and children 2007		Deaths in adults and children 2001	
Country	Estimate	[low estimate – high estimate]	Estimate	[low estimate – high estimate]	Estimate	[low estimate – high estimate]	Estimate	[low estimate – high estimate]
Lebanon	0.1	[<0.1 – 0.2]	0.1	[<0.1 – 0.4]	<200	[<500]	<200	[<500]
Libyan Arab Jamahiriya	…	…	…	…	…	…	…	…
Morocco	0.1	[<0.1 – 0.2]	0.1	[<0.1 – 0.2]	<1000	[1500]	<500	[<1000]
Oman	…	…	…	…	…	…	…	…
Qatar	…	…	…	…	…	…	…	…
Saudi Arabia	…	…	…	…	…	…	…	…
Sudan	1.0	[0.6 – 1.5]	0.3	[0.2 – 0.5]	25 000	[17 000 – 32 000]	21 000	[9200 – 35 000]
Syrian Arab Republic	…	…	…	…	…	…	…	…
Tunisia	<0.1	[0.1]	0.1	[<0.1 – 0.2]	<200	[<500]	…	[<200]
Turkey	…	…	…	…	…	…	…	…
United Arab Emirates	…	…	…	…	…	…	…	…
Yemen	…	…	…	…	…	…	…	…
North America	0.7	[0.6 – 0.9]	0.6	[0.3 – 1.0]	23 000	[9100 – 55 000]	18 000	[8900 – 37 000]
Canada	0.2	[0.1 – 0.4]	0.4	[0.2 – 0.7]	<500	[<1000]	<200	[<500]
United States of America	0.3	[0.1 – 0.6]	0.7	[0.3 – 1.3]	22 000	[9000 – 54 000]	17 000	[8800 – 36 000]
Caribbean	0.4	[0.3 – 0.6]	0.5	[0.3 – 0.7]	14 000	[11 000 – 16 000]	15 000	[12 000 – 18 000]
Bahamas	1.5	[0.3 – 2.8]	3.2	[0.8 – 5.5]	<200	[<500]	…	[<1000]
Barbados	0.6	[0.3 – 1.1]	1.3	[0.5 – 2.3]	<100	[<200]	…	[<200]
Cuba	0.1	[<0.1 – 0.2]	0.1	[<0.1 – 0.2]	<100	[<500]	<100	[<200]
Dominican Republic	0.6	[0.3 – 0.9]	0.3	[0.1 – 0.4]	4100	[3000 – 5100]	4800	[3700 – 6400]
Haiti	1.4	[1.0 – 1.8]	0.6	[0.2 – 0.9]	7200	[5800 – 8900]	7500	[5700 – 9900]
Jamaica	0.9	[0.5 – 1.4]	1.7	[0.8 – 2.8]	1500	[<1000 – 2200]	1200	[<1000 – 1700]
Trinidad and Tobago	1.0	[0.6 – 1.6]	0.3	[0.1 – 0.5]	…	[<1000]	<1000	[<500]
Latin America	0.2	[0.1 – 0.3]	0.7	[0.4 – 0.9]	63 000	[49 000 – 98 000]	47 000	[36 000 – 100 000]
Argentina	0.3	[0.2 – 0.4]	0.6	[0.3 – 0.9]	7000	[3800 – 11 000]	3700	[2500 – 5500]
Belize	1.5	[0.8 – 2.4]	0.5	[0.2 – 0.9]	<200	[<500]	<200	[<500]
Bolivia	0.1	[<0.1 – 0.2]	0.2	[0.1 – 0.3]	<500	[<1000]	…	[<500]
Brazil	0.6	[0.3 – 0.9]	1.0	[0.6 – 1.5]	15 000	[9700 – 22 000]	9400	[3500 – 16 000]
Chile	0.2	[0.1 – 0.3]	0.3	[0.2 – 0.5]	1100	[<1000 – 1800]	…	[<1000]
Colombia	0.3	[0.2 – 0.5]	0.7	[0.3 – 1.0]	9800	[6000 – 15 000]	5800	[4000 – 8600]
Costa Rica	0.2	[0.1 – 0.4]	0.4	[0.2 – 0.7]	<200	[<500]	…	[<200]
Ecuador	0.2	[0.1 – 0.3]	0.4	[0.1 – 0.7]	1400	[<1000 – 2600]	<1000	[1400]
El Salvador	0.5	[<0.1 – 0.9]	0.9	[<0.1 – 1.8]	1700	[<1000 – 18 000]	1200	[<100 – 26 000]
Guatemala	1.5	[0.6 – 2.4]	…	[<0.1]	3900	[2500 – 5500]	2900	[1800 – 4300]
Guyana	1.7	[0.2 – 2.8]	0.5	[0.2 – 0.9]	<1000	[<500 – 1100]	1300	[<1000 – 2000]
Honduras	0.4	[0.1 – 0.9]	0.7	[0.1 – 1.6]	1900	[<1000 – 3700]	3200	[1000 – 9900]
Mexico	0.2	[0.1 – 0.3]	0.3	[0.2 – 0.6]	11 000	[6000 – 19 000]	9900	[6800 – 15 000]
Nicaragua	0.1	[<0.1 – 0.2]	0.3	[0.1 – 0.5]	<500	[<1000]	<200	[<500]
Panama	0.6	[0.3 – 0.9]	1.1	[0.5 – 1.7]	<1000	[1400]	<1000	[1300]
Paraguay	0.3	[0.2 – 0.7]	0.7	[0.3 – 1.3]	<1000	[<500 – 1800]	<500	[<1000]
Peru	0.3	[0.1 – 0.4]	0.5	[0.2 – 0.8]	3300	[2000 – 5000]	2900	[2000 – 4200]
Suriname	1.4	[0.7 – 2.8]	2.7	[1.2 – 5.2]	…	[<500]	<200	[<1000]
Uruguay	0.3	[<0.1 – 0.7]	0.6	[0.1 – 1.4]	<500	[<100 – 1700]	<500	[<100 – 4000]
Venezuela	…	…	…	…	…	…	…	…

ANNEX 1

	3. Orphans due to AIDS				4. HIV prevalence (%) in most-at-risk groups in capital city					
	Orphans (0–17) currently living 2007		Orphans (0–17) living in 2001		Injecting drug users		Female sex workers		Men who have sex with men	
Country	Estimate	[low estimate – high estimate]	Estimate	[low estimate – high estimate]	Year	HIV (%)	Year	HIV (%)	Year	HIV (%)
Lebanon	...	...	...	...	...	...	...	...	...	...
Libyan Arab Jamahiriya	...	...	...	...	...	...	...	...	...	...
Morocco	...	...	...	...	...	...	2007	2.6	...	...
Oman	...	...	...	...	...	...	...	...	...	...
Qatar	...	...	...	...	...	...	...	...	...	...
Saudi Arabia	...	...	...	...	...	...	...	...	...	...
Sudan	...	...	...	...	...	...	...	...	...	...
Syrian Arab Republic	...	...	...	...	...	...	...	...	...	...
Tunisia	...	...	...	...	...	...	2007[1]	0.0	...	...
Turkey	...	...	...	...	2007	1.5	2007	1.6	2007	1.8
United Arab Emirates	...	...	...	...	...	...	...	...	...	...
Yemen	...	...	...	...	...	...	...	...	...	...
North America	...	...	...	...	...	...	...	...	...	...
Canada	...	...	...	...	2007[1]	13.2	...	...	...	...
United States of America	...	...	...	...	...	...	...	...	...	...
Caribbean	...	...	...	...	...	...	...	...	...	...
Bahamas	...	...	...	...	...	...	...	...	2007	8.2
Barbados	...	...	...	...	...	...	...	...	...	...
Cuba	...	...	...	...	...	...	2006	0.1	2006	0.9
Dominican Republic	...	...	...	...	...	...	2006	2.7	2004	11.0
Haiti	...	...	...	...	...	...	2007	5.0	...	...
Jamaica	...	...	...	...	...	...	2004	9.1	...	...
Trinidad and Tobago	...	...	...	...	...	...	...	...	2004	20.4
Latin America	...	...	...	...	...	...	...	...	...	...
Argentina	...	...	...	...	2007	6.7	...	...	2007	10.9
Belize	...	...	...	...	...	...	...	...	...	...
Bolivia	...	...	...	...	...	...	2007	0.4	2007	21.5
Brazil	...	...	...	...	...	...	...	...	...	...
Chile	...	...	...	...	...	...	2006	0.9	...	...
Colombia	...	...	...	...	...	...	...	...	2007	10.8
Costa Rica	...	...	...	...	...	...	2006	0.2	...	...
Ecuador	...	...	...	...	...	...	...	...	2007	19.3
El Salvador	...	...	...	...	...	...	2007	3.9	2007	17.8
Guatemala	...	...	...	...	...	...	...	...	...	...
Guyana	...	...	...	...	...	...	2005	26.6	2005	21.3
Honduras	...	...	...	...	...	...	2006	3.0	2006	6.3
Mexico	...	...	...	...	2005	2.8	2005	5.5	2006	9.9
Nicaragua	...	...	...	...	...	...	...	...	...	...
Panama	...	...	...	...	...	...	...	...	...	...
Paraguay	...	...	...	...	2006	9.1	2006	4.3	...	...
Peru	...	...	...	...	...	...	2006	0.5	2006	10.8
Suriname	...	...	...	...	...	...	2006	24.1	2006	6.7
Uruguay	...	...	...	...	...	...	...	...	...	...
Venezuela	...	...	...	...	...	...	...	...	...	...

[1] This data were reported in the 2007 UNGASS report.

Annex

Country Progress Indicators

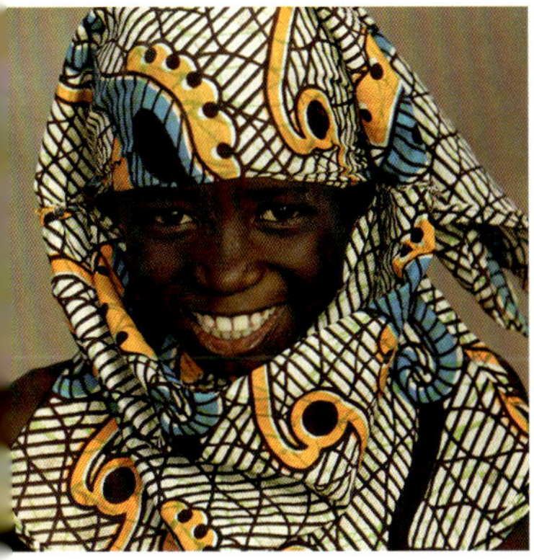

2

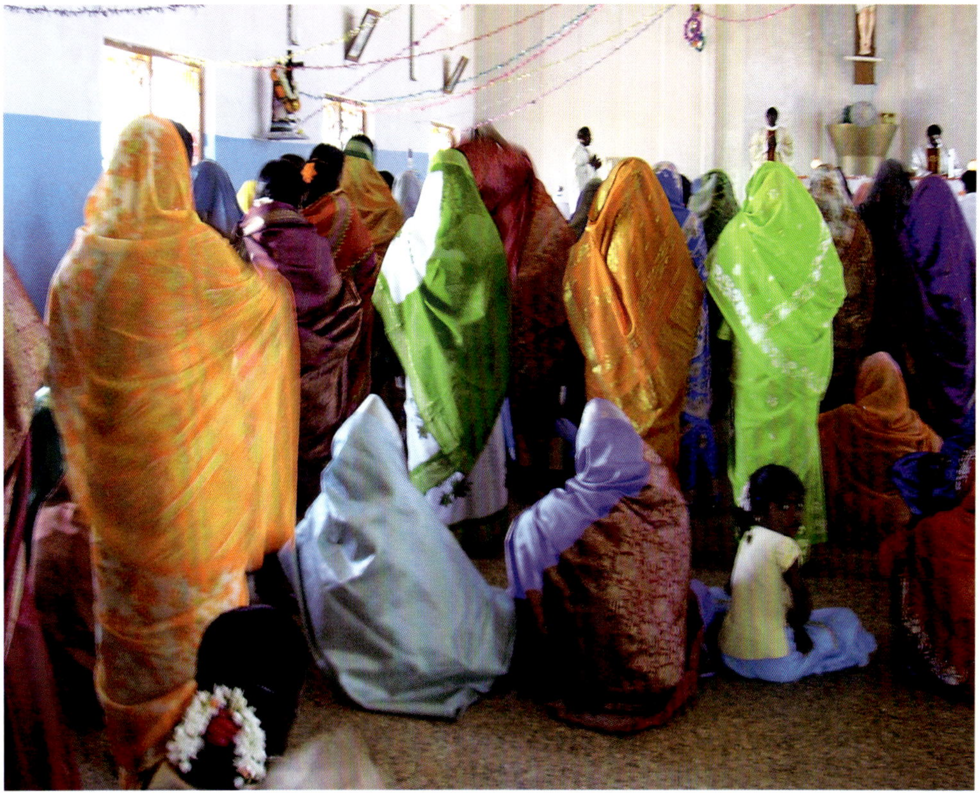

Annex 2

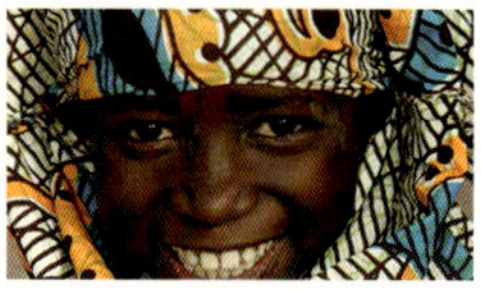

Country Progress Indicators

Country reporting and data validation

As of March 2008, 147 countries had reported on progress towards implementing the *Declaration of Commitment on HIV/AIDS* in their 2008 Country Progress Reports submitted to UNAIDS. Indicators reported were derived from the original UNGASS *Declaration of Commitment on HIV/AIDS* (2001). The data in the following tables reflect Country Progress Report data as well as information taken from other sources.

A comprehensive data review was undertaken by evaluation specialists at UNAIDS to check national reports for completeness, accuracy and harmonization with individual indicators. UNAIDS contacted 118 countries with follow-up data questions. Eighty per cent of questions regarding reported data were resolved through these communications. Data issues that were not resolved as of the publication date were not included in the data analyses summarized in this report. In addition a reconciliation process took place for data reported to UNAIDS, the Global Fund to Fight AIDS, Tuberculosis and Malaria; UNICEF; the US Government's President's Emergency Plan for AIDS Relief; WHO; and Measure Evaluation (data collected through the Demographic and Health Survey programme). As a result of discrepancies identified in this reconciliation, letters were sent to UNAIDS offices in 122 countries seeking clarification and resolution of outstanding data questions. Eighty-eight per cent of these 122 countries responded with clarifying information on coverage for antiretrovirals and prevention of mother-to-child transmission, and 50% responded to questions on other indicators. Only reconciled data values were used in the analyses discussed in this report.

The National Composite Policy Index (NCPI), a questionnaire that assesses progress in the development of national HIV policies and strategies, was validated through a separate process. Two evaluation specialists checked NCPI reports for internal consistency and completeness of the response. Confusing or illogical values were corrected; countries were contacted in cases of substantial missing data and multiple, non-consolidated NCPI submissions. Overall, UNAIDS contacted 34 countries to resolve data issues relating to the NCPI to which 31 countries responded. As there are over 200 data points for each country NCPI data are not included in Appendix B, but are available alongside individual country reports on the UNAIDS website. Validated data from 130 UN member states were included in the analyses summarized in this report.

Data tables

The following tables present data submitted to UNAIDS in Country Progress Reports, as a part of the monitoring of progress towards the *Declaration of Commitment.* To allow the reader to examine changes over time, where indicators and methods were consistent across reporting years, all available data from previous years are provided. Where possible the year that the data were collected was differentiated from the year of reporting. The percentages and numbers in the tables are given rounded to the nearest whole number. Some of the Country Progress Report data were still under review with countries at the time of production of this Annex. Where this is the case, it has been explicitly footnoted in the indicator data tables.

Where no data are available for a particular country for a given indicator, that country has been excluded from the relevant data table. Countries may not have submitted data for a given indicator either because no data was available with which to construct the indicator according to the UNGASS definition or because the country chose not to report on the indicator as it was considered not relevant to the county's epidemic.

Values printed in the table are those endorsed by countries. In some instances these values differ from those originally submitted as a result of the reconciliation process. As such, some values in these data tables may differ from those published in individual Country Progress Reports.

Where there were no data reported by a country for a specific indicator but data were available from another source, such as the Demographic and Health Survey, these data were included in the tables and are not necessarily the official data provided by the national governments. Where this was the case, the data source and year were clearly noted in the indicator data table and the specific indicator definition used is described and a reference for the source provided in the Notes Section following this Annex. These tables have been compiled and produced from the various data sources by staff at UNAIDS headquarters in Geneva who cannot take responsibility for the accuracy of the data from the original source.

Indicators

Since the first UNGASS progress report *Follow-up to the 2001 UNGASS: Progress Report on the Global Response to HIV/AIDS*, 2003 was compiled, core indicators for reporting have been consolidated and refined in each round of reporting, in collaboration with global partners and the UNAIDS Monitoring and Evaluation Reference Group (MERG), the international standards setting group for monitoring and evaluation. Revisions made to the UNGASS indicators since the last round of reporting are summarised below (Table 1). Instructions on how the indicators were constructed are available on the UNAIDS website in the document: *UNGASS Monitoring the Declaration of Commitment on HIV/AIDS: Guidelines on the Construction of Core Indicators (April 2007).*

In the previous round of UNGASS reporting, indicators were grouped into two categories according to the nature of the epidemic. The distinction between a generalized epidemic indicator set and a concentrated/low prevalence epidemic set has not been made for this round of reporting. This is due to the fact that epidemics do not fit neatly into simple dichotomous classifications. In 2006, for example, some countries with a generalized epidemic and a relatively high prevalence recognized that sub-epidemics in most-at-risk populations—sex workers, injecting drug users and men who have sex with men—were important in their epidemic and that prevention programmes for these populations were an essential element of their national response. Rightly, these countries chose to report on the indicators for these populations in addition to the generalized indicator set.

For this round of reporting all countries, regardless of their economic or epidemiological status, were requested to report on all indicators, where appropriate. Countries were expected to consider each indicator in light of the individual dynamics of their epidemic. When countries choose not to report on a particular indicator, they were asked to provide an explanation as to why they chose not to report, to allow for an analysis that differentiates between an absence of data and the inapplicability of particular indicators to particular country situations.

Table 1 Revisions to the UNGASS indicators since the previous round of reporting.

2005	2007	Comments on changes
National Commitment and Action Indicators		
Amount of national funds disbursed by governments in low- and middle-income countries	AIDS spending, by financing source	Definition changed
National Composite Policy Index	National Composite Policy Index	Questions added
Percentage of transfused blood units screened for HIV	Percentage of donated blood units screened for HIV in a quality-assured manner	Changed from transfused blood to donated blood. Added a second part to the indicator on the proportion of blood screened according to standard operating procedures and quality assurance
Percentage of women and men with advanced HIV infection receiving antiretroviral combination therapy	Percentage of adults and children with advanced HIV infection receiving antiretroviral combination therapy	Included children
Percentage of HIV-positive pregnant women receiving a complete course of antiretroviral prophylaxis to reduce the risk of mother-to-child transmission	Percentage of HIV-positive pregnant women who received antiretrovirals to reduce the risk of mother-to-child transmission	Definition changed
	Percentage of estimated HIV-positive incident Tuberculosis cases that received treatment for Tuberculosis and HIV	Indicator added to core list
	Percentage of women and men aged 15–49 who received an HIV test in the last 12 months and who know their results	Indicator added to core list
Percentage of most-at-risk populations who received HIV testing in the last 12 months and who know the results	Percentage of most-at-risk populations who received an HIV test in the last 12 months and who know their results	No changes
Percentage of most-at-risk populations reached by prevention programmes	Percentage of most-at-risk populations reached with HIV prevention programmes	Definition changed
Percentage of orphans and vulnerable children whose households received free basic external support in caring for the child	Percentage of orphaned and vulnerable children whose households received free basic external support in caring for the child	No changes
Percentage of schools with teachers who have been trained in life skills-based HIV/AIDS education and who taught it during the last academic year	Percentage of schools that provided life skills-based HIV education within the last academic year	Definition changed
Percentage of large enterprises/companies that have HIV/AIDS workplace policies and programmes		Removed from the core indicator list; incorporated in the NCPI
Percentage of women and men with sexually transmitted infections at health care facilities who are appropriately diagnosed, treated and counselled		Removed from the core indicator list; under revision for 2010 reporting

Knowledge and Behaviour Indicators		
Ratio of current school attendance among orphans to that among non-orphans, aged 10–14	Current school attendance among orphans and non-orphans aged 10–14	Ratio calculation no longer required
Percentage of young women and men aged 15–24 who both correctly identify ways of preventing the sexual transmission of HIV and who reject major misconceptions about HIV transmission	Percentage of young people aged 15–24 who both correctly identify ways of preventing the sexual transmission of HIV and who reject major misconceptions about HIV transmission	Suggest the replacement of the two misconception questions with local versions, where appropriate
Percentage of most-at-risk populations who both correctly identify ways of preventing the sexual transmission of HIV and who reject major misconceptions about HIV transmission	Percentage of most-at-risk populations who both correctly identify ways of preventing the sexual transmission of HIV and who reject major misconceptions about HIV transmission	Suggest the replacement of the two misconception questions with local versions, where appropriate
Percentage of young women and men who have had sex before the age of 15	Percentage of young women and men aged 15–24 who have had sex before the age of 15	Age range expanded
Percentage of young women and men aged 15–24 who have had sex with a non-marital, non-cohabiting sexual partner in the last 12 months	Percentage of women and men aged 15–49 who have had sex with more than one partner in the last 12 months	Age range expanded, definition changed
Percentage of young women and men aged 15–24 reporting the use of a condom the last time they had sex with a non-marital, non-cohabiting sexual partner	Percentage of women and men aged 15–49 who have had more than one sexual partner in the past 12 months who report the use of a condom during their last sexual intercourse	Age range expanded, definition changed
Percentage of female and male sex workers reporting the use of a condom with their most recent client	Percentage of female and male sex workers reporting the use of a condom with their most recent client	No changes
Percentage of men reporting the use of a condom the last time they had anal sex with a male partner	Percentage of men reporting the use of a condom the last time they had anal sex with a male partner	No changes
Percentage of injecting drug users who have adopted behaviours that reduce transmission of HIV, i.e. who both avoid sharing equipment and use condoms, in the last 12 months (for countries where injecting drug use is an established mode of HIV transmission)	Percentage of injecting drug users who report using a condom the last time they had sex	Composite indicator divided into component indicators (part 1)
	Percentage of injecting drug users who report using sterile injecting equipment the last time they injected	Composite indicator divided into component indicators (part 2)
Impact indicators		
Percentage of young women and men aged 15–24 who are HIV infected	Percentage of young women and men aged 15–24 who are HIV infected	No changes
Percentage of most-at-risk populations who are HIV infected	Percentage of most-at-risk populations who are HIV infected	No changes
Percentage of adults and children with HIV still alive 12 months after initiation of antiretroviral therapy	Percentage of adults and children with HIV known to be on treatment 12 months after initiation of antiretroviral therapy	Definition changed
Percentage of infants born to HIV-infected mothers who are infected	Percentage of infants born to HIV-infected mothers who are infected	Remains in core set but calculated at UNAIDS/ Geneva

Challenges in monitoring most-at-risk populations

Ensuring country-level representative samples and establishing a global response information system regarding programme coverage and risk behaviours for the most at risk populations presents significant technical and ethical challenges. Methods are being developed to try to achieve representative sampling of these hard-to-reach populations (e.g. respondent-driven sampling). While these methods are being refined, it is recognized that countries may not be able to attest to the representativeness of samples used for surveys of most-at-risk populations. The data from such behavioural surveillance surveys (BSS) which are often obtained from urban convenience samples in programme catchment areas, are likely to produce a bias when measuring service coverage and risk behaviours. Thus, countries were advised to report data for these indicators using the most recent survey of most-at-risk populations that has been reviewed and endorsed by technical experts within the country, such as monitoring and evaluation technical working groups or national research councils.

During the global data analysis a number of methodological differences among countries were observed in the approach for data collection on most-at-risk populations. These differences mostly relate to group definitions, measurement tools and time period applied for the data collection. All recognized differences are systematically presented in the footnotes provided in the tables.

On a country-level, it is important to interpret these indicator data along side the country reported NCPI, which provides an overview of the policy environment and programmatic response regarding most at risk populations in a given country, from both the perspective of the government as well as nongovernmental groups and civil society.

National Composite Policy Index

The NCPI questionnaire is completed through a review of relevant documents and through interviewing people most knowledgeable about the topics covered. One part[1] of the NCPI is completed by government officials, while another part[2] is completed by representatives from civil society and bi/multi-lateral organizations. The recommended consultative process for completing the NCPI aims to foster a conducive environment for inclusion of both government and nongovernment perspectives in the consolidated NCPI response submitted by the government as part of the UNGASS report. However, this is not always respected. The regional report on 2006 UNGASS data of the Caribbean noted that 'it is not always clear whose response prevails in case of discrepancies of opinions' (Reference: Keeping score: AIDS responses in the Caribbean: a consolidated analysis based on Caribbean reports submitted to the UNGASS 2006, p.25). To ensure full independence of the government and nongovernment responses, the government in Rwanda, for example, deliberately did not participate in the consensus meeting where the civil society NCPI responses were consolidated [Rwanda UNGASS Report, 2008]. On the whole, NCPI responses provided by the government are often more optimistic than those provided by nongovernment respondents. Where available, NCPI data on both perspectives were provided throughout the report.

1 Government officials complete questions on the national strategic plan, political support, and key policies and strategies of HIV programmes.

2 Nongovernment representatives complete questions on the country's human rights context in relation to HIV; civil society involvement in the HIV response; and key policies and strategies of HIV programmes.

Notes on specific indicators

1. AIDS Spending

As the national and international response to AIDS continues to scale up, it is increasingly important to accurately track in detail: i) how funds are spent at the national level and ii) where the funds originate. The data are used to measure national commitment and action, which is an important component of the UNGASS *Declaration of Commitment on HIV/AIDS*. In addition, the data help national-level decision-makers monitor the scope and effectiveness of their programmes. When aggregated across multiple countries, the data also help the international community evaluate the status of the global response. This piece of strategic information supports the coordination role of the National AIDS Authority in each country and provides the basis for resource allocation and improved strategic planning processes.

Since different countries can choose among different methodologies and tools to monitor the flow of AIDS funding—i.e. National AIDS Spending Assessments (NASA), AIDS sub-account of the National Health Accounts (NHA) and ad hoc Resource Flows Surveys—the National Funding Matrix includes a spreadsheet that allows financial data from any of these three methodologies to be easily entered, reviewed and reported. A "crosswalk" between NASA and NHA has been achieved for the AIDS health expenditures so there is now no difference between any of these tools to track AIDS-health expenditures; NASA simply provides more detail on expenditures on activities performed outside the health system, such as social mitigation, education, justice and other activities. A similar alignment process was undertaken for the UNFPA/UNAIDS/Netherlands Interdisciplinary Demographic Institute Resource Flows Project.

The purpose of this indicator is to collect accurate and consistent data on how funds are spent at the national level and where those funds are sourced

Definition: Domestic and international AIDS spending by categories and financing sources

This indicator is measured using a National AIDS Spending Assessment (NASA), which documents actual expenditures classified by eight AIDS Spending Categories and by financing source, including public expenditure from its own sources (i.e. government revenues such as taxes) and from international sources:

1. Prevention
2. Care and treatment
3. Orphans and vulnerable children[3]
4. Programme management and administration strengthening
5. Incentives for human resources
6. Social protection and social services (excluding orphans and vulnerable children)
7. Enabling environment and community development
8. Research (excluding operations research included under programme management).

Three main groups of financing sources:

1. Domestic public
2. International
3. Domestic private (optional for UNGASS reporting).

ANNEX 2

[3] In the context of resource needs estimates and AIDS Spending Assessments, vulnerable children are defined as those that have at least one parent who is alive but seriously ill (mainly because of HIV) and unable to take care of them.

2. Government HIV and AIDS Policies

National Composite Policy Index

The purpose of the National Composite Policy Index is to assess progress in the development and implementation of national-level HIV and AIDS policies and strategies.

The composite index covers the following broad areas of policy, strategy and programme implementation:

Part A- completed by government respondents

1. Strategic plan
2. Political support
3. Prevention
4. Treatment, care and support
5. Monitoring and evaluation

Part B- completed by civil society respondents

1. Human rights
2. Civil society involvement
3. Prevention
4. Care and support

3. Blood Safety

The purpose of this indicator is to assess progress in ensuring a safe blood supply. The indicator applies to all countries and it is measured annually using the WHO Global Database on Blood Safety protocol.

Indicator definition and components:

Definition: Percentage of donated blood units screened for HIV in a quality-assured manner.

Numerator: Number of donated blood units screened for HIV in blood centres/blood screening laboratories that have both: (1) followed documented standard operating procedures and (2) participated in an external quality assurance scheme

Denominator: Total number of blood units donated

4. HIV Treatment: Antiretroviral Therapy

The purpose of this indicator is to assess the progress of countries in providing antiretroviral combination therapy to adults and children with advanced HIV infection. The indicator is applicable to all countries and data for the numerator is collected continuously (monthly or quarterly) with the denominator estimated.

Indicator definition and components:

Definition: Percentage of adults and children with advanced HIV infection receiving antiretroviral therapy.

Numerator: Number of adults and children with advanced HIV infection who are currently receiving antiretroviral therapy in accordance with the nationally approved treatment protocol (or WHO/UNAIDS standards) at the end of the reporting period.

Denominator: Estimated number of adults and children with advanced HIV infection.

Notes on Methodology: all analysis of this indicator completed for the *Global Report*, including quoted country figures, reflect numerators which have gone through a tri agency reconciliation (UNAIDS/WHO/UNICEF) process and denominators which have been estimated directly from the UNAIDS/WHO Reference group on Estimates, Modelling and Projections methodology (Spectrum).

The reconciliation process ensured all agencies reported the same country endorsed figure which was the most recent and met the definition of people with advanced HIV currently on treatment. Every effort was made in cases of discrepancy across the three agencies to obtain approval from the country on a final indicator value. In cases where this was not possible, the country reported value has been footnoted.

For data representing 2007, some countries did not report data as of December 2007. In these instances the data were projected to December to reflect a consistent time period.[4]

The estimated denominators from UNAIDS/ WHO Reference group on Estimates, Modelling and Projections methodology were used for all analysis and quoted figures in the text to ensure consistency. The country reported denominators are included in Annex 2.

5. Prevention of Mother-to-Child Transmission

In the absence of any preventative interventions, infants born to and breastfed by HIV-infected women have roughly a one-in-three chance of acquiring infection themselves. This can happen during pregnancy, during labour and delivery or after delivery through breastfeeding. The risk of mother-to-child transmission can be significantly reduced through the complementary approaches of antiretroviral prophylactic regimes for the mother with or without prophylaxis to the infant, implementation of safe delivery practices and use of safe alternatives to breastfeeding. Antiretroviral prophylaxis followed by exclusive breastfeeding may also reduce the risk of vertical transmission when breastfeeding is limited to the first six months.

The purpose of this indicator is to assess progress in preventing vertical transmission of HIV

Indicator definition and components:

Definition: Percentage of HIV-infected pregnant women who received antiretrovirals to reduce the risk of mother-to-child transmission

Numerator: Number of HIV-infected pregnant women who received antiretrovirals during the last 12 months to reduce mother-to-child transmission

Denominator: Estimated number of HIV-infected pregnant women in the last 12 months

All analysis of this indicator completed for the *Global Report*, including quoted country figures, reflect numerators which have gone through a tri agency reconciliation (UNAIDS/ WHO/UNICEF) process and denominators which have been estimated directly from the UNAIDS/WHO Reference group on Estimates, Modelling and Projections methodology (Spectrum).

The reconciliation process ensured all agencies reported the same country endorsed figure which was the most recent and met the definition of HIV-infected women receiving antiretroviral drugs over the last 12 months, and thus reflect a full year. Every effort was made in cases of discrepancy across the three agencies to obtain approval from the country on a final indicator value. In cases where this was not possible, the country reported value has been footnoted in Annex 2.

For data representing 2007, some countries did not report data reflecting 12 months and in these instances the data were projected in order to reflect consistent time period.[5]

The estimated denominators from UNAIDS/ WHO Reference group on Estimates, Modelling and Projections methodology were used for all analysis and quoted figures in the text to ensure consistency. The country reported denominators are included in Annex 2.

6. Co-management of Tuberculosis and HIV Treatment

Tuberculosis (TB) is one of the commonest causes of morbidity and mortality in people living with HIV, even those on antiretroviral therapy. Intensified tuberculosis case-finding and access to quality diagnosis and treatment of tuberculosis in accordance with international/ national guidelines is essential for improving

4 Method for projection – all values reported that represent time earlier than December 2007 are projected taking the last two reported data points and calculating the growth per month, which is then used to project to December 2007.

5 Method for projection – all values reported that represent less than 12 month period are projected taking the number of HIV positive pregnant women on antiretrovirals per month and dividing by the number of months the data represents and multiplying by 12 months.

the quality and quantity of life for people living with HIV. A measure of the percentage of HIV-positive tuberculosis cases that access appropriate treatment for their tuberculosis and HIV is important.

The purpose of this indicator is to assess progress in detecting and treating tuberculosis in people living with HIV

Indicator definition and components:

Definition: Percentage of estimated HIV-positive incident Tuberculosis cases that received treatment for Tuberculosis and HIV

Numerator: Number of adults with advanced HIV infection who are currently receiving antiretroviral combination therapy in accordance with the nationally approved treatment protocol (or WHO/UNAIDS standards) and who were started on Tuberculosis treatment (in accordance with national Tuberculosis programme guidelines) within the reporting year

Denominator: Estimated number of incident Tuberculosis cases in people living with HIV

7. HIV Testing in the General Population

In order to protect themselves and to prevent infecting others, it is important for individuals to know their HIV status. Knowledge of one's status is also a critical factor in the decision to seek treatment.

The purpose of this indicator is to assess progress in implementing HIV testing and counselling

Indicator definition and components:

Definition: Percentage of women and men aged 15–49 who received an HIV test in the last 12 months and who know their results

Numerator: Number of respondents aged 15–49 who have been tested for HIV during the last 12 months and who know their results

Denominator: Number of all respondents aged 15–49

A number of countries chose to report on this indicator using data obtained through HIV testing programmes. These data are not comparable to data obtained through general population based surveys, and are footnoted in the data table.

8. HIV Testing in Most-at-risk Populations

In order to protect themselves and to prevent infecting others, it is important for members of most-at-risk populations to know their HIV status. Knowledge of one's status is also a critical factor in the decision to seek treatment. This indicator should be calculated separately for each population that is considered most-at-risk in a given country: sex workers, injecting drug users, and men who have sex with men.

The purpose of this indicator is to assess progress in implementing HIV testing and counselling among most-at-risk populations.

Indicator definition and components:

Definition: Percentage of most-at-risk populations who received an HIV test in the last 12 months and who know their results

Numerator: Number of most-at-risk population respondents who have been tested for HIV during the last 12 months and who know the results

Denominator: Number of most-at-risk population included in the sample

9. Most-at-risk Populations: Prevention Programmes

Most-at-risk populations are often difficult to reach with HIV prevention programmes. However, in order to prevent the spread of HIV among these populations as well as into the general population, it is important that they access these services. This indicator should be calculated separately for each population that is considered most-at-risk in a given country: sex workers, injecting drug users, men who have sex with men.

The purpose of this indicator is to assess progress in implementing HIV prevention programmes for most-at-risk populations

Indicator definition and components:

Definition: Percentage of most-at-risk populations reached with HIV prevention programmes

Numerator: Number of most-at-risk population respondents who replied "yes" to both (all three for injecting drug users) of the following questions

1. *Do you know where you can go if you wish to receive an HIV test?*
2. *In the last twelve months, have you been given condoms?*
3. *(Injecting drug users) In the last twelve months, have you been given sterile needles and syringes?*

Denominator: Total number of respondents surveyed

10. Support for Children Affected by HIV and AIDS

As the number of orphaned and vulnerable children continues to grow, adequate support to families and communities needs to be assured. In practice, care and support for orphaned children comes from families and communities. As a foundation for this support, it is important that households are connected to additional support from external sources.

The purpose of this indicator is to assess progress in providing support to households that are caring for orphaned and vulnerable children aged 0-17.

Indicator definition and components:

Definition: Percentage of orphaned and vulnerable children aged 0–17 whose households received free basic external support in caring for the child

Numerator: Number of orphaned and vulnerable children who live in households that received at least one of four types of support for each child

Denominator: Total number of orphaned and vulnerable children aged 0–17

For the purposes of this indicator and in accordance with UNICEF definitions (see reference below), an orphan is defined as a child below the age of 18 that has lost one or both parents.

A child made vulnerable by HIV is below the age of 18 and:

- i.) has lost one or both parents; or
- ii.) has a chronically ill parent (regardless of whether the parent lives in the same household as the child); or
- iii.) lives in a household where, in the last 12 months, at least one adult died and was sick for three of the four months before he or she died; or
- iv.) lives in a household where at least one adult was seriously ill for at least three of the past 12 months.

A number of countries chose to report on this indicator using data obtained through HIV testing programmes. These data are not comparable to data obtained through general population based surveys, and are footnoted in the data table.

11. Life Skills-based HIV Education in Schools

Life skills-based education is an effective methodology that uses participatory exercises to teach behaviours to young people that help them deal with the challenges and demands of everyday life. It can include decision-making and problem-solving skills, creative and critical thinking, self-awareness, communication and interpersonal relations. It can also teach young people how to cope with their emotions and causes of stress. When adapted specifically for HIV education in schools, a life skills-based approach helps young people understand and assess the individual, social and environmental factors that raise and lower the risk of HIV transmission. When properly implemented, it can have a positive effect on behaviours, including delay in sexual debut and reduction in number of sexual partners.

The purpose of this indicator is to assess progress towards implementation of life skills-based HIV education in all schools.

Indicator definition and components:

Definition: Percentage of schools that provided life skills-based HIV education in the last academic year

Numerator: Number of schools that provided life skills-based HIV education in the last academic year

Denominator: Number of schools surveyed

12. Orphans: School Attendance

AIDS is claiming ever growing numbers of adults just at the time in their lives when they are forming families and bringing up children. As a result, orphan prevalence is rising steadily in many countries, while fewer relatives within the prime adult ages mean that orphaned children face an increasingly uncertain future. Orphanhood is frequently accompanied by prejudice and increased poverty, factors that can further jeopardize children's chances of completing school education and may lead to the adoption of survival strategies that increase vulnerability to HIV. It is important therefore to monitor the extent to which AIDS support programmes succeed in securing the educational opportunities of orphaned children.

The purpose of this indicator is to assess progress towards preventing relative disadvantage in school attendance among orphans versus non-orphans.

Indicator definition and components:

Definition: Current school attendance among orphans and non-orphans aged 10–14

Part A: Current school attendance rate of orphans aged 10-14

Numerator: Number of children who have lost both parents and who attend school

Denominator: Number of children who have lost both parents

Part B: Current school attendance rate of children aged 10–14 both of whose parents are alive and who live with at least one parent

Numerator: Number of children both of whose parents are alive, who are living with at least one parent and who attend school

Denominator: Number of children both of whose parents are alive who are living with at least one parent

13. Young People: Knowledge about HIV Prevention

HIV epidemics are perpetuated through primarily sexual transmission of infection to successive generations of young people. Sound knowledge about HIV and AIDS is an essential pre-requisite—albeit, often an insufficient condition—for adoption of behaviours that reduce the risk of HIV transmission.

The purpose of this indicator is to assess progress towards universal knowledge of the essential facts about HIV transmission.

Indicator definition and components:

Definition: Percentage of young people aged 15–24 who both correctly identify ways of preventing the sexual transmission of HIV and who reject major misconceptions about HIV transmission

Numerator: Number of respondents aged 15–24 years who gave the correct answer to all five of the following questions:

1. *Can the risk of HIV transmission be reduced by having sex with only one uninfected partner who has no other partners?*
2. *Can a person reduce the risk of getting HIV by using a condom every time they have sex?*
3. *Can a healthy-looking person have HIV?*
4. *Can a person get HIV from mosquito bites?*
5. *Can a person get HIV by sharing food with someone who is infected?*

Denominator: Number of all respondents aged 15–24

ANNEX 2

14. Most-at-risk Populations: Knowledge about HIV Prevention

Concentrated epidemics are generally driven by sexual transmission or use of contaminated injecting equipment. Sound knowledge about HIV and AIDS is an essential prerequisite if people are going to adopt behaviours that reduce their risk of infection. This indicator should be calculated separately for each population that is considered most-at-risk in a given country: sex workers, injecting drug users, men who have sex with men.

The purpose of this indicator is to assess progress in building knowledge of the essential facts about HIV transmission among most-at-risk populations.

Indicator definition and components:

Definition: Percentage of most-at-risk populations who both correctly identify ways of preventing the sexual transmission of HIV and who reject major misconceptions about HIV transmission

Numerator: Number of most-at-risk population respondents who gave the correct answer to all five of the following questions:

1. *Can the risk of HIV transmission be reduced by having sex with only one uninfected partner who has no other partners?*
3. *Can a person reduce the risk of getting HIV by using a condom every time they have sex?*
3. *Can a healthy-looking person have HIV?*
4. *Can a person get HIV from mosquito bites?*
5. *Can a person get HIV by sharing food with someone who is infected?*

Denominator: Number of most-at-risk population respondents who gave answers, including "don't know", to all five questions

15. Sex Before the Age of 15

A major goal in many countries is to delay the age at which young people first have sex and discourage premarital sexual activity because it reduces their potential exposure to HIV. There is also evidence to suggest that first having sex at a later age reduces susceptibility to infection per act of sex, at least for women.

The purpose of this indicator is to assess progress in increasing the age at which young women and men aged 15–24 first have sex

Indicator definition and components:

Definition: Percentage of young women and men aged 15-24 who have had sexual intercourse before the age of 15

Numerator: Number of respondents (aged 15–24 years) who report the age at which they first had sexual intercourse as under 15 years

Denominator: Number of all respondents aged 15–24 years

16. Higher-risk Sex

The spread of HIV largely depends upon unprotected sex among people with a high number of partnerships. Individuals who have multiple partners (concurrently or sequentially) have a higher risk of HIV transmission than individuals that do not link into a wider sexual network.

The purpose of this indicator is to assess progress in reducing the percentage of people who have higher-risk sex.

Indicator definition and components:

Definition: Percentage of women and men aged 15–49 who have had sexual intercourse with more than one partner in the last 12 months

Numerator: Number of respondents aged 15–49 who have had sexual intercourse with more than one partner in the last 12 months

Denominator: Number of all respondents aged 15–49

17. Condom Use During Higher-risk Sex

Condom use is an important measure of protection against HIV, especially among people with multiple sexual partners.

The purpose of this indicator is to assess progress towards preventing exposure to HIV through unprotected sex with non-regular partners.

Indicator definition and components:

Definition: Percentage of women and men aged 15-49 who had more than one partner in the past 12 months who used a condom during their last sexual intercourse

Numerator: Number of respondents (aged 15–49) who reported having had more than one sexual partner in the last 12 months who also reported that a condom was used the last time they had sex

Denominator: Number of respondents (15–49) who reported having had more than one sexual partner in the last 12 months

18. Sex Workers: Condom Use

Various factors increase the risk of exposure to HIV among sex workers, including multiple, non-regular partners and more frequent sexual intercourse. However, sex workers can substantially reduce the risk of HIV transmission, both from clients and to clients, through consistent and correct condom use.

Note: countries with generalized epidemics may also have a concentrated sub-epidemic among sex workers. If so, it would be valuable for them to calculate and report on this indicator for this population.

The purpose of this indicator is to assess progress in preventing exposure to HIV among sex workers through unprotected sex with clients.

Indicator definition and components:

Definition: Percentage of female and male sex workers reporting the use of a condom with their most recent client

Numerator: Number of respondents who reported that a condom was used with their last client in the last 12 months

Denominator: Number of respondents who reported having commercial sex in the last 12 months

19. Men Who Have Sex with Men: Condom Use

Condoms can substantially reduce the risk of the sexual transmission of HIV. Consequently, consistent and correct condom use is important for men who have sex with men because of the high risk of HIV transmission during unprotected anal sex. In addition, men who have anal sex with other men may also have female partners, who could become infected as well. Condom use with their most recent male partner is considered a reliable indicator of longer-term behaviour.

Note: Countries with generalized epidemics may also have a concentrated sub-epidemic among men who have sex with men. If so, it would be valuable for them to calculate and report on this indicator for this population.

The purpose of this indicator is to assess progress in preventing exposure to HIV among men who have unprotected anal sex with a male partner.

Indicator definition and components:

Definition: Percentage of men reporting the use of a condom the last time they had anal sex with a male partner

Numerator: Number of respondents who reported that a condom was used the last time they had anal sex

Denominator: Number of respondents who reported having had anal sex with a male partner in the last six months

20. Injecting Drug Users: Condom Use

Safer injecting and sexual practices among injecting drug users are essential, even in countries where other modes of HIV transmission predominate, because: (i) the risk of HIV transmission from contaminated injecting equipment is extremely high; and (ii) injecting drug users can spread HIV (e.g. through sexual transmission) to the wider population.

The purpose of this indicator is to assess progress in preventing sexual transmission of HIV

Indicator definition and components:

Definition: Percentage of injecting drug users reporting the use of a condom the last time they had sexual intercourse

Numerator: Number of respondents who reported that a condom was used the last time they had sex

Denominator: Number of respondents who report having had sexual intercourse in the last month

21. Injecting Drug Users: Safe Injecting Practices

Safer injecting and sexual practices among injecting drug users are essential, even in countries where other modes of HIV transmission predominate, because: (i) the risk of HIV transmission from contaminated injecting equipment is extremely high; and (ii) injecting drug users can spread HIV (e.g. through sexual transmission) to the wider population.

Note: countries with generalized epidemics may also have a concentrated sub-epidemic among injecting drug users. If so, it would be valuable for them to calculate and report on this indicator for this population.

The purpose of this indicator is to assess progress in preventing injecting drug use-associated HIV transmission.

Indicator definition and components:

Definition: Percentage of injecting drug users reporting the use of sterile injecting equipment the last time they injected

Numerator: Number of respondents who report using sterile injecting equipment the last time they injected drugs

Denominator: Number of respondents who report injecting drugs in the last month

24. HIV Treatment: Survival After 12 Months on Antiretroviral Therapy

One of the goals of any antiretroviral therapy programme is to increase survival among infected individuals. As antiretroviral therapy is scaled up in countries around the world, it is also important to understand why and how many people drop out of treatment programmes. These data can be used to demonstrate the effectiveness of those programmes and highlight obstacles to expanding and improving them.

The purpose of this indicator is to assess progress in increasing survival among infected adults and children by maintaining them on antiretroviral therapy.

Indicator definition and components:

Definition: Percentage of adults and children with HIV known to be on treatment 12 months after initiation of antiretroviral therapy

Numerator: Number of adults and children who are still alive and on antiretroviral therapy at 12 months after initiating treatment

Denominator: Total number of adults and children who initiated antiretroviral therapy who were expected to achieve 12-month outcomes within the reporting period, including those who have died since starting antiretroviral therapy, those who have stopped antiretroviral therapy, and those recorded as lost to follow-up at month 12.

Revisions were made to this indicator to reflect minimal survival only. For this reason the indicator may reflect lower survival rate than the maximum survival definition which excludes individuals who stopped antiretroviral therapy, died, or were lost to follow-up. In cases where it is known a reported data value is not reflecting this definition, this information has been footnoted in the annex tables.

All analysis of this indicator completed for the *Global Report*, including quoted country figures, reflect numerators which have gone through a bi agency reconciliation (UNAIDS/WHO) process.

The reconciliation process ensured all agencies reported the same country endorsed figure which was the most recent and met the definition of minimum 12 month survival of one cohort. Every effort was made in cases of discrepancy between the two agencies to obtain approval from the country on a final indicator value. In cases where this was not possible, the country reported value has been footnoted in Annex 2.

Countries that provided reports on the implementation of the Declaration of Commitment (n=147)

High income

Antigua and Barbuda
Barbados
Bahamas
Cyprus
Estonia
Israel
Qatar
Slovenia
Trinidad and Tobago
Australia
Belgium
Canada
Switzerland
Germany
Spain
Finland
United Kingdom of Great Britain and Northern Ireland
Greece
Ireland
Japan
Netherlands
New Zealand
Sweden

Caribbean

Haiti
Cuba
Dominican Republic
Jamaica
Dominica
Grenada
Saint Kitts and Nevis
Saint Lucia
Saint Vincent and the Grenadines

East Asia

Mongolia
China

Eastern Europe and Central Asia

Kyrgyzstan
Tajikistan
Uzbekistan
Armenia
Azerbaijan
Bosnia and Herzegovina
Belarus
Georgia
Moldova
Ukraine
Bulgaria
Croatia
Kazakhstan
Lithuania
Latvia
Romania
Russian Federation

Latin America

Bolivia
Colombia
Ecuador
Guatemala
Guyana
Honduras
Nicaragua
Peru
Paraguay
Suriname
El Salvador
Argentina
Brazil

Belize
Chile
Costa Rica
Mexico
Panama
Uruguay

North Africa and Middle East

Sudan
Algeria
Jordan
Morocco
Tunisia
Lebanon
Turkey

Oceania

Papua New Guinea
Fiji
Micronesia, Federated States of
Marshall Islands
Tuvalu
Palau

South and South East Asia

Afghanistan
Bangladesh
India
Cambodia
Lao People's Democratic Republic
Nepal
Pakistan
Viet Nam
Indonesia
Iran, Islamic Republic of
Sri Lanka
Philippines
Thailand
Malaysia

Sub-Saharan Africa

Burkina Faso
Burundi
Benin
Democratic Republic of the Congo
Central African Republic
Côte d'Ivoire
Eritrea
Ethiopia
Ghana
Gambia
Guinea
Guinea-Bissau
Kenya
Comoros
Madagascar
Mali
Mauritania
Malawi
Mozambique
Niger
Nigeria
Rwanda
Sierra Leone
Senegal
Somalia
Sao Tome and Principe
Chad
Togo
United Republic of Tanzania
Uganda
Zambia
Zimbabwe
Angola
Congo, Republic of the
Cameroon
Cape Verde
Lesotho
Namibia
Swaziland
Botswana
Gabon
Mauritius
Seychelles
South Africa

Western and Central Europe

Albania
The former Yugoslav Republic of Macedonia
Hungary
Montenegro
Poland
Serbia

UNGASS indicator 1. Country Reports of Domestic and International AIDS Spending by service categories and financing sources.

Region/Reporting Country	Year of the expenditure	Total reported Domestic Public and International Expenditure (Million US Dollars)	Share by financing source					Total HIV Expenditures in selected services (Million US Dollars)		
								Prevention		
			Domestic Public (%)	International				Total for Prevention	Communication for social and behavioral change	Voluntary counseling and testing
				Bilaterals (%)	Multilaterals		All other international sources or not specified (%)			
					Global Fund (%)	UN and all other Multilaterals (%)				
Caribbean										
Antigua and Barbuda	2006	$0.157	65.9%	25.4%	8.7%	0.0%	0.0%	NA/NR	NA/NR	NA/NR
Antigua and Barbuda[1]	2007	$0.160	100.0%	NA/NR	NA/NR	NA/NR	NA/NR	NA/NR	NA/NR	NA/NR
Aruba[1]	2005	$0.010	100.0%	NA/NR	NA/NR	NA/NR	NA/NR	NA/NR	NA/NR	NA/NR
Aruba[1]	2006	$0.010	100.0%	NA/NR	NA/NR	NA/NR	NA/NR	NA/NR	NA/NR	NA/NR
Aruba[1]	2007	$0.010	100.0%	NA/NR	NA/NR	NA/NR	NA/NR	NA/NR	NA/NR	NA/NR
Bahamas[1]	2006	$2.145	71.6%	NA/NR	NA/NR	NA/NR	28.4%	$0.005	NA/NR	NA/NR
Barbados[1]	2006	$7.073	98.0%	NA/NR	NA/NR	NA/NR	2.0%	NA/NR	NA/NR	NA/NR
Cuba	2007	$41.927	80.9%	0.0%	19.1%	0.0%	0.0%	$6.385	$5.584	$0.801
Dominican Republic[1]	2007	$13.737	44.0%	NA/NR	NA/NR	NA/NR	56.0%	$4.121	NA/NR	NA/NR
Grenada[1]	2006	$1.050	NA/NR	NA/NR	NA/NR	NA/NR	NA/NR	NA/NR	NA/NR	NA/NR
Haiti	2006	$70.284	0.6%	67.3%	24.0%	6.50%	1.55%	$12.597	$1.882	$3.427
Jamaica	2005	$11.306	54.5%	5.8%	39.7%	NA/NR	NA/NR	NA/NR	NA/NR	NA/NR
Jamaica	2006	$10.362	65.9%	5.2%	28.9%	NA/NR	NA/NR	NA/NR	NA/NR	NA/NR
Jamaica	2007	$14.749	62.5%	2.0%	35.5%	NA/NR	NA/NR	NA/NR	NA/NR	NA/NR
Saint Lucia	2006	$1.000	21.4%	0.0%	7.8%	46.7%	24.10%	$0.604	$0.105	$0.014
Saint Lucia	2007	$0.772	21.6%	0.0%	13.9%	64.6%	0.0%	$0.446	$0.202	$0.042
Trinidad and Tobago	2006	$12.148	95.6%	0.0%	0.0%	4.4%	0.0%	$5.626	$3.218	$0.118
Turks and Caicos Islands	2006	$0.958	100.0%	NA/NR	NA/NR	NA/NR	NA/NR	NA/NR	NA/NR	NA/NR
Turks and Caicos Islands	2007	$1.109	100.0%	NA/NR	NA/NR	NA/NR	NA/NR	NA/NR	NA/NR	NA/NR
East Asia										
China	2006	$138.927	77.1%	4.6%	17.5%	0.8%	0.0%	$0.927	$0.927	NA/NR
China[2]	2007	$124.116	100.0%	NA/NR	NA/NR	NA/NR	NA/NR	$48.078	$46.392	$0.897
Japan	2006	$68.135	100.0%	0.0%	0.0%	0.0%	0.0%	$4.130	NA/NR	NA/NR
Mongolia	2007	$3.377	7.3%	23.6%	36.0%	19.2%	14.0%	$1.946	$0.179	$0.184
Eastern Europe & Central Asia										
Armenia	2007	$2.476	16.2%	7.3%	55.7%	20.8%	0.0%	$1.296	$0.101	$0.197
Azerbaijan	2007	$2.220	65.7%	0.0%	34.3%	NA/NR	0.0%	$0.851	NA/NR	$0.851
Belarus	2006	$13.133	68.19%	0.0%	28.53%	2.25%	1.03%	$9.745	$0.491	$0.977
Bulgaria	2005	$7.778	35.40%	0.0%	57.71%	6.89%	0.0%	$3.758	$0.336	$0.627
Bulgaria	2006	$6.604	48.8%	0.0%	43.0%	8.2%	0.0%	$3.114	$0.440	$0.491
Bulgaria	2007	$6.659	50.8%	0.0%	43.4%	5.9%	0.0%	$2.877	$0.418	$0.552
Croatia	2006	$8.424	73.8%	0.0%	23.0%	2.3%	0.9%	$3.743	NA/NR	$0.442
Georgia	2006	$5.263	10.9%	19.3%	56.5%	13.3%	0.0%	$2.563	$0.058	$0.066

ANNEX 2

UNGASS indicator 1. Country Reports of Domestic and International AIDS Spending by service categories and financing sources.

Total HIV Expenditures in selected services (Million US Dollars)

Prevention			Care and Treatment		Orphans and Vulnerable Children	Programme Support			Other HIV Expenditures
Programs for sex workers and their clients for MSM and programme for harm reduction for IDUs	Condom social marketing, public and commercial sector condom provision and female condom	Prevention of mother to child transmission	Total for Care and Treatment	Anti-retroviral therapy		Total for Program and management support	Programme management, planning and coordination	Monitoring and Evaluation[4]	
NA/NR	NA/NR	NA/NR	NA/NR	NA/NR	NA/NR	NA/NR	NA/NR	NA/NR	NA/NR
NA/NR	NA/NR	NA/NR	NA/NR	NA/NR	NA/NR	NA/NR	NA/NR	NA/NR	NA/NR
NA/NR	NA/NR	NA/NR	NA/NR	NA/NR	NA/NR	NA/NR	NA/NR	NA/NR	NA/NR
NA/NR	NA/NR	NA/NR	NA/NR	NA/NR	NA/NR	NA/NR	NA/NR	NA/NR	NA/NR
NA/NR	NA/NR	NA/NR	NA/NR	NA/NR	NA/NR	NA/NR	NA/NR	NA/NR	NA/NR
NA/NR	NA/NR	NA/NR	$0.704	$0.408	NA/NR	$0.145	$0.115	$0.001	$1.290
NA/NR	NA/NR	NA/NR	NA/NR	NA/NR	NA/NR	NA/NR	NA/NR	NA/NR	NA/NR
NA/NR	NA/NR	NA/NR	$32.604	$11.314	NA/NR	$0.176	$0.176	NA/NR	$2.762
NA/NR	NA/NR	NA/NR	$3.434	NA/NR	NA/NR	$2.473	NA/NR	NA/NR	$3.709
NA/NR	NA/NR	NA/NR	NA/NR	NA/NR	NA/NR	NA/NR	NA/NR	NA/NR	NA/NR
$0.914	$0.818	$3.288	$31.192	$13.910	$2.450	$20.286	$10.159	$4.639	$3.759
NA/NR	NA/NR	NA/NR	NA/NR	NA/NR	NA/NR	NA/NR	NA/NR	NA/NR	NA/NR
NA/NR	NA/NR	NA/NR	NA/NR	NA/NR	NA/NR	NA/NR	NA/NR	NA/NR	NA/NR
NA/NR	NA/NR	NA/NR	NA/NR	NA/NR	NA/NR	NA/NR	NA/NR	NA/NR	NA/NR
$0.001	$0.103	$0.010	$0.066	$0.015	$0.052	$0.080	$0.048	$0.025	$0.198
$0.005	$0.050	$0.001	$0.077	$0.029	$0.075	$0.139	$0.051	$0.086	$0.036
$0.651	$0.170	$0.113	$3.989	$1.184	$0.131	$1.778	$1.405	$0.054	$0.624
NA/NR	NA/NR	NA/NR	NA/NR	NA/NR	NA/NR	NA/NR	NA/NR	NA/NR	NA/NR
NA/NR	NA/NR	NA/NR	NA/NR	NA/NR	NA/NR	NA/NR	NA/NR	NA/NR	NA/NR
NA/NR	NA/NR	NA/NR	$1.012	NA/NR	$0.505	$7.300	$4.781	$2.329	$129.153
NA/NR	NA/NR	NA/NR	$56.583	$43.669	NA/NR	$17.362	$0.947	$4.502	$2.093
NA/NR	NA/NR	NA/NR	$9.389	NA/NR	NA/NR	$17.398	NA/NR	NA/NR	$37.218
$0.312	$0.291	$0.076	$0.205	$0.010	$0.016	$0.801	$0.453	$0.198	$0.409
$0.154	$0.016	$0.045	$0.392	$0.098	$0.004	$0.287	$0.188	$0.099	$0.498
NA/NR	NA/NR	NA/NR	$0.500	$0.417	NA/NR	$0.411	$0.411	NA/NR	$0.458
NA/NR	$0.233	$0.366	$1.443	$0.823	$0.084	$0.854	$0.233	$0.221	$1.007
$0.842	NA/NR	NA/NR	$2.689	$1.614	NA/NR	$0.561	$0.337	$0.135	$0.770
$0.588	$0.122	NA/NR	$2.585	$1.955	NA/NR	$0.363	$0.218	$0.087	$0.543
$0.597	NA/NR	NA/NR	$2.932	$2.025	NA/NR	$0.348	$0.209	$0.084	$0.501
$0.509	NA/NR	NA/NR	$4.354	NA/NR	NA/NR	$0.328	$0.125	$0.080	NA/NR
$1.025	$0.079	$0.225	$0.839	$0.552	NA/NR	$1.036	$0.206	$0.088	$0.824

UNGASS indicator 1. Country Reports of Domestic and International AIDS Spending by service categories and financing sources.

Region/Reporting Country	Year of the expenditure	Total reported Domestic Public and International Expenditure (Million US Dollars)	Share by financing source					Total HIV Expenditures in selected services (Million US Dollars)		
				International				Prevention		
			Domestic Public (%)	Bilaterals (%)	Multilaterals		All other international sources or not specified (%)	Total for Prevention	Communication for social and behavioral change	Voluntary counseling and testing
					Global Fund (%)	UN and all other Multilaterals (%)				
Kazakhstan	2007	$17.959	70.0%	1.3%	27.3%	0.6%	0.7%	$3.392	$0.111	NA/NR
Kyrgyzstan	2006	$7.917	8.8%	8.7%	38.7%	43.8%	0.0%	$6.469	$0.049	$0.088
Latvia[1]	2006	$5.748	98.7%	NA/NR	NA/NR	NA/NR	1.3%	$0.996	$0.032	$0.186
Republic of Moldova	2007	$8.186	26.9%	19.0%	17.1%	31.9%	5.1%	$6.292	$0.903	$0.325
Romania	2006	$76.088	93.1%	0.0%	5.4%	1.4%	0.0%	$5.239	NA/NR	NA/NR
Russian Federation[1]	2006	$304.835	83.4%	0.0%	11.6%	0.3%	4.7%	$61.749	NA/NR	NA/NR
Tajikistan	2006	$5.211	5.7%	19.4%	36.6%	19.8%	18.5%	$2.509	$0.173	$0.140
Ukraine	2005	$39.414	42.9%	17.1%	32.9%	5.5%	1.7%	$7.442	$0.025	$0.373
Ukraine	2006	$55.417	50.8%	8.2%	36.3%	3.1%	1.6%	$17.067	$0.197	$0.715
Latin America										
Argentina	2006	$149.527	96.7%	0.1%	2.9%	0.2%	0.2%	$24.855	$2.141	$3.011
Bolivia	2005	$1.833	9.6%	44.7%	21.4%	NA/NR	24.2%	$0.918	$0.182	NA/NR
Bolivia	2006	$4.025	9.1%	16.6%	51.6%	3.0%	19.8%	$1.242	$0.228	NA/NR
Bolivia	2007	$3.183	16.9%	40.7%	16.5%	5.7%	20.1%	$1.252	$0.209	NA/NR
Brazil[1]	2006	$565.186	99.5%	0.1%	0.0%	0.3%	0.0%	$34.159	$9.903	$2.455
Chile	2005	$54.070	83.6%	0.0%	16.4%	0.0%	0.0%	$9.472	$0.555	$0.430
Colombia	2006	$97.645	98.91%	0.0%	0.92%	0.14%	0.0%	$34.662	$2.799	$0.031
Costa Rica	2006	$11.271	89.6%	0.0%	9.1%	0.8%	0.6%	$3.418	$0.707	NA/NR
Ecuador[1]	2005	$2.951	88.9%	0.0%	4.2%	6.8%	0.0%	$0.545	$0.013	$0.250
Ecuador[1]	2006	$10.209	31.9%	0.0%	61.8%	4.6%	1.7%	$2.942	$0.052	$0.489
Ecuador[1]	2007	$7.473	42.8%	0.0%	38.6%	3.7%	14.8%	$2.413	$0.022	$0.435
El Salvador	2006	$33.128	82.0%	1.3%	8.4%	7.7%	0.6%	$9.691	$1.483	$1.135
Guatemala[1]	2005	$19.142	66.4%	NA/NR	NA/NR	NA/NR	33.6%	NA/NR	NA/NR	NA/NR
Guatemala[1]	2006	$18.957	65.0%	NA/NR	NA/NR	NA/NR	35.0%	NA/NR	NA/NR	NA/NR
Honduras	2006	$14.354	28.9%	23.5%	28.5%	4.4%	14.5%	$6.183	$0.430	$0.943
Mexico[1]	2005	$176.052	99.2%	0.1%	0.0%	0.0%	0.7%	$40.663	$0.291	$2.950
Panama	2006	$14.164	97.3%	0.0%	0.0%	2.7%	0.0%	$0.438	NA/NR	$0.038
Paraguay	2006	$1.018	75.5%	0.0%	0.0%	17.2%	7.3%	$0.234	NA/NR	$0.111
Paraguay	2007	$2.326	47.8%	0.0%	31.2%	11.2%	9.7%	$0.796	NA/NR	$0.154
Peru	2005	$21.875	41.33%	6.63%	34.06%	2.86%	15.12%	$5.115	$0.063	NA/NR
Peru	2006	$32.387	41.07%	1.72%	32.0%	1.74%	23.47%	$4.769	$0.197	NA/NR
Peru	2007	$28.008	44.5%	3.6%	21.8%	4.4%	25.7%	$9.060	$0.978	NA/NR
Uruguay[1]	2005	$6.245	94.9%	NA/NR	NA/NR	NA/NR	5.1%	$0.770	$0.030	$0.162
Uruguay[1]	2006	$5.731	93.3%	NA/NR	NA/NR	NA/NR	6.7%	$0.852	$0.081	$0.168

UNGASS indicator 1. Country Reports of Domestic and International AIDS Spending by service categories and financing sources.

Total HIV Expenditures in selected services (Million US Dollars)

Prevention			Care and Treatment		Orphans and Vulnerable Children	Programme Support			Other HIV Expenditures
Programs for sex workers and their clients for MSM and programme for harm reduction for IDUs	Condom social marketing, public and commercial sector condom provision and female condom	Prevention of mother to child transmission	Total for Care and Treatment	Anti-retroviral therapy		Total for Program and management support	Programme management, planning and coordination	Monitoring and Evaluation[4]	
$0.030	$0.899	NA/NR	$2.400	$2.066	NA/NR	$11.850	$0.158	$0.181	$0.317
$0.610	$0.016	NA/NR	$0.847	$0.169	$0.033	$0.470	$0.355	$0.030	$0.098
$0.338	NA/NR	$0.028	$4.400	$4.400	NA/NR	$0.352	$0.352	NA/NR	NA/NR
$0.332	NA/NR	$0.231	$0.680	$0.456	NA/NR	$1.137	$0.185	$0.337	$0.078
NA/NR	NA/NR	NA/NR	$57.796	NA/NR	NA/NR	$0.322	NA/NR	NA/NR	$12.732
NA/NR	NA/NR	NA/NR	$96.798	NA/NR	$32.610	$18.636	NA/NR	NA/NR	$95.041
$0.285	$0.105	$0.030	$0.144	$0.114	$0.020	$0.335	$0.144	$0.095	$2.203
$3.174	NA/NR	$0.837	$15.751	$2.416	$0.952	$7.678	$3.342	$0.991	$7.591
$7.267	NA/NR	$0.529	$23.289	$5.352	$0.901	$10.434	$2.675	$0.356	$3.727
$0.544	$1.034	$4.842	$107.280	$58.897	$1.272	$6.915	$1.682	$0.659	$9.206
$0.006	$0.004	$0.001	$0.483	$0.247	NA/NR	$0.266	$0.102	$0.038	$0.166
$0.002	$0.002	$0.004	$1.881	$1.664	NA/NR	$0.653	$0.239	$0.100	$0.248
$0.028	$0.044	$0.001	$0.766	$0.450	NA/NR	$0.868	$0.526	$0.090	$0.297
$0.405	$7.440	$5.155	$470.055	$438.384	$0.148	$25.403	$19.971	$4.899	$35.420
$0.108	$0.983	$1.919	$40.429	$36.318	NA/NR	$2.204	$1.554	$0.276	$1.966
NA/NR	$6.967	$2.132	$62.074	$36.541	$0.035	$0.774	$0.774	NA/NR	$0.100
NA/NR	$0.080	NA/NR	$7.681	$4.141	$0.057	$0.072	NA/NR	$0.011	$0.042
NA/NR	NA/NR	$0.011	$1.661	$1.468	$0.019	$0.534	$0.033	NA/NR	$0.191
NA/NR	$0.027	$0.534	$3.986	$1.932	$0.003	$1.201	$0.095	$0.102	$2.078
$0.013	$0.283	$0.188	$3.125	$2.358	NA/NR	$0.376	$0.118	$0.146	$1.559
$0.055	$1.450	$1.019	$20.867	$7.551	$0.399	$1.024	$0.510	$0.335	$1.147
NA/NR	NA/NR	NA/NR	NA/NR	NA/NR	NA/NR	NA/NR	NA/NR	NA/NR	NA/NR
NA/NR	NA/NR	NA/NR	NA/NR	NA/NR	NA/NR	NA/NR	NA/NR	NA/NR	NA/NR
$0.499	$0.305	$0.420	$4.204	$2.420	$0.030	$3.687	$1.659	$1.145	$0.250
$5.227	$3.369	$4.472	$122.333	$103.396	$0.036	$12.404	$3.737	$1.149	$0.615
$0.073	NA/NR	$0.011	$13.425	$13.422	$0.012	$0.206	$0.071	NA/NR	$0.083
NA/NR	$0.020	$0.059	$0.481	$0.163	NA/NR	$0.009	$0.005	$0.004	$0.294
$0.088	$0.036	$0.091	$0.683	$0.374	NA/NR	$0.168	$0.045	$0.063	$0.679
$1.128	$0.808	$0.555	$13.168	$7.806	NA/NR	$0.543	$0.311	$0.225	$3.049
$0.798	$0.763	$0.970	$20.738	$13.858	NA/NR	$0.688	$0.286	$0.378	$6.192
$1.935	$1.781	$1.428	$12.448	$3.163	$0.090	$0.948	$0.491	$0.436	$5.461
$0.042	$0.079	$0.073	$4.237	$3.816	NA/NR	$0.135	NA/NR	$0.014	$1.103
$0.037	$0.069	$0.052	$3.549	$3.074	NA/NR	$0.196	NA/NR	$0.015	$1.135

UNGASS indicator 1. Country Reports of Domestic and International AIDS Spending by service categories and financing sources.

Region/Reporting Country	Year of the expenditure	Total reported Domestic Public and International Expenditure (Million US Dollars)	Share by financing source					Total HIV Expenditures in selected services (Million US Dollars)		
								Prevention		
			Domestic Public (%)	International				Total for Prevention	Communication for social and behavioral change	Voluntary counseling and testing
				Bilaterals (%)	Multilaterals		All other international sources or not specified (%)			
					Global Fund (%)	UN and all other Multilaterals (%)				
Middle East & North Africa										
Algeria	2006	$3.674	30.9%	0.0%	65.2%	3.9%	0.0%	$1.561	$0.038	$0.046
Jordan	2007	$2.697	5.1%	NA/NR	NA/NR	NA/NR	94.9%	NA/NR	NA/NR	NA/NR
Lebanon	2007	$2.735	30.5%	36.2%	0.0%	17.1%	16.2%	$1.445	$0.050	$0.055
Morocco	2006	$6.900	33.0%	9.8%	32.5%	11.9%	12.8%	$2.996	NA/NR	NA/NR
Morocco	2007	$8.833	30.5%	3.4%	54.5%	8.4%	3.2%	$4.147	NA/NR	NA/NR
Sudan, North[1]	2007	$15.985	8.8%	0.0%	57.9%	33.4%	0.0%	$8.923	$1.024	$0.731
Sudan, South[1]	2006	$0.260	NA/NR	NA/NR	NA/NR	100.0%	NA/NR	NA/NR	NA/NR	NA/NR
Sudan, South[1]	2007	$1.313	NA/NR	NA/NR	NA/NR	100.0%	NA/NR	$0.518	$0.259	$0.152
Turkey[1]	2006	$54.175	92.3%	0.0%	3.2%	4.6%	0.0%	$27.657	$0.145	$0.055
Turkey[1]	2007	$56.472	89.3%	0.0%	3.5%	7.2%	0.0%	$25.265	$0.087	$0.089
Oceania										
Australia	2006	$101.415	100.0%	0.0%	0.0%	0.0%	0.0%	$1.898	$0.079	NA/NR
Marshall Islands	2007	$0.123	100.0%	0.0%	0.0%	0.0%	0.0%	NA/NR	NA/NR	NA/NR
Palau	2007	$0.333	16.4%	0.0%	10.7%	0.0%	72.9%	$0.148	$0.005	$0.026
South & South East Asia										
Cambodia	2006	$44.179	13.7%	42.5%	21.5%	19.2%	3.2%	$19.948	$0.685	$2.587
Indonesia	2006	$56.577	26.6%	47.7%	18.5%	7.2%	0.0%	$23.180	$3.765	$0.128
Iran (Islamic Republic of)	2006	$32.778	90.8%	0.0%	5.9%	3.3%	0.0%	$20.483	NA/NR	NA/NR
Lao People's Democratic Republic[1]	2006	$4.676	0.5%	NA/NR	NA/NR	NA/NR	99.5%	NA/NR	NA/NR	NA/NR
Lao People's Democratic Republic[1]	2007	$5.824	0.4%	NA/NR	NA/NR	NA/NR	99.6%	NA/NR	NA/NR	NA/NR
Nepal[1]	2006	$8.897	2.4%	46.5%	12.7%	14.4%	24.0%	$6.120	$0.289	$0.281
Pakistan	2007	$5.077	36.1%	0.0%	0.0%	59.8%	4.1%	$3.597	NA/NR	NA/NR
Philippines	2005	$6.842	18.9%	35.6%	28.7%	15.2%	1.7%	$3.187	$0.566	$0.064
Philippines	2006	$7.686	34.6%	40.8%	8.0%	15.5%	1.0%	$4.936	$2.362	$0.085
Sri Lanka	2007	$1.706	99.4%	0.0%	NA/NR	0.6%	0.0%	$0.011	NA/NR	NA/NR
Thailand	2007	$199.645	82.7%	0.5%	16.0%	0.8%	0.0%	$28.186	$0.188	$5.497
Viet Nam[1]	2006	$47.156	10.5%	NA/NR	NA/NR	NA/NR	89.5%	NA/NR	NA/NR	NA/NR
Sub-Saharan Africa										
Angola[1]	2006	$27.724	100.0%	NA/NR	NA/NR	NA/NR	NA/NR	NA/NR	NA/NR	NA/NR
Angola[1]	2007	$47.494	82.14%	0.0%	5.87%	8.21%	3.78%	$23.687	$5.270	NA/NR
Benin[1]	2006	$25.931	NA/NR	NA/NR	NA/NR	NA/NR	NA/NR	NA/NR	NA/NR	NA/NR
Benin[1]	2007	$25.992	NA/NR	NA/NR	NA/NR	NA/NR	NA/NR	NA/NR	NA/NR	NA/NR
Botswana[1]	2005	$206.939	79.8%	NA/NR	NA/NR	NA/NR	20.2%	$28.346	$5.576	$8.062

UNGASS indicator 1. Country Reports of Domestic and International AIDS Spending by service categories and financing sources.

Total HIV Expenditures in selected services (Million US Dollars)

Prevention			Care and Treatment		Orphans and Vulnerable Children	Programme Support			Other HIV Expenditures
Programs for sex workers and their clients for MSM and programme for harm reduction for IDUs	Condom social marketing, public and commercial sector condom provision and female condom	Prevention of mother to child transmission	Total for Care and Treatment	Anti-retroviral therapy		Total for Program and management support	Programme management, planning and coordination	Monitoring and Evaluation[4]	
$0.088	$0.407	$0.027	$1.578	$1.044	NA/NR	$0.206	NA/NR	$0.172	$0.329
NA/NR	NA/NR	NA/NR	NA/NR	NA/NR	NA/NR	NA/NR	NA/NR	NA/NR	NA/NR
$0.298	$0.029	NA/NR	$0.850	$0.820	NA/NR	$0.243	$0.163	$0.080	$0.197
NA/NR	NA/NR	NA/NR	$2.673	NA/NR	NA/NR	$0.518	NA/NR	NA/NR	$0.713
NA/NR	NA/NR	NA/NR	$3.644	NA/NR	NA/NR	$0.708	NA/NR	NA/NR	$0.334
NA/NR	$0.792	$0.243	$1.479	$1.351	$0.095	$4.306	$3.469	$0.508	$1.182
NA/NR	NA/NR	NA/NR	NA/NR	NA/NR	$0.060	$0.100	$0.100	NA/NR	$0.100
NA/NR	NA/NR	$0.051	$0.234	$0.200	$0.100	$0.220	$0.150	$0.070	$0.240
$0.816	$0.085	$0.015	$25.085	$6.500	$0.070	$1.102	$0.332	$0.770	$0.261
$0.878	NA/NR	$0.040	$27.429	$8.012	$0.200	$1.175	$0.356	$0.750	$2.003
$1.345	NA/NR	NA/NR	$93.003	$93.003	NA/NR	NA/NR	NA/NR	NA/NR	$6.514
NA/NR	NA/NR	NA/NR	NA/NR	NA/NR	NA/NR	NA/NR	NA/NR	NA/NR	NA/NR
NA/NR	$0.015	$0.021	$0.016	$0.009	NA/NR	$0.117	$0.074	$0.032	$0.053
$0.626	$4.381	NA/NR	$9.603	$2.708	$2.019	$8.826	$4.494	$4.230	$3.784
$0.143	$0.260	$0.022	$14.074	$0.092	$0.046	$12.161	$0.941	$0.361	$7.116
NA/NR	NA/NR	NA/NR	$2.944	NA/NR	NA/NR	$4.509	NA/NR	NA/NR	$4.843
NA/NR	NA/NR	NA/NR	NA/NR	NA/NR	NA/NR	NA/NR	NA/NR	NA/NR	NA/NR
NA/NR	NA/NR	NA/NR	NA/NR	NA/NR	NA/NR	NA/NR	NA/NR	NA/NR	NA/NR
$2.227	$1.326	NA/NR	$1.122	$0.013	$0.022	$0.962	$0.460	$0.336	$0.671
NA/NR	NA/NR	NA/NR	$0.046	NA/NR	$0.149	$0.412	NA/NR	NA/NR	$0.873
$1.331	$0.360	NA/NR	$0.550	$0.394	$0.011	$2.109	$0.782	$1.135	$0.985
$1.531	$0.003	$0.062	$0.123	$0.008	$0.023	$1.814	$0.832	$0.883	$0.791
$0.001	NA/NR	NA/NR	NA/NR	NA/NR	NA/NR	NA/NR	NA/NR	NA/NR	$1.695
$1.029	$2.529	$3.542	$143.334	$93.625	$3.006	$19.449	$10.991	$5.896	$5.669
NA/NR	NA/NR	NA/NR	NA/NR	NA/NR	NA/NR	NA/NR	NA/NR	NA/NR	NA/NR
NA/NR	NA/NR	NA/NR	NA/NR	NA/NR	NA/NR	NA/NR	NA/NR	NA/NR	NA/NR
NA/NR	NA/NR	$1.700	$17.095	$6.225	NA/NR	$1.529	$1.529	NA/NR	$5.183
NA/NR	NA/NR	NA/NR	NA/NR	NA/NR	NA/NR	NA/NR	NA/NR	NA/NR	NA/NR
NA/NR	NA/NR	NA/NR	NA/NR	NA/NR	NA/NR	NA/NR	NA/NR	NA/NR	NA/NR
NA/NR	$4.538	$6.745	$102.796	$38.741	$39.698	$27.991	$24.542	$2.237	$8.108

UNGASS indicator 1. Country Reports of Domestic and International AIDS Spending by service categories and financing sources.

Region/Reporting Country	Year of the expenditure	Total reported Domestic Public and International Expenditure (Million US Dollars)	Share by financing source					Total HIV Expenditures in selected services (Million US Dollars)		
								Prevention		
			Domestic Public (%)	International				Total for Prevention	Communication for social and behavioral change	Voluntary counseling and testing
				Bilaterals (%)	Multilaterals		All other international sources or not specified (%)			
					Global Fund (%)	UN and all other Multilaterals (%)				
Botswana	2006	$143.406	91.3%	8.1%	0.3%	NA/NR	0.4%	$9.853	$0.208	$0.324
Botswana	2007	$229.458	88.8%	10.5%	0.2%	NA/NR	0.4%	$15.995	$0.404	$0.162
Burkina Faso	2006	$43.275	22.3%	32.3%	6.7%	29.3%	9.4%	$12.251	$0.125	$1.196
Cameroon[1]	2005	$43.174	10.2%	NA/NR	NA/NR	NA/NR	89.8%	NA/NR	NA/NR	NA/NR
Cameroon[1]	2006	$33.938	17.7%	NA/NR	NA/NR	NA/NR	82.3%	NA/NR	NA/NR	NA/NR
Cameroon[1]	2007	$37.826	25.4%	NA/NR	NA/NR	NA/NR	74.6%	NA/NR	NA/NR	NA/NR
Cape Verde[1]	2006	$0.800	100.0%	NA/NR	NA/NR	NA/NR	NA/NR	$0.209	NA/NR	NA/NR
Cape Verde[1]	2007	$1.791	100.0%	NA/NR	NA/NR	NA/NR	NA/NR	$0.856	$0.242	NA/NR
Central African Republic	2006	$14.694	4.3%	0.0%	13.4%	69.2%	13.1%	$2.032	NA/NR	NA/NR
Chad[1]	2006	$1.733	NA/NR	NA/NR	NA/NR	NA/NR	NA/NR	NA/NR	NA/NR	NA/NR
Chad[1]	2007	$5.108	NA/NR	NA/NR	NA/NR	NA/NR	NA/NR	NA/NR	NA/NR	NA/NR
Comoros[1]	2007	$0.150	100.0%	NA/NR	NA/NR	NA/NR	NA/NR	NA/NR	NA/NR	NA/NR
Congo	2007	$16.151	31.1%	7.6%	29.1%	32.2%	0.0%	$5.329	NA/NR	$0.563
Cote d'Ivoire	2005	$15.723	26.5%	37.6%	2.4%	26.8%	6.6%	$3.998	$0.037	$0.354
Cote d'Ivoire	2006	$39.130	12.0%	26.9%	0.8%	55.1%	5.2%	$9.174	$0.169	$0.907
Democratic Republic of the Congo[1]	2006	$41.033	NA/NR	29.7%	25.0%	39.0%	6.3%	$11.896	$1.110	$1.483
Eritrea	2005	$15.412	4.1%	4.3%	23.4%	68.2%	0.0%	NA/NR	NA/NR	NA/NR
Eritrea	2006	$7.183	9.7%	0.0%	66.4%	23.9%	0.0%	NA/NR	NA/NR	NA/NR
Eritrea	2007	$7.793	9.7%	0.0%	50.6%	39.7%	0.0%	NA/NR	NA/NR	NA/NR
Gabon	2007	$9.691	58.9%	0.3%	25.4%	11.5%	3.9%	$3.489	NA/NR	NA/NR
Gambia	2007	$16.931	92.7%	0.0%	7.3%	NA/NR	0.0%	$16.023	$0.007	$0.200
Ghana	2006	$22.982	21.4%	7.9%	39.6%	2.3%	28.8%	$7.198	$3.659	$0.454
Guinea-Bissau	2006	$2.859	0.0%	2.9%	24.2%	69.8%	3.1%	$0.183	NA/NR	NA/NR
Guinea-Bissau	2007	$2.800	0.0%	7.3%	25.6%	63.7%	3.4%	$0.490	NA/NR	NA/NR
Lesotho	2006	$24.436	18.7%	28.5%	14.5%	30.3%	7.9%	$3.170	$0.224	$1.962
Madagascar	2007	$16.823	18.2%	14.0%	32.9%	34.9%	0.0%	$10.407	NA/NR	NA/NR
Malawi[1]	2005	$56.491	32.3%	0.0%	8.1%	NA/NR	59.5%	$5.758	$0.675	$0.618
Mali	2006	$26.773	32.3%	28.7%	22.2%	3.8%	13.0%	$11.740	$1.156	$0.069
Mauritius	2006	$1.501	70.7%	0.0%	0.0%	29.3%	0.0%	$0.506	$0.008	$0.045
Mozambique[7]	2005	$58.246	19.8%	41.5%	0.0%	30.9%	7.7%	$26.236	$3.594	$2.177
Mozambique[7]	2006	$95.505	15.0%	46.8%	0.7%	31.4%	6.2%	$31.555	$4.811	$2.413
Namibia[1]	2005	$79.122	48.73%	NA/NR	NA/NR	NA/NR	51.27%	NA/NR	NA/NR	NA/NR
Namibia[1]	2007	$130.500	50.80%	NA/NR	NA/NR	NA/NR	49.20%	$18.639	NA/NR	NA/NR
Niger	2006	$21.632	52.4%	6.6%	14.9%	26.0%	0.0%	$21.632	$19.982	$0.002

UNGASS indicator 1. Country Reports of Domestic and International AIDS Spending by service categories and financing sources.

Total HIV Expenditures in selected services (Million US Dollars)

Prevention			Care and Treatment		Orphans and Vulnerable Children	Programme Support			Other HIV Expenditures
Programs for sex workers and their clients for MSM and programme for harm reduction for IDUs	Condom social marketing, public and commercial sector condom provision and female condom	Prevention of mother to child transmission	Total for Care and Treatment	Anti-retroviral therapy		Total for Program and management support	Programme management, planning and coordination	Monitoring and Evaluation[4]	
NA/NR	$0.052	$4.305	$90.978	$33.150	$29.367	$13.007	$1.695	$0.457	$0.202
NA/NR	$0.017	$8.704	$140.364	$44.482	$51.442	$20.762	$2.498	$1.321	$0.895
$0.207	$2.692	$2.058	$14.323	$7.916	$1.931	$9.345	$4.726	$4.619	$5.425
NA/NR	NA/NR	NA/NR	NA/NR	NA/NR	NA/NR	NA/NR	NA/NR	NA/NR	NA/NR
NA/NR	NA/NR	NA/NR	NA/NR	NA/NR	NA/NR	NA/NR	NA/NR	NA/NR	NA/NR
NA/NR	NA/NR	NA/NR	NA/NR	NA/NR	NA/NR	NA/NR	NA/NR	NA/NR	NA/NR
NA/NR	NA/NR	NA/NR	NA/NR	NA/NR	NA/NR	$0.590	$0.465	$0.125	NA/NR
NA/NR	NA/NR	NA/NR	$0.254	NA/NR	$0.016	$0.665	$0.588	$0.077	NA/NR
NA/NR	NA/NR	NA/NR	$5.596	NA/NR	$4.858	$1.217	NA/NR	NA/NR	$0.990
NA/NR	NA/NR	NA/NR	NA/NR	NA/NR	NA/NR	NA/NR	NA/NR	NA/NR	NA/NR
NA/NR	NA/NR	NA/NR	NA/NR	NA/NR	NA/NR	NA/NR	NA/NR	NA/NR	NA/NR
NA/NR	NA/NR	NA/NR	NA/NR	NA/NR	NA/NR	NA/NR	NA/NR	NA/NR	NA/NR
$0.009	$1.456	$0.326	$5.607	$4.967	$0.626	$4.524	$3.733	$0.187	$0.066
$0.005	$2.623	$0.591	$5.968	NA/NR	$2.141	$2.323	$1.895	$0.428	$1.291
$0.004	$3.462	$2.191	$22.502	$1.873	$2.815	$3.027	$2.026	$0.715	$1.611
$0.018	$1.619	$0.805	$9.026	$4.018	$4.271	$13.065	$9.142	$2.019	$2.775
NA/NR	NA/NR	NA/NR	NA/NR	NA/NR	NA/NR	NA/NR	NA/NR	NA/NR	NA/NR
NA/NR	NA/NR	NA/NR	NA/NR	NA/NR	NA/NR	NA/NR	NA/NR	NA/NR	NA/NR
NA/NR	NA/NR	NA/NR	NA/NR	NA/NR	NA/NR	NA/NR	NA/NR	NA/NR	NA/NR
$0.004	$0.195	NA/NR	$2.544	$1.828	$0.708	$2.468	$0.423	$0.523	$0.481
NA/NR	$0.116	$0.191	$0.062	NA/NR	$0.077	$0.145	$0.006	$0.116	$0.625
$0.017	$0.768	NA/NR	$15.784	$4.297	NA/NR	NA/NR	NA/NR	NA/NR	NA/NR
NA/NR	NA/NR	NA/NR	$0.246	NA/NR	NA/NR	NA/NR	NA/NR	NA/NR	$2.430
NA/NR	NA/NR	NA/NR	$1.160	NA/NR	$0.006	NA/NR	NA/NR	NA/NR	$1.144
NA/NR	$0.225	$0.291	$4.834	$1.192	$3.967	$5.180	$3.143	$0.443	$7.286
NA/NR	NA/NR	NA/NR	$0.323	NA/NR	$0.199	$4.023	NA/NR	NA/NR	$1.872
NA/NR	$0.125	$0.021	$27.490	NA/NR	$1.009	$5.523	$2.614	$0.821	$16.712
$0.340	$0.170	$0.222	$3.022	$1.331	$0.820	$6.327	$2.627	$0.515	$4.864
$0.166	NA/NR	$0.023	$0.304	$0.304	$0.456	$0.198	$0.184	$0.014	$0.037
$0.305	$2.488	$2.558	$12.939	$6.718	$4.101	$10.509	$8.799	$1.491	$4.460
$0.140	$2.627	$4.935	$35.489	$19.422	$7.273	$14.573	$10.561	$2.145	$6.616
NA/NR	NA/NR	NA/NR	NA/NR	NA/NR	NA/NR	NA/NR	NA/NR	NA/NR	NA/NR
NA/NR	NA/NR	NA/NR	$74.574	NA/NR	NA/NR	$14.871	NA/NR	NA/NR	$22.416
NA/NR	NA/NR	NA/NR	NA/NR	NA/NR	NA/NR	NA/NR	NA/NR	NA/NR	NA/NR

UNGASS indicator 1. Country Reports of Domestic and International AIDS Spending by service categories and financing sources.

Region/Reporting Country	Year of the expenditure	Total reported Domestic Public and International Expenditure (Million US Dollars)	Share by financing source: Domestic Public (%)	International: Bilaterals (%)	International: Multilaterals: Global Fund (%)	International: Multilaterals: UN and all other Multilaterals (%)	International: All other international sources or not specified (%)	Total HIV Expenditures in selected services (Million US Dollars), Prevention: Total for Prevention	Prevention: Communication for social and behavioral change	Prevention: Voluntary counseling and testing
Nigeria[3]	2006	$19.141	56.2%	0.3%	28.9%	14.6%	0.0%	NA/NR	NA/NR	NA/NR
Nigeria[3]	2007	$19.141	56.2%	0.3%	28.9%	14.6%	0.0%	NA/NR	NA/NR	NA/NR
Rwanda[5]	2006	$84.742	5.1%	0.0%	15.3%	17.3%	62.3%	$20.651	$4.002	$4.656
Senegal[1]	2006	$11.935	48.5%	NA/NR	NA/NR	NA/NR	51.5%	NA/NR	NA/NR	NA/NR
Senegal[1]	2007	$17.815	47.8%	NA/NR	NA/NR	NA/NR	52.2%	NA/NR	NA/NR	NA/NR
Seychelles	2007	$0.146	87.1%	0.0%	0.0%	12.9%	0.0%	$0.146	NA/NR	NA/NR
Sierra Leone[1]	2006	$7.760	4.2%	NA/NR	NA/NR	NA/NR	95.8%	NA/NR	NA/NR	NA/NR
Sierra Leone[1]	2007	$5.619	4.2%	NA/NR	NA/NR	NA/NR	95.8%	NA/NR	NA/NR	NA/NR
Somalia[1]	2006	$12.203	NA/NR	NA/NR	NA/NR	NA/NR	NA/NR	NA/NR	NA/NR	NA/NR
Somalia[1]	2007	$9.812	NA/NR	0.0%	59.9%	36.2%	3.9%	NA/NR	NA/NR	NA/NR
South Africa[6]	2006	$575.680	74.0%	7.1%	14.0%	3.4%	1.5%	NA/NR	NA/NR	NA/NR
South Africa[6]	2007	$621.623	77.3%	4.0%	13.0%	3.2%	2.6%	NA/NR	NA/NR	NA/NR
Swaziland	2006	$49.113	39.8%	5.8%	31.0%	9.7%	13.6%	$8.301	$2.900	$2.243
Tanzania	2005	$266.371	40.6%	7.1%	14.2%	3.1%	35.0%	$82.399	$1.295	$4.961
Tanzania[1]	2006	$323.501	NA/NR	NA/NR	NA/NR	NA/NR	NA/NR	NA/NR	NA/NR	NA/NR
Togo	2006	$8.435	11.9%	3.9%	65.2%	10.5%	8.5%	$6.320	$1.245	$1.584
Togo	2007	$11.793	13.3%	4.4%	53.2%	11.8%	17.4%	$8.632	$1.790	$1.688
Uganda	2005	$202.419	6.1%	77.3%	4.4%	4.8%	7.4%	$37.841	$12.707	$12.006
Zambia	2006	$189.930	15.3%	60.9%	12.9%	7.0%	3.9%	$47.062	$5.118	$8.254
Zimbabwe[1]	2005	$89.432	16.4%	71.9%	0.0%	11.7%	0.0%	NA/NR	NA/NR	NA/NR
Zimbabwe[1]	2006	$129.517	49.0%	32.4%	0.0%	18.6%	0.0%	NA/NR	NA/NR	NA/NR
Western and Central Europe										
Albania	2005	$2.377	46.7%	0.0%	0.0%	0.0%	53.3%	NA/NR	NA/NR	NA/NR
Poland	2007	$42.786	100.0%	0.0%	0.0%	0.0%	0.0%	$4.400	$0.271	$0.154
Switzerland	2006	$18.506	100.0%	0.0%	0.0%	0.0%	0.0%	$5.747	$3.448	NA/NR
The former Yugoslav Republic of Macedonia	2005	$3.627	46.4%	0.0%	37.1%	13.24%	3.30%	$2.939	$0.173	$0.281

UNGASS indicator 1. Country Reports of Domestic and International AIDS Spending by service categories and financing sources.

Total HIV Expenditures in selected services (Million US Dollars)

Prevention			Care and Treatment		Orphans and Vulnerable Children	Programme Support			Other HIV Expenditures
Programs for sex workers and their clients for MSM and programme for harm reduction for IDUs	Condom social marketing, public and commercial sector condom provision and female condom	Prevention of mother to child transmission	Total for Care and Treatment	Anti-retroviral therapy		Total for Program and management support	Programme management, planning and coordination	Monitoring and Evaluation[4]	
NA/NR	NA/NR	NA/NR	NA/NR	NA/NR	NA/NR	NA/NR	NA/NR	NA/NR	NA/NR
NA/NR	NA/NR	NA/NR	NA/NR	NA/NR	NA/NR	NA/NR	NA/NR	NA/NR	NA/NR
NA/NR	$0.657	$2.089	$25.500	$6.337	$7.034	$25.311	$18.412	$0.358	$6.247
NA/NR	NA/NR	NA/NR	NA/NR	NA/NR	NA/NR	NA/NR	NA/NR	NA/NR	NA/NR
NA/NR	NA/NR	NA/NR	NA/NR	NA/NR	NA/NR	NA/NR	NA/NR	NA/NR	NA/NR
NA/NR	NA/NR	NA/NR	NA/NR	NA/NR	NA/NR	NA/NR	NA/NR	NA/NR	NA/NR
NA/NR	NA/NR	NA/NR	NA/NR	NA/NR	NA/NR	NA/NR	NA/NR	NA/NR	NA/NR
NA/NR	NA/NR	NA/NR	NA/NR	NA/NR	NA/NR	NA/NR	NA/NR	NA/NR	NA/NR
NA/NR	NA/NR	NA/NR	NA/NR	NA/NR	NA/NR	NA/NR	NA/NR	NA/NR	NA/NR
NA/NR	NA/NR	NA/NR	NA/NR	NA/NR	NA/NR	NA/NR	NA/NR	NA/NR	NA/NR
NA/NR	NA/NR	NA/NR	NA/NR	NA/NR	NA/NR	NA/NR	NA/NR	NA/NR	NA/NR
NA/NR	NA/NR	NA/NR	NA/NR	NA/NR	NA/NR	NA/NR	NA/NR	NA/NR	NA/NR
NA/NR	$0.713	$0.344	$9.384	$6.244	$15.027	$6.866	$3.136	$0.963	$9.535
$0.044	$1.735	$3.499	$63.340	$8.031	NA/NR	$48.277	$24.976	$0.108	$72.355
NA/NR	NA/NR	NA/NR	NA/NR	NA/NR	NA/NR	NA/NR	NA/NR	NA/NR	NA/NR
$0.083	$0.093	$0.153	$0.552	$0.247	$0.164	$1.033	$0.622	$0.144	$0.365
$0.113	$0.681	$0.239	$0.862	$0.386	$0.257	$1.471	$0.936	$0.225	$0.571
$0.079	$0.154	$5.705	$85.149	$59.231	$13.716	$44.878	$12.906	$10.855	$20.835
$0.117	$1.385	$17.864	$89.306	$38.992	$8.300	$27.052	$5.441	$5.898	$18.211
NA/NR	NA/NR	NA/NR	NA/NR	NA/NR	NA/NR	NA/NR	NA/NR	NA/NR	NA/NR
NA/NR	NA/NR	NA/NR	NA/NR	NA/NR	NA/NR	NA/NR	NA/NR	NA/NR	NA/NR
NA/NR	NA/NR	NA/NR	NA/NR	NA/NR	NA/NR	NA/NR	NA/NR	NA/NR	NA/NR
$2.881	NA/NR	$0.709	$38.022	$36.650	$0.013	$0.019	NA/NR	$0.017	$0.332
NA/NR	NA/NR	NA/NR	NA/NR	NA/NR	NA/NR	$1.264	$0.805	$0.460	$11.494
$2.071	$0.016	NA/NR	$0.107	$0.039	NA/NR	$0.395	$0.256	$0.082	$0.186

Notes:

"NA/NR" means that data was either "Not Applicable", "Not Reported"; occasionally that the expenditure was $0 but not sufficiently clarified in the country reports

This annex reflects the country reports and clarifications received as of May 27th 2008

1 These figures are preliminary and under revision, because of the need to assure that they are comprehensive, or because there was inadequate time for clarifications, differences in the reference period, or countries stated these to be partial estimates.

2 For 2007, the amount of International Spending was not yet available for China, therefore only Public Domestic Funding is reflected here

3 Nigeria reported for two years (2006 and 2007). The expenditure was therefore split in two and distributed equally over the two years; Spending data from PEPFAR not included.

4 This category labeled "Monitoring and Evaluation" includes operational research, serosurveillance, HIV drug resistance surveillance and information technology.

5 Bilateral sources do not include US$ 28.8 million from PEPFAR which were reported as part of "All other international" sources.

6 Spending data from PEPFAR not included.

7 It includes bilateral spending from US-AID but not Center for Disease Control (CDC) funding.

UNGASS indicator 3.
Percentage of donated blood units screened for HIV in a quality-assured manner

Country (or territory)	Indicator Value[1]
Afghanistan	39
Algeria	100
Antigua and Barbuda	33
Argentina	100
Armenia	100
Australia	100
Austria	100[2]
Bahamas	100
Bahrain	100[2]
Barbados	100
Belarus	100
Belgium	100
Belize	100
Benin	99
Bhutan	50[2]
Bolivia	88
Bosnia and Herzegovina	0
Botswana	100
Bulgaria	100
Burkina Faso	66
Burundi	100
Cambodia	97
Canada	100
Cape Verde	61
Central African Republic	76
Chad	100
China	100
Colombia	100
Comoros	100
Congo, Republic of the	100
Costa Rica	100
Côte d'Ivoire	100
Croatia	86
Cuba	100
Cyprus	100
Czech Republic	100[2]
Democratic Republic of the Congo	47
Dominica	100

UNGASS indicator 3.
Percentage of donated blood units screened for HIV in a quality-assured manner

Country (or territory)	Indicator Value[1]
Dominican Republic	100
Ecuador	100
El Salvador	100
Eritrea	100
Estonia	100
Ethiopia	100
Fiji	100
Finland	100
Gabon	100
Georgia	0
Germany	100
Ghana	100
Grenada	91
Guatemala	100
Guinea	53
Guinea-Bissau	100
Guyana	100
Haiti	100
Honduras	46
Hungary	100
India	100
Iran, Islamic Republic of	100
Ireland	100
Israel	100
Jamaica	100
Japan	100
Jordan	100
Kazakhstan	95
Kenya	100
Kuwait	100[2]
Kyrgyzstan	88
Lao People's Democratic Republic	100
Latvia	100
Lebanon	100
Lesotho	100
Lithuania	100
Luxembourg	100[2]
Madagascar	99

**UNGASS indicator 3.
Percentage of donated blood units screened for HIV in a quality-assured manner**

Country (or territory)	Indicator Value[1]
Malawi	99
Malaysia	100
Maldives	0[2]
Mali	94
Malta	100[2]
Marshall Islands	100
Mauritania	100
Mauritius	100
Mexico	100
Moldova	74
Mongolia	72
Montenegro	100
Morocco	100
Mozambique	36
Namibia	100[2]
Nepal	100
Netherlands	100[2]
New Zealand	100
Nicaragua	90
Niger	100
Nigeria	100
Norway	100[2]
Pakistan	87
Palau	100
Panama	100
Papua New Guinea	100
Paraguay	95
Peru	99
Poland	100[2]
Republic of Korea	100[2]
Romania	100
Rwanda	100
Saint Kitts and Nevis	100
Saint Lucia	100
Saint Vincent and the Grenadines	100
Samoa	100[2]
Sao Tome and Principe	0
Senegal	78

**UNGASS indicator 3.
Percentage of donated blood units screened for HIV in a quality-assured manner**

Country (or territory)	Indicator Value[1]
Serbia	100
Seychelles	100
Sierra Leone	100
Singapore	100
Slovenia	100
South Africa	100
Spain	100
Sri Lanka	42
Suriname	100
Swaziland	100
Sweden	100
Switzerland	100
Tajikistan	97
Thailand	99
Timor-Leste	58[2]
Togo	85
Trinidad and Tobago	100
Tunisia	100
Turkey	100
Uganda	100
Ukraine	0
United Kingdom of Great Britain and Northern Ireland	100
United Republic of Tanzania	100
Uruguay	100
Zambia	100
Zimbabwe	100

1 Report date 2007, but data collection can vary from 2005-2007
2 Data provided by WHO Department of Blood Transfusion Safety

UNGASS indicator 4. Percentage of adults and children with advanced HIV infection receiving antiretroviral therapy (ART)						
Country (or territory)	2004		2005		2006	
	All persons receiving ART treatment[1]	Percentage of persons with advanced HIV receiving antiretroviral therapy, using WHO/UNAIDS methodology (Low-High)	All persons receiving ART treatment[1]	Percentage of persons with advanced HIV receiving antiretroviral therapy, using WHO/UNAIDS methodology (Low-High)	All persons receiving ART treatment[4]	Percentage of persons with advanced HIV receiving antiretroviral therapy, using WHO/UNAIDS methodology (Low-High)
Albania	50	...	...	...	45[6]	...
Algeria	...	...	424	13 [6-24]	588[6]	14 [7-26]
Andorra	...	...	...		24[6]	...
Angola	3000	9 [2–16]	3000	8 [3-13]	6514[5]	16 [6-23]
Antigua and Barbuda	0	...	40	60[13]	114	...
Argentina	29500	70 [52->95]	30127	65 [49-90]	35211	71 [55->95]
Armenia	...	0[12]	29	6 [4-8]	47	8 [5-12]
Azerbaijan	...	0[12]	...	...	7	1[13]
Bahamas	...	...	...	...	1252	48 [34-67]
Bangladesh	5	<1 [<1–1]	5	<1 [<1-<1]	59[3]	3 [2-5]
Barbados	333	39 [29–52]	582	65 [48-86]	623	67 [50-90]
Belarus	33	<1 [<1–1]	120	3 [2-4]	638	15 [11-22]
Belgium	...	94[12]	...	...	6450[6]	67 [39->95]
Belize	178	20 [12–35]	180	19 [12-33]	435[3]	42 [27-68]
Benin	2000	13 [11–17]	4673	28 [23-36]	7634[3]	42 [35-53]
Bhutan	5	...[2]	5	...[2]	19[6]	...[2]
Bolivia	130	7 [5–10]	300	16 [11-22]	382	18 [13-25]
Bosnia and Herzegovina	13	10[12]	29	...	19[5]	...
Botswana	37000	44 [37–54]	59946	64 [55-76]	79490	76 [66-88]
Brazil	154000	74 [64–88]	174000	80 [69-95]	174270[5]	78 [68-94]
Bulgaria	90	45	187	...	196	...
Burkina Faso	3000	7 [6–10]	8214	19 [15-25]	14079	31 [25-39]
Burundi	3000	6 [5–8]	6416	13 [10-18]	8048	17 [13-23]
Cambodia	5000	14 [11–18]	12396	34 [28-44]	20131	54 [45-66]
Cameroon	14000	9 [7–11]	23820	14 [11-18]	28403	16 [13-21]
Canada	...	...	...	...	21000[6]	...
Cape Verde	...	...	215	...	223	...
Central African Republic	1000	3 [2–3]	1647	4 [3-5]	2782	6 [5-8]
Chad	300	1 [<1-1]	5275	11 [6-18]	5500	11 [7-16]
Chile	9000	>95 [74–>95]	6964	67 [51-89]	7782	68 [52-90]
China	9000	7 [5–11]	19282	13 [9-20]	31140[6]	19 [12-29]
Colombia	12000	28 [19–40]	13000	27 [19-39]	17540	34 [24-48]
Comoros	200	...[2]	...	...	5	>95[13]
Congo, Republic of the	464	2 [1–2]	2967	11 [9-14]	3186	12 [10-15]
Costa Rica	2000	>95 [83–>95]	2717	>95 [88->95]	2866	>95 [75->95]
Côte d'Ivoire	5000	3 [2–4]	18533	10 [8-13]	36348	19 [16-25]
Croatia	204	>95[12]	247	...	291[5]	...
Cuba	2000	>95 [>95–>95]	2079	>95 [>95->95]	1711	>95 [76->95]

UNGASS indicator 4. Percentage of adults and children with advanced HIV infection receiving antiretroviral therapy (ART)

2007

Persons on treatment				Country reported total number of persons receiving ART treatment	Month and year of country reported value	Number of persons receiving ART treatment at the end of 2007[4]	Percentage of persons with advanced HIV receiving antiretroviral therapy, using WHO/UNAIDS methodology (Low-High)	Total need estimated using UNAIDS/WHO methodology (Low-High)[18]	Total country reported need
Male	Female	Both sexes <15 years	Both sexes >15 years						
...	...	12	62	74	Dec 07	74	...	...	...
...	...	45	884	929	Oct 07	993[3]	20 [10-36]	4900 [2700-10000]	...
...	...	...	...	...	...	...	...	...	...
...	...	363[8]	10877[8]	11540	Dec 07	11540	25 [11-35]	47000 [33000-110000]	45287
14	16	...	...	30	Sep 07	148[3]	...	...	161
22557	15685	3654	34588	38242	Dec 07	38242	73 [57->95]	53000 [38000-67000]	38242
52	26	4	74	78	Dec 07	78	12 [8-17]	660 [<500-1000]	860
...	...	0	81	81	Dec 07	81	14 [6-24]	580 [<500-1300]	...
577	667	98	1146	1244	Sep 07	1244	43 [31-64]	2900 [1900-4100]	2083
...	...	...	...	178	Dec 07	178	7 [4-12]	2400 [1500-4000]	1125
358[7]	302[7]	17[15]		660	Jun 07	660[7]	73 [56->95]	980 [730-1300]	772
655	229	69	815	884	Dec 07	884	20 [14-29]	4300 [3000-6200]	1210
...	...	...	...	...	...	...	...	10000 [6100-18000]	...
263	295	65	493	558	Dec 07	558	49 [32-76]	1100 [740-1700]	4131
...	...	542	9223	9765	Dec 07	9765	49 [41-60]	20000 [16000-24000]	21706
10	8	0	18	18	Dec 07	18	...[2]	<100 [<100-<100]	...
345	151	22	474	496	Dec 07	496	22 [16-30]	2300 [1700-3100]	1055
22	8	1	29	30	Dec 07	30	...	...	30
32623[8]	50795[8]	9496[8]	73922[8]	92932	Dec 07	92932	79 [69->95]	120000 [100000-130000]	110000
109057	71943	6815	174185	181000	Dec 07	181000	80 [69->95]	230000 [190000-260000]	...
150	71	3	218	221	Dec 07	221	...	...	...
5084	10804	629[14]	15259	15888	Sep 07	16938[3]	35 [29-43]	48000 [39000-58000]	47942
3486	7408	1198	9696	10894	Dec 07	10894	23 [18-31]	47000 [35000-59000]	23532
13118	13546	2541	24123	26664	Dec 07	26664	67 [57-80]	40000 [34000-47000]	29200
16036	29781	1694	44123	45817	Dec 07	45817	25 [21-32]	180000 [140000-220000]	86453
...	...	...	...	...	...	...	...	...	...
125	166	23	268	291	Dec 07	291	...	...	1028
3215	4822	380[14]	5876[10]	8037	Sep 07	9591[3]	21 [18-27]	45000 [36000-54000]	36920
2738	4662	148	7252	7400	Dec 07	7400	13 [9-18]	55000 [41000-79000]	21000
8495	1728	...	...	10223	Dec 07	10223	82 [64->95]	12000 [9100-16000]	9023
19245[8,10]	15148[8,10]	766[8]	33846[8]	35112	Dec 07	35112	...	...	...
...	...	3[15]	...	...	...	...	...	54000 [39000-78000]	...
4	3	1	6	7	Dec 07	7	...[2]	<100 [<100-<100]	8
1886	2830	462	4254	4716	Sep 07	4956[3]	17 [14-21]	29000 [23000-35000]	11895
...	...	...	...	2952	Dec 07	2952[6]	>95 [64->95]	2800 [1600-4600]	3060
12349[8]	22525[8]	1785[8]	33089[8]	46007	Sep 07	51812[3]	28 [23-35]	190000 [150000-230000]	165448
...	...	...	...	310	Jun 07	322[3]	...	...	...
...	...	17	3089	3106	Dec 07	3106	>95 [>95->95]	1400 [760-2500]	1887

UNGASS indicator 4. Percentage of adults and children with advanced HIV infection receiving antiretroviral therapy (ART)						
Country (or territory)	2004		2005		2006	
	All persons receiving ART treatment[1]	Percentage of persons with advanced HIV receiving antiretroviral therapy, using WHO/UNAIDS methodology (Low-High)	All persons receiving ART treatment[1]	Percentage of persons with advanced HIV receiving antiretroviral therapy, using WHO/UNAIDS methodology (Low-High)	All persons receiving ART treatment[4]	Percentage of persons with advanced HIV receiving antiretroviral therapy, using WHO/UNAIDS methodology (Low-High)
Cyprus	...	...	...	...	...	...
Czech Republic	270	34 [18–57]	322	37 [19-62]	570[6]	60 [32->95]
Democratic Republic of the Congo	4000	4 [3–5]	7721	7 [6-9]	17561	15 [13-19]
Djibouti	200	6 [4–9]	350	9 [6-13]	598[3]	14 [11-20]
Dominica	5	...	21	37[13]	37	...
Dominican Republic	1000	5 [4–7]	2582	12 [10-17]	5001	24 [19-31]
Ecuador	1000	16 [9–28]	1567	23 [14-41]	1745[3]	24 [14-43]
Egypt	58	4 [3–5]	200	11 [8-16]	205[6]	10 [7-14]
El Salvador	2000	23 [2–76]	2873	31 [3-65]	4712	46 [6-75]
Equatorial Guinea	5	<1 [<1–<1]	5	<1 [<1-<1]	414[3]	14 [10-19]
Eritrea	50	<1 [<1–<1]	563	6 [4-10]	1175	12 [8-19]
Estonia	76	12 [4–33]	201	19 [7-48]	495	33 [15-76]
Ethiopia	11000	4 [3–5]	20477	7 [6-9]	53720	18 [15-23]
Fiji	...	...	...	...	...	...
Finland	...	95[12]	...	...	450[6]	54[13]
France	...	...	...	...	...	64[13]
Gabon	2000	20 [13–31]	2000	17 [12-26]	5278	39 [28-56]
Gambia	150	9 [5–19]	150	8 [5-16]	400[3]	19 [11-38]
Georgia	83	8[12]	140	>95[13]	267	69[13]
Germany	...	95[12]	...	...	27000[6]	...
Ghana	2000	3 [2–3]	4328	5 [4-7]	9882[3]	12 [9-15]
Greece	...	...	...	...	3426	...
Grenada	...	...	...	...	33	...
Guatemala	4000	24 [17–37]	5632	32 [22-46]	6030	31 [22-44]
Guinea	1000	7 [5–11]	2101	13 [9-19]	4699	26 [19-36]
Guinea-Bissau	...	...	62	2 [1-2]	349	9 [6-13]
Guyana	500	12 [8–17]	1200	29 [19-41]	1569	37 [26-51]
Haiti	3000	10 [8–13]	6896	22 [17-28]	8796	26 [21-33]
Honduras	3000	27 [11–53]	4305	39 [19-70]	4674	41 [22-66]
Hungary	300	20 [11–33]	402	24 [14-39]	412	22 [13-37]
India	28000	3 [2–7]	51888	6 [4-11]	90597	10 [7-16]
Indonesia	3000	19 [8–>95]	3520	14 [7-69]	5100	15 [7-41]
Iran, Islamic Republic of	...	...	420	3 [2-4]	525[3]	3 [2-5]
Iraq	...	...	75	...	0[6]	...
Israel	...	...	...	...	2431	61[13]
Jamaica	500	7 [5–11]	1456	20 [14-29]	2633	33 [25-48]
Japan	...	...	...	...	48	...
Jordan	40	21[12]	45	...	45[6]	...

ANNEX 2

UNGASS indicator 4. Percentage of adults and children with advanced HIV infection receiving antiretroviral therapy (ART)

2007

Persons on treatment				Country reported total number of persons receiving ART treatment	Month and year of country reported value	Number of persons receiving ART treatment at the end of 2007[4]	Percentage of persons with advanced HIV receiving antiretroviral therapy, using WHO/UNAIDS methodology (Low-High)	Total need estimated using UNAIDS/WHO methodology (Low-High)[18]	Total country reported need
Male	Female	Both sexes <15 years	Both sexes >15 years						
117	34	1	150	151	Dec 07	151	...	...	154
...	...	...	...	570	Jun 07	570[6]	56 [30->95]	1000 [590-1900]	...
...	...	1632[15]	...	14678	Jun 07	28925[3]	24 [20-29]	[99000-150000]	347490
343	362	25	680	705	Dec 07	705[6]	16 [12-21]	4500 [3300-5900]	...
9[7]	28[7]	2	37	39	Dec 07	39	...	...	53
3661	3803	589	7610	8199	Dec 07	8199	38 [31-48]	22000 [17000-27000]	21780
...	...	252	2962	3214	Dec 07	3214	42 [25-71]	7600 [4500-13000]	7632
...	...	18[15]	...	209	Dec 07	209[6]	9 [7-13]	2200 [1600-3100]	...
2136[10]	2315[10]	693[10]	3758[10]	5773	Dec 07	5773	51 [9-74]	11000 [7800-63000]	4840
...	...	...	...	859	Sep 07	985[3,6]	31 [23-43]	3100 [2300-4300]	...
...	...	65	1236	1301	Dec 07	1301	13 [9-20]	10000 [6700-15000]	12940
...	...	...	...	772	Dec 07	772	38 [19-81]	2000 [960-4100]	...
40138	50074	4534	85678	90212	Dec 07	90212	29 [25-36]	310000 [250000-370000]	258284
...	...	1	27	28	Dec 07	28[6]	... [2]	<200 [<100-<200]	...
...	...	...	...	...	...	...	...	1000 [600-1800]	...
...	...	...	...	...	...	...	...	88000 [51000-140000]	...
2886	3487	73	6300	6373	Dec 07	6373	42 [30-60]	15000 [11000-21000]	14598
...	...	...	...	423	Sep 07	431[3]	18 [12-37]	2300 [1200-3700]	4787
239	95	15	319	334	Nov 07	343[3]	... [2]	<500 [<200-<500]	476
...	...	...	...	...	...	...	...	35000 [20000-64000]	...
...	...	576	12781	13357	Dec 07	13357	15 (13-19)	87000 (69000–110000)	74060
...	...	...	...	...	...	...	...	6400 [3500-11000]	...
24[7]	21[7]	2	45	47	Dec 07	47	...	...	129
...	...	597	7215	7812	Dec 07	7812	37 [28-51]	21000 [15000-28000]	11113
2296	2932	307	4921	5228	Sep 07	5660[5]	27 [21-37]	21000 [15000-27000]	23250
321	569	41	849	890	Dec 07	890	20 [13-30]	4400 [2900-6600]	3171
894	1071	162	1803	1965	Dec 07	1965	45 [33-61]	4300 [3200-6000]	3240
6240	8274	439	...	14514	Dec 07	14514	41 [33-51]	36000 [29000-43000]	27738
...	...	751	4829	5580	Dec 07	5580	47 [29-71]	12000 [7900-19000]	9916
381	71	7	445	452	Dec 07	452	22 [13-38]	2000 [1200-3600]	...
73061[8]	40888[8]	8887[8]	114133[8]	158020	Dec 07	158020	...[9]	...	...
...	...	19[15]	...	...	...	6600[6]	15 [8-28]	43000 [23000-84000]	...
697	132	21	808	829	Sep 07	945[3]	5 [4-7]	19000 [13000-26000]	8730
0	0	0	0	0	Dec 07	0	...	...	...
...	...	...	...	...	...	...	...	2400 [1200-6100]	...
...	...	336[15]	...	3637	Dec 07	3637	43 [32-60]	8500 [6000-11000]	6000
...	...	...	...	...	...	...	...	6300 [4600-7200]	...
42	11	4	49	53	Dec 07	53	...	...	...

UNGASS indicator 4. Percentage of adults and children with advanced HIV infection receiving antiretroviral therapy (ART)

Country (or territory)	2004		2005		2006	
	All persons receiving ART treatment[1]	Percentage of persons with advanced HIV receiving antiretroviral therapy, using WHO/UNAIDS methodology (Low-High)	All persons receiving ART treatment[1]	Percentage of persons with advanced HIV receiving antiretroviral therapy, using WHO/UNAIDS methodology (Low-High)	All persons receiving ART treatment[4]	Percentage of persons with advanced HIV receiving antiretroviral therapy, using WHO/UNAIDS methodology (Low-High)
Kazakhstan	7	<1 [<1–5]	240	23 [12-62]	326	23 [13-39]
Kenya	29000	6 [5–8]	65773	14 [12-19]	125026	27 [22-36]
Kiribati	...	...	...	...	...	...
Kyrgyzstan	...	...	46	... [2]	47	23[13]
Lao People's Democratic Republic	104	... [2]	104	... [2]	479	94 [48->95]
Latvia	202	25 [9–38]	235	19 [9-29]	301[6]	18 (10–27)
Lebanon	...	...	200	28 [11-54]	213	25 [10-46]
Lesotho	3000	4 [3–5]	8400	11 [9-14]	17667[3]	22 [18-29]
Liberia	...	...	397	5 [2-8]	796[3]	10 [4-14]
Libyan Arab Jamahiriya	100	...	450	...	...	...
Lithuania	37	55[12]	55	... [2]	75[5]	79[13]
Luxembourg	...	...	...	... [2]	312[6]	... [2]
Madagascar	6	<1 [<1–<1]	6	<1 [<1-<1]	92[3]	3 [2-5]
Malawi	13183	5 [4–7]	29087	11 [9-14]	59980	21 [18-27]
Malaysia	2700	23 [16–33]	2700	19 [13-26]	...	...
Maldives	...	...	...	... [2]	1[6]	... [2]
Mali	808	4 [3–5]	7038	28 [22-38]	11508	42 [33-54]
Malta	...	...	...	...	...	...
Marshall Islands	...	...	...	...	...	...
Mauritania	39	2 [1–4]	...	...	256	8 [5-15]
Mauritius	120	...	120	18 [8-40]	243	24 [13-42]
Mexico	29000	45 [31–67]	30624	45 [31-64]	39295	54 [38-77]
Micronesia, Federated States of	...	...	...	0[13]	...	...
Moldova	120	8[12]	222	... [2]	262	48[13]
Mongolia	...	...	...	...	2	13[13]
Montenegro	...	...	...	...	26	...
Morocco	465	13 [9–19]	880	22 [14-31]	1370	29 [20-42]
Mozambique	7000	3 [2–3]	19854	7 [5-9]	40891[3]	12 [10-16]
Myanmar	2000	3 [2–4]	3500	5 [3-7]	5295[3]	7 [5-10]
Namibia	9000	22 [17–28]	29200	62 [50-80]	33593	64 [52-81]
Nauru	...	...	...	... [2]	...	...
Nepal	75	<1 [<1–<1]	75	<1 [<1-<1]	541[3]	3 [2-4]
Netherlands	...	>95[12]	...	...	...	...
Nicaragua	33	3 [1–4]	163	13 [4-19]	387	26 [9-38]
Niger	...	...	609	5 [3-6]	1168	8 [6-11]
Nigeria	13000	2 [<1–3]	41224	6 [3-9]	95008	13 [8-19]
Oman	100	...	225	...		...
Pakistan	100	<1 [<1–1]	132	<1 [<1-1]	167[3]	<1 [<1-1]

UNGASS indicator 4. Percentage of adults and children with advanced HIV infection receiving antiretroviral therapy (ART)									
2007									
Persons on treatment				Country reported total number of persons receiving ART treatment	Month and year of country reported value	Number of persons receiving ART treatment at the end of 2007[4]	Percentage of persons with advanced HIV receiving antiretroviral therapy, using WHO/UNAIDS methodology (Low-High)	Total need estimated using UNAIDS/WHO methodology (Low-High)[18]	Total country reported need
Male	Female	Both sexes <15 years	Both sexes >15 years						
283	159	71	371	442	Dec 07	442	23 [14-36]	1900 [1200-3200]	1078
60200[8]	111800[8]	15090[8]	156910[8]	177000	Dec 07	177000	38 [31-48]	[370000-570000]	407000
...	...	...	...	5	Dec 07	5	...	...	...
67	20	26	61	87	Dec 07	87	14 [8-26]	610 [<500-1100]	345
427	273	36	664	700	Dec 07	700	>95 [59->95]	690 [<200-1200]	1182
...	...	...	...	323	May 07	323	15 (9–22)	2200 [1500-3400]	...
192	54	9	237	246	Dec 07	246	26 [11-45]	940 [550-2300]	432
7582	14128	1553	20157	21710	Dec 07	21710	26 [21-33]	85000 [66000-100000]	84791
...	...	92[15]	...	1414	Dec 07	1414[6]	17 [9-23]	8500 [6100-17000]	...
...	...	...	...	1000	Dec 07	1000[6]	...	...	...
81	17	1	97	98	Dec 07	98	18 [8-31]	550 [<500-1200]	131
...	...	...	...	...	...	...	...[2]	<500 [<500-770]	...
...	...	...	...	138	Dec 07	138	4 [3-7]	3200 [2000-5400]	1206
51204[8,11]	79284[8,11]	10238[8,11,14]	120250[8,11]	100649	Dec 07	100649	35 [29-42]	290000 [240000-340000]	252720
...	...	500[15]	...	6590	Oct 07	6762[3]	35 [24-49]	20000 [14000-28000]	13080
...	...	...	...	...	...	1[6]	...[2]	<100 [<100-<100]	...
4369	7803	579	11593	12172	Nov 07	12398[3]	41 [32-51]	30000 [24000-38000]	31198
...	...	...	...	65	Jun 07	65[6]	...[2]	<500 [<500-640]	...
...	...	...	...	1	Dec 07	1	...	...	...
469	370	23	816	839	Dec 07	839	23 [13-40]	3600 [2100-6300]	1627
...	...	...	...	321	Dec 07	321	22 [14-32]	1500 [1000-2400]	1200
...	...	...	...	...	...	...	...	76000 [54000-110000]	...
...	...	...	...	1	Dec 07	1	...	...	...
261	203	19	445	464	Dec 07	464	58 [43-86]	800 [540-1100]	856
3	0	0	3	3	Dec 07	3	...[2]	<100 [<100-<100]	26
...	...	1[15]	...	...	...	...	...	...	...
867	781	58	1590	1648	Dec 07	1648	31 [21-44]	5300 [3700-7900]	2230
32990	52832	6320	79502	85822	Nov 07	89592[3]	24 [20-31]	370000 [290000-460000]	294986
6634	4466	...	...	11100	Dec 07	11100	15 [11-20]	76000 [55000-100000]	...
13783	25939	5283	34439	52316	Dec 07	52316	88 [73->95]	59000 [48000-72000]	56239
...	...	...	...	...	...	0[6]	...	...	...
762	478	51	1189	1240	Sep 07	1432[3]	7 [5-11]	20000 [13000-30000]	19200
...	...	...	...	7919	Apr 07	7919[6]	61 [36->95]	13000 [7100-22000]	...
336	186	45	477	522	Dec 07	522	30 [11-43]	1700 [1200-4700]	1233
723	751	62[14]	1412	1474	Oct 07	1536[3]	10 [7-13]	16000 [12000-22000]	8929
40643[8,10]	65429[8,10]	15345[8,10]	61381[8,10]	145392	Sep 07	197000[3]	26 [17-36]	750000 [550000-1100000]	...
200	60	...	...	260	Dec 07	260[6]	...	...	...
415	135	21	529	550	Dec 07	550	3 [2-4]	20000 [13000-34000]	7400

UNGASS indicator 4. Percentage of adults and children with advanced HIV infection receiving antiretroviral therapy (ART)						
Country (or territory)	2004		2005		2006	
	All persons receiving ART treatment[1]	Percentage of persons with advanced HIV receiving antiretroviral therapy, using WHO/UNAIDS methodology (Low-High)	All persons receiving ART treatment[1]	Percentage of persons with advanced HIV receiving antiretroviral therapy, using WHO/UNAIDS methodology (Low-High)	All persons receiving ART treatment[4]	Percentage of persons with advanced HIV receiving antiretroviral therapy, using WHO/UNAIDS methodology (Low-High)
Palau	...	...	...	33[13]	2	...
Panama	2000	33 [25–44]	2765	43 [33-57]	2835	42 [32-54]
Papua New Guinea	171	7 [6–9]	320	10 [9-12]	1098	26 [22-31]
Paraguay	300	10 [5–18]	640	18 [10-32]	1026[3]	25 [13-43]
Peru	2000	12 [9–16]	6410	35 [26-47]	8424	42 [31-54]
Philippines	71	4[12]	...	...	170	24 [17-35]
Poland	2000	35 [20–59]	2707	39 [22-66]	3072	38 [21-64]
Romania	6000	82 [70–>95]	6116	77 [66->95]	6790	81 [69->95]
Russian Federation	3000	4 [2–7]	5000	5 [2-7]	14681	10 [6-15]
Rwanda	7000	10 [9–13]	19289	29 [24-36]	34636	52 [45-63]
Saint Kitts and Nevis	24	...	32	...	39	...
Saint Lucia	20	...	50	81[13]	50	...
Saint Vincent and the Grenadines	32	...	64	>95[13]	80[3]	...
Samoa	...	...	...	...	...	...
Sao Tome and Principe	...	...	17	...	51	...
Senegal	1600	26 [18–38]	4200	54 [40-75]	5500	57 [44-75]
Serbia	317	11 [6–19]	580	19 [9-32]	608	18 [9-31]
Seychelles	43	...	43	...	82	...
Sierra Leone	...	...	210	2 [1-4]	1416	12 [7-19]
Slovakia	65	95[12]	65	...	96[6]	...
Slovenia	...	...	...	...	147	...
Solomon Islands	...	...	...	...	...	...
Somalia	...	...	35	<1 [<1-1]	111	2 [1-4]
South Africa	55000	4 [3–6]	206718	15 [12-20]	324754[3]	21 [17-28]
Spain	...	92[12]	...	...	77500[6]	...
Sri Lanka	25	4 [3–6]	25	4 [3-5]	69	10 [7-14]
Sudan	400	<1 [<1–<1]	400	<1 [<1-<1]	...[17]	...
Suriname	220	25 [12–63]	391	36 [20-70]	460	35 [22-60]
Swaziland	6000	14 [12–17]	13006	27 [23-34]	18493[3]	35 [30-42]
Sweden	...	95[12]	...	...	2800	74[13]
Syrian Arab Republic	468	...	60	...		...
Tajikistan	...	0[12]	5	<1 [<1-7]	37	4 [2-10]
Thailand	50000	21 [15–30]	81158	34 [26-47]	112196[3]	46 [35-62]
The former Yugoslav Republic of Macedonia	2	20[12]	7	...	11	...
Togo	2000	6 [4–8]	6545	18 [14-23]	6993	18 [14-23]
Trinidad and Tobago	1000	28 [19–43]	1700	46 [30-70]	2113	53 [36-78]
Tunisia	...	...	229	31 [21-45]	298	33 [23-46]
Turkey	250	...	344	...	685	...

UNGASS indicator 4. Percentage of adults and children with advanced HIV infection receiving antiretroviral therapy (ART)									
2007									
Persons on treatment				Country reported total number of persons receiving ART treatment	Month and year of country reported value	Number of persons receiving ART treatment at the end of 2007[4]	Percentage of persons with advanced HIV receiving antiretroviral therapy, using WHO/UNAIDS methodology (Low-High)	Total need estimated using UNAIDS/WHO methodology (Low-High)[18]	Total country reported need
Male	Female	Both sexes <15 years	Both sexes >15 years						
1	2	0	3	3	Dec 07	3	...	...	3
...	...	167	...	3994	Dec 07	3994	56 [43-71]	7200 [5600-9300]	6500
1037	1213	185	2065	2250	Dec 07	2250	38 [33-45]	5900 [5000-6800]	6348
678[7]	271[7]	104	949	1053	Nov 07	1056[3]	22 [12-37]	4800 [2900-8800]	3066
...	...	322[10]	7721[10]	10860	Dec 07	10860[6]	48 [36-62]	23000 [17000-30000]	...
134	202	4	332	336	Dec 07	336	31 [22-45]	1100 [740-1500]	600
2 392	990	118	3264	3382	Dec 07	3382[6]	36 [20-62]	9300 [5500-17000]	4390
3231[10]	3187[10]	196	6304	6500	Dec 07	6500	73 [62->95]	8900 [5400-10000]	6418
...	...	...	...	31094	Dec 07	31094	16 [10-25]	190000 [120000-300000]	33365
17980[8]	30089[8]	4350[8]	43719[8]	48069	Dec 07	48569	71 [62-84]	68000 [58000-78000]	...
...	...	...	...	...	...	53[6]	...	...	...
40	32	2	70	72	Sep 07	78[3]	...	...	384
...	...	...	...	...	...	104[6]	...	...	...
...	...	...	...	6	Dec 07	6[6]	...	...	...
27	47	2	72	74	Dec 07	74	...	...	300
2220	4479	384	6315	6699	Dec 07	6699	56 [44-70]	12000 [9600-15000]	10465
...	...	...	...	628	May 07	628	17 (8-30)	3700 [2100-7700]	...
...	...	...	...	...	...	94	...	...	...
...	...	...	...	2649	Dec 07	2649	20 (13-30)	13000 [9000-20000]	596
79[10]	17[10]	0	98	98	Jun 07	98	...	...	...
...	...	...	...	157	Jul 07	157	...	...	...
...	...	...	...	3	Dec 07	3[6]	...	...	...
86	125	5	206	211	Dec 07	211	3 [2-6]	6300 [3500-11000]	5284
73882[8,16]	130401[8,16]	32060[8,10]	339671[8,10]	428951	Sep 07	458951[3]	28 [22-36]	1700000 [1300000-2100000]	889000
...	...	...	...	...	...	...	...	100000 [54000-170000]	...
...	...	...	...	107	Dec 07	107	14 [10-20]	780 [540-1100]	776
...	...	...	...	...	Dec 07	...[17]	1 [1-2]	87000 [58000-120000]	...
...	...	58[10]	650[10]	729	Dec 07	729	46 [30-74]	1600 [980-2400]	...
7702	12908	2123	22412	24535	Dec 07	24535	42 [36-50]	59000 [49000-68000]	58249
...	...	...	...	...	...	...	...	4500 [2500-8100]	784
57	18	4	71	75	Dec 07	75[6]	...	...	...
57	29	4	82	86	Dec 07	86	6 [4-11]	1300 [750-2400]	79
...	...	6687[8]	126852[8]	143539	Sep 07	152974[3]	61 [47-81]	250000 [190000-320000]	252387
4	11	1	14	15	Dec 07	15	...	...	...
2793	5187	559	7421	7980	Dec 07	7980	19 [15-24]	41000 [33000-52000]	26232
...	...	...	...	2592	Dec 07	2592	58 [41-82]	4500 [3100-6300]	...
...	...	...	...	...	...	...	...	1000 [760-1500]	...
...	...	9[15]	...	...	...	...	...	...	...

ANNEX 2

UNGASS indicator 4. Percentage of adults and children with advanced HIV infection receiving antiretroviral therapy (ART)						
Country (or territory)	2004		2005		2006	
	All persons receiving ART treatment[1]	Percentage of persons with advanced HIV receiving antiretroviral therapy, using WHO/UNAIDS methodology (Low-High)	All persons receiving ART treatment[1]	Percentage of persons with advanced HIV receiving antiretroviral therapy, using WHO/UNAIDS methodology (Low-High)	All persons receiving ART treatment[4]	Percentage of persons with advanced HIV receiving antiretroviral therapy, using WHO/UNAIDS methodology (Low-High)
Uganda	44000	12 [9–15]	74869	21 [16-26]	96294[3]	27 [22-33]
Ukraine	1000	2 [2–3]	3450	5 [4-7]	4777	6 [5-8]
United Kingdom of Great Britain and Northern Ireland	...	92[12]	...	...	36000[5]	>95[13]
United Republic of Tanzania	3000	<1 [<1–<1]	21543	5 [4-6]	60342	14 [12-18]
United States of America	...	...	...	70[13]	...	...
Uruguay	900	48 [8->95]	1427	64 [14->95]	1495[6]	55 [17->95]
Uzbekistan	...	...	...	...	259[6]	30 [12-66]
Vanuatu	...	...	...	...	2[6]	...
Venezuela	9000	45 [8–79]	15417	64 [14->95]	...	53 [16-88]
Viet Nam	300	<1 [<1–1]	3000	6 [4-10]	8310	14 [9-23]
Yemen	...	...	...	...	0[6]	...
Zambia	20000	7 [6–9]	48585	16 [13-20]	82030	26 [22-32]
Zimbabwe	8000	1 [1–2]	24500	4 [3-5]	66920	11 [9-15]

1 Values for 2004 and 2005 are those reported by countries to WHO, unless otherwise noted. In certain cases when 2005 data were not available, 2004 values were used
2 Coverage figures are not calculated for countries with a need estimated to be less than 500
3 Country reported values are projected to December (see annex notes for methods)
4 Values reconciled between UNAIDS, WHO and UNICEF in consultations with countries unless otherwise noted
5 Country reported different value to UNAIDS: Angola = 7491; Bosnia and Herzegovina = 33; Brazil = 184252; Croatia = 73; Lithuania = 84; United Kingdom of Great Britain and Northern Ireland = 324000
6 No data received by UNAIDS, values were provided by WHO. Values are as of the end of December, with the exception of the following for 2006: Albania = Oct; Algeria = Nov; Belgium = April; Canada = Sep; Finland = Aug; Iraq = June; Jordan = Sep; Uruguay = Sep; Vanuatu = Oct; Yemen = Sep.
7 Data reflects adults only
8 The 2007 age and/or sex disaggregated values do not include private sector data and therefore do not add up to the total which do include private sector data
9 Epidemiological estimates were under review at the time of publication
10 Disaggregated data may not add up to reported total since sex and age information maybe missing for some patients. Please note that this data may not accurately represent national sex and age distribution for ART treatment as missing data may not be evenly distributed across sex and age.
11 Country reported cumulative figures which do not account for attrition, people lost to follow-up or people who died
12 Different source: 2003 value reported by country to UNAIDS for UNGASS report 2004
13 Different source: value reported to UNAIDS only
14 Country reported data value differs from that reported to UNICEF
15 Value reported to UNICEF for Dec, with exception of Jamaica and Liberia, which were reported for September
16 For South Africa, the country reported value for males is 167278 and females is 204452
17 Data values were reported separately for North Sudan and South Sudan: North Sudan Dec 2006 = 807, Dec 2007 = 775 ; South Sudan Dec 2006 = 161, Sep 2007 = 303
18 The total need estimates are presented in rounded numbers. However, unrounded numbers were used in the calculation of coverage rates, global and regional totals, so there may be minor discrepancies between these presented figures and those calculated using unrounded estimates

UNGASS indicator 4. Percentage of adults and children with advanced HIV infection receiving antiretroviral therapy (ART)

2007									
Persons on treatment				Country reported total number of persons receiving ART treatment	Month and year of country reported value	Number of persons receiving ART treatment at the end of 2007[4]	Percentage of persons with advanced HIV receiving antiretroviral therapy, using WHO/UNAIDS methodology (Low-High)	Total need estimated using UNAIDS/WHO methodology (Low-High)[18]	Total country reported need
Male	Female	Both sexes <15 years	Both sexes >15 years						
30 943[10]	52606[10]	8532	102700	111232	Sep 07	115348[3]	33 [27-40]	350000 [290000-430000]	312000
4111	3546	908	6749	7657	Dec 07	7657	8 [7-11]	91000 [69000-120000]	21770
...	...	...	...	...	...	...	...	35000 [20000-58000]	...
30100[10]	53346[10]	11176	124520	135696	Dec 07	135696	31 [26-38]	440000 [360000-530000]	1867918
...	...	...	...	...	...	...	...	780000 [440000-1300000]	...
...	...	...	...	1776	Dec 07	1776	56 [23->95]	3100 [1700-7800]	1970
...	...	225[15]	...	...	...	319[6]	24 [9-51]	1400 [630-3500]	...
...	...	...	...	2	Dec 07	2[6]	...	...	...
...	...	...	...	...	...	15417[6]	44 [17-75]	35000 [21000-89000]	...
6872[10]	2118[10]	789	14180	14969	Sep 07	17354[3]	26 [17-42]	67000 [41000-110000]	49960
69	38	1	106	107	Dec 07	107[6]	...	...	...
65648[8]	83551[8]	11602[8]	137597[8]	149199	Dec 07	151199	46 [40-56]	330000 [270000-380000]	370000
32377[8,10]	52837[8,10]	8237[8,10]	77479[8,10]	97692	Dec 07	97692	18 [15-23]	570000 [440000-690000]	260000

ANNEX 2

UNGASS Indicator 5. Percentage of HIV-positive pregnant women who received antiretrovirals to reduce the risk of mother-to-child transmission

Country (or territory)	2004		2005		2006
	Number of HIV positive pregnant women receiving antiretrovirals[1]	Percentage of HIV positive pregnant women receiving antiretrovirals, using WHO/UNAIDS methodology (Low-High)[2]	Number of HIV positive pregnant women receiving antiretrovirals[1]	Percentage of HIV positive pregnant women receiving antiretrovirals, using WHO/UNAIDS methodology (Low-High)[2]	Number of HIV positive pregnant women receiving antiretrovirals[1]
Afghanistan	...	...	...	...	0
Algeria	...	...	...	...	18[5]
Angola	...	...	...	2 [2-3]	1923
Antigua and Barbuda	...	...	...	50[5]	4[3,5]
Argentina	...	55[4]	...	[94->95]	2120
Armenia	...	3[4]	...	...	5
Australia	...	...	...	...	...
Azerbaijan	...	...	...	...	1
Bahamas	...	...	...	...	95[5]
Bangladesh	...	...	...	...	5
Barbados	...	...	...	90[5]	37
Belarus	119	[83->95]	...	...	158
Belize	...	70[4]	38	[18-47]	57
Benin	...	...	1214	27 [23-31]	2378
Bhutan	...	...	...	...	3
Bolivia	...	...	...	...	27[5]
Bosnia and Herzegovina	...	...	...	...	0[5]
Botswana	10508	89 [82->95]	7543	64 [59-70]	12994
Brazil	7233	[60->95]	6771	[56->95]	6510
Bulgaria	...	...	...	...	1[5]
Burkina Faso	398	5 [4-6]	937	11 [9-13]	1615
Burundi	374	4 [3-6]	524	6 [5-9]	1112[3]
Cambodia	159	[6-9]	228	[10-15]	312
Cameroon	4200	11 [10-13]	3592	10 [9-12]	7588[3]
Cape Verde	...	...	12	...	43[3]
Central African Republic	243	2 [2-3]	803	7 [7-8]	1943
Chad	...	...	193	1 [<1-2]	254[3]
Chile	...	...	...	...	139[5]
China	118	[1-3]	135	[1-3]	650
Colombia	...	...	...	...	112[3]
Comoros	...	...	...	...	0
Congo, Republic of the	312	7 [6-8]	1093	23 [20-28]	325
Costa Rica	...	...	...	...	21[3]
Côte d'Ivoire	...	...	2543	8 [7-9]	2773
Croatia	...	...	...	...	3[5]
Cuba	...	...	...	...	34[5]
Czech Republic	...	...	...	...	15
Democratic Republic of the Congo	846	2 [2-3]	1725	5 [4-6]	3422[3]
Djibouti	49	6 [5-8]	16	2 [2-3]	52[5]
Dominica	...	...	...	>95[5]	1[5]

UNGASS Indicator 5. Percentage of HIV-positive pregnant women who received antiretrovirals to reduce the risk of mother-to-child transmission						
2006	2007					
Percentage of HIV positive pregnant women receiving antiretrovirals, using WHO/ UNAIDS methodology (Low-High)[2]	Number of HIV positive pregnant women receiving antiretrovirals[6]	Percentage of HIV positive pregnant women receiving antiretrovirals, using WHO/UNAIDS methodology (Low-High)[2]	Low	High	Total number of HIV positive pregnant women, as estimated via UNAIDS/WHO methodology (Low-High)[13]	Total number of HIV positive pregnant women as reported to UNAIDS[12]
...	0	...				...
[3-12]	19	[3-12]	<200	660	... [<200-660]	0
11 [9-14]	1645	9 [7-13]	13000	22000	18000 [13000-22000]	22332
83[5]	4[7]	...		...	...	5
[94->95]	2193	[93->95]	1200	2400	... [1200-2400]	2530
[16-38]	6	[19-45]	<100	<100	... [<100-<100]	6
...	28	...	<100	<100	... [<100-<100]	33
[<1-4]	6	[4-17]	<100	<200	... [<100-<200]	...
>95 [86->95]	77[7]	>95 [68->95]	<100	<200	<100 [<100-<200]	76
[1-5]	...	...	<200	<500	... [<200-<500]	...
[>95->95]	20	[73->95]	<100	<100	... [<100-<100]	21
[>95->95]	127	[90->95]	<100	<200	... [<100-<200]	144
[26-69]	55	[24-64]	<100	<500	... [<100-<500]	57
53 [45-61]	1830	40 [35-47]	3900	5300	4500 [3900-5300]	1158
[44->95]	...	–	<100	<100	... [<100-<100]	...
[11-20]	34[5]	[12-13]	<200	<500	... [<200-<500]	763
0[5]	0[5]	...	...	...	...	1
>95 [>95->95]	12419	>95 [>95->95]	10000	12000	11000 [10000-12000]	...
[55->95]	6188	[49->95]	5600	13000	... [5600-13000]	12535
...	1[5]	...	...	...	...	...
19 [16-23]	1480	18 [15-22]	6800	10000	8300 [6800-10000]	18495
14 [10-20]	1102	14 [11-22]	5100	10000	7800 [5100-10000]	18010
[14-22]	505	[25-41]	1200	2000	... [1200-2000]	4509
22 [18-30]	7516[7]	22 [18-34]	22000	42000	34000 [22000-42000]	67875
31[5]	51	...	...	...	...	99
18 [16-20]	3714[7]	34 [30-38]	9800	12000	11000 [9800-12000]	36093
1 [1-2]	...	1 [1-2]	10000	22000	18000 [10000-22000]	...
[28-57]	117	[12-23]	<500	500	... [<500-500]	117
[6-15]	593	[6-14]	4300	11000	... [4300-11000]	787
[3-7]	144	[4-9]	1600	3700	... [1600-3700]	184
0	0	0	<100	<100	... [<100-<100]	4
7 [6-9]	240[8]	5 [4-7]	3400	5400	4400 [3400-5400]	1617
[9-27]	...	[9-25]	<100	<500	... [<100-<500]	37
9 [8-11]	3240[7]	12 [9-16]	21000	34000	28000 [21000-34000]	21977
>95[5]	2	...	...	...	...	3
[33->95]	41	[37->95]	<100	<200	... [<100-<200]	35
[84->95]	...	...	<100	<100	... [<100-<100]	...
9 [8-11]	3435	9 [8-10]	33000	46000	38000 [33000-46000]	68865
...	...	...	610	1000	820 [610-1000]	...
>95[5]	1	...	...	...	...	1

UNGASS Indicator 5. Percentage of HIV-positive pregnant women who received antiretrovirals to reduce the risk of mother-to-child transmission

Country (or territory)	2004		2005		2006
	Number of HIV positive pregnant women receiving antiretrovirals[1]	Percentage of HIV positive pregnant women receiving antiretrovirals, using WHO/UNAIDS methodology (Low-High)[2]	Number of HIV positive pregnant women receiving antiretrovirals[1]	Percentage of HIV positive pregnant women receiving antiretrovirals, using WHO/UNAIDS methodology (Low-High)[2]	Number of HIV positive pregnant women receiving antiretrovirals[1]
Dominican Republic	968	[38-61]	676	[27-43]	738
Ecuador	...	...	223	[30-94]	213[3]
Egypt	...	...	...	...	...
El Salvador	...	...	144	[11-36]	193[3]
Equatorial Guinea	...	...	...	...	103[5]
Eritrea	61	3 [2-4]	88	4 [3-5]	75
Estonia	...	...	...	...	...
Ethiopia	1390	2 [2-2]	2341	4 [3-4]	2330
Fiji	...	...	...	25[5]	5
Gabon	...	...	90	4 [3-5]	89
Gambia	...	...	87	[11-37]	103
Georgia	7	[47->95]	15	[7-21]	15[3]
Germany	...	...	...	80[5]	225[5]
Ghana	196	1 [1-1]	1078	7 [7-8]	1239
Greece	...	...	...	...	18[5]
Grenada	...	...	...	...	5[5]
Guatemala	11	[<1-<1]	111	[1-3]	167[3]
Guinea	146	3 [2-3]	77	1 [1-2]	486
Guinea-Bissau	...	...	...	20[5]	195[3]
Guyana	73	[14-42]	112	[22-74]	144
Haiti	620	13 [11-16]	800	17 [14-20]	991
Honduras	...	...	198	[18-54]	200
Hungary	...	...	...	...	0[5]
India	4289	[4-7]	2279	[2-4]	7007[3]
Indonesia	15	[<1-2]	4	[<1-<1]	40[5]
Iran, Islamic Republic of	...	...	...	...	19[5]
Jamaica	323	[52->95]	300	[48->95]	371[3]
Japan	...	...	...	...	29[5]
Jordan	...	...	...	...	0
Kazakhstan	37	[19-66]	47	[16-69]	80[3]
Kenya	21069	25 [22-29]	19403	24 [21-28]	37130
Kyrgyzstan	...	...	...	...	9
Lao People's Democratic Republic	2	[2-17]	11	[9-30]	24[5]
Latvia	...	...	...	...	37[5]
Lesotho	821	6 [6-7]	1811	14 [13-16]	2005[3]
Liberia	3	<1 [<1-<1]	130	5 [4-6]	76
Lithuania	1	[3-13]	...	...	2[5]
Madagascar	...	...	8	[1-3]	7[3]
Malawi	2719	4 [3-4]	5076	7 [6-8]	9231
Malaysia	141	[9-21]	...	...	170

UNGASS Indicator 5. Percentage of HIV-positive pregnant women who received antiretrovirals to reduce the risk of mother-to-child transmission

2006	2007					
Percentage of HIV positive pregnant women receiving antiretrovirals, using WHO/UNAIDS methodology (Low-High)[2]	Number of HIV positive pregnant women receiving antiretrovirals[6]	Percentage of HIV positive pregnant women receiving antiretrovirals, using WHO/UNAIDS methodology (Low-High)[2]	Low	High	Total number of HIV positive pregnant women, as estimated via UNAIDS/WHO methodology (Low-High)[13]	Total number of HIV positive pregnant women as reported to UNAIDS[12]
[32-54]	795	[36-65]	1200	2200	... [1200-2200]	1649
[28-87]	268	[34->95]	<500	800	... [<500-800]	347
...	5	[2-2]	<200	<500	... [<200-<500]	...
[17-48]	130	[12-32]	<500	1100	... [<500-1100]	130
14 [11-20]	–	...	530	940	710 [530-940]	...
3 [2-5]	168[7]	7 [4-11]	1600	4000	2500 [1600-4000]	3578
...	...	...	<100	<200	<100 [<100-<200]	...
4 [3-4]	4888	7 [7-8]	58000	74000	66000 [58000-74000]	75420
[60-76]	7	[82->95]	<100	<100	... [<100-<100]	7
4 [3-5]	494	21 [14-32]	1600	3500	2300 [1600-3500]	2570
[13-44]	133[7]	[17-58]	<500	800	... [<500-800]	709
[40->95]	22	[41->95]	<100	<100	... [<100-<100]	25
[40->95]	...	...	<200	590	... [<200-590]	...
9 [8-10]	2896	21 [18-24]	12000	16000	14000 [12000-16000]	19918
[14-45]	21	[16-69]	<100	<200	... [<100-<200]	21
50[5]	7	...	...	...	...	10
[2-5]	373	[5-12]	3200	8100	... [3200-8100]	2270
8 [6-10]	679[7]	11 [8-14]	5000	8600	6200 [5000-8600]	1722
13 [9-19]	349	24 [17-34]	1000	2100	1500 [1000-2100]	3716
[29->95]	...	...	<200	<500	... [<200-<500]	...
20 [17-24]	1107[9]	22 [18-26]	4200	6100	5100 [4200-6100]	5224
[18-64]	220	[19-79]	<500	1200	... [<500-1200]	...
0[5]	1	[2-8]	<100	<100	... [<100-<100]	1
[8-16]	8816	[10-24]	37000	92000	... [37000-92000]	86121
[<1-2]	89	[2-4]	2100	5300	... [2100-5300]	...
[1-2]	22	[1-2]	940	1800	... [940-1800]	220
[58->95]	292[7]	[45->95]	<500	640	... [<500-640]	171
[49-62]	...	...	<100	<100	... [<100-<100]	...
...	2[10]	...	...	...	...	0
[23->95]	126	[30->95]	<100	<500	... [<100-<500]	210
48 [42-56]	52858[7]	69 [61-80]	66000	86000	76000 [66000-86000]	105000
[8-27]	3	[2-8]	<100	<200	... [<100-<200]	197
[14-42]	24	[9-36]	<100	<500	... [<100-<500]	235
[34-78]	37	[33-75]	<100	<200	... [<100-<200]	38
16 [15-18]	3966	32 [29-36]	11000	14000	12000 [11000-14000]	12750
3 [2-3]	224	7 [6-9]	2400	3900	3100 [2400-3900]	...
[6-25]	9	[27->95]	<100	<100	... [<100-<100]	10
[1-3]	25	[3-9]	<500	760	... [<500-760]	1521
13 [11-15]	23158	32 [28-36]	64000	82000	73000 [64000-82000]	71847
[9-23]	183	[9-24]	770	2000	... [770-2000]	158

UNGASS Indicator 5. Percentage of HIV-positive pregnant women who received antiretrovirals to reduce the risk of mother-to-child transmission

Country (or territory)	2004		2005		2006
	Number of HIV positive pregnant women receiving antiretrovirals[1]	Percentage of HIV positive pregnant women receiving antiretrovirals, using WHO/UNAIDS methodology (Low-High)[2]	Number of HIV positive pregnant women receiving antiretrovirals[1]	Percentage of HIV positive pregnant women receiving antiretrovirals, using WHO/UNAIDS methodology (Low-High)[2]	Number of HIV positive pregnant women receiving antiretrovirals[1]
Mali	87	[1-1]	415	[4-6]	656
Mauritania	...	...	10	[1-4]	12[3]
Mauritius	...	>95[4]	...	...	23[5]
Mexico	...	...	...	...	146[3]
Moldova	31	[56->95]	32	...	62
Mongolia	...	...	...	...	1
Montenegro	...	...	...	...	0
Morocco	...	...	...	...	...
Mozambique	3117	3 [3-4]	8490	9 [8-11]	12150
Myanmar	274	[4-8]	629	[9-18]	993
Namibia	1126	12 [10-14]	4055	43 [36-52]	6022[3]
Nepal	...	...	...	...	35
New Zealand	...	...	...	...	8[5]
Nicaragua	...	...	29	[11-31]	26
Niger	0	0	57	[1-3]	214[3]
Nigeria	1050	<1 [<1-<1]	532	<1 [<1-<1]	6168[3]
Pakistan	...	...	...	...	8
Panama	...	...	...	...	153[5]
Papua New Guinea	46	5 [5-6]	46	4 [4-4]	31
Paraguay	...	...	47	[6-20]	73[3]
Peru	161	[10-20]	188	[11-22]	560[3]
Philippines	...	...	...	...	2[5]
Poland	...	...	...	...	62[3]
Romania	21	[6-11]	...	<1[5]	75
Russian Federation	5601	[55->95]	5709	[54->95]	6224[3]
Rwanda	4141	35 [31-40]	5782	51 [45-58]	7768
Saint Kitts and Nevis	...	...	...	...	...
Saint Lucia	...	...	...	20[5]	3[5]
Saint Vincent and the Grenadines	...	...	...	62[5]	17[5]
Sao Tome and Principe	2	...	8	...	11[5]
Senegal	...	...	57	[1-2]	212[5]
Serbia	5	[4-15]	6	[5-17]	2
Seychelles	...		...	>95[5]	5[5]
Sierra Leone	17	<1 [<1-<1]	57	1 [1-2]	354
Singapore	...	...	...	...	...
Somalia	...	...	...	3[5]	5
South Africa	32541	15 [13-17]	75077	34 [29-40]	111357[3]
Sri Lanka	...	...	...	...	1[3]
Suriname	33	[22-67]	...	...	35
Swaziland	592	5 [4-5]	4780	36 [33-40]	8221

UNGASS Indicator 5. Percentage of HIV-positive pregnant women who received antiretrovirals to reduce the risk of mother-to-child transmission						
2006	2007					
Percentage of HIV positive pregnant women receiving antiretrovirals, using WHO/ UNAIDS methodology (Low-High)[2]	Number of HIV positive pregnant women receiving antiretrovirals[6]	Percentage of HIV positive pregnant women receiving antiretrovirals, using WHO/UNAIDS methodology (Low-High)[2]	Low	High	Total number of HIV positive pregnant women, as estimated via UNAIDS/WHO methodology (Low-High)[13]	Total number of HIV positive pregnant women as reported to UNAIDS[12]
[6-10]	1018	[10-15]	6800	11000	... [6800-11000]	8570
[2-5]	45	[6-20]	<500	770	... [<500-770]	800
[8-28]	19	[6-23]	<100	<500	... [<100-<500]	60
[3-7]	...	...	2000	4900	... [2000-4900]	...
[50->95]	73	[51->95]	<100	<200	... [<100-<200]	86
[10-56]	0	0	<100	<100	... [<100-<100]	13
...	1	...	...	...	...	...
...	42	[8-18]	<500	550	... [<500-550]	544
13 [11-15]	44975	46 [39-56]	81000	120000	97000 [81000-120000]	150995
[14-31]	1280	[18-43]	2900	7100	... [2900-7100]	...
65 [54-79]	...	64 [53-80]	7600	11000	9400 [7600-11000]	...
[2-4]	36	[2-4]	990	2300	... [990-2300]	1800
[57->95]	9[5]	[61->95]	<100	<100	... [<100-<100]	...
[9-27]	43	[15-44]	<100	<500	... [<100-<500]	174
[5-10]	1006[7]	[20-47]	2100	5000	... [2100-5000]	6710
3 [3-5]	12278	7 [5-10]	130000	240000	190000 [130000-240000]	...
[<1-<1]	5	[<1-<1]	1500	3700	... [1500-3700]	...
[32-65]	71[7]	[14-29]	<500	510	... [<500-510]	377
2 [2-2]	84	4 [4-5]	1800	2100	1900 [1800-2100]	3621
[9-30]	141[7]	[17-57]	<500	830	... [<500-830]	374
[33-64]	502	[28-56]	890	1800	... [890-1800]	...
[1-2]	1	[<1-<1]	<200	<500	... [<200-<500]	2
[26-87]	63	[26-85]	<100	<500	... [<100-<500]	63
[23-45]	68	[22-42]	<200	<500	... [<200-<500]	70
[57->95]	6419	[59->95]	4500	11000	... [4500-11000]	...
71 [62-81]	6485[7]	60 [51-71]	9100	13000	11000 [9100-13000]	...
>95[5]	...	...	...	...	...	...
64[5]	11	...	...	...	...	14
85[5]	...	...	...	...	...	...
9[5]	22	...	...	...	...	90
[4-8][5]	264	[4-9]	3000	6300	... [3000-6300]	385
[2-6]	...	[2-5]	<100	<200	... [<100-<200]	...
>95[5]	...	...	...	...	...	...
8 [6-11]	919	21 [15-29]	3100	6200	4400 [3100-6200]	520
...	12[7]	[24-72]	<100	<100	... [<100-<100]	...
[0-1]	11	[1-2]	510	1700	... [510-1700]	2865
50 [43-60]	127164[7]	57 [49-69]	180000	260000	220000 [180000-260000]	290000
[1-3]	1	[1-3]	<100	<100	... [<100-<100]	55
[20-61]	...	[18-57]	<100	<200	... [<100-<200]	...
62 [57-69]	8772	67 [60-74]	12000	15000	13000 [12000-15000]	13178

UNGASS Indicator 5. Percentage of HIV-positive pregnant women who received antiretrovirals to reduce the risk of mother-to-child transmission

Country (or territory)	2004		2005		2006
	Number of HIV positive pregnant women receiving antiretrovirals[1]	Percentage of HIV positive pregnant women receiving antiretrovirals, using WHO/UNAIDS methodology (Low-High)[2]	Number of HIV positive pregnant women receiving antiretrovirals[1]	Percentage of HIV positive pregnant women receiving antiretrovirals, using WHO/UNAIDS methodology (Low-High)[2]	Number of HIV positive pregnant women receiving antiretrovirals[1]
Sweden	...	...	...	...	31[5]
Tajikistan	...	...	4	[1-7]	4
Thailand	5020	[34-68]	5081	[34-71]	4305[3]
Timor-Leste	...	...	...	...	...
Togo	180	2 [2-3]	720	9 [7-11]	910
Trinidad and Tobago	...	...	...	71[5]	173[5]
Tunisia	...	...	...	...	0
Turkey	...	...	...	...	4
Uganda	7907	9 [8-10]	12073	15 [13-17]	19991
Ukraine	2817	[53-91]	2168	[36-63]	2517
United Kingdom of Great Britain and Northern Ireland	...	...	...	...	1065[5]
United Republic of Tanzania	1800	2 [2-2]	6202	6 [6-7]	14758
Uruguay	...	>95[4]	...	19[5]	53
Uzbekistan	...	...	...	...	...
Venezuela	...	...	...	...	310
Viet Nam	...	...	368	[6-16]	1385
Yemen	...	...	...	...	...
Zambia	12983	18 [16-20]	14071	19 [17-22]	25578
Zimbabwe	5534	8 [7-8]	8461	13 [12-14]	10127

1 Values provided by UNICEF, unless otherwise noted. Data reflect a 12 month period, unless otherwise noted
2 All values rounded to nearest integer. Ranges are presented for countries with low and concentrated epidemics
3 Value differs from that reported to UNAIDS in 2008
4 2003 value used to represent 2004, as reported by country to UNAIDS for UNGASS 2004
5 Value reported to UNAIDS
6 All data reflect values representing 12 month period ending December 2007 which have been reconciled between reporting country and UNAIDS/WHO/UNICEF, unless otherwise noted
7 Data not representing a 12 month period have been projected to create a 12 month value (see annex notes for methods). Reported values are shown in the table below:

Countries for which the numbers of HIV-infected pregnant women who received ARVs for PMTCT are projected		
Country	**Date and month of reported value**	**Reported value**
Cameroon	Jan 07–Oct 07	6 263
Central African Republic	Jan 07–Jun 07	1 857
Côte d'Ivoire	Jan 07–Jul 07	1 890
Eritrea	Jan 07–Oct 07	140
Gambia	Jan 07–Sep 07	100
Guinea	Jan 07–Sep 07	509
Jamaica	Jan 07–Jun 07	146
Kenya	Jan 07–Jun 07	26 429
Myanmar	Jan 07–Oct 07	1 067
Niger	Jan 07–Jun 07	503
Panama	Jan 07–Sep 07	53
Paraguay	Jan 07–Nov 07	129
Rwanda	Jan 07–Nov 07	5 945
South Africa	Jan 07–Sep 07	95 373
Sweden	Jan 07–Sep 07	23

UNGASS Indicator 5. Percentage of HIV-positive pregnant women who received antiretrovirals to reduce the risk of mother-to-child transmission

2006	2007					
Percentage of HIV positive pregnant women receiving antiretrovirals, using WHO/ UNAIDS methodology (Low-High)[2]	Number of HIV positive pregnant women receiving antiretrovirals[6]	Percentage of HIV positive pregnant women receiving antiretrovirals, using WHO/UNAIDS methodology (Low-High)[2]	Low	High	Total number of HIV positive pregnant women, as estimated via UNAIDS/WHO methodology (Low-High)[13]	Total number of HIV positive pregnant women as reported to UNAIDS[12]
[21-66]	31[7,11]	[21-63]	<100	<200	... [<100-<200]	31
[1-6]	9	[2-11]	<100	<500	... [<100-<500]	438
[29-63]	9352	[62->95]	6400	15000	... [6400-15000]	6196
...	2	...	...	...	...	...
11 [9-14]	705	9 [7-11]	6300	10000	8000 [6300-10000]	10329
[47->95]	137	[37-78]	<200	<500	... [<200-<500]	...
0	1	[1-3]	<100	<100	... [<100-<100]	...
>95	...	...	...	...	...	...
25 [22-28]	26484	34 [29-39]	68000	92000	78000 [68000-92000]	91000
[40-69]	3046	[45-79]	3800	6700	... [3800-6700]	3293
[76->95]	48[5,9]	[3-14]	<500	1600	... [<500-1600]	487
15 [14-16]	31863	32 [29-35]	91000	110000	100000 [91000-110000]	114800
[22-79]	...	[20-76]	<100	<500	... [<100-<500]	...
[3-19]	95	[11-68]	<200	830	... [<200-830]	...
[8-25]	...	[7-24]	1300	4600	... [1300-4600]	...
[22-60]	744	[12-31]	2400	6400	... [2400-6400]	5352
...	2	...	...	...	...	...
35 [31-39]	35314	47 [41-52]	68000	86000	76000 [68000-86000]	90252
17 [16-19]	15381	29 [27-32]	48000	57000	52000 [48000-57000]	16769

8 Country reported 274 for Jan-Dec 2007

9 Country reported 1066 for Jan-Dec 2007

10 Country reported 0 for Jan-Dec 2007

11 Represents Stockholm only

12 Country reported need may not always represent the estimated number of HIV positive pregnant women. In some cases it may refer to the number of identified HIV positive pregnant women or other definition not necessarily representative of national need number. Please refer to country's specific progress report for more information: http://data.unaids.org/pub/Report/2008

13 The estimates are given in rounded numbers. However, unrounded numbers were used in the calculation of coverage rates, global and regional totals, so there may be minor discrepancies between these presented figures and those calculated using unrounded estimates

UNGASS indicator 6. Percentage of estimated HIV-positive incident TB cases that received treatment for TB and HIV

Country (or territory)	2007	
	Adults treated	Percentage of patients treated
Afghanistan	2	<1
Algeria[1]	82	87
Argentina	415	55
Armenia[1]	15	59
Azerbaijan	3	4
Bahamas	26	81
Barbados	2	100
Belarus	136	72
Belize	9	69
Benin	157	31
Bolivia	60	41
Bulgaria[2]	32	
Burkina Faso	199	1
Cape Verde	3	3
Central African Republic	3671	15
China	901	13
Costa Rica	13	100
Côte d'Ivoire	994	10
Croatia	3	100
Cuba	46	90
Dominica	1	100
Dominican Republic[1]	322	115
DR Congo	162	<1
Ecuador	150	40
El Salvador	63	100
Ethiopia	2658	13
Fiji	2	40
Finland	0	
Gabon	521	13
Georgia	34	71
Grenada[2]	0	
Guatemala	109	33
Guinea	245	61
Haiti	61	5
Honduras	383	71
Hungary[3]	7	<1
India	19400	23
Iran	52	20
Jamaica	18	72
Japan	10	83
Jordan	0	
Kazakhstan	76	33
Latvia	27	57
Lebanon[1]	3	148
Lithuania	5	38
Malawi	18910	70
Malaysia	72	33
Mauritania[1,4]	95	86
Mauritius	3	16
Mexico	806	78
Morocco	88	73
Mozambique[1]	1008	4
Nepal[1]	321	46
Nicaragua	13	14
Niger	197	1
Nigeria	28625	56
Panama	270	5
Papua New Guinea	320	35
Paraguay	20	14
Peru	93	11
Philippines	99	49
Poland[1]	70	176
Republic of Moldova	23	10
Russian Federation[1,4]	463	39
Saint Kitts & Nevis	2	100
Saint Lucia	2	50
Sao Tome & Principe[2]	0	
Senegal	319	15
Seychelles	11	100
Slovenia[2]	0	
Somalia	14	2
South Africa[3]	159382	50
St Vincent & Grenadines	4	100
Tajikistan	6	8
TFYR Macedonia[2]	2	
Thailand[1]	2260	23
Togo[1]	44	2
Turkey[2]	47	
Ukraine	411	15
UR Tanzania	188	12
Uruguay	20	25
Viet Nam	390	15
Zambia	21103	35

1 Estimate of denominator provided by WHO (Global Tuberculosis Control Report 2008)
2 No denominator is available
3 Denominator is the total number of TB cases reported in 2007
4 For Mauritania, data available for 2 year period only, thus indicator for 2007 assumes cases evenly spread over each year. For Russian Federation, data reported from 4 geographical regions only – Ulyanovskaya oblast, Saratovskaya oblast, Tverskaya oblast, and Altayskiy kray

UNGASS indicator 7. Percentage of women and men aged 15-49 who received an HIV test in the last 12 months and who know their results

Country (or territory)	Country reported value							Most recent DHS		
	Survey year	Male	Female	Both sexes				Survey year	Male	Female
		15-49	15-49	15-19	20-24	25-49	15-49		15-49	15-49
Afghanistan	2007						27			
Algeria	2006	0	1	0	1[1]	1	1			
Angola	2006	7	4				5			
Antigua and Barbuda	2006						25			
Argentina	2005		8	4	12					
Barbados	2006	97[1]	99[1]				99[1]			
Belarus	2007	26	33	26	35	31	31			
Belgium		8	9		5	10	9			
Belize	2006	10	20				15			
Benin	2006	12	15	7	17	15	14	2006	5	7
Bolivia	2007	87[1]	87[1]	86[1]	88[1]	87[1]	87[1]			
Bosnia and Herzegovina	2006		0	0	0	0				
Burkina Faso	2007	18	23	15	28	27	21			
Burundi	2007	91[1]	93[1]	91[1]	92[1]	93[1]	92[1]			
Cambodia	2006	5	3	2	6	4	4	2005	5	3
Cameroon	2004	7	5	3	6	6	5	2004	7	5
Canada	2006						32			
Cape Verde	2005	10	10	3	13	13	10	2005	10	10
Central African Republic	2006	15	17	10	19	17	16			
Chad	2004	2	1	0	1	1	1	2004	2	1
Chile	2007	22	35	8	33	48	28			
China	2006	2	2				2			
Colombia	2007	11[2]	27[2]				19[2]			
Congo, Republic of the	2005	3	3	1	4	4	3	2005	3	3
Costa Rica	2007	8[1]	7[1]			80[1]	12[1]			
Côte d'Ivoire	2005	3	4	2	3	4	3	2005	3	4
Cuba	2006	28	32	17	32	32	30			
Democratic Republic of the Congo	2007	4	4	2	5	5	4	2007	4	4
Dominican Republic	2007	19	21	8	22	23	20	2007	19	21
Ecuador	2007		11	7	13	12				
Eritrea	2007						6			
Ethiopia	2005	2	2				2	2005	2	2
Gabon	2007	50[1]	64[1]	33[1]	54[1]	62[1]	59[1]			
Gambia	2005	8	12				10			
Germany	2007	14	11				13			
Ghana	2006							2006	3	4
Greece	2007	13	11	5	9	16	12			
Grenada	2006	6	13	3	19	10	10			
Guinea	2005	3	1	1	2	2	2	2005	3	1
Guinea-Bissau	2006		5							
Guyana	2005	10	11	7	17	11	11	2005	10	11
Haiti	2006	5	8	3	8	8	7	2005	5	8

UNGASS indicator 7. Percentage of women and men aged 15-49 who received an HIV test in the last 12 months and who know their results

Country (or territory)	Country reported value							Most recent DHS		
	Survey year	Male	Female	Both sexes				Survey year	Male	Female
		15-49	15-49	15-19	20-24	25-49	15-49		15-49	15-49
Honduras	2006	21[1]	23[1]				23[1]			
Hungary	2007	0	0				0			
India	2006	1	1	0	2	2	1	2006	1	1
Israel				16	14	14	15			
Jamaica	2004	12	19			17	16			
Japan	2006						98[1]			
Kazakhstan	2007	4	5	2	4	5	7			
Kenya	2003	8	7	4	9	7	14	2003	8	7
Lesotho	2005	5	6	2	7	8	6	2004	5	6
Lithuania	2007	24[1]	20[1]			24[1]	24[1]			
Madagascar	2004	1[3]	0[3]					2004	1	<1
Malawi	2007						11[1]	2004	8	7
Malaysia	2007						75[1]			
Mali	2006	3	7	2	4	3	5	2006	10	7
Marshall Islands	2006	56[1]	67[1]	67[1]	50[1]		60[1]			
Mauritania	2007	10	3				5			
Mauritius	2004				3[1]	2[1]	2[1]			
Mexico	2006						1[1]			
Moldova	2007	6	11	3	10	10	8			
Montenegro	2006		3	1	4	3				
Morocco	2007	6[1]	4[1]	3[1]	6[1]		5[1]			
Mozambique	2004	2	2	3	3	2	2	2003	3	2
Namibia	2007	18	29	9	26	27	23	2006	18	29
Nicaragua	2007		5	2	4	7	5			
Niger	2006	4	2	2	2	3	2			
Nigeria	2005	9	8	3	8	11	9			
Palau	2006		16[1]	27[1]	20[1]	14[1]				
Philippines	2003	2						2003		1
Poland	2007						1[1]			
Russian Federation	2007	30[1]	38[1]	20[1]	35[1]	37[1]	34[1]			
Rwanda	2005	11	12	4	16	13	11	2005	11	12
Saint Kitts and Nevis	2006					10[1]	10[1]			
Saint Lucia	2007	34[1]	39[1]				36[1]			
Saint Vincent and the Grenadines	2006	8	12	6	12	12	10			
Senegal	2005	2	1	1	1	1	1	2005	1	2
Seychelles	2006	100[1]	100[1]	100[1]	100[1]	100[1]	100[1]			
Sierra Leone	2007	8[1]	9				9[1]			
Singapore	2007	9	7	0	13	8	8			
Somalia	2004	5[1]	3[1]				4[1]			
South Africa	2006	90[1]	90[1]	90[1]	90[1]	90[1]	90[1]			
Spain	2003						25			
Sri Lanka	2007	0[1]	0[1]	0[1]	0[1]	0[1]	0[1]			

UNGASS indicator 7. Percentage of women and men aged 15-49 who received an HIV test in the last 12 months and who know their results

Country (or territory)	Country reported value							Most recent DHS		
	Survey year	Male	Female	Both sexes				Survey year	Male	Female
		15-49	15-49	15-19	20-24	25-49	15-49		15-49	15-49
Suriname	2006		30							
Swaziland	2007	9	22	6	18	21	16	2007	9	22
Switzerland	2007	7	7	5	7	7	7			
Tajikistan	2007	4[1]	2[1]	2[1]	5[1]		3[1]			
Thailand	2006	16	22	16	22	19	19			
The former Yugoslav Republic of Macedonia	2006		3	2	3	3				
Togo	2007	16	15	10	17	17	16			
Trinidad and Tobago	2006						8[1]			
Turkey	2006	100[1]	100[1]	100[1]	100[1]	100[1]	100[1]			
Uganda	2006	10	12				12	2006	10	12
Ukraine	2007	11[1]	20[1]	12[1]	19[1]	16[1]	16[1]			
United Kingdom of Great Britain and Northern Ireland	2006	1[1]	3[1]				2[1]			
United Republic of Tanzania	2007						36	2004	7	6
Uruguay	2007	20	19	15	20	20	20			
Viet Nam	2005	3	2	1	3	3	2	2005	3	2
Zambia	2007	12	19	10	19	17	15	2007	12	19
Zimbabwe	2006	7	7	4	9	7	7	2006	7	7

[1] Methodology not harmonized with UNGASS 2008 guidelines
[2] 14-26 years
[3] 15-24 years

UNGASS indicator 8. Percentage of most-at-risk populations that have received an HIV test in the last 12 months and who know their results[1]

	Sex Workers				Injecting Drug Users				Men who have Sex with Men	
UNGASS	2005	2007			2005	2007			2005	2007
Country (or territory)	All	All	Male	Female	All	All	Male	Female	All	All
Afghanistan		11[5]		11		6				
Algeria					15					
Angola		42[5]		42						
Argentina	36		38	65		47	43	62	96	98
Armenia	33	18[5]		18	21	23	23	13	42	5
Australia		63[5]		63		57[4]				50
Bahamas										61
Bangladesh	2[5]	6	8	5	3	3[6]	3			6
Barbados		73[4,5]		73[4]						
Belarus	49	63[5]		63	39	49	49	49	55	53
Belgium										62[3]
Benin		30[5]		30						
Bolivia		78[4]	85[4]	78[4]						100[4]
Bosnia and Herzegovina		96[2,4]				53[6]	53			10[2,4]
Bulgaria		53[5]		53		38	36	52		29
Burkina Faso		94[4,5]		94[4]						
Burundi	38	38[2,5]		38[2]						
Cambodia		68[5]		68						58
Cameroon		32[2,5]		32[2]						
Canada						59				43[4]
Chile										37
China		29[5]		29		41	40	45		33
Colombia		82	71	85						61
Congo, Republic of the	3								8	
Costa Rica										43
Cuba		36	38	32						33
Côte d'Ivoire		51[5]		51						57[4]
Democratic Republic of the Congo		37[2,5]		37[2]						
Dominican Republic		64[2,5]		64[2]						
Ecuador				87[4]						50[4]
El Salvador		96[5]		96						55
Eritrea		78								
Estonia		52[5]		56		62	63	60		27[4]
Ethiopia		97[5]		97						
Gabon		54	33	55						
Georgia	24	33[5]		33	6	9[6]	9		27	30[2]
Germany										18
Ghana		39								25
Greece										39
Guatemala		93[5]		93						64

UNGASS indicator 8. Percentage of most-at-risk populations that have received an HIV test in the last 12 months and who know their results[1]

	Sex Workers				Injecting Drug Users				Men who have Sex with Men	
UNGASS	2005	2007			2005	2007			2005	2007
Country (or territory)	All	All	Male	Female	All	All	Male	Female	All	All
Guinea		58[5]		58						
Guyana		64		64						44
Haiti		71								48
Honduras		71[5]		71						40
Hungary						8				
India				34						
Indonesia	15	31	52	25	18	36	36	42	15	32
Iran, Islamic Republic of		20[5]		20	9	23	23	16		
Jamaica	43	43[5]		43						
Japan										38
Kazakhstan		70[5]		70		42	41	49		38
Kenya		12[2]								40
Kyrgyzstan		53[5]		53		34	32	43		70
Lao People's Democratic Republic	9									5
Latvia						61	62	60		
Lebanon		24[4]	11[4]	25[4]		4[4]	2[4]	50[4]		14[4]
Lithuania		50[5]		50		64	60	81		28
Madagascar		49[5]		49						
Malawi		69[5]		69						
Malaysia		100[3,4]				100[4]				100
Mali		7								
Mauritania		100[4,5]		100[4]						15[4]
Mauritius		30[2]				20[2]	24[2]	0[2]		16[2]
Mexico		72	63	76		31[2]	28[2]	48[2]		54
Moldova		31[5]	.	31		34	33	38		38
Mongolia	67	53[5]		53					23	60
Montenegro		73[4,5]		73[4]						81[4]
Morocco		51[5]		51	13	13	13	11		
Nepal		40	52	37		21[6]	21			30
Niger		38[5]		38						
Nigeria		38[5]		38		23	23	33		30
Pakistan		4	4	5			4[4]			
Panama	77	55	59	52					45	76
Papua New Guinea		47[5]		47						42
Paraguay		100[5]	100	100		100	100	100		100
Peru				54[4]						21
Philippines		12[5]		12		4	4	15		16
Poland						<1				<1
Romania	36	35[5]		35	36	16[4]	17[4]	10[4]		47
Russian Federation		61[5]		61		46	44	50		32

UNGASS indicator 8. Percentage of most-at-risk populations that have received an HIV test in the last 12 months and who know their results[1]

	Sex Workers				Injecting Drug Users				Men who have Sex with Men	
UNGASS	2005	2007			2005	2007			2005	2007
Country (or territory)	All	All	Male	Female	All	All	Male	Female	All	All
Rwanda		65[5]		65						
Saint Lucia						100[4]	100[4]	100[4]		
Sao Tome and Principe		72[4,5]		72[4]						
Senegal		70[5]		70					11	
Serbia									53	
Sierra Leone		79	75							
Singapore				100						47
Spain		67[2,4,5]				68[2,4]	67[2,4]	72[2,4]		49[3]
Sri Lanka		43[5]		43						14
Suriname		62	75	59						
Swaziland		94[4,5]		94[4]						
Sweden		34[4]	100[4]	33[4]		84[4]	83[4]	86[4]		41
Switzerland			38			60	59	61		31
Tajikistan		29[5]		29		24	23	30		
Thailand		53	54	52						35
The former Yugoslav Republic of Macedonia	67	47	87	39	32	44	42	53	7	56
Togo		40	22	89						
Tunisia				100[4]						35[3]
Turkey	26	97	100	97		8	11	0		31
Ukraine	32	46[5]		46	27	29	29	30	25	27
United Kingdom of Great Britain and Northern Ireland										17[2]
Uzbekistan		19[5]		19		18	18	18		25
Viet Nam		15[5]		15		11[6]	11			16
Zambia		17	14	23						

1 Report date 2007, but data collection can vary from 2005-2007
2 Data collection started before 2005
3 Data collection period not defined
4 Methodology not harmonized with UNGASS 2008 guidelines
5 Females only
6 Males only

UNGASS indicator 9. Percentage of most-at-risk populations reached with HIV prevention programmes[1]

UNGASS	2007						
Country (or territory)	Sex Workers			Injecting Drug Users			Men who have Sex with Men
	All	Male	Female	All	Male	Female	
Afghanistan	11[3]	9[3]	11[3]				
Angola	17						
Argentina			82				98
Armenia	41[4]		41	54	55	44	10
Bahamas							48
Bangladesh	54	47	57	82	82	90	13
Belarus	86[4]		86	56	54	61	90
Benin	60[4]		60				
Bulgaria	77[4]		77	47	45	60	30
Burkina Faso	37	15	59				
Burundi	72[2,4]		72[2]				
Cameroon	70[2,4]		70[2]				
China	46[4]		46	25	25	25	38
Comoros	59[4]		59				
Costa Rica							26
Cuba	60	59	65				56
Côte d'Ivoire							100[3]
Ecuador			76				49
El Salvador	73						62
Eritrea	88[3,4]		88[3]				
Estonia							56
Gabon	29	27	29				
Georgia				17[5]	17		
Greece							19
Guatemala	93[4]		93				75
Guinea	92[4]		92				
Guyana	28[4]		28				17
Honduras	23[4]		23				24
Indonesia	40	60	34	45	44	55	40
Jamaica	60						
Kazakhstan	71[3]			44[3]			48[3]
Kyrgyzstan	89[3,4]		89[3]	78[3]	78[3]	78[3]	77[3]
Latvia				47	45	53	
Lebanon	<1[3]	11[3]	22[3]				15[3]
Lithuania	43[4]		43				40
Malawi	69		69				
Malaysia	86[4]						100[3]
Mexico	36	55	28	5	5	4	18
Moldova	96		96	89	89	89	86
Mongolia	64						67
Morocco	49[4]		49				
Nepal	42	56	39	78[5]	78		47

UNGASS indicator 9. Percentage of most-at-risk populations reached with HIV prevention programmes[1]							
UNGASS	2007						
Country (or territory)	Sex Workers			Injecting Drug Users			Men who have Sex with Men
	All	Male	Female	All	Male	Female	
Pakistan	3[3]	3[3]	2[3]		16[3]		
Panama	76	73	78				89
Papua New Guinea	31[4]		31				10
Paraguay	18						
Peru			80				44
Philippines	14[4]		14	14	13	28	19
Romania							59
Russian Federation	39			24	33	21	17
Sao Tome and Principe	80[3,4]		80[3]				
Sierra Leone	73[4]		73				
Singapore			100[3]				
Swaziland	77[3,4]		77[3]				
Sweden	50[3]	100[3]	55[3]	27	26	30	
Tajikistan	60[4]		60	25	21	41	
Togo	76	75	81				
Turkey	42[4]		42		22	30	19
Ukraine	69[4]		69	46	45	50	50
Viet Nam	65[3,4]		65[3]	43[3]	43[3]		26
Zambia	63[2,4]		63[2]				

1 Report date 2007, but data collection can vary from 2005-2007
2 Data collection started before 2005
3 Methodology not harmonized with UNGASS 2008 guidelines
4 Females only
5 Males only

ANNEX 2

UNGASS indicator 10. Percentage of orphaned and vulnerable children aged 0-17 whose households received free basic external support in caring for the child

Country (or territory)	2005		Country reported value for 2007		Most recent DHS (or MICS)	
	Survey year	Coverage	Survey year	Coverage	Survey year	Coverage
Benin			2006	69[1]		
Botswana	2004	34				
Burkina Faso			2007	5[1]		
Burundi			2006	50[1]		
Cameroon			2006	9	2006[3]	9
Central African Republic			2006	20[2]	2007	8
Costa Rica			2006	100[1]		
Côte d'Ivoire			2006	9[1]	2005	9
Croatia			2007	100[1]		
Democratic Republic of Congo					2007	9
Dominican Republic			2007	4[1]		
Ethiopia	2004	4	2004	4		
Finland				99		
Gabon			2007	10		
Ghana			2006	2[1]		
Guinea			2007	17[1]		
Guinea-Bissau			2006	8	2006[3]	8
Haiti			2006	5	2005	5
Kenya		10				
Lesotho	2004	25				
Madagascar	2003	7				
Malawi			2006	53[2]	2006[3]	19
Mali	2005	39	2007	45[1]		
Namibia			2007	17	2006	17
Nigeria			2007	10[1]		
Rwanda			2005	13	2005	13
Saint Lucia			2007	69[1]		
Senegal			2007	44[1]		
Seychelles			2006	100[1]		
Sierra Leone			2005	1	2005	1
South Africa			2007	67[1]		
Swaziland			2007	41	2007	41
Togo		10	2006	60[2]	2006[3]	6
Turkey			2006	100[1]		
Uganda			2006	11	2006	11
United Republic of Tanzania			2006	51[1]		
Zambia	2005	13	2007	16	2007	16
Zimbabwe			2006	31	2006	31

[1] Methodology not harmonized with UNGASS 2008 guidelines
[2] Differs from value provided by UNICEF
[3] Source is the Multiple Indicator Cluster Survey (UNICEF MICS)

UNGASS indicator 11. Percentage of schools that provided life skills-based HIV education in the last academic year

Country (or territory)	2007
Angola	1
Antigua and Barbuda	13
Azerbaijan	19
Bahamas	72
Barbados	41
Belarus	79
Bosnia and Herzegovina	24
Botswana	100
Bulgaria	6
Burkina Faso	1
Burundi	64
Cambodia	26
Cape Verde	100
Central African Republic	15
Chad	4
Comoros	15
Congo, Republic of the	82
Costa Rica	100
Croatia	5
Cuba	71
Côte d'Ivoire	1
Democratic Republic of the Congo	0
Dominica	100
Dominican Republic	1
El Salvador	4
Eritrea	26
Ethiopia	70
Finland	95
Gabon	35
Gambia	33
Germany	50
Ghana	58
Grenada	0
Honduras	39
Indonesia	10
Iran, Islamic Republic of	0
Jamaica	24
Kazakhstan	72
Lao People's Democratic Republic	32
Mexico	27
Moldova	93
Namibia	79

UNGASS indicator 11. Percentage of schools that provided life skills-based HIV education in the last academic year

Country (or territory)	2007
Nepal	6
Nicaragua	8
Niger	8
Nigeria	34
Pakistan	6
Papua New Guinea	25
Romania	64
Russian Federation	82
Saint Lucia	91
Saint Vincent and the Grenadines	87
Sao Tome and Principe	100
Serbia	1
Seychelles	100
South Africa	96
Swaziland	51
Togo	0
Turkey	100
Ukraine	57
Zambia	60
Zimbabwe	100

UNGASS indicator 12. Current school attendance among orphans and among non-orphans aged 10-14 (ratio of orphans to non-orphans)					
Country (or territory)	2003	2005		2007	
	Ratio	Survey year	Ratio	Survey year	Ratio
Angola	0.90			2001	0.90
Argentina				2005	1.03
Benin				2006	0.85
Bolivia				2003	0.74[1]
Botswana	0.99				
Burkina Faso				2007	0.87
Burundi	0.70			2005	0.85
Cambodia				2006	0.83
Cameroon	0.94			2006	0.89
Central African Republic	0.91			2006	0.96
Chad	0.96			2004	1.03
Colombia				2005	0.85[1]
Comoros	0.59				
Congo, Republic of the				2005	1.12
Croatia				2007	1.00[2]
Cuba				2005	1.00[2]
Côte d'Ivoire	0.83			2005	1.21[3]
Democratic Republic of the Congo	0.72			2007	0.77[1]
Equatorial Guinea	0.95				
Eritrea				2002	0.83[1]
Ethiopia	0.60			2004	
Finland					>0.99
Gabon	0.98			2007	1.14
Gambia	0.85			2006	0.87
Ghana	0.93			2006	1.04[4]
Guinea	1.13			2005	0.73[1]
Guinea-Bissau	1.03			2006	0.97
Guyana				2005	0.95[1]
Haiti				2000	0.87[1]
India				2006	0.72[1]
Indonesia				2002	0.84[1]
Jamaica				2005	
Kenya	0.74	2005	0.97	2003	0.95[1]
Lesotho	0.87			2007	0.95
Madagascar	0.65	2003	0.80	2004	0.83
Malawi	0.93	2004	0.97		
Mali	0.72				
Mozambique	0.47			2004	0.80
Namibia	0.92	2005	0.97	2007	1.00
Nicaragua				2007	0.88
Niger	1.07			2006	0.67
Nigeria	0.87			2007	0.86[2]

UNGASS indicator 12. Current school attendance among orphans and among non-orphans aged 10-14 (ratio of orphans to non-orphans)					
Country (or territory)	2003	2005		2007	
	Ratio	Survey year	Ratio	Survey year	Ratio
Papua New Guinea				2007	0.86
Peru				2006	
Rwanda	0.80			2005	0.82
Saint Lucia				2007	1.76[2]
Senegal	0.74			2007	1.25[2]
Sierra Leone	0.71			2005	0.83
Somalia	0.65			2006	0.78
South Africa	0.95			2007	0.81[2]
Sudan	0.96				
Swaziland	0.91			2007	0.97
Thailand				2006	0.93
Togo	0.96			2007	0.94
Turkey				2007	0.70[2]
Uganda	0.95			2000	0.95
United Republic of Tanzania	0.74			2007	0.64
Zambia	0.87	2005	0.17	2005	1.02[2]
Zimbabwe	0.85			2006	0.95

1 Demographic and Health Survey value provided by MEASURE DHS (www.measuredhs.com)
2 Data collection method differs from the UNGASS recommended methodology
3 Differs from value provided by UNICEF
4 Multiple Indicator Cluster Survey based on small denominators, typically 25-49 unweighted cases

UNGASS indicator 13. Percentage of young women and men aged 15-24 who both correctly identify ways of preventing the sexual transmission of HIV and who reject major misconceptions about HIV transmission

Country (or territory)	2003	2005			Country reported value for 2007				Most recent DHS (or MICS)		
	Females 15-24	Survey year	Males 15-24	Females 15-24	Survey year	Males 15-24	Females 15-24	Both sexes 15-24	Survey year	Males	Females
Albania	<1								2005[1]		6
Algeria					2006		16	16	2006[1]		13
Angola			43	35	2006	25	21	23			
Antigua and Barbuda					2005			48			
Argentina					2005	83	89	86			
Armenia					2007	42	34	36	2005	15	23
Azerbaijan	2								2006[1]	5	6
Bangladesh					2005	24	21	22	2006[1]		16
Belarus					2007	70	65	68	2005[1]		34
Belize					2006	26	26	26			
Benin			11	8	2006	35	16	20	2006	35	16
Bolivia	22								2003	18	15
Bosnia and Herzegovina					2006		44		2005[1]		48
Botswana	28										
Bulgaria					2006	18	21	19			
Burkina Faso					2007	45	46	45	2003	23	15
Burundi	24	2004	4	4	2005		31		2005[1]		30
Cambodia	37				2006	45	49	47	2005	45	50
Cameroon	16	2004	34	27	2006		32	32	2004	34	27
Cape Verde					2005	37	38	38	2005	36	36
Central African Republic	5				2006	31	22	24	2006[1]	27	17
Chad	5				2004	20	8	11	2004	19	7
Chile					2007						
China					2007	50	55	42			
Comoros	10								2000[1]		18
Congo, Republic of the					2005	22	10	13	2005	35	26
Costa Rica					2006	43	42	42			
Côte d'Ivoire	16				2005	28	18	22	2005	28	18
Croatia					2006	16	25	20			
Cuba	52				2006	55	61	58	2000[1]		30
Cyprus					2007	10	11	10			
Democratic Republic of the Congo					2006	29	22	26	2007	21	15
Djibouti									2006[1]		18
Dominican Republic	33				2007	34	41	37	2007[1]	34	41
Ecuador					2006	31	27	29			
Equatorial Guinea	4								2000[1]		4
Eritrea									2002		37
Estonia					2007	28	37	32			
Ethiopia					2005	33	21	24	2005	33	20
Finland								85			
Gabon					2007	58	60	59			
Gambia	15				2005	34	25	29	2006[1]		39

ANNEX 2

UNGASS indicator 13. Percentage of young women and men aged 15-24 who both correctly identify ways of preventing the sexual transmission of HIV and who reject major misconceptions about HIV transmission

Country (or territory)	2003	2005			Country reported value for 2007				Most recent DHS (or MICS)		
	Females 15-24	Survey year	Males 15-24	Females 15-24	Survey year	Males 15-24	Females 15-24	Both sexes 15-24	Survey year	Males	Females
Georgia					2005		4				
Germany					2007						
Ghana		2003	40	36					2006	33	25
Greece					2007	27	23	25			
Grenada					2006	43	40	41			
Guatemala					2002	10	9	9			
Guinea					2007	20	12	16	2005	23	17
Guinea-Bissau	8				2006		18		2006		18
Guyana	36				2005	34	44	39	2005	47	53
Haiti	14				2006	40	32	35	2005	40	34
Honduras					2005	39	89	77	2006		30
India					2006	33	24	28	2006	36	20
Indonesia	7										
Iraq									2006[1]		3
Jamaica					2004	23	47	35	2005[1]		60
Japan					2004						
Kazakhstan					2007	18	20	19	2006[1]		22
Kenya	26	2005	80	58					2003	47	34
Kyrgyzstan					2006	30	33	32	2006[1]		20
Latvia					2007	3	3	3			
Lesotho	18								2004	19	27
Madagascar		2003	16	19	2006	46	45	45	2004	16	19
Malawi	34	2005	36	24					2004	36	24
Mali					2006	22	18	20	2006	22	18
Marshall Islands					2006	8	4	6	2007	39	27
Mauritius					2004			22			
Mexico					2002	18	18				
Moldova	19				2006	26	27	26	2005		
Mongolia	32	2005	3	5	2005	17	15	16	2005[1]		35
Montenegro					2006				2006[1]		30
Morocco					2007				2003		12
Mozambique					2004	39	25	28	2003	33	20
Namibia					2007	62	65	63	2006	62	65
Nepal					2006	44	28	32	2006	44	28
Nicaragua					2007		81	81	2001		22
Niger	5				2006	16	13	14	2006	16	13
Nigeria					2005	25	20	23	2003	21	18
Palau					2006		27				
Peru					2006			55	2007		19
Philippines									2003	18	12
Russian Federation					2007	33	35	34			
Rwanda	23				2005	54	51	52	2005	54	51

UNGASS indicator 13. Percentage of young women and men aged 15-24 who both correctly identify ways of preventing the sexual transmission of HIV and who reject major misconceptions about HIV transmission

Country (or territory)	2003	2005			Country reported value for 2007				Most recent DHS (or MICS)		
	Females 15-24	Survey year	Males 15-24	Females 15-24	Survey year	Males 15-24	Females 15-24	Both sexes 15-24	Survey year	Males	Females
Saint Kitts and Nevis					2006			52			
Saint Lucia					2006	61	57	59			
Saint Vincent and the Grenadines					2006	59	40	49			
Sao Tome and Principe	11				2006				2006[1]		44
Senegal					2005	24	19	22	2005	26	21
Serbia					2006	20	21	20	2006[1]		42
Seychelles					2003	59	67	63			
Sierra Leone	16				2007				2005[1]		17
Singapore					2007	15	20	17			
Somalia		2004	13	8	2006		4	4	2006[1]		4
South Africa	20										
Sri Lanka					2007	10	7	8			
Suriname	27				2006		41	41	2006[1]		41
Swaziland	27				2007	52	52	52	2007	52	52
Syrian Arab Republic									2006[1]		7
Tajikistan					2007	11	11	11	2005[1]		3
Thailand					2006	47	33	40	2005[1]		46
The former Yugoslav Republic of Macedonia					2007	19	26	22	2005[1]		27
Togo	20				2007	59	44	51	2006[1]		28
Trinidad and Tobago	33				2007			56	2006[1]		28
Tunisia						26	29	27			
Turkey					2007	35	39	37			
Tuvalu					2005						
Uganda	28				2006	38	32	33	2006	38	32
Ukraine					2007	39	42	40	2007	43	42
United Republic of Tanzania	26								2004	40	45
Uruguay					2007	52	48	50			
Uzbekistan	3								2006[1]		31
Viet Nam	25				2005	50	42	46	2005	50	42
Zambia	26	2005	46	41	2007	37	34	35	2007	37	34
Zimbabwe		2003	56	54	2006	46	44	45	2006	46	44

[1] Source is the Multiple Indicator Cluster Survey (UNICEF MICS)

ANNEX 2

UNGASS indicator 14. Percentage of most-at-risk populations who both correctly identify ways of preventing the sexual transmission of HIV and who reject major misconceptions about HIV transmission [1]

	Sex Workers				Injecting Drug Users				Men who have Sex with Men	
UNGASS	2005	2007			2005	2007			2005	2007
Country (or territory)	All	All	Male	Female	All	All	Male	Female	All	All
Argentina	69		67[6]						56	
Armenia	49	54[4]		54	60	68	69	56	54	74
Bahamas										45
Bangladesh	23	31	30	31	14	20[5]	20		14	27
Barbados		37[3,4]		37[3]						
Belarus	24	50[4]		50	61	58	51	68	63	56
Benin									42	
Bosnia and Herzegovina						22[5]	22			
Bulgaria		35[4]		35		29	28	34		32
Burundi	4	44[2,4]		44[2]						
Cameroon		40[2,4]		40[2]						
China	24[4]	41			36	49	48	52	37	55
Congo, Republic of the	67								3	
Costa Rica									49	85
Côte d'Ivoire		32[4]		32						
Cuba		52	49	61						54
Democratic Republic of the Congo		30[2,4]		30[2]						
Ecuador				47[3]						59[3]
El Salvador		6								25
Estonia		83[3,4]		83[3]		75[3]	75[3]	74[3]		60[3]
Ethiopia		36[4]		36						
Gabon		24	13	25						
Georgia	1	4[4]		4	36	41[5]	41			0[2]
Greece										74
Guatemala		3[4]		3						33
Guinea		4[4]		4						
Guyana		63								67
Haiti		6[4]		6						36
Honduras		21[4]		21						21
India				38						
Indonesia	24	28	37	26	7	58	58	68	43	42
Iran, Islamic Republic of		8[4]		8		24	24	15		
Jamaica	26	26[4]		26						
Kazakhstan		63[4]		63		63	63	63		66
Kyrgyzstan	1	36[4]		36		64	62	69	7	89
Lao People's Democratic Republic	21									31[3]
Latvia						45	44	50		
Lithuania		24[4]		24						39
Madagascar		30								
Malaysia		78[2]				98[2]				

ANNEX 2

UNGASS indicator 14. Percentage of most-at-risk populations who both correctly identify ways of preventing the sexual transmission of HIV and who reject major misconceptions about HIV transmission [1]

	Sex Workers				Injecting Drug Users				Men who have Sex with Men	
UNGASS	2005	2007			2005	2007			2005	2007
Country (or territory)	All	All	Male	Female	All	All	Male	Female	All	All
Mali	90									
Mauritius		2[2,4]				62[2]				48[2]
Mexico		49	54	47						66
Moldova	35	58[4]		58	37	64	64	66	38	47
Mongolia		29[4]		29						23
Morocco	72				7					
Nepal	17	32	41	30	50	66[5]	66		27	45
Nigeria		33[4]		33		34	34	36		44
Pakistan		10[3]	21[3]	<1[3]			20			
Panama		91	91	92						78
Papua New Guinea		35[4]		35						71
Peru									73	40
Philippines		2		2		26	27	23		10
Romania	14	14[4]		14	18	30	24	63		45
Russian Federation		36[4]		36		46	47	43		26
Rwanda		36[4]		36						
Saint Lucia						13[3]	10[3]	33[3]		
Sao Tome and Principe				72						
Senegal		41[4]		41						
Sri Lanka		10[4]		10						20
Suriname		78	75	79						
Swaziland		46[4]		46[4]						
Sweden		46	100	45						
Tajikistan		41[4]		41		46	45	51		
Thailand		28	23	29		49				25
The former Yugoslav Republic of Macedonia	10	47	67	43	27	34	32	47	34	41
Togo		45	46	42						
Turkey	22									
Ukraine	8	48[4]		48	21	47	47	45	49	47
Viet Nam	24	35[4]		35	34	38[3,5]	38[3]			55[3]
Zambia		41	41	42						

1 Report date 2007, but data collection can vary from 2005-2007
2 Data collection started before 2005
3 Methodology not harmonized with UNGASS 2008 guidelines
4 Females only
5 Males only
6 Transgender

ANNEX 2

UNGASS indicator 15. Percentage of young women and men aged 15-24 who have had sexual intercourse before the age of 15

Country (or territory)	2005			Country reported value for 2007				Most recent DHS (or MICS)		
	Survey year	Males	Females	Survey year	Males	Females	Both sexes 15-24	Survey year	Males	Females
Angola		47	24	2006	36	28	32			
Antigua and Barbuda				2006			25			
Argentina				2005	27	19	23			
Armenia				2007	11	<1	3	2005	3	<1
Azerbaijan								2006	1	1
Bangladesh				2005	4	1	2			
Barbados		36	26							
Belarus				2007	8	4	5			
Belize				2006	11	6	9			
Benin		16	9	2006	13	12	12	2006	13	12
Bosnia and Herzegovina				2006		1		2006[1]		<1
Bulgaria				2006	13	7	10			
Burkina Faso				2007	3	7	6	2003	4	7
Burundi		14	6	2005		3		2005[1]		3
Cambodia		<1	<1	2006	<1	1	1	2005	<1	1
Cameroon	2004	23	35	2006		14		2006[1]		14
Cape Verde				2005	41	24	30	2005	41	24
Central African Republic	2004	10	10	2006	20	33	30	2006	13	25
Chad				2004	19	39	35	2004	10	26
Chile				2006	12	6	9			
Colombia				2007			37	2005		13
Congo, Republic of the	2003	10	10	2005	27	24	24	2005	27	24
Costa Rica				2006	15	7	11			
Cuba				2006	33	15	24			
Cyprus				2007	15	1	8			
Côte d'Ivoire	2004	13	15	2005	15	19	18	2005	15	19
Democratic Republic of the Congo				2006	31	23	28	2007	18	18
Dominican Republic				2007	24	33	29	2007	24	15
Ecuador				2004		10				
El Salvador				2003	54	21	27			
Eritrea								2002		13
Estonia				2007	10	11	10			
Ethiopia		40	42	2005	2	16	12	2005	2	16
Fiji				2007			50			
Gabon				2007	38	14	25	2000	42	24
Gambia				2006		5		2006[1]		5
Georgia				2005		2	2			
Germany				2006	10	12	11			
Ghana								2006	4	6
Greece				2007	35	7	24			
Grenada				2006	32	20	25			
Guatemala				2002	20	9	11	1999		10

UNGASS indicator 15. Percentage of young women and men aged 15-24 who have had sexual intercourse before the age of 15										
Country (or territory)	2005			Country reported value for 2007				Most recent DHS (or MICS)		
	Survey year	Males	Females	Survey year	Males	Females	Both sexes 15-24	Survey year	Males	Females
Guinea	2005	16	18	2007	20	31	25	2005	17	22
Guinea-Bissau				2006		22				
Guyana				2005	30	12	21	2005	13	9
Haiti				2006	43	15	23	2005	43	15
Honduras				2005	19	11	13	2006		11
India				2006	2	4	3	2006	2	10
Iran, Islamic Republic of				2005						
Jamaica				2004						
Japan				2004	8	9	9			
Kazakhstan				2007	20	3	9			
Kenya	2005	20	17	2003	29	14	21	2003	29	14
Kyrgyzstan				2007	9	<1	5	2006[1]		0
Latvia				2007	16	9	12			
Lebanon				2004			4			
Lesotho	2004	27	14	2005	12	6	8	2004	13	6
Lithuania				2006	22	10	16			
Madagascar	2003	22	31	2006	33	39	36	2004	9	15
Malawi				2006				2004	14	15
Mali				2006	5	25	6	2006	5	25
Marshall Islands				2006	17	10	14	2007	27	14
Mauritania				2007		14	14			
Mauritius				2004	3	1	2			
Mexico				2005	4	4	4			
Moldova	2005	34	24	2006	8	1	4	2005	9	1
Mongolia	2005	3	<1	2005	3	<1	1			
Montenegro				2007	4	2	3	2006[1]		<1
Morocco				2007	8	1	5			
Mozambique				2004	26	28	28	2003	26	28
Namibia				2007	18	7	12	2006	18	7
Nepal								2006	4	7
Nicaragua				2007		14	14	2001		12
Niger				2006	8	39	25	2006	5	30
Nigeria	2005	5	15	2005	5	15	10	2003	7	21
Pakistan				2006	1	<1				
Palau				2006		5				
Papua New Guinea				2007	4	4	4			
Peru				2007		6		2007		6
Philippines								2003	2	1
Romania				2006	17	3	10			
Russian Federation	2004	17	8	2007	12	3	7			
Rwanda				2005	13	4	7	2005	13	4
Saint Kitts and Nevis				2006	36	10	22			

UNGASS indicator 15. Percentage of young women and men aged 15-24 who have had sexual intercourse before the age of 15

Country (or territory)	2005			Country reported value for 2007				Most recent DHS (or MICS)		
	Survey year	Males	Females	Survey year	Males	Females	Both sexes 15-24	Survey year	Males	Females
Saint Lucia				2006	32	20	26			
Saint Vincent and the Grenadines	2005	63	37	2006	31	14	22			
Sao Tome and Principe				2006						
Senegal				2005	12	9	10	2005	12	9
Sierra Leone				2005	25		25			
Singapore				2007	3	2	2			
South Africa				2005	5	12	8			
Spain				2003	18	11	15			
Sri Lanka				2007			3			
Suriname				2006			8			
Swaziland				2007	5	7	6	2007	5	7
Sweden				2007	15	21	19			
Switzerland				2007	10	7	8			
Tajikistan				2006	1	<1	1			
Thailand		11	7	2006	21	5	13			
The former Yugoslav Republic of Macedonia				2007	8	1	5	2006[1]		<1
Togo				2007	13	10	11	1998	<1	19
Trinidad and Tobago				2007			12			
Tunisia					7	<1	4			
Turkey				2007						
Turkmenistan								2000		<1
Uganda				2006	12	16	15	2006	12	16
Ukraine				2007	7	3	5	2007	2	1
United Kingdom of Great Britain and Northern Ireland				2001	14	12	13			
United Republic of Tanzania				2005	10	13	11	2004	9	12
Uruguay				2007	25	10	18			
Uzbekistan								1996		1
Viet Nam				2005	1	<1	<1	2005	<1	1
Zambia				2007	16	14	15	2007	16	14
Zimbabwe		9	8	2006	5	5	5	2006	4	5

[1] Source is the Multiple Indicator Cluster Survey (UNICEF MICS)

ANNEX 2

UNGASS indicator 16. Percentage of women and men aged 15-49 who have had sexual intercourse with more than one partner in the last 12 months

Country (or territory)	2003[1]					2005[1]				
	Survey year	Males	Females	Both sexes		Survey year	Males	Females	Both sexes	
		15-49	15-49	15-24	25-49		15-49	15-49	15-24	25-49
Angola										
Antigua and Barbuda										
Armenia	2000	9	<1	4	4	2005	9	<1	6	3
Azerbaijan										
Bangladesh										
Belarus										
Belize										
Benin	1996		2			2001	22	1	7	8
Bolivia						2003	15	1	10	7
Bosnia and Herzegovina										
Burkina Faso	1999	13	1	9	6	2003	15	1	5	9
Burundi										
Cambodia	2000		<1			2005	6	<1	2	4
Cameroon	1998	41	10	25	25	2004	31	6	15	22
Canada										
Cape Verde						2005	36	3	19	19
Central African Republic										
Chad	1997	19	1	11	8	2004	17	1	6	10
Chile										
Colombia	2000		3			2005		3		
Comoros										
Congo, Republic of the						2005	24	7	15	16
Costa Rica										
Cuba										
Cyprus										
Côte d'Ivoire	1998	33	5	19	19	2005	24	4	12	15
Democratic Republic of the Congo										
Dominican Republic	1996	16	2	4	6	2002	23	2	13	13
Estonia										
Ethiopia	2000	7	1	3	5	2005	2	<1	1	2
Gabon	2000	24	14	20	18					
Gambia										
Germany										
Ghana						2003	10	1	4	7
Greece										
Grenada										
Guatemala										
Guinea	1999	26	4	15	15	2005	25	2	11	14
Guinea-Bissau										
Guyana						2005	7	1	6	3

UNGASS indicator 16. Percentage of women and men aged 15-49 who have had sexual intercourse with more than one partner in the last 12 months

Country reported value for 2007							Most recent DHS (or MICS)		
Survey year	Males	Females	Both sexes				Survey year	Males	Females
	15-49	15-49	15-49	15-19	20-24	25-49		15-49	15-49
2006	51	25	38	54	46	26			
2006			55						
							2005	9	<1
							2006	6	<1
2005	18		18	25	25	14			
2007	33	14	21	27	32	15			
2006	13[2]	4[2]	8[2]						
2006	12	35	17	62	30	8	2006	28	
							2003	15	1
2006		8		4	11				
2007	14	1	7	2	6	9	2006[4]		1[2]
							2005[4]		1[2]
2006	6	<1	3	1	4	3	2005	6	<1
2004	40	8	18	17	20	17	2006[4]		5[2]
2006			13						
2005	69	43	52	86	71	36	2005	36	3
2006	24[2]	6[2]	11[2]	6	14				
2004	17	1	8	4	9	10	2004	17	1
2006	12	2	7	6	14	6			
2007		4[3]			35[3]		2005	<1	3
2003	24	4	11			9			
2005	28	8	14	19	16	13	2005	24	7
2006	37	35	39						
2006	35	10	23	22	29	22			
2007	25	6	15						
2005	31	4	16	15	18	16	2005	24	4
2007	22	4	9	10	11	9	2007	17	3
2007	30	4	17	22	25	16	2007	24	3
2007	23	19	21	17	26				
2005	3	<1	2	1	2	2	2005	2	<1
2007	51	38	43	53	36	43			
2006		1[2]					2006[4]		1[2]
2007	35	22	29						
2006	22[2]	40[2]	26[2]				2006	8	1
2007	33	8	20	22	48	18			
2006	30	13	21	19	30	16			
2002	13		13	34	19	8			
2005	25	2	8	6	10	8	2005	25	2
2006				5	7		2006[4]		6[2]
2005	9	1	5				2005	7	1

UNGASS indicator 16. Percentage of women and men aged 15-49 who have had sexual intercourse with more than one partner in the last 12 months										
Country (or territory)	2003[1]					2005[1]				
	Survey year	Males	Females	Both sexes		Survey year	Males	Females	Both sexes	
		15-49	15-49	15-24	25-49		15-49	15-49	15-24	25-49
Haiti	2000	24	1	11	13	2005	23	1	11	13
Honduras						2006		1		
India						2006	1	<1	1	1
Jamaica										
Kazakhstan										
Kenya	1998	24	3	16	11	2003	12	2	7	7
Kyrgyzstan										
Lebanon										
Lesotho						2004	21	8	11	16
Lithuania										
Madagascar						2004	17	3	11	9
Malawi	2000	15	1	6	9	2004	9	1	4	6
Mali	1996	13				2001	17	1	5	11
Marshall Islands										
Mauritius										
Mexico										
Moldova						2005	11	1	9	4
Mongolia										
Montenegro										
Morocco										
Mozambique						2003	30	5	18	17
Namibia	2000	16	2	9	10					
Nepal	2001	3								
Nicaragua	2001		1							
Niger	1998	10	1	7	5					
Nigeria						2003	15	2	5	10
Palau										
Papua New Guinea										
Peru	1996	23	<1	4	9	2000		<1		
Philippines						2003	6			
Poland										
Russian Federation										
Rwanda	2000	2	<1	1	2	2005	3	<1	1	2
Saint Kitts and Nevis										
Saint Lucia										
Saint Vincent and the Grenadines										
Senegal						2005	13	1	4	10
Serbia										
Seychelles										
Sierra Leone										

UNGASS indicator 16. Percentage of women and men aged 15-49 who have had sexual intercourse with more than one partner in the last 12 months

Country reported value for 2007							Most recent DHS (or MICS)		
Survey year	Males	Females	Both sexes				Survey year	Males	Females
	15-49	15-49	15-49	15-19	20-24	25-49		15-49	15-49
2006	23	1	12	7	16	13	2005	23	1
2005	16	1	4				2006	<1	1
2006	8	2	5	6	9	4	2006	1	<1
2004	48	11	29						
2007	25	5	15	9	23	15			
2003	12	2	5	3	6	5	2003	12	2
2007	28	2	15	10	21		2006[4]		<1[2]
2004	24	4	17						
2005	30	11	16				2004	21	8
2007	43	26	41	<1	<1	41			
2004	20	3	7				2004	17	3
2005	1	1	1	2	1	1	2004	9	1
2006	23	2	5	5	4	1	2006	15	1
2006	23	18	21	19	30		2007	7	3
2004	9	1	5	4	5	6			
2003	8				6	9			
2007	16	2	8	11	19	5	2005	11	1
2005	54		54						
							2005[4]		<1[2]
2007	37	2	19	14	27				
2004	52	24	29	60	34	19	2003	30	5
2007	16	3	9	10	15	7	2006	11	2
							2006	2	<1
2007		2	2	1	2	2			
2006	9	1	2	5	4	2	2006	12	1
2005	19	2	10	3	10	14	2003	15	2
2006		9		36	13	5			
2007	13	2	8	6	11	7			
2006	33	12					2007		1
							2003	6	
2005	8	5	7						
2006	20	9	15	16	26	13			
2005	3	<1	2	<1	1	2	2005	3	<1
2006	53	19	36						
2007	42	25	35						
2006	25	10	17	13	32	9			
2005	25	4	8	7	11	7	2005	13	1
2006	42	11	26	32	24	<1	2005[4]		3[2]
2003	23	11	17						
2005	9	36	21						

UNGASS indicator 16. Percentage of women and men aged 15-49 who have had sexual intercourse with more than one partner in the last 12 months										
Country (or territory)	2003[1]					2005[1]				
	Survey year	Males	Females	Both sexes		Survey year	Males	Females	Both sexes	
		15-49	15-49	15-24	25-49		15-49	15-49	15-24	25-49
Singapore										
South Africa										
Spain										
Sri Lanka										
Suriname										
Swaziland										
Sweden										
Switzerland										
Tajikistan										
Thailand										
Togo	1998	21	3	13	13					
Trinidad and Tobago										
Turkey										
Turkmenistan	2000		<1							
Uganda	1995	8	1	5	4	2001	18	2	6	12
Ukraine										
Uzbekistan										
United Kingdom of Great Britain and Northern Ireland										
United Republic of Tanzania	1999	29	9	17	20	2004	23	3	10	15
Uruguay										
Viet Nam						2005	14	2	6	9
Zambia	1996	27	4	18	12	2002	21	2	10	13
Zimbabwe	1999	13	2	6	8	2006	9	1	4	6

1 Data provided by MEASURE DHS
2 15-24 years
3 25-64 years only
4 Source is the Multiple Indicator Cluster Survey (UNICEF MICS)

UNGASS indicator 16. Percentage of women and men aged 15-49 who have had sexual intercourse with more than one partner in the last 12 months									
Country reported value for 2007							Most recent DHS (or MICS)		
Survey year	Males	Females	Both sexes				Survey year	Males	Females
	15-49	15-49	15-49	15-19	20-24	25-49		15-49	15-49
2007	7	2	4	2	10	4			
2005	3	18	10	18	15	8			
2003	27	13	20						
2007	3	<1	2	1	1	3			
2006			3						
2007	14	2					2007	14	2
2007	23	23	23	33	34	11			
2007	18	10	14	25	26	10			
2006			6	3	9				
2006	18	1	9	24	18	7			
2007	26	6	16	10	22	17	2006[4]		3[2]
2007	94	79	85						
2007		15	15	19	20	11			
							2000		<1
2006	21	2	12	3	9	16	2006	21	2
2007	21	7	14	18	23	11	2007	13	2
							2006[4]		<1[2]
2001	25	15	20	30	35	16			
2006	20	5	13	46			2004	23	3
2007	23	11	17	28	35	11			
2005	1	<1	<1	<1	1	<1	2005	14	2
2007	14	1	7	3	7	9	2007	14	1
2006	14	1	7	7	9	6	2006	9	1

ANNEX 2

UNGASS indicator 17. Percentage of women and men aged 15-49 who had more than one sexual partner in the past 12 months reporting the use of a condom during their last sexual intercourse

Country (or territory)	2003[1]					2005[1]				
	Survey year	Male 15-49	Females 15-49	Both sexes		Survey year	Males 15-49	Females 15-49	Both sexes	
				15-24	25-49				15-24	25-49
Albania										
Angola										
Antigua and Barbuda										
Argentina										
Armenia	2000	32				2005	58			
Azerbaijan										
Bangladesh										
Belarus										
Benin	1996		13			2001	23	18	33	17
Bosnia and Herzegovina										
Burkina Faso	1999	55	36	56		2003	43	44	68	33
Burundi										
Cambodia						2005	41			
Cameroon	1998	23	13	27	17	2004	38	35	53	28
Canada										
Cape Verde						2005	69	57	78	59
Central African Republic										
Chad	1997	20	10	22	17	2004	20	7		
Chile										
Colombia	2000		22			2005		31		
Congo, Republic of the						2005	30	23		
Costa Rica										
Cuba										
Cyprus										
Côte d'Ivoire	1998	45	23	53	34	2005	38	41	59	26
Democratic Republic of the Congo										
Dominican Republic	1996	9	19	7	10	2002	35	33	45	27
Estonia										
Ethiopia	2000	20	11	43	10	2005	9			
Gabon	2000	40	26	41	29					
Gambia										
Germany										
Ghana						2003	22	33	39	
Greece										
Grenada										
Guatemala										
Guinea	1999	24	9	31	17	2005	24	20	38	17
Guinea-Bissau										
Guyana						2005	53	56		
Haiti	2000	21	30	30	16	2005	34	21	49	23

UNGASS indicator 17. Percentage of women and men aged 15-49 who had more than one sexual partner in the past 12 months reporting the use of a condom during their last sexual intercourse

Country reported value for 2007							Most recent DHS (or MICS)		
Survey year	Males 15-49	Females 15-49	Both sexes				Survey year	Males 15-49	Females 15-49
			15-49	15-19	20-24	25-49			
2005									
2006	46	18	32	26	40	31			
2006			87						
2005	48	44	46	48	44				
							2005	58	
2006							2006	26	<1
2005	35		35	42	31	36			
2007	62	60	61	76	68	49			
2006	25	42	32	31	36	29	2006	17	
2006		72		73	71				
2007	36	51	38	69	61	30	1999	55	36
2004	55	45	49						
2006	40	12	39	83	73	23	2005	41	
2006	55	41	48	61	62	43	2006[4]		68[5]
	23	16	19						
2005	72	46	58	70	61	47	2005	69	57
2006									
2004	20	7					2004	20	7
2006	30	18	28	32	34	25			
							2005		31
2005	43	21	30	24	29	35	2005	30	23
2006	15	11	13			12			
2006	41	33	39	72	53	30			
2007	63	53	61						
2005	52	34	44	47	45	42	2005	38	41
2007	26	16	21	16	26	21	2007	16	8
2007	42	33	37	54	44	34	2007	45	35
2007	64	55	61	61	64				
2005	52	24	43	38	47	34	2005	9	
2007	72[2]	70[2]	71[2]	65[2]	73[2]	71[2]			
							2006[4]		64[5]
2007			58						
2006	33	54					2006	38	35
2007	71	55	67	61	58	75			
2006	68	52		61	63				
2002				47	58	50			
2005	32	26	31	35	43	27	2005	24	20
							2006[4]		58[5]
2005	53	56	53				2005	53	56
2006	34	21	33	41	53	23	2005	34	21

UNGASS indicator 17. Percentage of women and men aged 15-49 who had more than one sexual partner in the past 12 months reporting the use of a condom during their last sexual intercourse

Country (or territory)	2003[1]					2005[1]				
	Survey year	Male 15-49	Females 15-49	Both sexes		Survey year	Males 15-49	Females 15-49	Both sexes	
				15-24	25-49				15-24	25-49
Honduras						2006		27		
India						2006	23	12		
Jamaica										
Kazakhstan										
Kenya	1998	36	18	38	30	2003	33	12	47	17
Kyrgyzstan										
Lebanon										
Lesotho						2004	41	19	47	26
Lithuania										
Madagascar						2004	9	2	12	6
Malawi	2000	14	15	26	7	2004	20	16	32	13
Mali	1996	34				2001	16	14	27	13
Marshall Islands										
Mauritania										
Mauritius										
Mexico										
Moldova						2005	45	22	56	28
Mongolia										
Morocco										
Mozambique						2003	19	14	38	10
Namibia	2000	65	45	72	56					
Nepal										
Nicaragua	2001		19							
Niger	1998	26	28							
Nigeria						2003	22	13	34	17
Palau										
Papua New Guinea										
Peru	2000		15							
Philippines						2003		22		
Rwanda	2000	28	30			2005	8	14		
Saint Kitts and Nevis										
Saint Lucia										
Saint Vincent and the Grenadines										
Sao Tome and Principe										
Senegal						2005	31	21	61	22
Serbia										
Sierra Leone										
Singapore										
South Africa										
Spain										

UNGASS indicator 17. Percentage of women and men aged 15-49 who had more than one sexual partner in the past 12 months reporting the use of a condom during their last sexual intercourse

Country reported value for 2007							Most recent DHS (or MICS)		
Survey year	Males 15-49	Females 15-49	Both sexes				Survey year	Males 15-49	Females 15-49
			15-49	15-19	20-24	25-49			
2006	38	32	37				2006		27
2006	67	62	66	61	68	66	2006	23	12
2004	67	53	64						
2007	82	82	82	88	93	77			
2003	33	12	30	48	47	17	2003	33	12
2007	81	75	80	85	78				
2004	72	67	72						
2004	41	19	34	49	40	26	2004	41	19
2007	46	20	44			44			
2004	13	5	8	8	8	8	2004	9	2
2004	47	30	38	35	47	33	2006[4]		45[5]
2006	38	17	20	19	29	34	2006	12	8
2006	19	15	18	17	19		2007	20	11
2007	10		10						
2004	44	46	44	50	43	43			
2003	20				78	14			
2007	48	60	49	45	50	52	2005	45	22
2005	34		34						
2007	61	75	62	63	61				
2003	19	14	18	28	28	10	2003	19	14
2007	74	66	68	79	76	60	2006	74	66
2006	54						2006	30	
2001		19					2001		19
2006	7	8					2006	7	8
2005	62	44	56	44	56	62			
2006		23				60			
2007	45	26	43	50	49	38			
2006			48	59	43		2007		31
2003	22						2003		22
2005	8	14	8				2005	8	14
2006			67						
2007	48	39	45						
2006	62	52	59	59	59				
2006		57[3]		60	59				
2005	62	37	52	39	51	59	2005	31	21
2006				73	78				
2007	11	26	37						
2007	51	0	42	50	14	51			
2005	67	47	64	80	72	56			
2003	50	42	46						

ANNEX 2

UNGASS indicator 17. Percentage of women and men aged 15-49 who had more than one sexual partner in the past 12 months reporting the use of a condom during their last sexual intercourse

Country (or territory)	2003[1]					2005[1]				
	Survey year	Male 15-49	Females 15-49	Both sexes 15-24	Both sexes 25-49	Survey year	Males 15-49	Females 15-49	Both sexes 15-24	Both sexes 25-49
Suriname										
Swaziland										
Switzerland										
Tajikistan										
Thailand										
Togo	1998	33	21	42	25					
Turkey										
Uganda	1995	18	8	24	9	2001	24	25		
Ukraine										
United Kingdom of Great Britain and Northern Ireland										
United Republic of Tanzania	1999	22	16	25	17	2004	29	21	37	23
Uruguay										
Viet Nam						2005	58			
Zambia	1996	31	18	36	23	2001	27	21	40	20
Zimbabwe	1999	40	46	56	30	2006	36	41	57	24

1 Data provided by MEASURE DHS
2 data from two cities only
3 female is 15-24 years only
4 Source is the Multiple Indicator Cluster Survey (UNICEF MICS)
5 15-24 years

UNGASS indicator 17. Percentage of women and men aged 15-49 who had more than one sexual partner in the past 12 months reporting the use of a condom during their last sexual intercourse									
Country reported value for 2007							Most recent DHS (or MICS)		
Survey year	Males 15-49	Females 15-49	Both sexes				Survey year	Males 15-49	Females 15-49
			15-49	15-19	20-24	25-49			
2006			49						
2007	56	57	56		62	51	2007	56	57
2007	62	52	58	83	61	48			
2006			65	53	69				
2006	53	14	51	63	49	50			
2007	73	69	73	72	76	71	1998	33	21
2007		58	53	52	71	45			
2006	42	41	42		30	41	2006	42	41
2007	75	61	72	77	64	72	2007	46	48
2001	10	5	7	15	15	5			
2005	50	38	44	38	41		2004	29	21
2007	69	65	68	76	81	56			
	1	0	0	0	1	0	2005	58	
2007	50	37	46	39	49	48	2007	28	33
2006	71	47	64	50	67	68	2006	36	41

ANNEX 2

UNGASS indicator 18. Percentage of female and male sex workers reporting the use of a condom with their most recent client[1]						
UNGASS	2005			2007		
Country (or territory)	All	Males	Females	All	Males	Females
Afghanistan				50[3,5]		50[3]
Angola				78[5]		78
Armenia	89	100	89	91[5]		91
Bangladesh	40	44	32	63	44	67
Barbados				80[5]		80
Belarus	77	100	77	76[5]		76
Benin				83[5]		83
Bolivia				88[4]	57[4]	88[4]
Bulgaria				95[5]		95
Burkina Faso	96			99	98	99
Burundi	74		74	74[2,5]		74[2]
Cambodia	96		96	99[5]		99
Cameroon				74[2,4,5]		74[2,4]
Canada					61[4]	80[4]
Cape Verde				74[5]		74
China			69	82[5]		82
Colombia				89	82	97
Comoros				59[5]		59
Costa Rica				92[5]		92
Côte d'Ivoire				96[5]		96
Croatia				86[2]		
Cuba				61	63	56
Democratic Republic of the Congo				61[2,5]		61[2]
Dominican Republic				96[2]		
Ecuador						95
El Salvador				96	89	97
Eritrea				76[5]		
Estonia				94[5]		94
Ethiopia				87[5]		84
Gabon				67	53	67
Georgia			95	94[5]		94
Ghana				98		
Guatemala				96	91	97
Guinea				100[5]		100
Guinea-Bissau						60
Guyana				89[5]		89
Haiti				90[5]		90
Honduras				68	71	66
India						88
Indonesia	55	48	56	69	72	68

UNGASS indicator 18. Percentage of female and male sex workers reporting the use of a condom with their most recent client[1]

UNGASS	2005			2007		
Country (or territory)	All	Males	Females	All	Males	Females
Iran, Islamic Republic of				55[5]		55
Jamaica	84			84		
Kazakhstan				97[5]		97
Kyrgyzstan	81			84[5]		84
Lao People's Democratic Republic	83	59	89			
Lebanon				34[4]	47[4]	34[4]
Lithuania				77[5]		77
Madagascar				79		
Malawi				69[5]		69
Malaysia				35[2]		
Mali				99[5]		99
Mauritius				100[2,5]		100[2]
Mexico				96	96	96
Moldova	98			93[5]		93
Mongolia	94	50	96	92[5]		92
Morocco	38		38	54[5]		54
Nepal	67			81	93	77
Niger				96[5]		96
Nigeria				98[5]		98
Pakistan	23	7	37	34	21	45
Panama	92	91	92	76	64	84
Papua New Guinea				94[5]		94
Paraguay				76	71	78
Peru					42	96
Philippines				65	50	65
Poland						46[2]
Romania			85	85[5]		85
Russian Federation	77			92[5]		92
Rwanda				87[5]		87
Sao Tome and Principe						60
Senegal	86		87	99[5]		99
Sierra Leone				68[5]		68
Singapore						99
Sri Lanka			65	89[5]		89
Suriname				70	79	68
Swaziland				98[5]		98
Sweden				22	100	20
Switzerland					72	
Tajikistan				75[5]		75
Thailand				96[4,5]		

UNGASS indicator 18. Percentage of female and male sex workers reporting the use of a condom with their most recent client[1]						
UNGASS	2005			2007		
Country (or territory)	All	Males	Females	All	Males	Females
The former Yugoslav Republic of Macedonia	86	88	84	78	93	75
Togo				78	76	84
Turkey				33[5]		33
Ukraine	80		80	86[5]		86
Uzbekistan				65[5]		65
Viet Nam	90		90	97[4,5]		97[4]
Zambia				81	72	82
Zimbabwe				4[4,6]	4[4]	

1 Report date 2007, but data collection can vary from 2005-2007
2 Data collection started before 2005
3 Data collection period not defined
4 Methodology not harmonized with UNGASS 2008 guidelines
5 Females only
6 Males only

UNGASS indicator 19. Percentage of men reporting the use of a condom the last time they had anal sex with a male partner[1]

UNGASS	2005	2007
Country (or territory)		
Argentina		91
Armenia	30	84
Australia		58[3,4]
Bahamas		69
Bangladesh	49	24
Belarus	62	67
Bulgaria		46
Cambodia		86
Chile		29
China	41	64
Colombia		80
Congo, Republic of the	23	
Costa Rica		71
Côte d'Ivoire		47
Croatia		53
Cuba		55
Dominican Republic		79[2]
Ecuador		63
El Salvador		83
Estonia		47
Fiji	20	
Georgia	54	
Germany		58
Ghana		48
Greece		89
Guatemala		78
Guyana		81
Haiti		73
Honduras		47
Indonesia	48	39
Japan		55
Kazakhstan		66
Kenya		75
Kyrgyzstan	68	81
Lao People's Democratic Republic		24[4]
Lebanon		39[4]
Lithuania		58
Mali		54
Mauritius		52[2]
Mexico		79

UNGASS indicator 19. Percentage of men reporting the use of a condom the last time they had anal sex with a male partner[1]

UNGASS	2005	2007
Country (or territory)		
Moldova	63	48
Mongolia	13	67
Nepal		74
Nigeria		53
Pakistan	8	24
Panama	84	86
Papua New Guinea		88[4]
Peru	46	47
Philippines		32
Poland		32[2,4]
Romania		73
Russian Federation	39	60
Saint Lucia		74
Senegal	45	55[2]
Slovenia		75[4]
Sri Lanka		61
Suriname		89
Sweden		42[4]
Switzerland		80[4]
Thailand		88
The former Yugoslav Republic of Macedonia	29	56
Togo		60
Trinidad and Tobago		47[2]
Turkey		37
Tuvalu		63
Ukraine	72	39
Uzbekistan		61
Viet Nam		61

1 Report date 2007, but data collection can vary from 2005-2007
2 Data collection started before 2005
3 Data collection period not defined
4 Methodology not harmonized with UNGASS 2008 guidelines

UNGASS indicator 20. Percentage of injecting drug users reporting the use a condom the last time they had sexual intercourse[1]

Country (or territory)	All	Males	Females
Argentina	64	63	65
Armenia	56	56	55
Australia	20[3]	20[3]	20[3]
Azerbaijan	18[2]		
Bangladesh	44	44	55
Belarus	59	57	65
Bosnia and Herzegovina	23[4]	23	
Bulgaria	19	18	28
Canada	43		
China	34[3]	32[3]	43[3]
Estonia	68	66	74
Georgia	48[4]	48	
Greece	48		
Indonesia	34	34	30
Iran, Islamic Republic of	33	33	30
Japan	65[4]	65	
Kazakhstan	37	37	36
Kyrgyzstan	11	11	9
Latvia	38	40	34
Lebanon	15[3]	15[3]	
Malaysia	5[2]		
Mauritius	13[2]	15[2]	0[2]
Mexico	29	27	38
Moldova	68	73	52
Morocco	13	12	21
Nepal	38[4]	38	
Nigeria	66	66	68
Pakistan		21	
Paraguay	33	33	36
Russian Federation	37	39	31
Sweden	25	28	19
Switzerland	50[3]	53[3]	42[3]
Tajikistan	36	33	47
Thailand	35		
The former Yugoslav Republic of Macedonia	51	51	51
Turkey	10	9	13
Ukraine	55	55	56
Uzbekistan	39	37	50
Viet Nam	36[3,4]	36[3]	

1 Report date 2007, but data collection can vary from 2005 to 2007
2 Data Collection period started before 2005
3 Methodology not harmonized with UNGASS 2008 guidelines
4 Males only

UNGASS indicator 21. Percentage of injecting drug users reporting the use of sterile injecting equipment the last time they injected [1]

Country (or territory)	All	Males	Females
Afghanistan	46		
Argentina	65	64	67
Armenia	95	95	93
Australia	71[4]		
Azerbaijan	77		
Bangladesh	34	34	74
Belarus	71	71	70
Bosnia and Herzegovina	25[5]	25	
Bulgaria	25	26	23
Canada	68[3,4]		
China	41	42	32
Georgia	93[5]	93	
Greece	67		
Indonesia	82[2]	82[2]	89[2]
Iran, Islamic Republic of	75	75	62
Japan	47[5]	47	
Kazakhstan	59	59	58
Kyrgyzstan	77	76	81
Latvia	90	87	96
Lebanon	60[4]	63[4]	0[4]
Malaysia	28[2]		
Mauritius	32[2]	32[2]	33[2]
Mexico	14	15	9
Moldova	96	96	95
Morocco	7	7	12
Nepal	96[5]	96	
Nigeria	89	89	86
Pakistan		28	
Paraguay	80	80	79
Philippines	48	47	63
Romania	28[2]	30[2]	17[2]
Russian Federation	82	83	81
Sweden	38	38	35
Switzerland	94[4]	95[4]	92[4]
Tajikistan	32	35	21
The former Yugoslav Republic of Macedonia	73	73	69
Turkey	10	9	13
Ukraine	84	85	81
Uzbekistan	23	23	25
Viet Nam	89[5]	89	

1 Report date 2007, but data collection can vary from 2005 to 2007
2 Data Collection period started before 2005
3 Data collection period undefined
4 Methodology not harmonized with UNGASS guidelines
5 Males only

UNGASS Indicator 24. Percentage of adults and children with HIV known to be on treatment 12 months after initiation of antiretroviral therapy[1]

Country (or territory)	2005					2007				
	Male	Female	Both sexes <15	Both sexes 15+	Total	Male	Female	Both sexes <15	Both sexes 15+	Total
Antigua and Barbuda						53	57			55[2]
Argentina										90
Armenia						80	100		84	84
Azerbaijan						57	43		86	86[3]
Bahamas						68	71	90	68	70
Barbados	93	94			93	93	96		95	95
Belarus						74	77	97	74	75
Benin										73
Bolivia						97	96	100	97	97
Bosnia and Herzegovina										100[3]
Botswana			92			82	86			85[4]
Bulgaria						89	93	33	97	91
Burkina Faso						77	71	77	73	73
Burundi						77	82	77	81	80
Cambodia								94	87	88
Cameroon						96	96	97	96	96
Cape Verde						93	86	100	88	89
Central African Republic						85	85	89	85	85
Chile										89
China						84	91	96	85	85
Colombia										76
Comoros						40	60	0	100	100[3]
Costa Rica										91
Côte d'Ivoire						86	91	82	90	89
Croatia						100	88	0	97	97
Cuba						96	96	100	96	96
Democratic Republic of the Congo						66	72	62	70	70
Djibouti										82
Dominican Republic								89	90	90
El Salvador										85
Eritrea										93
Ethiopia	90	86			89					70
Fiji								100	78	79
Finland										90
Gabon						50	62	63	58	58
Gambia										92
Georgia	85	100			88	71	86	75	71	75[5]
Germany						77	80			78
Greece						95	96	100	95	96
Grenada						83	100	100	83	88
Guatemala										91

UNGASS Indicator 24. Percentage of adults and children with HIV known to be on treatment 12 months after initiation of antiretroviral therapy[1]

Country (or territory)	2005					2007				
	Male	Female	Both sexes <15	Both sexes 15+	Total	Male	Female	Both sexes <15	Both sexes 15+	Total
Guinea-Bissau										62
Guyana						70	78	97	73	75
Haiti										84
Honduras										91
Hungary						99	98	83	99	99
India										80
Iran, Islamic Republic of						78	79	75	78	78
Jamaica									88	88
Japan										100
Jordan										98
Kazakhstan						72	61	8	73	68
Kenya										87
Kyrgyzstan						70	57	100	66	68
Lao People's Democratic Republic						90	90	93	90	90
Lebanon										100
Lesotho					82	74	75	79	73	74
Lithuania						54	71		58	58
Madagascar					100					94
Malawi					83					69
Malaysia										87
Mali						72	72	72	72	72
Marshall Islands							100		100	100[3]
Mauritania										92
Mauritius						84	90		85	85
Moldova						82	93	88	87	87
Mongolia						67			67	67[3]
Montenegro						75	20		60	60[3]
Morocco										93
Mozambique										97
Namibia					91[2]			82	69	71
Nepal										85
New Zealand										98
Nicaragua										100
Niger								36	47	47
Nigeria					98[6]			92	95	95
Pakistan										87
Palau						100	100		100	100[3]
Panama										96
Papua New Guinea						67	56	10	67	61
Paraguay						30	14	6	44	49
Peru						85	87	95	85	85

UNGASS Indicator 24. Percentage of adults and children with HIV known to be on treatment 12 months after initiation of antiretroviral therapy[1]

Country (or territory)	2005					2007				
	Male	Female	Both sexes <15	Both sexes 15+	Total	Male	Female	Both sexes <15	Both sexes 15+	Total
Philippines						96	96		96	96
Rwanda										91
Saint Kitts and Nevis										100
Saint Lucia					80	100	97	100	98	98
Saint Vincent and the Grenadines						43	80	50	63	62
Sao Tome and Principe						65	82	100	74	75
Senegal						79	94			89
Seychelles						62	43	100	53	55
Sierra Leone										81
South Africa										53
Sri Lanka										64
Suriname										80
Swaziland						63	65	65	64	64
Sweden										
Switzerland						92	84		89	89
Tajikistan						55	61		57	57
Thailand						85	85	88	85	85
The former Yugoslav Republic of Macedonia						43	50		44	44[3]
Togo						90	90	90	90	90
Tunisia						93	90			92
Turkey						26	16	3	24	23
Uganda										88
Ukraine	69	75	70	100	72	73	83	91	76	78
Uruguay										74
Viet Nam								93	81	82
Zambia						87	90	92	88	88
Zimbabwe										93

1 Data values represent 1 cohort with 12 month minimum survival, with patients lost to follow-up and death included in the denominator, unless otherwise noted
2 Represents cumulative survival
3 Represents <10 persons alive and still on ART in last 12 months
4 Reflects 24 month survival (Jan 2005-Dec 2006)
5 Represents 2006
6 Represents 8 month survival

REFERENCES

Chapter 1 | THE GLOBAL HIV CHALLENGE

Commission on AIDS in Asia (2008). *Redefining AIDS in Asia – crafting an effective response.* Oxford University Press, New Delhi.

May RM, Anderson RM (1979). Population biology of infectious diseases – Part II. *Nature*, 280:455–461.

McNeil DG (2007). *A time to rethink AIDS's grip.* New York Times, 25 November.

UNAIDS (2006). *Setting national targets for moving towards universal access.* Geneva, UNAIDS.

UNAIDS (2007). *Monitoring the Declaration of Commitment on HIV/AIDS: guidelines on construction of core indicators, 2008 reporting.* Geneva, UNAIDS.

UNAIDS et al. (2004). *National spending for HIV/AIDS.* Geneva, UNAIDS.

UNDP (2005). *Human development report.* New York, NY, UNDP.

UNICEF, UNAIDS, WHO (2008). *Children and AIDS: second stocktaking report.* New York, NY, UNICEF.

United Nations General Assembly (2006). *Political Declaration on HIV/AIDS.* No. A/60/262, adopted 2 June 2006.

WHO (2005). *Major causes of death worldwide among children under 5 years of age and neonates in the world, 2000–2003.* http://libdoc.who.int/publications/2005/9241562986_part4.pdf

Chapter 2 | STATUS OF THE GLOBAL HIV EPIDEMIC

Actuarial Society of South Africa (2005). *ASSA 2003 AIDS and demographic model.* Cape Town, Actuarial Society of South Africa.

Adimora AA et al. (2003). Concurrent partnerships among rural African Americans with recently reported heterosexually transmitted HIV infection. *Journal of Acquired Immune Deficiency Syndromes*, 34(4):423–439.

Adimora AA et al. (2004). Concurrent sexual partnerships among African Americans in the rural south. *Annals of Epidemiology*, 14(3):155–160.

Allen CF et al. (2006). Sexually transmitted infection use and risk factors for HIV infection among female sex workers in Georgetown, Guyana. *Journal of Acquired Immune Deficiency Syndromes*, 43(1):96–101.

Anderson BA, Phillips HE (2006). *Adult mortality (age 15–64) based on death notification data in South Africa: 1997-2004.* Pretoria, Statistics South Africa (Report No. 03-09-05).

Anonymous. (2006). India in the spotlight (editorial). *Lancet*, 367:1876 June 10.

Asamoah-Odei E, Garcia-Celleja JM, Boerma T (2004). HIV prevalence and trends in sub-Saharan: no decline and large subregional differences. *Lancet*, 364:35–40.

Balthasar H, Jeannin A, Dubois-Arber F (2005). *VIH/SIDA: augmentation des expositions au risque d'infection par le VIH chez les homes ayant des rapports sexuels avec des hommes: premiers résultats de Gay Survey 04.* Bull BAG (Report No. 48:891–895).

Bautista CT et al. (2006). Seroprevalence of and risk factors for HIV-1 infection among female commercial sex workers in South America. *Sexually Transmitted Infections*, 82(4):311–316.

Benotsch EG et al. (2004). Drug use and sexual risk behaviors among female Russian IDUs who exchange sex for money or drugs. *International Journal of STD and AIDS*, 15(5):343–347.

Boulos D et al. (2006). Estimates of HIV prevalence and incidence in Canada, 2005. *Canadian Communicable Disease Report*, 32:165–174.

Bradshaw D et al. (2004). Unabated rise in number of adult deaths in South Africa. *South African Medical Journal*, 94(4):278–279.

Brahmbhatt H et al. (2006). Mortality in HIV-infected and uninfected children of HIV-infected and uninfected mothers in rural Uganda. *Journal of Acquired Immune Deficiency Syndrome*, 41(4):504–508.

Bravo-Garcia E, Magis-Rodriquez C, Saavedra J (2006). *New estimates in Mexico: more than 180,000 people living with HIV.* XVI International AIDS Conference. 13–18 August. Toronto, Ontario (Abstract CDC0411).

Brucková M et al. (2007). HIV/AIDS in the Czech Republic, 2006. *Eurosurveillance Weekly Release*, 12(4).

Carael M et al. (2004). Sexual networks and HIV in four African populations: the use of a standardised behavioural survey with biological markers. In: Morris M, ed. *Network Epidemiology: a handbook for network survey design and data collection.* Oxford, Oxford University Press.

Caribbean Commission on Health and Development (2005). *Report of the Caribbean Commission on Health and Development for the 26th Meeting of the CARICOM Heads of Government: Overview.* 3–6 July, Saint Lucia

Caribbean Epidemiology Centre, PAHO, WHO (2004). *Status and trends, analysis of the Caribbean HIV/AIDS epidemic, 1982–2002.* Trinidad and Tobago. Caribbean Epidemiology Centre, PAHO, WHO.

Cayemittes M et al. (2006). *Enquête mortalité, morbidité et utilisation des services EMMUS-IV: Haïti 2005–2006.* Juillet. Pétion ville et Calverton, Institut Haïtien de l'Enfance et ORC Macro.

Central Bureau of Statistics [Kenya], Ministry of Health [Kenya] and ORC Macro (2004). *Kenya Demographic and Health Survey 2003.* Calverton. Central Bureau of Statistics [Kenya], Ministry of Health [Kenya] and ORC Macro.

Central Statistical Office [Swaziland] and Macro International Inc (2007). *Swaziland Demographic and Health Survey 2006–2007: preliminary report.* Calverton (June).

Centre d'Evaluation et de Recherche Appliquée (CERA) et Family Health International (2006). *Résultats préliminaires.* Enquêtes de Surveillance des Comportements. Haiti 2006, FHI BSS III.

Centro de Estudios Sociales y Demograficos et al. (2007). *Republica Dominicana Encuesta Demografica y de Salud 2007 Informe Preliminar.* Noviembre. Santo Domingo and Calverton.

Chandrasekaran P et al. (2006). Containing HIV/AIDS in India: the unfinished agenda. *Lancet Infectious Diseases*, 6(8):508–521.

Chen L et al. (2007). Sexual Risk Factors for HIV Infection in Early and Advanced HIV Epidemics in Sub-Saharan Africa: Systematic Overview of 68 Epidemiological Studies. *PLoS ONE*, 2(10):e1001.

Choi SYP, Cheung YW, Chen K (2006). Gender and HIV risk behaviour among intravenous drug users in Sichuan province, China. *Social Science and Medicine*, 62(7):1672–1684.

Coffee M, Lurie MN, Garnett GP (2007). Modelling the impact of migration on the HIV epidemic in South Africa. *AIDS*, 21(3):343–350.

Cohen J (2006). Up in smoke: epidemic changes course. *Science*, 313:487–488.

Commission on AIDS in Asia (2008). *Redefining AIDS in Asia: crafting an efffective response.* New Delhi, Oxford University Press.

Conselho Nacional de Combate ao HIV/SIDA (2006). *Relatório de actividades por 2005.* Maputo, Ministério de Saúde.

de Walque D (2007). Sero-discordant couples in five African countries: implications for prevention strategies. *Population and Development Review*, 33(3):501–523.

Department of Health [South Africa] (2007). *National HIV and syphilis antenatal prevalence survey, South Africa 2006.* Pretoria. Department of Health [South Africa].

Dodds JP et al. (2004). Increasing risk behaviour and high levels of undiagnosed HIV infection in a community sample of homosexual men. *Sexually Transmitted Infections*, 80:236–240.

Dorrington R et al. (2001). *The impact of HIV/AIDS on adult mortality in South Africa.* Medical Research Council (September) (http://www.mrc.ac.za/bod/, accessed 8 May 2008).

Dourado I et al. (2007). HIV-1 seroprevalence in the general population of Salvador, Bahia State, Northeast Brazil. *Cadernos de Saúde Pública*, 23(1):25–32.

Elrashied S (2006). *Prevalence, knowledge and related risky sexual behaviours of HIV/AIDS among receptive men who have sex with men (MSM) in Khartoum State, Sudan, 2005.* XVI International AIDS Conference. 13–18 August. Toronto, Ontario (Abstract TUPE0509).

EuroHIV (2006a). *HIV/AIDS surveillance in Europe: end-year report 2005.* Saint-Maurice, Institut de Veille Sanitaire (No 73).

EuroHIV (2006b). *HIV/AIDS surveillance in Europe: mid-year report 2005.* Saint-Maurice, Institut de Veille Sanitaire (No 72).

EuroHIV (2007a). *HIV/AIDS surveillance in Europe: mid-year report 2007, No 76.* Institut de Veille Sanitaire. Saint-Maurice (No 76) (http://www.eurohiv.org, accessed 8 May 2008).

EuroHIV (2007b). *HIV/AIDS surveillance in Europe: end-year report 2006, No 75.* Institut de Veille Sanitaire. Saint-Maurice (No 75) (http://www.eurohiv.org, accessed 8 May 2008).

Federal Ministry of Health [Nigeria] (2006). *The 2005 national HIV seroprevalence sentinel survey among pregnant women attending antenatal clinics in Nigeria: summary position paper.* Abuja (April). Federal Ministry of Health [Nigeria].

Fonseca ME et al. (2006). Os programas de reducao de danos ao uso de drogas no Brasil: caacterizacao preliminar de 45 programas. *Caderna de Saude Publica*, 2(4):761–770.

Gaillard EM et al. (2006). Understanding the reasons for decline of HIV prevalence in Haiti. *Sexually Transmitted Infections*, Supplement 82(1):14–20. April.

Garnett GP and Johnson AM (1997). Coining a new term in epidemiology: concurrency and HIV. *AIDS*, 11(5):681–683.

Gebre Y et al. (2006). *Tracking the course of the HIV epidemic through second generation surveillance in Jamaica: Survey of female sex workers.* XVI International AIDS Conference. 13–18 August. Toronto, Ontario (Abstract CDC0313).

Girault P et al. (2004). HIV, STIs and sexual behaviors among men who have sex with men in Phnom Penh, Cambodia. *AIDS Education and Prevention*, 6(1):31–44.

Gomes do Espirito Santo ME and Etheredge GD (2005). Male clients of brothel prostitutes as a bridge for HIV infection between high risk and low risk groups of women in Senegal. *Sexually Transmitted Infections*, 81:342–344.

Gorbach PM et al. (2006). Changing behaviors and patterns among Cambodian sex workers: 1997–2003. *Journal of Acquired Immune Deficiency Syndromes*, 42(2):242–247.

Gouws E et al. (2006). Short-term estimates of adult HIV incidence by mode of transmission: Kenya and Thailand as examples. *Sexually Transmitted Infections*, 82(Suppl. 3):iii5l–iii5.

Gouws E et al. (in press). Comparison of adult HIV prevalence from national population-based surveys and antenatal clinic surveillance in countries with generalized epidemics: implications for calibrating surveillance data. *Sexually Transmitted Diseases.* Supplement in press.

Gregson S et al. (2007). Critique of early models of the demographic impact of HIV/AIDS in sub-Saharan Africa based on contemporary empirical data from Zimbabwe. *Proceedings of the National Academy of Science*, Aug 30; 1776–1795.

Gupta A et al. (2006). Same-sex behavior and high rates of HIV among men attending sexually transmitted infection clinics in Pune, India, (1993–2002). *Journal of Acquired Immune Deficiency Syndromes*, 43(4):483–490.

Hallett TB et al. (2006). Declines in HIV prevalence can be associated with changing sexual behaviour in Uganda, urban Kenya, Zimbabwe and urban Haiti. *Sexually Transmitted Infections*, 82(Suppl. 1):i1-i8.

Halperin DT, Epstein H (2007). Why is HIV prevalence so severe in Southern Africa? The role of multiple concurrent partnerships and lack of male circumcision: implications for AIDS prevention. *Southern African Journal of HIV Medicine*, March:19–25.

Hamers FF et al (2006). HIV/AIDS in Europe: trends in EU-wide priorities. *Eurosurveillance*, 11(47).

Hamouda O et al. (2007). Epidemiology of HIV infections in Germany. *Bundesgesundheitsblatt*, 50(4):399–411.

Hauri AM, Armstrong GL, Hutin YJF (2004). The global burden of disease attributable to contaminated injections given in health care settings. *International Journal of STD and AIDS*, 15:7–16.

Heaton L, Fowler T, Palamuleni M (2006). *The HIV/AIDS epidemic in Malawi – putting the epidemic in context.* XVI International AIDS Conference. 13–18 August. Toronto, Ontario (Abstract CDC0062).

Helleringer S, Kohler HP (2007). Sexual network structure and the spread of HIV in Africa: evidence from Likoma Island, Malawi. *AIDS*, 21(17):2323–2332.

Hesketh T et al. (2006). *Risk behaviours in injecting drug users in Yunnan province, China: lessons for policy.* XVI International AIDS Conference. 13–18 August. Toronto, Ontario (Abstract CDD0591).

Hosegood V et al. (2007). The effects of high HIV prevalence on orphanhood and living arrangements of children in Malawi, Tanzania, and South Africa. *Population Studies* (Cambridge), 61(3):327–336.

IDES et al. (2005). *HIV, HBV, HCV prevalence related to sexual behavior and drug use in 200 injecting drug users in Montevideo, Uruguay.* Montevideo, Ministry of Health..

Inciardi JA, Syvertsen JL, and Surratt HL (2005). HIV/AIDS in the Caribbean Basin. *AIDS Care*, 17 (Suppl. 1): S9–S25.

Institute of Medical Research (2007). *"It's in Every Corner Now": A nationwide study of HIV, AIDS and STIs.* Gorokoa, Papua New Guinea Institute of Medical Research, Operational Research Unit.

Kengeya-Kayondo JF et al. (1995). Human immunodeficiency virus (HIV-1) seropositivity among children in a rural population of south-west Uganda: probable routes of exposure. *Annals of Tropical Paediatrics*, 15:115–120.

Kerrigan D et al. (2006). Environmental-structural interventions to reduce HIV/STI risk among female sex workers in the Dominican Republic. *American Journal of Public Health*, 96(1):120–125.

Kilani B et al. (2003). *Sero-epidemiology of HCV-HIV co-infection in Tunisia.* IAS Conference on HIV Pathogenesis and Treatment. 13–16 July. *Antiviral Therapy*, 8(Suppl. 1):S452–S453 (Abstract No. 952) (http://www.aegis.org/conferences/IASHIVPT/2003/952.html, accessed 8 May 2008).

Kintin FD et al. (2004). *Enquete de prevalence des IST/VIH et des comportements sexuels chez les travailleuses due sexe et leurs partenaires masculins a Ouagadougou, Burkina Faso.* Ouagadougou, Conseil national de lutte contre le sida et les IST, CIDA, CCSID (Novembre).

Kirungi WL et al. (2006). Trends in antenatal HIV prevalence in urban Uganda associated with uptake of preventive sexual behaviour. *Sexually Transmitted Infections*, 82(Suppl. 1):136–141.

Kiwanuka N et al. (2004). The incidence of HIV-1 associated with injections and transfusions in a prospective cohort, Rakai, Uganda. *AIDS*, 18(2):342–344.

Ladnaya NN (2007). The national HIV and AIDS epidemic and HIV surveillance in the Russian Federation. Presentation to Mapping the AIDS Pandemic meeting. June 30. Moscow.

Lagarde E et al. (2001). Concurrent sexual partnerships and HIV prevalence in five urban communities of sub-Saharan Africa. *AIDS*, 15(7):877–884.

Lee RK et al. (2006). *Risk behaviours for HIV among men who have sex with men in Trinidad and Tobago.* XVI International AIDS Conference. 13–18 August. Toronto, Ontario (Abstract CDD0366).

Liu H et al. (2006). Drug users: Potentially important bridge population in the transmission of sexually transmitted diseases, including AIDS, in China. *Sexually Transmitted Diseases*, 33(2):111–117.

Lu F et al. (2006). *HIV/AIDS epidemic in China: Increasing or decreasing?* XVI International AIDS Conference. 13–18 August. Toronto, Ontario (Abstract MOPE0462).

Lurie MN et al. (2003). Who infects whom? HIV-1 concordance and discordance among migrant and non-migrant couples in South Africa. *AIDS*, 17:2245–2252.

Magis C et al. (2006). *HIV prevalence and factors associated with the possession of condoms among male sex workers in two cities: Guadalajara and Mexico City, Mexico.* XVI International AIDS Conference. 13–18 August. Toronto, Ontario (Abstract CDC0336).

Maibani-Michie G and Yeka W (2005). *A Baseline Research for Poro Sapot Project: A Program for Prevention of HIV/AIDS among MSM in Port Moresby and FSW in Goroka and Port Moresby Papua New Guinea.* Papua New Guinea (IMR/FHI Research Report to USAID).

Malamba SS et al. (1994). Risk factors for HIV-1 infection in adults in a rural Ugandan community: a case-control study. *AIDS*, 8(2):253–257.

Marston M et al. (2007). Estimating 'net' HIV-related mortality and the importance of background mortality rates. *AIDS,* November 21(Suppl. 6):S65–S71.

Martínez GP, Elea NA, Chiu AM (2006). Epidemiology of HIV infection and acquired immune deficiency disease syndrome in Chile. *Revista Chilena Infectología*, 23(4):321–329.

Mason E (2006). Positioning paediatric HIV in the child survival agenda. Presentation to UNICEF–WHO consultation. January 11–13. New York, NY, UNICEF.

McFarland W, Mvere D, Katzenstein D (1997). Risk factors for prevalent and incident HIV infection in a cohort of volunteer blood donors in Harare, Zimbabwe: implications for blood safety. *AIDS*, 11(Suppl. 1):S97–S102.

Medical Research Council (2005). *South African national burden of disease study 2000.* Cape Town, Medical Research Council (http://www.mrc.ac.za/bod/reports.htm, accessed 8 May 2008).

Mejía A et al. (2006). *HIV seroprevalence and associated risk factors in men who have sex with men in the Villavicencio city, Colombia, 2005.* XVI International AIDS Conference. Toronto, Ontario (Abstract CDC0734).

Michelo C et al. (2006). Steep HIV prevalence declines among young people in selected Zambian communities: population-based observations (1995–2003). *BMC Public Health*, 10 November (http://www.biomedcentral.com/1471-2458/6/279, accessed 8 May 2008).

Mimouni B, Remaoun N (2006). *Etude du Lien Potentiel entre l'Usage Problématique de Drogues et le VIH/SIDA en Algérie 2004–2005.* Alger, Ministerie de education.

Ministère de la Santé [Maroc] (2007). *Surveillance sentinelle du VIH: Resultats 2006 et tendances de la séroprévalence du VIH.* Janvier. Rabat.

Ministère de la Santé du Mali (2006). *Résumé des résultats de l'enquête ISBS 2006.* Bamakó.

Ministère de la Santé et de l'Hygiène Publique de la Côte d'Ivoire, CDC/RETRO–CI/MEASURE Evaluation (2007). *Enquête de surveillance sentinelle du VIH de 2005.* Abidjan.

Ministère de la Santé Publique et de la Population (2007). Etude de serosurveillance par methode sentinelle de la prevalence du VIH, de la syphilis, de l'hépatite B et de l'hépatite C chez les femmes enceintes en Haiti, 2006/2007. Juillet. Port au Prince.

Ministerio de la Protecciòn Social de Colombia y ONUSIDA Grupo Tematico (2006). *Infeccion por VIH y SIDA en Colombia, Estado del arte. 2000–2005.* Mayo. Bogota, Ministerio de la Proteccion Social de Colombia y ONUSIDA Gruupo Tematico.

Ministerio de Salud de Peru (2005). *Sentinel surveillance report.* Lima, Ministerio de Salud de Peru, Directorate of Epidemiology.

Ministerio de Salud de Peru (2006). *Análisis de la situación epidemiológica del VIH/SIDA en el Perú – Bases Epidemiológicas para la Prevención y el Control.* Lima (Noviembre).

Ministry of Health [Botswana] (2006). *2006 Botswana Second-Generation HIV/AIDS Surveillance Technical Report.* Gabarone.

Ministry of Health [Cambodia] (2006). *Report on HIV sentinel surveillance in Cambodia, 2003.* Phnom Penh (July). Ministry of Health [Cambodia].

Ministry of Health [China] (2006). *2005 update on the HIV/AIDS epidemic and response in China*. Beijing, Ministry of Health China, UNAIDS, WHO.

Ministry of Health [Egypt], USAID, Impact and FHI (2006). *HIV/AIDS Biological and Behavioral Surveillance Survey; Summary Report; Egypt 2006*. Cairo, National AIDS Programme.

Ministry of Health [Guyana] (2005). *Behavioural surveillance survey, Round I: 2003/2004 – Executive Summary*. Georgetown. Ministry of Health [Guyana].

Ministry of Health [Indonesia] and Statistics Indonesia (2007). *Risk behavior and HIV prevalence in Tanah Papua, 2006*. Jakarta. Ministry of Health [Indonesia] and Statistics Indonesia.

Ministry of Health [Kazakhstan] et al. (2005). Results of investigation of the real situation with drug abuse in Kazakhstan. Almaty (in Russian).

Ministry of Health [Kenya] (2005). *AIDS in Kenya, 7th edition*. Nairobi, National AIDS and STI Control Programme (NASCOP).

Ministry of Health [New Zealand] (2007). *AIDS – New Zealand*. February. Auckland (Issue 59) (http://www.moh.govt.nz/moh.nsf/indexmh/aids-nz-issue59, accessed 8 May 2008).

Ministry of Health [Pakistan] (2006). *Integrated biological and behavioural surveillance: A pilot study in Karachi and Rawalpindi, 2004–2005*. Islamabad, Ministry of Health.

Ministry of Health [Syria], UNODC, UNAIDS (2007). *Assessment on Drug Use and HIV in Syria*. Damascus (Draft Report, July). Ministry of Health [Syria], UNODC, UNAIDS.

Ministry of Health [Uganda], ORC Macro (2006). *Uganda HIV/AIDS Sero-behavioural Survey 2004/2005*. Kampala and Calverton (March). Ministry of Health [Uganda], ORC Macro.

Ministry of Health [Ukraine] (2007). *HIV infection in Ukraine: Information bulletin no. 27*. Kyiv, Ukraine. Ministry of Health [Ukraine].

Ministry of Health [Ukraine] (2008). *Ukraine: National Report on Monitoring Progress Towards the UNGASS Declaration of Commitment on HIV/AIDS (Reporting Period: January 2006 - December 2007)*. Kyiv, Ukraine. Ministry of Health [Ukraine].

Ministry of Health [Uzbekistan] (2007). *Strategic Programme of Response to HIV in the Republic of Uzbekistan for 2007–2011*. Tashkent. Ministry of Health [Uzbekistan].

Ministry of Health [Viet Nam] (2005). *HIV/AIDS estimates and projections 2005–2010*. Hanoi, General Department of Preventive Medicine and HIV/AIDS Control, Ministry of Health.

Ministry of Health [Viet Nam] (2006). *Results from the HIV/STI integrated biological and behavioural surveillance (IBBS) in Viet Nam, 2005–2006*. Hanoi. Ministry of Health [Viet Nam].

Ministry of Health [Zambia] (2005). *Zambia Antenatal Clinic Sentinel Surveillance Report, 1994–2004*. November. Ministry of Health [Zambia]. Lusaka. Ministry of Health [Zambia].

Ministry of Health and Child Welfare [Zimbabwe] (2007). *2006 ANC preliminary report*. Harare. Ministry of Health and Child Welfare [Zimbabwe].

Ministry of Health and Medical Education [Iran] (2005). *AIDS/HIV Surveillance Report*. September. Tehran, Centre for Disease Management.

Ministry of Health and Population [Malawi] (2005). *HIV and syphilis sero survey and national HIV prevalence estimates report*. Lilongwe, Ministry of Health and Population Malawi.

Ministry of Health and Social Security [Dominica] (2007). *HIV/AIDS epidemiology and information in Dominica*. Roseau. Ministry of Health and Social Security [Dominica].

Mishra V et al. (2007). HIV infection does not disproportionately affect the poorer in sub-Saharan Africa. *AIDS*, November 21(Suppl. 7):S17–S28.

Montano SM et al. (2005). Prevalences, genotypes and risk factors for HIV transmission in South America. *Journal of Acquired Immune Deficiency Syndromes*, 40(1):57–64.

Moreau-Gruet F, Dubois-Arber F, Jeannin A (2006). Long-term HIV/AIDS-related prevention behaviours among men having sex with men: Switzerland 1992–2000. *AIDS Care*, 18:35–43.

Morris M, Kretzschmar M (1997). Concurrent partnerships and the spread of HIV. *AIDS*, 11(5):641–648.

Mulder DW et al. (1996). Post-natal incidence of HIV-I infection among children in a rural Ugandan population: no evidence for transmission other than mother-to-child. *Tropical Medicine and International Health*, 1:81–85.

National AIDS Commission [Indonesia] (2006). *Country report on the follow up to the Declaration of Commitment on HIV/AIDS (UNGASS) 2004–2005*. Jakarta. National AIDS Commission [Indonesia].

National AIDS Commission [Malawi] (2007). *Report of the Malawi Triangulation Project: Synthesis of data on trends in the national and local HIV epidemic and the reach and intensity of prevention efforts*. Lilongwe, National AIDS Commission, WHO, University of California San Francisco, UNAIDS, United States Centers for Disease Control and Prevention (January).

National AIDS Control Council [Kenya] (2007). *National HIV prevalence in Kenya*. Nairobi (July). National AIDS Control Council [Kenya].

National AIDS Council Secretariat [Papua New Guinea] (2007). *The 2007 consensus report on the HIV epidemic in Papua New Guinea*. Port Moresby. National AIDS Council Secretariat [Papua New Guinea].

National AIDS Council Secretariat [Papua New Guinea] and National HIV/AIDS Support Project (2007). *HIV/AIDS Behavioural Surveillance Survey Within High Risk Settings Papua New Guinea: BSS Round 1, 2006*. Port Moresby. National AIDS Council Secretariat [Papua New Guinea] and National HIV/AIDS Support Project.

National AIDS Program [Argentina] (2005). *Epidemiological surveillance report*. Buenos Aires (December). National AIDS Program [Argentina]

National AIDS Program [Paraguay] (2006). *HIV/STI sentinel prevalence and behavioral study on clients of female sex workers and injecting drug users*. National AIDS Program Paraguay, PRONASIDA. Asunción.

National Centre for HIV/AIDS, Dermatology and STIs (2004). *HIV Sentinel Surveillance (HSS) 2003: trends results, and estimates*. Phnom Penh. National Centre for HIV/AIDS, Dermatology and STIs.

National Centre for HIV/AIDS, Dermatology and STIs (2007). *HIV sentinel surveillance (HSS) 2006/2007: results, trends and estimates*. Phnom Penh. National Centre for HIV/AIDS, Dermatology and STIs.

National Centre in HIV Epidemiology and Clinical Research (2007a). *Australian HIV Surveillance Report*, 23(1) January.

National Centre in HIV Epidemiology and Clinical Research (2007b). *HIV/AIDS, viral hepatitis and sexually transmissible infections in Australia Annual Surveillance Report 2007*. Sydney, NSW , National Centre in HIV Epidemiology and Clinical Research, The University of New South Wales. Canberra, ACT, Australian Institute of Health and Welfare.

National Institute of Health and Family Welfare, National AIDS Control Organisation (2007). *Annual HIV Sentinel Surveillance Country Report 2006*. New Delhi. National Institute of Health and Family Welfare, National AIDS Control Organisation.

Ndetei D (2004). *Study on the assessment of the linkages between drug abuse, injecting drug abuse and HIV/AIDS in Kenya: a rapid situation assessment 2004*. Nairobi, United Nations Office on Drugs and Crime.

Newell ML et al. (2004). Mortality of infected and uninfected infants born to HIV-infected mothers in Africa: a pooled analysis. *Lancet*, 364(9441):1236–1243.

Nguyen TA et al. (in press). Prevalence and risk factors associated with HIV infection among men having sex with men in Ho Chi Minh City, Vietnam. *AIDS and Behavior*, in press (June 27).

Notkola V, Timaeus IM, Siiskonen H (2004). Impact on mortality of the AIDS epidemics in northern Namibia assessed using parish registers. *AIDS*, 18:1061–1065.

Obermeyer CM (2006). HIV in the Middle East. *British Medical Journal*, 333:851–854.

Odek-Ogunde M (2004). *World Health Organization phase II drug injecting study: behavioural and seroprevalence (HIV, HBV, HCV) survey among injecting drug users in Nairobi*. Nairobi, WHO.

Okie S (2006). Fighting HIV—lessons from Brazil. *New England Journal of Medicine*, 354(19):1977–1981.

Over M et al. (2007). The economics of effective AIDS treatment in Thailand. *AIDS*, 21(Suppl. 4):S105–S116.

Pan American Health Organization (2007). *AIDS in the Americas: The evolving epidemic, response and challenges ahead.* Washington, DC. Pan American Health Organization.

Pando MA et al. (2006). Epidemiology of human immunodeficiency virus, viral hepatitis (B and C), *Treponema pallidum*, and human T-cell lymphotropic I/II virus among men who have sex with men in Buenos Aires, Argentina. *Sexually Transmitted Diseases*, 33(5):307–313.

Pasteur Scientific and Research Institute of Epidemiology (2005). *Epidemiological surveillance and monitoring of HIV in risk behaviour groups in Volgogradskaya Oblast.* Saint Petersburg. Pasteur Scientific and Research Institute of Epidemiology.

Pisani E et al. (2004). HIV, syphilis infection, and sexual practices among transgenders, male sex workers, and other men who have sex with men in Jakarta, Indonesia. *Sexually Transmitted Infections*, 80(6):536–540.

Population Division of the Department of Economic and Social Affairs of the United Nations Secretariat (2008). *World Population Prospects: The 2006 Revision and World Urbanization Prospects: The 2005 Revision* (http://esa.un.org/unpp, accessed 10 March 2008).

Population Services International (2007). *Assessment of key health behaviors, their determinants and exposure to preventive interventions among street-based sex workers in Samara and Saratov, Russian Federation.* Moscow, Population Services International.

Prestage G, et al. (2006). *Trends in unprotected anal intercourse among Sydney gay men.* XVI International AIDS Conference. 13–18 August. Toronto, Ontario (Abstract WEPE0721).

Programa Nacional de Prevención y control de las ITS/VIH/Sida (2006). *Actualización de la situación Nacional hasta el 31 de Dic 2006.* Diciembre. Dirección Nacional de Epidemiología, MINSAP. La Habana.

Public Health Agency of Canada (2006). *HIV and AIDS in Canada: surveillance report to June 30, 2006.* Ottawa (http://www.phac-aspc.gc.ca/aids-sida/publication/index.html#surveillance, accessed 8 May 2008).

Public Health Agency of Canada (2007). *HIV and AIDS in Canada. Selected surveillance tables to June 30, 2007.* Ottawa, Surveillance and Risk Assessment Division, Centre for Infectious Disease Prevention and Control, Public Health Agency of Canada (http://www.phac-aspc.gc.ca/aids-sida/publication/index.html#surveillance, accessed 8 May 2008).

Ramesh B et al. (2006). *Sex work typology and risk for HIV in female sex workers: findings from an integrated biological and behavioural assessment in the southern Indian state of Karnataka.* XVI International AIDS Conference. 13–18 August. Toronto, Ontario (Abstract WEAC0305).

Reid G, Kamarulzaman A, Sran SK (2007). Malaysia and harm reduction: the challenges and responses. *International Journal of Drug Policy*, 18(2):136–140.

Rhodes T et al. (2004). HIV transmission and HIV prevention associated with injecting drug use in the Russian Federation. *International Journal of Drug Policy*, 15(1):1–16.

Robert Koch Institut (2007). *Epidemiologisches Bulletin.* Berlin (5 October).

Rosinska M (2006). Current trends in HIV/AIDS epidemiology in Poland, 1999–2004. *Eurosurveillance*, 11(4–6):94–97.

Rossi D et al. (2006). The HIV/AIDS epidemic and changes in injecting drug use in Buenos Aires, Argentina. *Cadernos de Saúde Pública*, 22(4):741–750.

Sanchez JL et al. (2006). High HIV prevalence and risk factors among injection drug users in Tashkent, Uzbekistan, 2003–2004. *Drug and Alcohol Dependency*, 82(Suppl. 1):S15–S22.

Sanchez J et al. (2007). HIV-1, sexually transmitted infections, and sexual behavior trends among men who have sex with men in Lima, Peru. *Journal of Acquired Immune Deficiency Syndromes*, 44(5):578–585.

Sanders EJ et al. (2007). HIV-1 infection in high risk men who have sex with men in Mombassa, Kenya. *AIDS*, 21:2513–2520.

Sandoy IF et al. (2007). Associations between sexual behaviour change in young people and decline in HIV prevalence in Zambia. *BMC Public Health*, 23 April (http://www.biomedcentral.com/content/pdf/1471-2458-7-60.pdf, accessed 8 May 2008).

Scherbinska A (2006). *HIV infection in Ukraine: a review of epidemiological data.* XVI International AIDS Conference. 13–18 August. Toronto, Ontario (Abstract CDC0398).

Schmid GP et al. (2004). Transmission of HIV-1 infection in sub-Saharan Africa and effect of elimination of unsafe injections. *Lancet*, 363:482–488

Secretaría de Estado de Salud Pública y Asistencia Social de Republica Dominica (2005). *Encuestas de vigilancia del comportamiento sobre VIH/ SIDA/ ITS en RSX y HSH del Área V de Salud.* Enero. Santo Domingo.

Secretaría de Salud de Honduras et al. (2007a). *Estudio Centroamericano de vigilancia de comportamiento sexual y prevalencia de VIH/ITS en poblaciones vulnerables: Trabajadoras Sexuales.* Agosto. Tegucigalpa.

Secretaría de Salud de Honduras et al. (2007b). *Estudio Centroamericano de vigilancia de comportamiento sexual y prevalencia de VIH/ITS en poblaciones vulnerables: Hombres que tienen sexo con hombres (HSH).* Julio. Tegucigalpa.

Silva ACM, Barone AA (2006). Risk factors for HIV infection among patients infected with hepatitis C virus. *Revista de Saúde Pública*, 40(3):482–488.

Silverman JG et al. (2006). HIV prevalence and predictors among rescued sex-trafficked women and girls in Mumbai, India. *Journal of Acquired Immune Deficiency Syndrome*, 43(5):588–93.

Silverman JG et al. (2007). HIV prevalence and predictors of infection in sex-trafficked Nepalese girls and women. *Journal of the American Medical Association*, 298(5):536–342.

Smolskaya TT (2006). *Studying HIV prevalence and risks among men having sex with men in Moscow and Saint Petersburg.* Saint Petersburg, Saint Petersburg Scientific and Research Institute of Epidemiology and Microbiology named after Pasteur, World Health Organization.

Smolskaya TT et al. (2004). Sentinel HIV surveillance among risk groups in Azerbaijan, Moldova and Russian Federation. WHO Regional office for Europe.

Soto RJ et al. (2007). Sentinel surveillance of sexually transmitted infection/HIV and risk behaviours in vulnerable populations in 5 Central American countries. *Journal of Acquired Immune Deficiency Syndromes* 46(1):101–111.

Statistics Indonesia and Ministry of Health [Indonesia] (2006). *Situation of risk behaviour for HIV in Indonesia. Results of BSS 2004–2005.* Jakarta. Statistics Indonesia and Ministry of Health.

Statistics South Africa (2005). Mortality and causes of death in South Africa, 1997–2003: Findings from death notification. Pretoria (http://www.statssa.gov.za/publications/P03093/P03093.pdf, accessed 8 May 2008).

Statistics South Africa (2006). *Mortality and causes of death in South Africa, 2003 and 2004: Findings from death notification.* Pretoria, Statistics South Africa.

Statistics South Africa (2007). *Mid-year population estimates 2007.* Pretoria, Statistics South Africa (July, statistical release P0302).

Stover J et al. (2006). Projecting the demographic impact of AIDS and the number of people in need of treatment: updates to the Spectrum projection package. *Sexually Transmitted Infections*, 82(Suppl. 3):45-50 June.

Stover J et al. (in press). The Spectrum projection package: improvements in estimating mortality, ART needs, PMTCT impact and uncertainty bounds. *Sexually Transmitted Infections.* Supplement in press.

Sulliman FT, Ameerberg SAG, Dhannoo MI (2004). *Report of the rapid situation assessment and responses on drug use in Mauritius and Rodrigues.* Mauritius, Ministry of Health.

Taha TE et al. (2000). Association of HIV-1 load and CD4 lymphocyte count with mortality among untreated African children over one year of age. *AIDS*, 14(4):453–459 March.

Todd CS et al. (2007). HIV, Hepatitis C, and Hepatitis B infections and associated risk behavior in injection drug users in Kabul, Afghanistan. *Emerging Infectious Diseases*, 13(9):1327--1331.

Toro-Alfonso J and Varas-Díaz N (2008). *Identificación y descripción de conocimiento, actitudes, creencias y comportamientos de riesgo para la transmisión del VIH en población de homosexuales y hombres que tienen sexo con hombres en la República Dominicana.* USAID and Projecto Conecta. Santo Domingo.

Tuang NA et al. (2007). Human immunodeficiency virus (HIV) infection patterns and risk behaviours in different population groups and provinces in Viet Nam. *Bulletin of the World Health Organization*, 85(1):35–41.

Uganda Bureau of Statistics, Macro International Inc (2007). *Uganda Demographic and Health Survey 2006.* Calverton, MD. Uganda Bureau of Statistics, Macro International Inc.

UK Collaborative Group for HIV and STI Surveillance (2007). *Testing Times: HIV and other Sexually Transmitted Infections in the United Kingdom: 2007.* London, Health Protection Agency, Centre for Infections.

UNAIDS (2005). *Evidence for HIV decline in Zimbabwe: a comprehe nsive review of the epidemiological data.* Geneva (November). UNAIDS.

UNAIDS (2006). *Report on the global AIDS epidemic.* Geneva. UNAIDS.

UNAIDS Reference Group on Estimates, Modelling and Projections (2002). *Improving estimates and projections of HIV/AIDS* (http://www.epidem.org/Publications/Madrid%20report.pdf, accessed 24 April 2008).

UNAIDS Reference Group on Estimates, Modelling and Projections (2006). *Improving parameter estimation, projection methods, uncertainty estimation, and epidemic classification* (http://www.epidem.org/Publications/Prague2006report.pdf, accessed 24 April 2008).

UNODC (2005). *Afghanistan drug use survey 2005.* Kabul. UNODC.

US Centers for Disease Control and Prevention (2007). *HIV/AIDS surveillance report: Cases of HIV infection and AIDS in the United States and Dependent Areas, 2005.* Atlanta, Georgia, Centers for Disease Control and Prevention (Revised June 2007, Vol 17).

Van Griensven F et al. (2006). HIV prevalence among populations of men who have sex with men—Thailand, 2003 and 2005. *Morbidity and Mortality Weekly Report*, 55(31):844–848.

Wade AS et al. (2005). HIV infection and sexually transmitted infections among men who have sex with men in Senegal. *AIDS*, 19(18):2133–2140.

Wawer MJ et al. (1994). Incidence of HIV-1 infection in a rural region of Uganda. *British Medical Journal*, 308(6922):171–173.

Wawer MJ et al. (2005). Rates of HIV-1 transmission per coital act, by stage of HIV-1 infection, in Rakai, Uganda. *Journal of Infectious Diseases*, 191:1403–1409.

WHO (2006). *The World Health Report 2006 – working together for health.* Geneva (http://www.who.int/whr/2006/en/, accessed 8 May 2008). WHO.

WHO (2007). *HIV/AIDS in the South-East Asia region.* New Delhi, WHO Regional Office for South-East Asia (March) (http://www.searo.who.int/hiv-aids, accessed 8 May 2008).

Zamani S et al. (2005). Prevalence of and factors associated with HIV-1 infection among drug users visiting treatment centers in Tehran, Iran. *AIDS*, 19:709–716.

Zamani S et al. (2006). High prevalence of HIV infection associated with incarceration among community-based drug users in Tehran, Iran. *Journal of Acquired Immune Deficiency Syndromes*, 42(3):342–346.

Zulu KP, Bulawo ND, Zulu W (2006). *Understanding HIV risk behaviour among men who have sex with men in Zambia. XVI International AIDS* Conference. 13–18 August. Toronto, Ontario (Abstract WEPE0719).

Chapter 3 | ADDRESSING SOCIETAL CAUSES OF HIV RISK AND VULNERABILITY

Barker G, Ricardo C, Nascimento M (2007). *Engaging men and boys in changing gender-based inequity in health: evidence from programme interventions.* Geneva, World Health Organization.

Bärnighausen T et al. (2007). The socioeconomic determinants of HIV incidence: evidence from a longitudinal, population-based study in rural South Africa. *AIDS,* 21(Suppl. 7):S29–S38.

Blumenthal SJ (2008). *Women, HIV/AIDS and stigma: results from a national survey.* (http://www.amfar.org/binary-data/AMFAR_PDF/pdf/000/000/181-1.pdf, accessed 10 April 2008).

Bott S, Morrison A, Ellsberg M (2005). *Preventing and responding to gender-based violence in middle and low-income countries: a global review and analysis.* Washington DC, World Bank (World Bank Policy Research Working Paper, No. 3618).

Burns B, Mingat A, Rakotomalala R (2003). *Achieving universal primary education by 2015: a chance for every child.* Washington DC, World Bank.

Burris S, et al (2007). *Do Criminal Laws Influence HIV Risk Behavior? An Empirical Trial.* Temple University Legal Studies Research Paper No. 2007-03. Philadelphia. Arizona State Law Journal.

Canadian HIV/AIDS Legal Network, Open Society Institute, International HIV/AIDS Alliance (2008). *"Nothing about us without us": Greater, meaningful involvement of people who use illegal drugs: A public health, ethical and human rights imperative.* Canadian HIV/AIDS Legal Network, Open Society Institute, International HIV/AIDS Alliance, Toronto.

Carpano C, Izumi K, Mathieson K (2007). *Gender, property rights and livelihoods in the era of AIDS.* FAO Technical Consultation, Rome. UN Food and Agriculture Organization. 28–30 November.

CEDPA (2001). *Adolescent girls in India choose a better future: an impact assessment.* Washington DC, Centre for Development and Population Activities.

Chan J (2006). Criminal law and HIV transmission or exposure: 10 new cases. *HIV/AIDS Policy and Law Review,* 11:45–47.

Chen S, Ravallion M (2004). *How Have the World's Poorest Fared Since the Early 1980s?* Policy Research Working Paper no. WPS 3341, Washington DC, World Bank

Commission on the Social Determinants of Health (2007b). *Achieving health equity: from root causes to fair outcomes: interim statement.* Geneva, Commision on the Social Determinants of Health.

Deininger K (2003). Does cost of schooling affect enrollment by the poor? Universal primary education in Uganda. *Economics of Education Review,* 22(3):291–305.

Duvvury N, Knoess J (2005). *Gender based violence and HIV/AIDS in Cambodia: links, opportunities and potential responses.* Eschborn, Deutsche Gesellschaft fur Technische Zusammenarbeit.

Ford K et al. (2004). Voluntary HIV testing, disclosure, and stigma among injection drug users in Bali, Indonesia. *AIDS Education and Prevention,* 16(6):487–498.

Funders for Lesbian and Gay Issues (2007). *Lesbian, gay, bisexual, transgender and intersex grantmaking in the global South and East.* New York, Funders for Lesbian and Gay Issues.

Gable L et al. (2007). *Legal aspects of HIV/AIDS: a guide for law and policy reform.* Washington DC, World Bank.

García-Moreno C et al (2005). *WHO multi-country study on women's health and domestic violence against women: initial results on prevalence, health outcomes and women's responses.* Geneva, World Health Organization.

Gillespie S, Kadiyala S, Greener R (2007). Is poverty or wealth driving HIV transmission? *AIDS,* 21(Suppl. 7): S5–S16.

Global Coalition on Women and AIDS (2006a). *Keeping the promise: an agenda for action on women and AIDS.* Geneva, UNAIDS.

Global Coalition on Women and AIDS (2006b). *Economic security for women, fight AIDS.* Geneva, UNAIDS (Issue Brief 3).

GNP+, THT (2005). *Criminalisation of HIV transmission in Europe: a rapid scan of the laws and rates of prosecution for HIV transmission within signatory States of the European Convention of Human Rights.* The Global Network of people living with HIV/AIDS and Terrence Higgins Trust (http://www.gnpplus.net/criminalisation/rapidscan.pdf, accessed 25 April 2008).

Gupta, GR (2005). *Luncheon remarks on women and AIDS.* InterAction Forum. Washington DC, InterAction.

Hallman K (2004). *Socioeconomic disadvantage and unsafe sexual behaviours among young women and men in South Africa.* New York, Population Council (Policy Research Division Working Paper, No.190).

Hallman K (2005). Gendered socioeconomic conditions and HIV risk behaviors among young people in South Africa. *African Journal of AIDS Research*, 4(1):37–50.

Hargreaves JR, Boler T (2006). *Girl power: girls' education, sexual behaviour and AIDS in Africa.* Johannesburg, ActionAid International.

Hargreaves JR et al. (2008). Systematic review exploring time trends in the association between educational attainment and risk of HIV infection in sub-Saharan Africa. *AIDS*, 22:403–414.

Heywood MJ (2002). *Litigating AIDS: background, strategies and outcomes of the Treatment Action Campaign's (TAC) case to prevent mother-to-child HIV transmission in South Africa.* 14th International AIDS Conference July 7–12 Geneva, International AIDS Society.

Human Rights Watch (2006). *Rhetoric and risk: human rights abuses impeding Ukraine's fight against HIV/AIDS.* New York, Human Rights Watch.

Human Rights Watch (2007). *Hidden in the mealie meal: gender-based abuses and women's HIV treatment in Zambia.* New York, Human Rights Watch.

Insitutute of Medicine (2008). V*iolence Prevention in Low- and Middle-Income Countries: Finding a Place on the Global Agenda. Workshop Summary.* National Academies Press, Washington DC.

ICRW (2006a). *HIV/AIDS stigma: finding solutions to strengthen HIV/AIDS programs. August.* Washington DC, International Center for Research on Women.

ICRW (2006b). *Information bulletin: reducing women's and girls' vulnerability to HIV/AIDS by strengthening their property and inheritance rights.* May. Washington DC, International Center for Research on Women.

ICRW and Instituto Promundo (2007). *Engaging men and boys to achieve gender equality: how can we build on what we have learned?* Washington DC, International Center for Research on Women.

IPPF et al (2008a). *The people living with HIV stigma index: user guide.* London, International Planned Parenthood Federation.

IPPF et al (2008b). *The people living with HIV stigma index: questionnaire.* London, International Planned Parenthood Federation.

Jenkins C, Sarkar S (2007). *Interventions for HIV prevention and support for vulnerable populations: focus on Asia and the Pacific.* Bangkok, Alternate Visions.

Jewkes R et al (2007). *Evaluation of Stepping Stones: a gender transformative HIV prevention intervention.* Pretoria, South African Medical Research Council.

Jones P (2005). "A Test of Governance": rights-based struggles and the politics of HIV/AIDS policy in South Africa. *Political Geography,* 24(4):419–447.

Kaai S et al (2007). *Changes in stigma among a cohort of people on antiretroviral therapy: findings from Mombasa, Kenya.* Nairobi, Population Council (Horizons research summary).

Kruger V (2003). *MAP evaluation report.* Johannesburg, EngenderHealth.

Liu H et al. (2006). Understanding interrelationships among HIV-related stigma, concern about HIV infection, and intent to disclose HIV serostatus: a pretest-posttest study in a rural area of eastern China. *AIDS Patient Care and STDs*, 20(2):133–142.

Lopman B et al. (2007). HIV incidence and poverty in Manicaland, Zimbabwe: is HIV becoming a disease of the poor? *AIDS*, 21(Suppl. 7):S57–S66.

Ma W et al. (2007). Acceptance of and barriers to voluntary HIV counselling and testing among adults in Guizhou province, China. *AIDS*, 21(Suppl. 8):S129–135.

Mahendra VS et al (2006). *Reducing AIDS-related stigma and discrimination in Indian hospitals*. New Delhi, Population Council (Horizons final report).

Mahendra VS et al. (2007). Understanding and measuring HIV related stigma in healthcare settings: a developing country perspective. *Journal of Social Aspects of HIV/AIDS*, 4(2): 616-625.

Mann J and Tarantola D eds (1996). *AIDS in the world II: global dimensions, social roots and response*. New York, Oxford University Press.

Marmot MG (2006). Status syndrome: a challenge to medicine. *Journal of the American Medical Association*, 295:1304–1307.

McCrummen S (2007). Prevalence of rape in E. Congo described as worst in world. *Washington Post*, 9 September.

Medley A et al. (2004). Rates, barriers and outcomes of HIV sero-disclosure among women in developing countries: implications for prevention of mother-to-child transmission programmes. *Bulletin of the World Health Organization*, 82(4):299–307.

Mercy JA et al. (2008) Preventing Violence in Developing Countries: A Framework for Action, in Institute of Medicine, *Violence Prevention in Low- and Middle-Income Countries: Finding a Place on the Global Agenda, Workshop Summary*. National Academies Press, Washington DC.

Merson MH e al. (in press). The History and Challenge of HIV Prevention. *Lancet*.

Mills EA (2006). From the physical self to the social body: expressions and effects of HIV-related stigma in South Africa. *Journal of Community & Applied Social Psychology*, 16:498–503.

Mishra V et al. (2007). HIV infection does not disproportionately affect the poorer in sub-Saharan Africa. *AIDS*, 21(Suppl.7):S17–S28.

Nyblade L et al. (2003). *Disentangling HIV and AIDS stigma in Ethiopia, Tanzania and Zambia*. Washington DC, International Center for Research on Women.

Oanh KTH et al. (2008). *Improving hospital-based quality of care in Vietnam by reducing HIV-related stigma and discrimination*. New York, Population Council.

Open Society Institute (2006a). *Fostering enabling legal and policy environments to protect the health and human rights of sex workers*. Report of a meeting co-sponsored by the Sexual Health and Rights Project & Law and Health Initiative. Johannesburg, South Africa. June 22 -24 2006. New York, Open Society Institute.

Open Society Institute (2006b). *Sex worker health and rights: where is the funding? Sexual health and rights project*. New York, Open Society Institute.

Ottosson D (2007). *State-sponsored homophobia: a world survey of laws prohibiting same sex activity between consenting adults*. Brussels, International Lesbian and Gay Association.

Pardasani MP (2005). HIV prevention and sex workers: an international lesson in empowerment. *International Journal of Social Welfare*, 14:116–126.

Peacock D, Levack A (2004). The men as partners program in South Africa: reaching men to end gender-based violence and promote sexual and reproductive health. *International Journal of Men's Health*, Fall: 173-188.

Pearhouse R (2007). Legislation contagion: the spread of problematic new HIV laws in Western Africa. *HIV/AIDS Policy and Law Review*, 12:1–11.

Physicians for Human Rights (2007). *Epidemic of Inequality: Women's Rights and HIV/AIDS in Botswana & Swaziland*. Physicians for Human Rights, Cambridge (USA).

Piot P, Greener R, Russell S (2007). Squaring the circle: AIDS, poverty, and human development. *PLoSMedicine*, 4(10):e314.

Population Council (2006). *Reducing stigma and discrimination in hospitals: positive findings from India.* Washington DC, Population Council.

Population Reference Bureau (2007). *World population data sheet.* (http://www.prb.org/Datafinder.aspx, accessed 28 March 2008).

Pronyk J et al. (2006). Effect of a structural intervention for the prevention of intimate-partner violence and HIV in rural South Africa: a cluster randomised trial. *The Lancet*, 368:1973–1983.

Pulerwitz J et al. (2006). *Promoting more gender-equitable norms and behaviours among young men as an HIV/AIDS prevention strategy.* Washington DC, Population Council (Horizons final report).

Pulerwitz J, Barker G (2008). Measuring attitudes toward gender norms among young men in Brazil. *Men and Masculinities*, 10:322–338.

Raise Initiative (Reproductive Health Access, Information and Services in Emergencies) (2007). *Fact sheet: gender based violence* (http://www.raiseinitiative.org/library/pdf/fs_gbv.pdf, accessed 8 May 2008).

Reis C et al. (2005). Discriminatory attitudes and practices by health workers toward patients with HIV/AIDS in Nigeria. *PLoS Medicine*, 2(8): e246 (doi:10.1371/journal.pmed.0020246).

SADC (2006). Expert Think Tank Meeting on HIV Prevention in High Prevalence Countries in Southern Africa Report, Maseru, Lesotho, 10-12 May 2006. Southern African Development Community, Gaborone.

Shilts R (1987). *And the band played on: people, politics and the AIDS epidemic.* New York, St. Martin's Press.

Strickland R (2004). *To have and to hold: women's property and inheritance rights in the context of HIV/AIDS in sub-Saharan Africa.* Washington DC, International Centre Research on Women (ICRW Working Paper).

UNAIDS (2002). *Criminal law, public health and HIV transmission: a policy options paper.* Geneva, UNAIDS (UNAIDS Best Practice Collection).

UNAIDS (2003). *Fact sheet on stigma and discrimination.* Geneva, UNAIDS.

UNAIDS (2007a). *Practical guidelines for intensifying HIV prevention, towards universal access.* March. Geneva, UNAIDS.

UNAIDS (2007b). Presentation of policy guidance to address gender issues at the 20th meeting of the UNAIDS Programme Coordinating Board. 25–27 June 2007. Geneva. (http://data.unaids.org/pub/Presentation/2007/policy_guidance_address_gender_issues_item4_2_en.pdf, accessed 8 May 2008).

UNAIDS (2007c). *Report of the UNAIDS technical consultation on social change communication.* 2-3 August 2007. Geneva.

UNAIDS (2007d). *AIDS epidemic update 2007.* December. Geneva, UNAIDS.

UNAIDS (2008). *Reducing HIV Stigma and Discrimination: a critical part of national AIDS programmes, A resource for national stakeholders in the HIV response.* Geneva.

UNAIDS et al (2008). *Eliminating female genital mutilation: an interagency statement.* Geneva, World Health Organization.

UNESCO (2007) *Education for All for 2015: Will We Make It?* UNESCO, Paris.

UNICEF (2005). *Progress for children: a report card on gender parity and primary education (No.2).*UNICEF.

UNDP (2007). *Human development report 2007/2008.* New York, United Nations Development Program.

United Nations Office for the Coordination of Humanitarian Affairs (2005). *Broken bodies, broken dreams: violence against women exposed.* New York, UN Office for the Coordination of Humanitarian Affairs.

Verma R et al (2006). *Challenging and Changing Gender Attitudes among Young Men in Mumbai, India.* Reproductive Health Matters 2006;14(28):135–143

Weiser S et al. (2007). Food insufficiency is associated with high-risk sexual behavior among women in Botswana and Swaziland. *PLoS Medicine*, 4(10): e260.

Welbourn A (1995). *Stepping Stones: A training package on HIV/AIDS, gender issues, communication and relationship skills.* Strategies for Hope Trust, Oxford UK.

White RC, Carr R (2005). Homosexuality and HIV/AIDS stigma in Jamaica. *Culture, Health & Sexuality,* 7(4):347–359.

WHO (2007). *Engaging men and boys in changing gender-based inequity in health: evidence from programme interventions.* Geneva, World Health Organization.

Wolfe W et al. (2006). Effects of HIV-related stigma among an early sample of patients receiving antiretroviral therapy in Botswana. *AIDS Care,* 18(8):931–933.

World Vision (2008). Protecting women from HIV/AIDS via microenterprise development (MED). (http://www.worldvision.org/worldvision/appeals.nsf/stable/im_MED_Prod_Desc_v7, accessed 26 March 2008).

Chapter 4 | PREVENTING NEW HIV INFECTIONS

Aceijas C et al. (2004). Global coverage of injecting drug use and HIV infection among injecting drug users. *AIDS,* 18:1295–2203.

Akhmedov K et al. (2007). *Introduction of youth friendly services for most at risk adolescents in Uzbekistan: an emergency response to the fastest growing HIV epidemic in Central Asia.* 2007 Implementers Meeting: Scaling Up Through Partnerships. 16–19 June. Kigali, Rwanda.

Allen S et al. (2003). Sexual behavior of HIV discordant couples after HIV counseling and testing. *AIDS,* 17:733–740.

Auerbach JD, Hayes RJ, Kandathil SM. Overview of effective and promising interventions to prevent HIV infection. In: Ross DA, Dick B, Ferguson J, eds. (2006). *Preventing HIV/AIDS in young people: a systematic review of evidence from developing countries.* UNAIDS Inter-Agency Task Team on Young People. Geneva, World Health Organization.

Auvert B et al. (2005). Randomized, controlled intervention trial of male circumcision for reduction of HIV infection risk: the ANRS 1265 trial. *PLoS Medicine,* 2:e298.

Bailey RC et al. (2007). Male circumcision for HIV prevention in young men in Kisumu, Kenya: a randomised controlled trial. *Lancet,* 369:643–656.

Basu I et al. (2004). HIV prevention among sex workers in India. *Journal of Acquired Immune Deficiency Syndromes,* 36:845–852.

Bearinger LH et al. (2007). Global perspectives on the sexual and reproductive health of adolescents: patterns, prevention and potential. *Lancet,* 369:1220–1231.

Becquet R et al. (2005). Infant Feeding Practices before Implementing Alternatives to Prolonged Breastfeeding to Reduce HIV Transmission Through Breastmilk in Abidjan, Côte d'Ivoire. *J Trop Pediatr* 51 :351-355.

Biddlecom AE et al. (2007). *Protecting the next generation in sub-Saharan Africa: learning from adolescents to prevent HIV and unintended pregnancy.* New York, Guttmacher Institute.

Buchbinder SP et al. (2005). Sexual risk, nitrite inhalant use, and lack of circumcision associated with HIV seroconversion in men who have sex with men in the United States. *Journal of Acquired Immune Deficiency Syndromes,* 39:82–89.

CADRE (2007). *Concurrent sexual partnerships amongst young adults in South Africa: challenges for HIV prevention communication.* Johannesburg, Centre for AIDS Development, Research and Evaluation.

Cassels S, Clark SJ, Morris M (2008). Mathematical models for HIV transmission dynamics: tools for social and behavioral science research. *Journal of Acquired Immune Deficiency Syndromes,* 47:S34–S39.

Castilla J et al. (2005). Effectiveness of highly active antiretroviral therapy in reducing heterosexual transmission of HIV. *Journal of Acquired Immune Deficiency Syndromes,* 40:96–101.

Centers for Disease Control and Prevention (2005). HIV prevalence, unrecognized HIV infection, and HIV testing among men who have sex with men – five U.S. Cities, June 2004-April 2005. *Morbidity and Mortality Weekly Report*, 54:597–601.

Centers for Disease Control and Prevention (2006a). Youth risk behaviour surveillance – United States, 2005. *Morbidity and Mortality Weekly Report*, 55(SS-5):1–108.

Centers for Disease Control and Prevention (2006b). HIV prevalence among populations of men who have sex with men – Thailand, 2003 and 2005. *Morbidity and Mortality Weekly Report*, 55:844–848.

Chinaglia M et al. (2007). *Reaching truckers in Brazil with non-stigmatizing and effective HIV/STI services.* Washington DC, Population Council.

Clinton Global Initiative (2007). *Latest news for AIDS prevention education with migrant construction workers.* (http://commitments.clintonglobalinitiative.org/projects.htm?mode=progressreport&rid=43084&op=ViewArticle&articleId=227&blogId=232, accessed 23 March 2008).

Coates TJ et al. (2008). Behavioural science contributions to HIV prevention: insights from the past and directions for the future, Lancet *in press.*

Crepaz N et al. (2006). Do prevention interventions reduce HIV risk behaviours among people living with HIV? A meta-analytic review of controlled trials. *AIDS*, 20:143–157.

Darabi L et al. (2008). *Protecting the next generation in Uganda: new evidence on adolescent sexual and reproductive health needs.* New York, Guttmacher Institute.

De Cock K et al. (2000). Prevention of mother-to-child HIV transmission in resource-poor countries: translating research into policy and practice. *Journal of the American Medical Association*, 283:1175–1182.

de Walque D (2007). Sero-discordant couples in five african countries: implications for prevention strategies. *Population and Development Review*, 33:501–523.

Doherty T et al. (2007). Effectiveness of the WHO/UNICEF guidelines on infant feeding for HIV-positive women: results from a prospective cohort study in South Africa. *AIDS* 21:1791-1797.

Dolan K et al. (2007). HIV in prisons in low- and middle-income countries. *Lancet Infectious Diseases*, 7:32–41.

Donegan E et al. (1994). Transfusion transmission of retroviruses: human T-lymphotropic viruses types 1 and 2 compared with human immunodeficiency virus type 1. *Transfusion*, 34:478–483.

Donnelly J (2007). Saving the babies: a victory for Africa. *Boston Globe*, 27 August.

Dupas P (2006). *Relative risk and the market for sex: teenagers, sugar daddies and HIV in Kenya.* (http://ipc.umich.edu/edts/pdfs/DupasRelativeRisks.pdf, accessed 3 January 2008).

Emmanuel F, Archibald C, Altaf F (2006). *What drives the HIV epidemic among injecting drug users in Pakistan: a risk factor analysis.* XVI International AIDS Conference. 13–18 August. Toronto. (Abstract No. MOPE0524).

EuroHIV (2007). *HIV/AIDS surveillance in Europe, end-year report, 2006, No. 76.* Sant-Maurice, Institute de Veille Sanitaire (http://www.eurohiv.org, accessed 8 May 2008).

Fiellin DA, Green TC, Heimer R (2007). *Combating the twin epidemics of HIV/AIDS and addiction: opportunities for progress and gaps in scale. A report of the CSIS Task Force on HIV/AIDS.* Washington, Center for Strategic and International Studies.

Global Commission on International Migration (2005). *Migration in an interconnected world: new directions for action.* Geneva, Global Commission on International Migration.

Global HIV Prevention Working Group (2004). *HIV prevention in the era of expanded treatment access.* New York, Bill & Melinda Gates Foundation, Henry J. Kaiser Family Foundation.

Global HIV Prevention Working Group (2006). *New approaches to HIV prevention: accelerating research and ensuring future access.* New York, Bill & Melinda Gates Foundation, Henry J. Kaiser Family Foundation.

Gray RH et al. (2007). Male circumcision for HIV prevention in men in Rakai, Uganda: a randomized trial. *Lancet*, 369:657–666.

Gray RH, Wawer MJ (2007). Randomised trials of HIV prevention. *Lancet,* 370:200–201.

Gregson S et al. (2002). Sexual mixing patterns and sex differentials in teenage exposure to HIV infection in rural Zimbabwe. *Lancet,* 359:1896–1903.

Guay LA et al. (1999). Intrapartum and neonatal single-dose nevirapine compared with zidovudine for prevention of mother-to-child transmission of HIV-1 in Kampala, Uganda: HIVNET 012 randomised trial. *Lancet,* 354:795–802.

Hallett T et al. (2008). Understanding the impact of male circumcision interventions on the spread of HIV in southern Africa. *PLoS ONE* (In Press)

Hankins C (2008). Sex, drugs and gender? High time for lived experience to inform action. Editorial. *International Journal of Drug Policy,* 19:95–96.

Hendriksen ES et al. (2007). Predictors of condom use among young adults in South Africa: the Reproductive Health and HIV Research Unit National Youth Survey. *American Journal of Public Health,* 97:1241–1248.

Henry J Kaiser Family Foundation (2006). *AIDS at 25: An overview of major trends in the US epidemic.* Menlo Park, California, Henry J Kaiser Family Foundation (http://www.kff.org/hivaids/upload/7525.pdf, accessed 13 March 2008).

HIV Vaccines and Microbicides Resource Tracking Working Group (2007). *Building a Comprehensive Response: Funding for HIV Vaccines, Microbicides and Other New Prevention Options: 2000-2006.* HIV Vaccines and Microbicides Resource Tracking Group. Accessed 8 May 2008 at http://www.hivresourcetracking.org/content/RT_Report_Nov2007.pdf.

ICRW, Instituto Promundo (2007). *Engaging men and boys to achieve gender equality: how can we build on what we have learned?* Washington, International Center for Research on Women.

Institute of Medicine (2006). *Preventing HIV infection among injection drug users in high risk countries: an assessment of the evidence.* Washington, Institute of Medicine.

International Harm Reduction Development Program (2007). *Women, harm reduction and HIV.* New York, Open Society Institute.

ILO (2006). *HIV/AIDS and work: impact on children and youth, and response.* Geneva, International Labour Organization.

Kahn JG, Marseille E, Auvert B. (2006). Cost-effectiveness of male circumcision for HIV prevention in a South African setting. *PLoS Medicine,* 3:e517.

Kerrigan D et al. (2006). Environmental/structural interventions to reduce HIV/STI risk among female sex workers in the Dominican Republic. *American Journal of Public Health* 96:120–125.

Khan MR et al. (2007). Mobility and HIV-related sexual behavior in Burkina Faso. *AIDS & Behavior,* 12:202–212.

Kissin DM et al. (2008). Rapid HIV testing and prevention of perinatal HIV transmission in high-risk maternity hospitals in St. Petersburg, Russia. *American Journal of Obstetrics & Gynecology,* 198(2):183.e1–7.

Kuhn L et al. (2007). High uptake of exclusive breastfeeding and reduced early post-natal HIV transmission. *PLoS Medicine,* 2:e1363.

Lines R et al. (2006). *Needle exchange: lessons from a comprehensive review of international evidence and experience.* Toronto, Canadian HIV/AIDS Legal Network.

Manzi M et al. (2005). High acceptability of voluntary counselling and HIV-testing but unacceptable loss to follow up in a prevention of mother-to-child HIV transmission programme in rural Malawi: scaling-up requires a different way of acting. *Tropical Medicine and International Health* 10:1242-1250.

Marston C, King E (2006). Factors that shape young people's sexual behaviour: a systematic review. *Lancet,* 368:1581–1586.

Maticka-Tyndale E, Brouillard-Coyle C. The effectiveness of community interventions targeting HIV and AIDS prevention at young people in developing countries. In: Ross DA, Dick B, Ferguson J, eds. (2006). *Preventing HIV/AIDS in young people: a systematic review of evidence from developing countries.* UNAIDS Inter-Agency Task Team on Young People. Geneva, World Health Organization.

MEASURE DHS, 2008, Macro International, Inc. Calverton MD, USA.

Millett GA, Peterson JL(2007). The Known Hidden Epidemic: HIV/AIDS Among Black Men Who Have Sex with Men in the United States. *American Journal of Preventive Medicine* S31-S37.

Montefiori D et al. (2007). Antibody-based HIV-1 vaccines: recent developments and future directions. *PLoS Medicine,* 4:e348.

Morris CN, Ferguson AG (2006). Estimation of the sexual transmission of HIV in Kenya and Uganda on the trans-Africa highway: the continuing role for prevention in high risk groups. *Sexually Transmitted Infections* 82:368-371.

Nashkhoev M, Sergeyev B (2007). *AIDS in the Commonwealth of Independent States.* Monitoring the AIDS Pandemic Network. Washington, US Bureau of the Census.

National Research Council, Institute of Medicine, Panel on Transitions to Adulthood in Developing Countries (2005). *Growing Up Global: The Changing Transitions to Adulthood in Developing Countries.* Washington, National Academies Press.

Nelson R (2007). Female-initiated prevention strategies key to tackling HIV. *Lancet Infectious Diseases,* 7:183.

Oanh KTH (2007). *HIV/AIDS policy in Vietnam: a civil society perspective.* New York, Open Society Institute.

Osmond DH et al. (2007). Changes in prevalence of HIV infection and sexual risk behavior in men who have sex with men in San Francisco: 1997–2002. *American Journal of Public Health,* 97:1677–1683.

Padian NS et al. (2007). Diaphragm and lubricant gel for prevention of HIV acquisition in southern African women: a randomised controlled trial. *Lancet,* 370:251–261.

Pardasani M (2005). HIV Prevention and sex workers: An international lesson in empowerment. *International Journal of Social Welfare* 14:16-126.

Peltzer CI et al. (2007). Male circumcision, gender and HIV prevention in sub-Saharan Africa: a (social science) research agenda. *Journal of Social Aspects of HIV/AIDS,* 4 (3): 658-667.

Physicians for Human Rights (2007). *Success stories from the field: curbing the spread of HIV/AIDS among drug injectors. Innovative and effective programs in Brazil, India, Russia , and the China-Vietnam border.* Cambridge (USA), Physicians for Human Rights.

Piot P et al. (in press) Coming to terms with complexity: A call to action for HIV prevention. *Lancet.*

Population Council (2003). *Expanding workplace HIV/AIDS prevention activities for a highly mobile population: construction workers in Ho Chi Minh City* (http://www.popcouncil.org/horizons/ressum/wrkplc/vtnmcnstrwrkr/vtnmcnstrwrkr_intro.html, accessed 23 March 2008).

Population Council, USAID (2007). *Implementing STI/HIV prevention and care interventions for men who have sex with men in Dakar, Senegal.* Washington DC, Population Council, Horizons Project.

Robertson M et al. (2008). Efficacy Results from the STEP Study (Merck V520 Protocol 023/HVTN 502): A Phase II, Test-of-Concept Trial of the MRKAd5 HIV-1 Gag/Pol/Nef Trivalent Vaccine.. 15th conference on Retroviruses and Opportunistic Infections, Boston. USA.

SADC (2006). Expert Think Tank Meeting on HIV Prevention in High Prevalence Countries in Southern Africa Report, Maseru, Lesotho, 10-12 May 2006. Southern African Development Community, Gaborone.

Say L, Raine R (2007). A systematic review of inequalities in the use of maternal health care in developing countries: examining the scale of the problem and the importance of context. *Bulletin of the World Health Organization,* 85:733–820.

Schoofs M (2007). Challenge for AIDS fighters: circumcising Africans safely. *Wall Street Journal,* 7 September.

Southern African Migration Project (2005). *HIV/AIDS Population Mobility and Migration in Southern Africa : Towards a Research and Policy Agenda*. Geneva, International Organisation for Migration.

Steen R et al. (2006). Pursuing scale and quality in STI interventions with sex workers: initial results from Avahan India AIDS Initiative. *Sexually Transmitted Infections* 82:381–385.

Stover J et al. (2006). The global impact of scaling up HIV/AIDS prevention programs in low- and middle-income countries. *Science,* 311:1474–1476.

Stripipatana T et al. (2007). Site-specific interventions to improve prevention of mother-to-child transmission of human immunodeficiency virus programs in less developed settings. *American Journal of Obstetrics and Gynecology* 197:S107-S112.

Suarez et al. (2001). Influence of a partner's HIV Serostatus, use of highly active antiretroviral therapy, and viral load on the perceptions of sexual risk behavior in a community sample of men who have sex with men. *Journal of Acquired Immune Deficiency Syndromes,* 28:471–477.

Swartz L, Nkau DP (2004). *The impact of HIV/AIDS on the mining sector, with special emphasis on Southern African male migrant workers.*Bangkok, UNDP South East Asia HIV and Development Programme, Committee for International Cooperation in National Research on Demography.

Teeraratkul A et al. (2005). Evaluating programs to prevent mother-to-child HIV transmission in two large Bangkok hospitals, 1999-2001. *Journal of Acquired Immune Deficiency Syndromes* 38:208-212.

Templeton D, Hogben M (2007). *Circumcision not protective against HIV seroconversion in homosexual men.* 17th Meeting of the International Society for Sexually Transmitted Diseases. Seattle. 30 July 2007. (Abstract No. 215).

Thai AIDS Treatment Action Group, Human Rights Watch (2007). *Deadly denial: barriers to HIV/AIDS treatment for people who use drugs.* New York. Bangkok, November 19:17(C)

Tonwe-Gold B et al. (2007). Antiretroviral Treatment and Prevention of Peripartum and Postnatal HIV Transmission in West Africa: Evaluation of a Two-Tiered Approach. *PloS Medicine* 4:e257.

TRC (2008). *International coordination and information service for drug substitution patients seeking to travel abroad.* Travel Resource Center (www.indro-online.de/nia.htm, accessed 14 April 2008).

UNAIDS (2001). *Working with men for HIV prevention and care.* Geneva, UNAIDS (UNAIDS Best Practice Collection).

UNAIDS (2005). *Intensifying HIV prevention: UNAIDS policy position paper.* Geneva, UNAIDS.

UNAIDS (2006a). *Evidence for HIV decline in Zimbabwe: a comprehensive review of the epidemiological data.* UNAIDS, Geneva.

UNAIDS (2006b) *Report on the global AIDS epidemic.* UNAIDS, Geneva.

UNAIDS (2006c). *High Coverage Sites: HIV Prevention among Injecting Drug Users in Transitional and Developing Countries, Case Studies.* UNAIDS Best Practice Collection.

UNAIDS (2007a). *Practical guidelines for intensifying HIV prevention: towards universal access.* Geneva, UNAIDS.

UNAIDS (2007b). *AIDS epidemic update.* Geneva, UNAIDS.

UNAIDS (2007c). *Financial resources required to achieve universal access to HIV prevention, treatment, care and support.* Geneva, UNAIDS.

UNAIDS (2007d). *Ethical considerations in biomedical HIV prevention trials: UNAIDS/WHO guidance document.* Geneva, UNAIDS.

UNAIDS, AVAC (2007). *Good participatory practice guidelines for biomedical HIV prevention trials.* Geneva, UNAIDS.

UNAIDS, WHO (2007). *New data on male circumcision and HIV prevention: policy and programme implications.* UNAIDS/WHO Technical Consultation, Male Circumcision and HIV Prevention: Research Implications for Policy and Programming. 6–8 March 2007. Montruex, Switzerland.

UN Commission on Narcotic Drugs (2008). *World situation with regard to drug abuse: report of the Secretariat.* UN Economic and Social Council, 51st session. 10–14 March, 2008. Vienna.

UNDP (2007). *Human development report.* New York, United Nations Development Programme.

Underhill K, Montgomery P, Operario D (2007). Sexual abstinence only programmes to prevent HIV infection in high income countries: systematic review. *BMJ* 335:248–252.

UNFPA (2003). *The state of the world population, 2003. Making one billion count: investing in adolescents' health rights.* New York, United Nations Population Fund.

UNICEF, UNAIDS, WHO (2008). *Children and AIDS: Second stocktaking report.* New York, UNICEF.

UNICEF (2008). *State of the world's children 2008.* New York, UNICEF.

UNODC (2007). *World drug report 2007.* UNODC, Vienna.

United Nations (2006). *International migration and development* http://www.un.org/esa/population/migration/hld/index.html, accessed 29 May 2008

Vernazza P et al. (2008). Les personnes sérepositives ne souffrant d'aucune autre MST et suivant un traitement antiretroviral efficace ne transmettent pas le VIH par voie sexuelle []. *Bulletin des medicins Suisse* 89:165–169.

Vu BN et al. (2008). Male sexuality in Vietnam: the case of male-to-male sex. *Sexual Health,* 5:83–88.

Watson-Jones D et al. (2008). Effect of herpes simplex suppression on incidence of HIV among women in Tanzania. *New England Journal of Medicine,* 358:1560–1571.

Wawer MJ et al. (2005). Rates of HIV-1 transmission per coital act by stage of HIV-1 infection, in Rakai, Uganda. *Journal of Infectious Diseases,* 191:1403–1409.

Wegbreit J et al. (2006). Effectiveness of HIV prevention strategies in resource-poor countries: tailoring the intervention to the context. *AIDS,* 20:1217–1235.

Wellings K et al. (2006). Sexual behaviour in context: a global perspective. *Lancet,* 368:1706–1728.

Were WA et al. (2006). Undiagnosed HIV infection and couple HIV discordance among household members of HIV-Infected people receiving antiretroviral therapy in Uganda. *Journal of Acquired Immune Deficiency Syndromes,* 43:91–95.

White RG (2003). Commentary: What can we make of an association between human immunodeficiency virus prevalence and population mobility? *International Journal of Epidemiology,* 32:753–754.

WHO (2006a). Demand for male circumcision rises in a bid to prevent HIV. *Bulletin of the World Health Organization* 84:505-508.

WHO et al. (2006b). *Preventing HIV/AIDS in young people: a systematic review of the evidence from developing countries,* WHO Technical Report Series No. 938. August. World Health Organization, Geneva.

WHO (2006c). *HIV and Infant Feeding Technical Consultation Held on behalf of the Inter-Agency Task Team (IATT) on Prevention of HIV Infections in Pregnant Women, Mothers and their Infants.* Consensus statement, 25-27 October. World Health Organization, Geneva.

WHO (2006d). *Antiretroviral Drugs for Treating Pregnant Women and Preventing HIV Infection in Infant: Towards Universal Access, Recommendations for a Public Health Approach.* World Health Organization, Geneva.

WHO (2007). *HIV/AIDS in the South-East Asia region.* Martch. New Delhi, WHO Regional Office for South-East Asia (http://www.searo.who.int/hiv-aids, accessed 8 May 2008).

Williams BG et al. (2006). The potential impact of male circumcision on HIV in sub-Saharan Africa. *PLoS Medicine,* 3(7):e262.

World Association for Sexual Health (2008). *Sexual health for the millennium: a declaration and technical document.* Minneapolis (USA), World Association for Sexual Health.

Zaba B et al. (2004). Age at first sex: understanding recent trends in African demographic surveys. *Sexually Transmitted Infections,* 80(Supp. II):ii28-ii35.

Chapter 5 | TREATMENT AND CARE

Abgrail S et al. (2006). Switch from a first virologically effective protease inhibitor-containing regimen to a regimen containing efavirenz, nevirapine or abacavir. *AIDS* 20:2099-2106.

Agence France Press (2008). 'Unacceptable' Delay in Detecting Brazil AIDS Cases: Official. 14 February.

Anglican United Nations Office (2007). *Working Together: The Anglican Response to HIV & AIDS in Africa.* Anglican United Nations Office, Geneva.

Antiretroviral Therapy in Lower Income Countries Collaboration, ART Cohort Collaboration Groups (2006). Mortality of HIV-1-infected patients in the first year of antiretroviral therapy: comparison between low-income and high-income countries. *Lancet* 367:817-824.

Arah OA, Ogbu UC, Okeke CE (2008). Too Poor to Leave, Too Rich to Stay: Developmental and Global Health Correlates of Physician Migration to the United States, Canada, Australia, and the United Kingdom. *Am J Pub Health* 98:148-154.

Aspeling HE, van Wyk NC (2008). Factors associated with adherence to antiretroviral therapy for the treatment of HIV-infected women attending an urban care facility. *Int J Nurs Pract* 14:3-10.

Barreto CC et al. (2006). Trends in antiretroviral drug resistance and clade distribution among HIV-1 infected blood donors in Sao Paulo, Brazil. *J Acquir Immune Defic Syndr* 41:338-341.

Badri M et al. (2006). Cost-effectiveness of Highly Active Antiretroviral Therapy in South Africa. *Plos Medicine* January 3: e4

Basu S et al. (2007). Prevention of nosocomial transmission of extensively drug-resistant tuberculosis in rural South Africa district hospitals: an epidemiological modeling study. *Lancet* 370:1500-1507.

Beck E et al. (2006). National adult antiretroviral therapy guidelines in resource-limited countries: concordance with 2003 WHO guidelines? *AIDS* 2006;20:1497-1502.

Beck E et al. (2008a). Treatment Outcome and Cost-effectiveness of different HAART regimens in the UK 1996-2002. *Int J STD & AIDS* (in press).

Beck E, Walensky RP (2008b). The Outcome and Impact of Ten Years of HAART, in *A Decade of HAART* (Zuniga JM et al., eds.). Oxford University Press, Oxford, UK, in press.

Becquet R et al. (2006). Complementary feeding adequacy in relation to nutritional status among early weaned breastfed children who are born to HIV-infected mothers: ANRS 1201/1202 Ditrame Plus, Abidjan, Cote d'Ivoire. *Pediatrics* 117:e701-e710.

Bolton-Moore C et al (2007). Clinical outcomes and CD4 cell response in children receiving antiretroviral therapy at primary health care facilities in Zambia. *Journal of the American Medical Association* 298:1888-1899.

Bong C et al (2007). Risk factors for early mortality in children on adult fixed-dose combination antiretroviral treatment in a central hospital in Malawi. *AIDS* 21:1805-1810.

Bryce J et al. (2008). Maternal and child undernutrition: effective action at national level. *Lancet* DOI:10.1016/S0140-6736(07)61694-8 (early online publication).

Burman WJ et al. (2008). The Impact of Episodic CD4 Cell Count-Guided Antiretroviral Therapy on Quality of Life. *J Acquir Immune Defic Syndr* 47:185-193.

Catalan J et al. (2005). *Mental Health and HIV/AIDS: Psychotherapeutic Interventions in Antiretroviral (ARV) Therapy (for second level care).* World Health Organization, Geneva.

Cazanave C et al. (2008). Reduced bone mineral density in HIV-infected patients: prevalence and associated factors. *AIDS* 22:395-402.

Centers for Disease Control and Prevention (2002). Number of Persons Tested for HIV – United States, 2002. *MMWR* 53:1110-1113.

Centers for Disease Control and Prevention (2005). *Coinfection with HIV and Hepatitis C: Fact Sheet.* Accessed 9 February 2008 at http://www.cdc.gov/hiv/resources/factsheets/coinfection.htm.

Chaisson RE, Martinson NA (2008). Tuberculosis in Africa – Combating an HIV-Driven Crisis. *New Eng J Med* 358;1089-1092.

Clotet B et al. (2007). Efficacy and safety of darunavir-ritonavir at week 48 in treatment-experienced patients with HIV-1 infection in POWER 1 and 2: a pooled subgroup analysis of data from two randomized trials. *Lancet* 369:1169-1178.

Dalal RP et al. (2008). Characteristics and Outcomes of Adult Patients Lost to Follow-Up at an Antiretroviral Treatment Clinic in Johannesburg, South Africa. *J Acquir Immune Defic Syndr* 47:101-107.

De Baets AJ et al. (2005). Pediatric Human Immunodeficiency Virus Screening in an African District Hospital. *Clin Diagn Lab Immunol* 12:86-92.

Delfraissy JF et al. (2008). Lopinavir/ritonavir monotherapy or plus zidovudine and lamivudine in antiretroviral/naïve HIV-infected patients. *AIDS* 22:385-393.

Dhir AA et al. (2008). Spectrum of HIV/AIDS related cancers in India. *Cancer Causes Control* 19:147-153.

Dippenaar H, Marston J (2008). *The status of palliative care for children in the Motheo District of the Free State*. Unpublished.

Dowdy DW et al. (2006). The potential impact of enhanced diagnostic techniques for tuberculosis driven by HIV: a mathematical model. *AIDS* 20:751-762.

Egger M (2007). Outcome of antiretroviral therapy in resource-limited and industrialized countries. Conference on Retroviruses and Opportunistic Infections, Los Angeles USA.

EronJ et al. (2006). The KLEAN study of fosamprenavir-ritonavir versus lopinavir-ritonavir, each in combination with abacavir-lamuvudine, for initial treatment of HIV infection over 48 weeks: a randomized non-inferiority trial. *Lancet* 368:476-482.

Este JA, Telenti A (2007). HIV entry inhibitors. *Lancet* 370:81-88.

Ethiopia Federal Ministry of Health (2007). *Millennium AIDS Campaign Ethiopia, November 2006-August 2007.*

EuroHIV (2007). *HIV/AIDS surveillance in Europe: end-year report 2006, No 75*. Institut de Veille Sanitaire. Saint-Maurice. Available at http://www.eurohiv.org

Family Health International (2007). *Primary health care services increased with integration of basic HIV care.* Accessed 23 March 2008 at www.fhi.org/en/HIVAIDS/country/Rwanda.

Fassinou P et al (2004). Highly active antiretroviral therapies among HIV-1-infected children in Abidjan, Côte d'Ivoire. *AIDS* 18:1905-1913.

Fellay J et al. (2001). Prevalence of adverse events associated with potent antiretroviral treatment: Swiss HIV Cohort Study. *Lancet* 358:1322-1327.

Fidler S et al. (2008). Primary HIV infection: to treat or not to treat? *Curr Opin Infect Dis* 21:4-10.

Food and Nutrition Technical Assistance (2004a). *HIV/AIDS: A Guide for Nutritional Care and Support.* Academy for Educational Development, Washington DC.

Food and Nutrition Technical Assistance (2004b). *Food and Nutrition Implications of Antiretroviral Therapy in Resource Limited Settings.* Technical Note No. 7. Academy for Educational Development, Washington DC.

Freeman MC et al. (2005). Integrating mental health in global initiatives for HIV/AIDS. *Brit J Psychiatry* 187:1-3.

Friis H (2005). *Miconutrients and HIV infection: a review of current evidence, Consultation on Nutrition and HIV/AIDS in Africa.* World Health Organization, Geneva, 10-13 April.

Gandhi NR et al. (2006). Extensively drug-resistant tuberculosis as a cause of death in patients co-infected with tuberculosis and HIV in a rural area of South Africa. *Lancet* 368:1575-1580.

George E et al (2007). Antiretroviral Therapy for HIV-1-Infected Children in Haiti. *Journal of Infectious Diseases* 195:1411-1418.

Gillespie S, Kadiyala S (2005). *HIV/AIDS and Food and Nutrition Security: From Evidence to Action.* International Food Policy Research Institute, Washington DC.

Gimbel S et al. (2007). *Rolling out ART in Mozambique 2003-2006: Task Shifting and Decentralization.* 2007 HIV/AIDS Implementers Meeting, Kigali, Rwanda, June. Abstract No. 90.

Girardi E, Sabin CA, Monforte AD (2007). Late Diagnosis of HIV Infection: Epidemiologic Features, Consequences and Strategies to Encourage Earlier Testing *J Acquir Immune Defic Syndr* 46(Supp. 1):S3-S8.

Global Business Coalition on HIV/AIDS (2007). *Case Study – Anglo Coal South Africa.* 23 February. Accessed 8 February 2008 at http://www.businessfightsaids.org/live/cases/cases.php?id=40.

Global Fund to Fight AIDS, Tuberculosis and Malaria (2007a). *Global Fund Investments Deliver AIDS Treatment to 1.4 Million People.* Global Fund to Fight AIDS, Tuberculosis and Malaria, Geneva. Press Release, 30 November.

Global Fund to Fight AIDS, Tuberculosis and Malaria (2007b). *Press release.* 12 November.

Global Fund to Fight AIDS, Tuberculosis and Malaria (2008). *Monthly Progress Update – 31 January 2008.* Accessed 23 March 2008 at http://www.theglobalfund.org/en/files/publications/basics/progress_update/progressupdate.pdf.

Gray A (2004). *Access to Medicines and Drug Regulation in Developing Countries: A Resource Guide for DFID.* UK Department for International Development, London.

Grinsztejn B et al. (2007). Safety and efficacy of the HIV-1 integrase inhibitor raltegravir (MK-0518) in treatment-experienced patients with multidrug-resistant virus: a phase II randomized controlled trial. *Lancet* 369:1261-1269.

Grulich AE et al. (2007). Incidence of cancers in people with HIV/AIDS compared with immunosuppressed transplant recipients: a meta-analysis. *Lancet* 370:59-67.

Harling G, Wood R, Beck EJ (2005). Efficiency of Intervention in HIV Infection, 1994-2004. *Disease Management and Health Outcomes* 13: 371-394

Hegarty AM, Chaudhry SI, Hodgson TA (2008). Oral healthcare for HIV-infected patients: an international perspective. *Expert Opin Pharmacother* 9:387-404.

Heiden D et al. (2007). Cytomegalovirus Retinitis: The Neglected Disease of the AIDS Pandemic. *PLoS Med* 4:e334.

Hicks PL et al. (2007). The impact of illicit drug use and substance abuse treatment on adherence to HAART. *AIDS Care* 19:1134-1140.

Hoffman CJ, Thio CL (2007). Clinical implications of HIV and hepatitis B co-infection in Asia and Africa (2007) *Lancet Infectious Diseases* 7:402-409.

Hopewell PC et al. (2006). International standards for tuberculosis care. *Lancet Infect Dis* 6:710-725.

Human Rights Watch, Thai AIDS Treatment Action Group (2007a). *Barriers to HIV/AIDS Treatment for People Who Use Drugs in Thailand.*

Human Rights Watch (2007b). *Hidden in the Mealie Meal: Gender-Based Abuses and Women's HIV Treatment in Zambia.* Human Rights Watch, New York.

International Narcotics Control Board (1989). *Report of the International Narcotics Control Board for 1989: demand for and supply of opiates for medical and scientific needs.* United Nations, Vienna

International Treatment Preparedness Coalition (2007). *Missing the Target #5: Improving AIDS Drug Access and Advancing Health Care for All.* December.

International Union of Superiors General (2008). *In Loving Service: Catholic Religious Institutes of men and women addressing HIV and AIDS through communities of care and prevention, findings of a global survey.* Unpublished draft, February.

Isaac R et al. (2008). Declines in dietary macronutrient intake in persons with HIV infection who develop depression. *Public Health Nutr* 11:124-131.

Janssens B et al (2007). Effectiveness of Highly Active Antiretroviral Therapy in HIV-Positive Children: Evaluation at 12 Months in a Routine Program in Cambodia. *Pediatrics* 120:e1134-e1140.

Johnson M et al. (2006). 96-week comparison of once-daily atazanavir/ritonavir and twice-daily lopinavir/ritonavir in patients with multiple virologic failures. *AIDS* 20:711-718.

Jones CY et al. (2006). Micronutrient levels and HIV disease status in HIV-infected patients on highly active antiretroviral therapy in the Nutrition for Healthy Living cohort. *J Acquir Immune Defic Syndr* 43:475-482.

Lange JMA (2006). Antiretroviral treatment and care of HIV, in *The HIV Pandemic: local and global implications* (Beck E et al., eds.). Oxford University Press, Oxford, UK.

Lazzarin A et al. (2007). Efficacy and safety of TMC125 (etravirine) in treatment-experienced HIV-1-infected patients in DUET-2: 24-week results from a randomized, double-blind, placebo-controlled trial. *Lancet* 370:39-48.

Lohse N et al. (2007). Survival of Persons with and without HIV Infection in Denmark, 1995-2005. *Ann Intern Med* 146;87-95.

MacArthur RD et al. (2006). A comparison of three highly active antiretroviral treatment strategies consisting of non-nucleoside reverse transcriptase inhibitors, protease inhibitors, or both in the presence of nucleoside reverse transcriptase inhibitors as initial therapy (CPCRA 058 FIRST Study): a long-term randomized trial. *Lancet* 368:2125-2135.

Makombe SD et al. (2007). A national survey of the impact of rapid scale-up of antiretroviral therapy on health-care workers in Malawi: effects on human resources and survival. *Bull World Health Organ* 85:851-857.

Malawi National AIDS Commission (2007). *InfoBrief 2: 200 HTC Week.*

Marston M et al. (2005). Estimating the net effect of HIV on child mortality in African populations affected by generalized HIV epidemics. *J Acquir Immune Defic Syndr* 38:219-227.

Marston B, De Cock KM (2004). Multivitamins, Nutrition and Antiretroviral Therapy for HIV Disease in Africa. *New England Journal of Medicine* 351:78-80.

MEASURE DHS, 2008. Macro International, Inc. , Calverton MD.

Miller G (2006). The Unseen: Mental Illness's Global Toll. *Science* 311:458-461.

Mills EJ et al. (2006). Adherence to antiretroviral therapy in sub-Saharan Africa and North America: A meta-analysis. *JAMA* 296:679-690.

Moore A, Morrison SJ (2007). *Health Worker Shortages Challenge PEPFAR Options for Strengthening Health Systems.* Task Force on HIV/AIDS. Center for Strategic and International Studies, Washington D.C. September.

Newell ML et al. (2004). Mortality of infected and uninfected infants born to HIV-infected mothers in Africa: a pooled analysis. *Lancet* 364:1236-1243.

New York City Department of Health and Mental Hygiene (2005). *HIV/AIDS Epidemiology Program Fourth Quarter Report.* 3:1-4. October.

New York City Department of Health and Mental Hygiene (2007). *HIV Epidemiology& Field Services Semi-Annual Report.* October.

Niel Malan DR et al. (2008). Efficacy and Safety of Atazanavir, With or Without Ritonavir, as Part of Once-Daily Highly Active Antiretroviral Therapy Regimens in Antiretroviral-Naïve Patients. *J Acquir Immune Defic Syndr* 47:161-167.

Nunn AS et al. (2007). Evolution of Antiretroviral Drug Costs in Brazil in the Context of Free and Universal Access to AIDS Treatment. *PLoS Med* 4:e305.

Nyirenda M et al. (2007). Mortality levels and trends by HIV serostatus in rural South Africa. *AIDS* 21 (Supp. 6): S73-S79.

Obermeyer CM, Osborn M (2007). The Utilization of Testing and Counseling for HIV: A Review of the Social and Behavioral Evidence. *Am J Pub Health* 97:1762-1774.

O'Brien DP et al (2006). In resource-limited settings good early outcomes can be achieved in children using adult fixed-dose combination antiretroviral therapy. *AIDS* 20:1955-1960.

Ormassen V et al. (2007). HIV related and non-HIV related mortality before and after the introduction of highly active antiretroviral therapy (HAART) in Norway compared to the general population. *Scand J Infect Dis* 39:51-57.

Palmer S et al. (2008). Low-leel viremia persists for at least 7 years in patients on suppressive antiretroviral therapy. *PNAS* 105;3879-3884.

Panel on Antiretroviral Guidelines for Adults and Adolescents (2008). *Guidelines for the use of antiretroviral agents in HIV-1-infected adults and adolescents.* US Department of Health and Human Services, Washington.

Patel K et al. (2008). Long-term effectiveness of highly active antiretroviral therapy on the survival of children and adolescents with HIV infection: a 10-year follow-up study. *Clin Infect Dis* 46:507-515.

Patel V (2007). Mental health in low- and middle-income countries. *Brit Med Bull* doi:10.1093/bmb/ldm010 (advance online publication).

Pence BW et al. (2007). Psychiatric illness and virologic response in patients initiating highly active antiretroviral therapy. *J Acquir Immune Defic Syndr* 44:159-166.

Phillips AN et al. (2007). Risk of extensive virologic failure to the three original antiretroviral drug classes over long-term follow-up from the start of therapy in patients with HIV infection: an observational cohort study. *Lancet* 370:1923-1928.

Phillips EJ, Malial SA (2008). Pharmacogenetics and the potential for the individualization of antiretroviral therapy. *Curr Opin Infect Dis* 21:16-24.

Prendergast A et al. (2007). International perspectives, progress, and future challenges of paediatric HIV infection. *Lancet* 370:68-80.

President's Emergency Plan for AIDS Relief (2008). *The Power of Partnerships: Fourth Annual Report to Congress on PEPFAR.*

Puthankit T et al. (2007). Hospitalization and Mortality among HIV-Infected Children after Receiving Highly Active Antiretroviral Therapy. *Clin Infect Dis* 44:599-604.

Reddi A et al. (2007). Preliminary outcomes of a paediatric highly active antiretroviral therapy cohort from KwaZulu-Natal, South Africa. *BMC Paediatrics* 7:13.

Rouet F et al. (2008). Frequent occurrence of chronic hepatitis B virus infection among West African HIV type-1-infected children. *Clin Infect Dis* 46:361-366.

Sanders E (2008). New life for African patients: Thanks to US funding, antiviral drugs are available to those too poor to afford them. *Los Angeles Times.* 15 February.

Samb B et al. (2007). Rapid Expansion of the Health Workforce in Response to the HIV Epidemic. *New Eng J Med* 2007;357:2510-2514.

Sherman GG. Matsebula TC, Jones SA (2005). Is early HIV testing of infants in poorly resourced prevention of mother-to-child transmission programmes affordable? *Trop Med & Int Health* 10:1108-1113.

Smit C et al. (2006). Effective therapy has altered the spectrum of cause-specific mortality following HIV seroconversion. *AIDS* 20:741-749.

Smit C et al. (2008). Risk of Hepatitis-Related Mortality Increased Among Hepatitis C Virus/HIV-Coinfected Drug Users Compared with Drug Users Infected Only With Hepatitis C Virus: A 20-Year Prospective Study. *J Acquir Immune Defic Syndr* 47:221-225.

Srithanaviboonchai K et al. (2008). Novel low-cost assay for the monitoring of CD4 counts in HIV-infected individuals. *J Acquir Immun Defic Syndr* 47:135-139.

Steen TW et al. (2007). Two and a Half Years of Routine HIV Testing in Botswana. *J Acquir Immune Defic Syndr* 44:484-488.

Strategies for Management of Antiretroviral Therapy (SMART) Study Group et al. (2006). CD4+ count-guided interruption of antiretroviral treatment. *New Eng J Med* 355:2283-2296.

Steinbrook R (2007). Closing the Affordability Gap for Drugs in Low-Income Countries. *New Eng J Med* 357:1996-1999.

Sulkowski MS, Benhamou Y (2007). Therapeutic issues in HIV/HCV-co-infected patients. *J Viral Hep* 14:371-386.

Tegger MK et al. (2008). The Effect of Mental Illness, Substance Use and Treatment for Depression on the Initiation of Highly Active Antiretroviral Therapy among HIV-Infected Individuals. *AIDS Patient Care and STDs* 22:233-243.

Thomas CF, Limper AH (2004). Pneuomocystic pneumonia. *New Eng J Med* 350:2487-2498.

UK Collaborative HIV Cohort Study (2008). Are previous treatment interruptions associated with higher viral rebound rates in patients with viral suppression? *AIDS* 22:349-356.

UNAIDS (2007a). *Financing Resources Required to Achieve Universal Access to HIV Prevention, Treatment, Care and Support.* UNAIDS, Geneva.

UNAIDS (2007b). *Report on the progress on follow-up support to countries in their national target setting towards universal access.* 20th Meeting of the UNAIDS Programme Coordinating Board, Geneva, 25-27 June, Provisional agenda item 4.1. UNAIDS, Geneva.

UNAIDS (2007c). *AIDS epidemic update.* UNAIDS, Geneva.

UNAIDS, WHO (2007). *Guidance on Provider-Initiated HIV Testing and Counseling in Health Facilities.* World Health Organization, Geneva.

UNITAID (2008). *Fact Sheet.* Accessed 8 March 2008 at http://www.unitaid.eu/images/action/factsheet.pdf.

UNDP (2007). *Human Development Report 2007/2008.* United Nations Development Program, New York.

Walensky RP et al. (2006). The survival benefits of AIDS treatment in the United States. *J Infect Dis* 194;11-19.

Walzer A et al. (2006). Determinants of survival without antiretroviral therapy after infancy in HIV-1-infected Zambian children in the CHAP Trial. *J Acquir Immune Def Syndr* 42:637-645.

Wang H et al. (2007). Self-Reported Adherence to Antiretroviral Treatment among HIV-Infected People in Central China. *AIDS Patient Care STDS* (Epub ahead of print).

Wang X, Wu Z (2007). Factors associated with adherence to antiretroviral therapy among HIV/AIDS patients in rural China. *AIDS* 21(Supp. 8):S149-S155.

Weinstock HS et al. (2004). The Epidemiology of Antiretroviral Drug Resistance among Drug-Naïve HIV-1-Infected Persons in 10 US Cities. *JID* 189:2174-2180.

Weiser SD et al. (2006). Routine HIV Testing in Botswana: A Population-Based Study on Attitudes, Practices and Human Rights Concerns. *PLoS Med* 3:e261.

Whalen C et al. (1995). Accelerated course of human immunodeficiency virus infection after tuberculosis. *Am J Respir Crit Care Med* 151:129-135.

WHO (2008a). *Global Tuberculosis Control 2008: Surveillance, Planning, Financing.* World Health Organization, Geneva.

WHO (2008b). The methadone fix. *Bulletin of the World Health Organization* 86:164-165.

WHO (2008c). *Anti-tuberculosis drug resistance in the world – Report No. 4, The WHO/IUATLD global project on anti-tuberculosis drug resistance surveillance.* World Health Organization, Geneva.

WHO (2007a). *Prioritizing second-line antiretroviral drugs for adults and adolescents: a public health approach, Report of a WHO Working Group meeting.* World Health Organization, Geneva, 21-22 May.

WHO (2007b). *Tuberculosis Care and TB-HIV Co-management: Integrated Management of Adolescent and Adult Illness (IMAI).* World Health Organization, Geneva.

WHO (2007c). *TB/HIV Facts at a Glance.* World Health Organization, Geneva. Accessed 9 February 2008 at http://www.who.int/tb/challenges/hiv/facts/en/index.html.

WHO (2007d). *Global Tuberculosis Control: Surveillance, Planning, Financing.* World Health Organization, Geneva.

WHO (2007e). *Task Shifting to Tackle Health Workers Shortages.* World Health Organization, Geneva.

WHO (2007f). *Appreciating assets: mapping, understanding, translating and engaging religious health assets in Zambia and Lesotho.* World Health Organization, Geneva.

WHO (2006a). *Antiretroviral Therapy for HIV Infection in Adults and Adolescents: Recommendations for a Public Health Approach.* World Health Organization, Geneva.

WHO (2006b). *Report on the WHO/UNAIDS meeting on forecasting ARV needs up to 2010.* World Health Organization, Geneva.

WHO (2006c). *Antiretroviral Therapy for HIV Infection in Infants and Children: Towards Universal Access, Recommendations for a public health approach.* World Health Organization, Geneva.

WHO (2006d). *Working together for health.* World Health Organization, Geneva.

WHO (2004). *Interim policy on collaborative TB/HIV activities.* World Health Organization, Geneva.

WHO (2003). *Nutrient requirements for people living with HIV/AIDS : Report of a technical consultation.* World Health Organization, Geneva.

WHO, UNAIDS, PEPFAR (2008). *Task shifting. Global recommendations and guidelines.* World Health Organization, Geneva.

WHO, UNICEF, UNAIDS (2007). *Towards universal access: scaling up priority HIV/AIDS interventions in the health sector, Progress report, April 2007.* World Health Organization, Geneva.

Wiedle PJ et al. (2006). Adherence to antiretroviral therapy in a home-based AIDS care programme in rural Uganda. *Lancet* 368:1587-1594.

Wilson I et al. (2005). Quality of HIV care provided by nurse practitioners, physician assistances,and physicians. *Ann Intern Med* 143:729-737.

Chapter 6 | MITIGATING THE EPIDEMIC'S IMPACT

Asia Development Bank, UNAIDS (2004). *Asia-Pacific's Opportunity: Investing to Avert an HIV/AIDS Crisis.* ADB/UNAIDS Study Series.

Barnett T (2004). *HIV/AIDS, Nutrition and Food Security: Looking to Future Challenges,* in *The Macroeconomics of HIV/AIDS.* International Monetary Fund, Washington DC.

Beegle K (2003). *Labor effects of adult morality in Tanzanian households.* Policy Research Working Paper No. 3062. World Bank.

Bell C, Devarajan S, Gersbach H (2004). Thinking About the Long-Run Economic Costs of AIDS, in *The Macroeconomics of HIV/AIDS.* International Monetary Fund, Washington DC.

Bhorat H, Kanbur R (2005). *Poverty and Well-Being in Post-Apartheid South Africa.* DPRU Working Paper No. 05/101. Accessed 3 March 2008 at http://papers.ssrn.com/sol3/papers.cfm?abstract_id=982805.

Birdsall N, Hamoudi A (2004). AIDS and the Accumulation and Utilization of Human Capital in Africa, in *The Macroeconomics of HIV/AIDS.* International Monetary Fund, Washington DC.

Bollinger L, Stover J, Riwa P (1999). *The economic impact of AIDS in Tanzania.* Policy Working Paper. Policy Project.

Chapoto A, Jayne TS, Mason N (2007). Security of widows' access to land in the era of HIV/AIDS: Panel survey evidence from Zambia. Food Security Research Project – Zambia, Ministry of Agriculture & Cooperatives, Agriculture Consultative Forum, Michigan State University.

Chapoto A, Jayne TS (2005). *Socio-economic characteristics of Individuals affected by AIDS-related Prime-age Mortality in Zambia.* Lusaka, Zambia, Food Security Research Project.

Chirambo K (2007). AIDS, Politics and Governance: Preliminary results on the impact of HIV/AIDS on the electoral process in Namibia, Malawi, Senegal, South Africa, Tanzania and Zambia. Presented to the University of Warwick/UNDP Conference on 'Governance of HIV/AIDS Responses: Making Participation and Accountability Count.'

Collins DL, Leibbrandt M (2007). The financial impact of HIV/AIDS on poor households in South Africa. *AIDS* 21(Supp. 1):S75-S81.

Commission on AIDS in Asia (2008). *Redefining AIDS in Asia – Crafting an effective response.*

Connelly D et al (2007). Prevalence of HIV infection and median CD4 counts among health care workers in South Africa. *S Afr Med J* 97:115-120.

Dinkelman T, Lam D, Leibbrandt M (2007). Household and community income, economic shocks and risky sexual behavior of young adults: evidence from the Cape Area Panel Study 2002 and 2005. *AIDS* 21(Supp. 1): S49-S56.

Dorward AR, Mwale IM (2004). Labor Market and Wage Impacts of HIV/AIDS in Rural Malawi, in *The Macroeconomics of HIV/AIDS.* International Monetary Fund, Washington DC.

Fourie I (2005). *The Impact of HIV/AIDS on the South African Mining Industry.* LBMA Precious Metals Conference, Johannesburg. Accessed 4 March 2008 at http://www.lbma.org.uk/conf2005/2f.fourie_LBMA2005.pdf.

Garrett L (2005). *HIV and National Security: Where Are the Links?* Council on Foreign Relations, New York.

Gillespie S, Kadiyala S (2005). *HIV/AIDS and Food and Nutrition Security: From Evidence to Action.* International Food Policy Research Institute, Washington DC.

Gillespie S et al (2007). Investigating the empirical evidence for understanding vulnerability and the associations between poverty, HIV infection and AIDS impact. *AIDS* 2007;21(Supp. 1):S1-S4.

Global Coalition on Women and AIDS (2006). *Support Women Caregivers.* Issue Brief No. 5. UNAIDS, Geneva.

Global Fund Partnership Forum (2006). *Site visit, 30 June 2006 – Philanjalo Hospice.* Global Fund to Fight AIDS, Tuberculosis and Malaria. Accessed 24 March 2006 at http://www.theglobalfund.org/en/about/forum/2006/philanjalo/.

Global Fund to Fight AIDS, Tuberculosis and Malaria (2008). *Monthly Progress Update – 31 January 2008.* Accessed 6 March 2008 at http://www.theglobalfund.org/en/files/publications/basics/progress_update/progressupdate.pdf.

Greener R (2004). The Impact of HIV/AIDS on Poverty and Inequality, in *The Macroeconomics of HIV/AIDS.* International Monetary Fund, Washington DC.

Haacker M (2004a). HIV/AIDS: The Impact on the Social Fabric and the Economy, in *The Macroeconomics of HIV/AIDS.* International Monetary Fund, Washington DC.

Haacker M (2004b). The Impact of HIV/AIDS: The Impact on Government Finance and Public Services, in *The Macroeconomics of HIV/AIDS.* International Monetary Fund, Washington DC.

International Center for Research on Women (2007). *Women's Property Rights as an AIDS Response: Lessons from Community Interventions in Africa.* International Center for Research on Women, Washington DC.

International Treatment Preparedness Coalition (2007) *Missing the Target #5: Improving AIDS Drug Access and Advancing Health Care for All.* Treatment Monitoring and Advocacy Project, San Francisco USA.

IRIN News (2006). *Swaziland: The vital but underestimated role of AIDS caregivers.* 9 May. Accessed 24 March 2008 at http://www.irinnews.org/report.aspx?reportid=58966.

Jayne TS et al (2004). HIV/AIDS and the Agricultural Sector in Eastern and Southern Africa: Anticipating the Consequences, in *The Macroeconomics of HIV/AIDS.* International Monetary Fund, Washington DC.

Karlan D, Ashraf N, Yin W (2007). *Female Empowerment: Impact of a Commitment Savings Product in the Philippines.* Working Paper No. 106. Center for Global Development, Washington DC.

Kim JC et al (2007). Understanding the Impact of a Microfinance-Based Intervention on Women's Empowerment and the Reduction of Intimate Partner Violence in South Africa. *Am J Pub Health* 97:1794-1802.

Mermin J et al. (2008). Mortality in HIV-infected Ugandan adults receiving antiretroviral treatment and survival of their HIV-uninfected children: a prospective cohort study. *Lancet* 371:752-759.

Mishra V et al (2007). The socioeconomic determinants of HIV incidence: evidence from a longitudinal, population-based study in rural South Africa. *AIDS* 2007;21(Supp. 1):S29-S38.

Pal K et al (2005). Can Low Income Countries Afford Basic Social Protection? First Results of a Modeling Exercise. International Labour Organization, Geneva.

Piot P, Greener R, Russell S (2007). Squaring the Circle: AIDS, Poverty and Human Development. *PLoS Med* 4:e314.

Preston-Whyte et al (2007). Revealing the full extent of households' experiences of HIV and AIDS in rural South Africa. *Soc Sci Med* 65(6):1249-1259

Pronyk PM et al (2007). *The role of structural factors in explaining variations in community HIV prevalence: a study in rural South Africa.* Acornhoek, South Africa, Rural AIDS and Development Action Resource Programme, Accessed 12 May 2008 at http://web.wits.ac.za/NR/rdonlyres/87874FDD-0C41-4945-A28B-9AEAFD027283/0/Pronyk_IMAGE_Structural_Factors_IMAGE_Working_Paper_1.pdf.

Pronyk PM et al (2006). Effect of a structural intervention for the prevention of intimate-partner violence and HIV in rural South Africa: a cluster randomised trial. *Lancet* 368:1973-1983.

Reuters (2008). 'Malawi to Raise Pay of Civil Servants with HIV.' 7 January.

Rosen S et al (2006). *The Impact of AIDS on Government Service Delivery: The Case of the Zambian Wildlife Authority.* Health and Development Discussion Paper No. 8. Center for International Health and Development, Boston University School of Public Health, Boston.

Secretary-General's Task Force on Women, Girls and HIV/AIDS in Southern Africa (2004). *Facing the Future Together.*

Simon J et al (2007). Early effects of antiretroviral therapy on work performance: Results from a cohort study of Kenyan agricultural workers. Center for International Health and Development, Boston University School of Public Health. Accessed 26 September 2007 at http://www.hivimplement/agenda/pdf/E1/E1%20Simon%abstract%20811.ppt.pdf.

Swaminathan H, Bhatla N, Chakraborty S (2007). *Women's Property Rights as an AIDS Response: Emerging Efforts in South Asia.* International Center for Research on Women, Washington DC.

Thirumurthy H, Zivin JF, Goldstein M (2007). *AIDS Treatment and Intrahousehold Resource Allocations: Children's Nutrition and School in Kenya.* Working Paper No. 105. Center for Global Development, Washington DC.

UNAIDS (2006). *AIDS, Security and Humanitarian Response.* 19th Meeting of the UNAIDS Programme Coordinating Board, Lusaka, Zambia, 6-8 December. UNAIDS, Geneva. Available at http://data.unaids.org/pub/Report/2006/20061101_PCB_Security_and_Humanitarian_Response_en.pdf.

UNDP (2007). *Human Development Report 2007/2008.* United Nations Development Programme, New York.

UNDP (2005) *Human Development Report.* UNDP, New York.

UNESCO, UNHCR (2007). *Educational responses to HIV and AIDS for refugees and internally displaced persons: Discussion paper for decision-makers.* UNESCO, Paris.

UNHCR (2007). *Statistical year book 2006: Trends in Displacement, Protection and Solutions.* Office of United Nations High Commissioner on Refugees, Geneva.

UNICEF (2007a). *The Impact of Social Cash Transfers on Children Affected by HIV and AIDS.* UNICEF, New York.

UNICEF (2007b). *State of the World's Children.* UNICEF, New York.

UNICEF, UNAIDS, WHO (2008). *Children and AIDS: Second Stocktaking Report.* UNICEF, New York.

United States President's Emergency Plan for AIDS Relief (2007). *Latest Results.* Accessed 6 March 2008 at http://www.pepfar.gov/about/c19785.htm.

Webb D (2007). From the individual to the system: the coming of age of programmes for orphans and vulnerable children. *Exchange on HIV/AIDS, sexuality and gender* 2:1-4.

WHO/UNICEF/WHO (2006). *Epidemiological Fact Sheets on HIV/AIDS and Sexually Transmitted Infections: Uganda*. World Health Organization, Geneva. December.

Zambia Central Board of Health, Center for International Health and Development (Boston University School of Public Health) (2004). *The Costs of HIV/AIDS Among Professional Staff in the Zambian Public Health Sector.* Zambian Central Board of Public Health, Lusaka.

Chapter 7 | WHERE DO WE GO FROM HERE?

Attawell K, Dickinson C (2007). *An independent assessment of progress on the implementation of the global task team recommendations in support of national AIDS responses.* Twentieth meeting of the UNAIDS Programme Coordinating Board (Item UNAIDS/PCB(20)/CRP4).

Center for Global Development (2007). *Does the IMF constrain health spending in poor countries? Evidence and an agenda for action.* Washington DC, Center for Global Development (Report of the Working Group on IMF Programs and Health Spending).

Centro Nacional para la Prevención y control del SIDA, Ministry of Health [Mexico] (2008). *Country Report 2008 to monitor progress in the implementation of the Declaration of Commitment (DoC): HIV spending indicator*

Gouws E et al. (2006). Short term estimates of adult HIV incidence by mode of transmission: Kenya and Thailand as examples. *Sexually Transmitted Infections,* 82(Suppl. 3):iii51-iii55.

Hayes S et al. (2007). *Decentralized funding in response to the AIDS Pandemic: An opportunity for promoting good governance in Africa* (Report prepared for the United Nations

Development Program, the University of Warwick Center for the Study of Regionalization, and Globalization Conference: Governance of HIV and AIDS Responses).

McDougal JS et al. (2006). Comparison of HIV type 1 incidence observed during longitudinal follow-up with incidence estimated by cross-sectional analysis using the BED Capture enzyme immunoassay. *AIDS Research and Human Retroviruses,* 22:945–952.

Office of US Global AIDS Coordinator et al. (2008). *The power of partnerships: The US President's emergency plan for AIDS relief, 2008 annual report to Congress.* Washington DC, US State Department.

Ofosu-Korentang B, Annan J (2005). *District Planning and Implementation Strategy Note and Guide.* UNDP, New York.

Organisation of African Unity (2001). *Abuja declaration on HIV/AIDS, tuberculosis and other related diseases.* African Summit on HIV/AIDS, Tuberculosis and Other Related Diseases. 24–27 April. Abuja, Nigeria (http://www.un.org/ga/aids/pdf/abuja_declaration.pdf, accessed 17 March 2008).

Samb B et al. (2007). Rapid expansion of the health workforce in response to the HIV epidemic. *New England Journal of Medicine,* 357:2510–2514.

Stover J et al. (2006). The global impact of scaling up HIV/AIDS prevention programs in low- and middle-income countries. *Science,* 311:1474–1476.

UNAIDS (2006). *Report on the global AIDS epidemic.* UNAIDS, Geneva.

UNAIDS (2007a). *Le Maroc: une réponse nationale à VIH.* Geneva, UNAIDS (UNAIDS Best Practice Collection).

UNAIDS (2007b). *Towards universal access to prevention, treatment and care: experiences and challenges from the Mbeya region in Tanzania—a case study.* Geneva, UNAIDS (UNAIDS Best Practice Collection).

UNAIDS (2007c). *Financial resources required to achieve universal access to HIV prevention, treatment, care and support.* Geneva, UNAIDS (http://data.unaids.org/pub/Report/2007/20070925_advocacy_grne2_en.pdf).

UNAIDS (2008). *The socioeconomic impact of the HIV/AIDS epidemic.* Geneva (AIDS Financing and Economics Division working paper), UNAIDS, Geneva.

UNAIDS Zambia (2006). *Joint United Nations programme on support on AIDS 2007–2010,* UNAIDS, Lusaka, Zambia.

UNDP (2007). *Human Development Report.* New York, United Nations Development Program.

UNDP Bureau for Development Policy, HIV/AIDS Group, Democratic Governance Group (2007). *Decentralized responses to HIV/AIDS: An analysis of local government responses.* New York, United Nations Development Program.

World Bank (2007). *The Africa multi-country AIDS program 2000–2006: Results of the World Bank's response to a development crisis.* Washington DC, World Bank.

PHOTOGRAPHY CREDITS

Foreword

Page 9 UNAIDS/O.O'Hanlon

Chapter 1 | THE GLOBAL HIV CHALLENGE

Page 11 UNAIDS/P.Virot (top left), UNAIDS/P.Virot (bottom right)
Page 16 UNAIDS
Page 26 UNAIDS

Chapter 2 | STATUS OF THE GLOBAL HIV EPIDEMIC

Page 29 UNAIDS/A.Dutta (top left), UNAIDS/O.O'Hanlon (bottom right)
Page 40 UNAIDS/P.Virot
Page 56 UNAIDS/P.Virot

Chapter 3 | ADDRESSING SOCIETAL CAUSES OF HIV RISK AND VULNERABILITY

Page 63 UNAIDS/S.Drakborg (top left), UNAIDS/S.Drakborg (bottom right)
Page 73 UNAIDS/A.Dutta
Page 82 UNAIDS/P.Virot
Page 86 UNAIDS
Page 93 UNAIDS

Chapter 4 | PREVENTING NEW HIV INFECTIONS

Page 95 UNAIDS/P.Virot (top left), UNAIDS/P.Virot (bottom right)
Page 101 UNAIDS/O.O'Hanlon
Page 104 UNAIDS
Page 109 UNAIDS/Tango Photo/P.Carrera
Page 112 UNAIDS
Page 114 UNAIDS/ILO/J.Maillard
Page 116 UNAIDS

Chapter 5 | TREATMENT AND CARE

Page 129 UNAIDS/P.Virot (top left), UNAIDS/P.Virot (bottom right)
Page 133 UNAIDS
Page 137 UNAIDS/WHO/S.Torfin
Page 155 UNAIDS/W.Phillips

Chapter 6 | MITIGATING THE EPIDEMIC'S IMPACT

Page 159 UNAIDS/S.Montanari (top left), UNAIDS/C.Sattlberger (bottom right)
Page 164 UNAIDS/A.Gutman
Page 173 UNAIDS
Page 174 UNAIDS/A.Gutman

Chapter 7 | WHERE DO WE GO FROM HERE?

Page 187	UNAIDS/P.Virot (top left), UNAIDS/P.Virot (bottom right)
Page 195	UNAIDS
Page 197	UNAIDS
Page 204	UNAIDS/P.Virot
Page 208	UNAIDS/A.Dutta

Annex 1 | HIV AND AIDS ESTIMATES AND DATA, 2007 AND 2001

Page 211	UNAIDS/L.Rahn (top left), UNAIDS/P.Virot (bottom right)

Annex 2 | COUNTRY PROGRESS INDICATORS

Page 235	UNAIDS/P.Virot (top left), UNAIDS/S.Montanari (bottom right)

Disclaimer: Photographs in this report do not necessarily represent the situation, opinions, or beliefs of the persons depicted, and in no way imply their HIV status.